Dupuytren's Disease
Biology and Treatment

Editorial Advisory Board

Chairman:

Douglas W. Lamb FRCS
Princess Margaret Rose Orthopaedic Hospital
Fairmilehead, Edinburgh, UK

Nicholas Barton FRCS
Department of Hand Surgery, University Hospital,
Queen's Medical Centre, Nottingham, UK

W. Bruce Connolly FRCS FRACS FACS
Hand Unit, Sydney Hospital, Macquarie Street,
Sydney, New South Wales, Australia

Lee W. Milford Jr BS MS MD
The Campbell Clinic, Madison Avenue,
Memphis, Tennessee, USA

Volumes already published

The Interphalangeal Joints
William H. Bowers

The Paralysed Hand
Douglas W. Lamb

Unsatisfactory Results in Hand Surgery
R. M. McFarlane

Fractures of the Hand and Wrist
N. J. Barton

Volumes in preparation

The Thumb
James W. Strickland

Microsurgical Procedures
Viktor E. Meyer and Michael J. M. Black

Joint Replacement in the Upper Limb
William A. Souter

Congenital Malformations of the Hand and Forearm
Dieter Buck-Gramcko

Skin Cover in the Injured Hand
David M. Evans

Fingertip and Nailbed Injuries
Guy Foucher

The Painful Hand
K. Wynn-Parry

Tumours of the Hand and Upper Limb
G. Bogumill and E. Fleegler

THE HAND AND UPPER LIMB   Volume 5

Dupuytren's Disease
Biology and Treatment

EDITED BY

R. M. McFarlane MD MSc FRCS(C)
Professor of Surgery and Chief, Division of Plastic Surgery,
Faculty of Medicine, The University of Western Ontario
and Victoria Hospital, London, Ontario, Canada

D. A. McGrouther MSc MD(Hons) FRCS FRCS(G)
Professor of Plastic and Reconstructive Surgery,
University College Hospital,
London, UK

M. H. Flint MB BS (London) FRCS FRACS
Career Fellow, Medical Research Council, New Zealand;
Director, Connective Tissue Research Group,
Department of Surgery, University of Auckland, New Zealand

FOREWORD BY
H. Graham Stack FRCS
Consultant in Hand Surgery, Regional Plastic
Surgery Centre, St Andrew's Hospital, Billericay,
Essex; Hunterian Professor, Royal College of
Surgeons of England

CHURCHILL LIVINGSTONE
EDINBURGH LONDON MELBOURNE AND NEW YORK 1990

CHURCHILL LIVINGSTONE
Medical Division of Longman Group UK Limited

Distributed in the United States of America by
Churchill Livingstone Inc., 1560 Broadway, New York,
N.Y. 10036, and by associated companies, branches
and representatives throughout the world.

© Longman Group UK Limited 1990

All rights reserved; no part of this publication may be
reproduced, stored in a retrieval system, or transmitted in
any form or by any means, electronic, mechanical,
photocopying, recording or otherwise, without either the
prior written permission of the Publishers (Churchill
Livingstone, Robert Stevenson House, 1–3 Baxter's Place,
Leith Walk, Edinburgh EH1 3AF) or a licence permitting
restricted copying in the United Kingdom issued by the
Copyright Licensing Agency Ltd, 33–34 Alfred Place,
London WC1E 7DP.

First published 1990

ISBN 0 443 03818 X

British Library Cataloguing in Publication Data
Dupuytren's disease.
  1. Man. Hands. Dupuytren's contracture
  I. McFarlane, Robert II. Flint, M. H.
  III. McGrouther, D. A. (Duncan Angus)
  617.397

Library of Congress Cataloging in Publication Data
Dupuytren's disease/edited by R. M. McFarlane,
  M. H. Flint, D. A. McGrouther; foreword by G. Stack.
    p.   cm.
    Includes bibliographical references.
    ISBN 0-443-03818-X
    1. Dupuytren's contracture. I. McFarlane, Robert M.
II. Flint, M. H. III. McGrouther, D. A.
    [DNLM: 1. Dupuytren's Contracture. WE 830 D988]
RD778.5.D87 1990
617.5′75 — dc20
DNLM/DLC
for Library of Congress   89-70803

Produced by Longman Singapore Publishers (Pte) Ltd.
Printed in Singapore.

Foreword

Dupuytren's contracture (or disease) remains one of the most enigmatic problems in hand surgery, and it is therefore fitting that from time to time a book is dedicated to a review of progress and the up-to-date position.

This book, presented by R. M. McFarlane, M. H. Flint and D. A. McGrouther, contains many ideas which were first presented at one of the two meetings of the Dupuytren Group, originally convened in Vienna by Hanno Millesi, and continued in London, Ontario under the chairmanship of Bob McFarlane. The basis of both meetings was a number of reports of personal progress and opinions on various aspects of the problem, but at the centre were reports dealing with the biological basis and biochemistry of connective tissues.

The main difficulty in understanding this work for the uninvolved clinician is that so much has been discovered and consequently the terminology has changed to such an extent that nothing that went before is now recognizable. Thus the newly interested reader will have to change from thinking about mucopolysaccharides to glycosaminoglycans. This progress has come recently, probably from the stimulation of scientists in other disciplines by the surgeons, and by the surgeons co-operating in the chemical and immunological research. There has also been a great deal of cross-stimulation through international co-operation that has developed since the war through the formation of Hand Societies. Our start came from Sir Archibald McIndoe, founder member of the British (First) Hand Club; one of his assistants, Tord Skoog, wrote the first post-war review of the condition in 1948.

It was Harvey Allen in Chicago who pointed out to me the spiralling of the nerve around the strands, also mentioned by Iselin, Hueston and Gosset, all in slightly different situations in the hand. Littler has emphasized the involvement of the digital vessels in the neurovascular bundles, as well as the digital nerves (Fig. 1).

Then in 1963 John Hueston's book *Dupuytren's Contracture* was published, and it was this book, combined with stimulation from Norman Capener, that led to my opportunity to work in Hans Landsmeer's laboratory in Leiden, where Raoul Tubiana's associate, J. M. Thomine, also visited. Jean Gosset was involved at that time and co-operative discussions ensued in Paris at GEM (Group Etude de la Main) and SICOT meetings.

Further work by McFarlane and McGrouther has made much progress in the elucidation of the anatomical arrangements. The explanation of involvement of the skin remains a problem, although some of us regard it as the involvement of those fascial components which are responsible for the thickness of the integument in the palmar region.

Surgical technique has changed in the direction of less extensive, more careful operations and more rational release of contractures as a result of better understanding of the anatomy. This has led to better understanding of the nerve displacements, with fewer nerves being damaged as a result. The neurovascular bundle which contains the nerve is held by a condensation of the fascial layers fixed in the region of the base of the proximal phalanx. When the finger is flexed by the contracture, this brings the nerve forward into the palm, and the nerve therefore has to pass directly forward from behind the transverse fibres of the palmar fascia

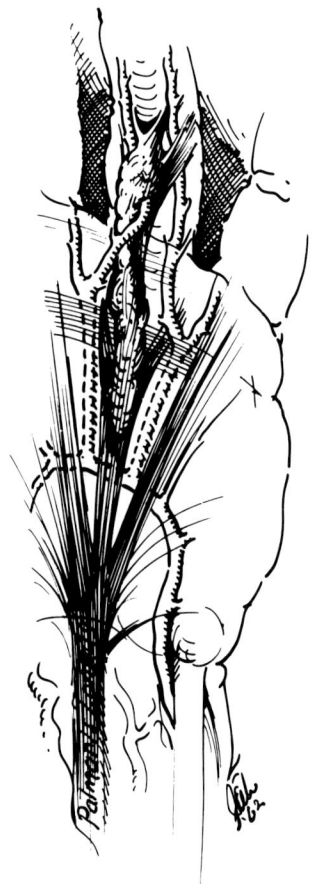

Fig. 1 Relationship of hypertrophied palmar and digital fascia to neurovascular bundle, (accompanying nerve not shown). Resection of fascia demands exquisite care to prevent nerve damage. The finger with the cut nerve is far more disabled that the one moderately flexed by fascial contracture. The triangular component of the palmar aponeurosis shown is the area most frequently involved in the *maladie de Dupuytren*.

before turning over the contracted strand to pass distally into the finger.

Preservation of the blood supply to the skin should lead to less skin necrosis. The work of Charles McCash (1964) has emphasized the great regenerative capability of the skin.

More recently the spotlight has turned to the chemical and pathological aspects of the disease. Glimcher, Flint and Bailey and their co-workers have made important contributions to this field, and it is from this and from the work on immunology that more progress is to be expected. Research is now directed to the chemistry of the collagens, and to the special cells, the 'contracting fibroblasts', which appear to modulate this. It is my opinion that this research has a very good chance of leading us to discover the nature of the collagen changes, and how or whether the special cell, the contracting fibroblast, or 'tractoblast' (Schultz) is responsible. Perhaps a variable enzyme, with a genetic background, is at fault.

I cannot hope to expound on all the aspects of the problem here, so I appeal to all interested persons to find and understand the writings of all the other contributors and to support them in their search for the answer, even by joining in.

The sources I have mentioned are the ones which have been milestones in my own contribution. I leave you to find your own among the others.

Graham Stack

Acknowledgement
The original of Figure 1 was given to me by Bill Littler, and is reproduced with his permission, and that of Little Brown & Company.

Preface

We have brought together in this volume scientists and clinicians who have a common interest in Dupuytren's disease (DD). Some of these writers have already met on two occasions, in Vienna in 1983 at a meeting organized by Hanno Millesi, and at a second colloquium organized by Robert McFarlane in London, Ontario in 1985. At these meetings, the current views of connective tissue biology and pathology as well as surgery pertaining to DD were discussed at length. The new and sometimes divergent views discussed at these meetings stimulated us to collect this information in book form. We felt that is was important to re-appraise the original scientific record. In a field of which the literature spans at least 150 years in numerous European languages, the ravages of time, wars, and inaccurate translation and misquotation have gradually distorted the truth. To remedy this, David Elliot enlisted the help of linguists and translators to consolidate the scientific record and has unearthed in the libraries of Edinburgh, Manchester, London, Paris, and Washington a number of surprising new references. The historical perspective is humbling when one appreciates what has been reported then lost, and later hailed as new information. We believe that this comprehensive bibliography of early reports will be invaluable to future scholars.

Traditionally DD has been classified as one of the group of fibromatoses, but extrapolation of recent connective tissue research indicates that many facets of the 'disease' are explicable as biological phenomena. In Section 1, connective tissue biology, biochemistry, and pathology relevent to DD are reviewed. The authors have been able to demonstrate the dynamic nature of DD and have sought to explain the inter-relationships of the progressive biological events ranging from changes in the uninvolved palmar fascia to disabling contracture of the fingers.

In Section 2, the embryology and anatomy of the fascial structures in the hand are described. The relationship of the palmar fascia to the development of the palmar lesion is defined. The pathological anatomy of the fascias of the finger, the radial and ulnar sides of the hand and the extensor surface have been discussed separately. A standardized terminology is presented and the relevance of these anatomical structures to the surgeon is stressed.

Much has been deduced about the nature of the disease from epidemiological studies. Section 3 is devoted to a review of knowledge gained from surveys of Western and Oriental patients, and in the select group of patients operated on. The association of DD with disease, work, injury, and genetic, immunological and diathesic factors provides a fuller picture.

In Section 4 the biological aspects of the aetiology and pathogenesis are discussed from a personal viewpoint by the editors.

The many possibilities of treatment are presented in Section 5 with special consideration given to the management of the skin, the fascia, and the proximal interphalangeal joint. We have drawn on a widespread panel of well known hand surgeons who provide their methods of treatment. Rehabilitation, complications, and results are discussed.

In this triumvirate of editors each has his own viewpoint, background and training. Coming as we do from the Old World and the New, the north and the south, the east and the west, we each live in different social and economic conditions and amongst different races. Being influenced by these different environments, we have tried to consolidate what is known as well as present opinion, what is new yet factual about the *maladie de Dupuytren*.

Finally, we must apologize to our willing contributors who have dispensed their wisdom with great generosity. Anxious to prevent the problems of repetation inherent in a multi-author volume, the editors have drastically pruned the tree of knowledge and made necessary sacrifices to ensure the continuity of the text. We hope that this encourages its further growth.

R. M. McFarlane
D. A. McGrouther
M. H. Flint

Acknowledgements

We are grateful to the following for permission to use material previously published elsewhere:

The editors are grateful to Anne B. Redfern for permission to use line drawings.

Chapter 4
Figure 4.7 is from Skalli et al 1989a Myofibroblasts from diverse pathological settings are heterogeneous in their content of actin isoforms and intermediate filament proteins. Laboratory Investigation (Manuscript L1-8483) (in press) © US & Canadian Academy of Pathology Inc.

Chapter 5
The author of this chapter has used Figure 4 from Delbruck A. et al 1988 Journal of Clinical Chemistry and Clinical Biochemistry 26: 7-14 and Figures 3 and 4 from Delbruck A. et al 1981 Journal of Clinical Chemistry and Clinical Biochemistry 19 © Walter de Gruyter & Co., Berlin.

Chapter 8
Figures 8.1, 8.9, 8.12, 8.13, 8.14 and 8.15 are from Tomasek J. J., Schultz R. J., Haaksma C. J. (1987) Extracellular matrix-cytoskeletal connections at the surface of the specialized contractile fibroblast (myofibroblast) in Dupuytren's disease. Journal of Bone and Joint Surgery 69A: 1400-1407 by kind permission of The Journal of Bone and Joint Surgery, Boston, Massachusetts, USA.

Figures 8.2A & B are from Tomasek J. J., Hay E. D., Fujiwara K. (1982) Collagen modulates cell shape and cytoskeleton of embryonic corneal and fibroma fibroblasts: Distribution of actin, α-actinin, and myosin. Developmental Biology 92: 107-122 © Academic Press, Orlando, Florida.

Figures 8.3A & B, 8.4A & B, 8.5 and 8.6 are from Tomasek J. J., Schultz R. J., Episalla C. W., Newman S. A. (1986) The cytoskeleton and extracellular matrix of the Dupuytren's disease 'myofibroblast': An immunofluourscence study of a nonmuscle cell type. Journal of Hand Surgery 11A: 365-371 © C. V. Mosby Company.

Chapter 19
Figures 19.2, 19.3, 19.4, 19.5, 19.6, 19.7 are from The Hand vols 8, 9 and 10 by kind permission of the Editor.

Figure 19.1 is taken from Acta Chirurgica Scandinavica 1972 vol 138(7): 698 by kind permission of the Assistant Editor.

Chapter 23
Figures 23.3 and 23.4 are from Noble et al (1984) Journal of Bone and Joint Surgery 66B: 323-324 by kind permission of the Editor and publishers.

Figure 23.5 is from Kennedy et al (1982) Postgraduate Medical Journal 58: 482 by kind permission of the authors and MacMillan Press Ltd.

Figure 23.6 is from Critchley et al (1976) Journal of Neurology, Neurosurgery and Psychiatry 39: 501 by kind permission of the authors, the Editor and the publishers.

Other acknowledgements for borrowed material have been made in the individual illustration captions in the text. In the event of an acknowledgement having been inadvertently overlooked, the publishers should like to be informed so that they can insert the appropriate information at the first opportunity.

Contributors

M. A. Badalmente PhD
Associate Professor, Director of Electron Microscopy and Neuromuscular Research, Department of Orthopaedic Surgery, State University of New York, Stony Brook School of Medicine, New York, USA

A. J. Bailey MA PhD ScD FRSC
Professor, Head of Laboratory, Agricultural and Food Research Council, AFRC Institute of Food Research, Bristol Laboratory, Langford, Bristol, UK

N. J. Barton MA FRCS
Consultant Orthopaedic Surgeon, Department of Hand Surgery, University Hospital, Queen's Medical Centre, Nottingham, UK

P. Bedeschi MD
Professor of Orthopaedics and Director, Department of Orthopaedic Surgery, University Medical Centre, Modena 41000, Italy

J. S. Botz HNC
Research Assistant, Division of Plastic Surgery, Victoria Hospital, London, Ontario, Canada

W. E. Burkhalter MD
Vice Chairman and Professor, Department of Orthopaedics and Rehabilitation Chief, Hand Surgery, University of Miami School of Medicine, Miami, Florida, USA

P. M. Byron MD
Formerly Clinical Director of Primary Care, Hand Rehabilitation Center, Philadelphia, USA

K. A. Caughell BSc MSc MB BCh
Former Resident in Plastic Surgery, The University of Western Ontario, London, Ontario, Canada

J. Colville FRCS (Ed) FRCSI
Consultant Plastic Surgeon, Royal Victoria Hospital and Ulster Hospital, Belfast, N. Ireland

A. F. Delbrück MD
Professor, Head of Laboratory Services and Institute of Clinical Chemistry LL, Med. Hochschule, Hanover, W. Germany

M. Egawa MD
Nishinomaya City, Hyogo Pref, Japan

T. Egawa MD (Deceased)

M. H. Flint MBBS FRCS FRACS
Director, Connective Tissue Research Group, Department of Surgery, School of Medicine, University of Auckland, New Zealand

G. Gabbiani MD
Professor of Pathology, Department of Pathology, University Medical Centre, Geneva, Switzerland

M. J. Glimcher MD
Harriet M. Peabody Professor of Orthopaedic Surgery; Director, Laboratory for the Study of Skeletal Disorders and Rehabilitation, The Children's Hospital and Harvard Medical School, Boston, Massachusetts, USA

R. I. Gonzalez MD FACS
Plastic Surgeon, San Mateo, California, USA

E. Gurr Privat Dozent Dr. rer. nat
Head Laboratory Services, Municipal Hospital 'Links der Weser', Bremen, W. Germany

E. J. Hall-Findlay BSc MD FRCS (C)
Chief of Staff, Mineral Springs Hospital, Banff, Alberta, Canada

A. Horiki MD
Director of Horiki Orthopaedic Clinic, Osaka Pref, Japan

J. T. Hueston BA MD MS FRCS FRACS
Consultant Plastic Surgeon, Royal Melbourne Hospital, Australia

L. C. Hurst MD
Associate Professor and Associate Chairman, Chief of Hand Surgery, Department of Orthopaedics, State University of New York, Stony Brook School of Medicine, New York, USA

F. Iselin MD
Director, Hand Surgery Center, Paris W, France

R. M. McFarlane MD MSc FRCS(C)
Professor of Surgery and Chief, Division of Plastic Surgery, Faculty of Medicine, The University of Western Ontario and Victoria Hospital, London, Ontario, Canada

D. A. McGrouther MSc MD(Hons) FRCS FRCS(G)
Professor of Plastic and Reconstructive Surgery, University College Hospital, London, UK

E. J. Mackin PT
Director of Hand Therapy, Hand Rehabilitation Center, Philadelphia, USA; Editor, *Journal of Hand Therapy*

S. W. Meagher AB MD
Senior Instructor in Surgery, Tufts University Medical School, Boston, Massachusetts, USA

O. A. Mikkelson MD
Chief Division of Rheumasurgery, Hospital of Rheumatic Diseases; Attending Surgeon, The County Hospital, Haugesund, Norway

J. P. Moermans MD
Service Chirugie, University Hospital Brugmann, Brussels, Belgium

B. Nagay MD
Professor of Surgery, Head, 1st General and Hand Surgery Clinic, Pomeranian Medical Academy, Szczecin, Poland

H. M. Peabody MD
Professor of Orthopaedic Surgery, Harvard Medical School, Boston, USA

C. A. Poole BSc (Hons) PhD
Senior Research Fellow, School of Medicine, Department of Surgery, University of Auckland, New Zealand

E. A. Rosenthal MD
Director Hand Surgery Service, Baystate Medical Center, Springfield, Massachusetts; Active Staff, Mercy Hospital: Associate Clinical Professor of Orthopedic Surgery, Tufts University School of Medicine, Assistant Clinical Professor of Orthopedic Surgery, University of Connecticut School of Medicine, USA

V. Salvi MD
Professor, L. D. in Clinica Ortopedica, Chief of the Department of Orthopaedic Surgery, Traumatology and Hand Surgery, Ospedale Civile, Cuorgne, Italy

R. J. Schultz MD
Professor and Chairman, Department of Orthopaedic Surgery and Rehabilitation, University of South Florida, USA

W. Schurch MD FRCP(C)
Associate Professor of Pathology, Department of Pathology, University of Montreal, Montreal, Canada

H. Senrui MD
Active Member of Japan Society of Hand Surgery

D. T. Shum, MB FRCP(C) Diplomate, American Board of Pathology
Staff Pathologist, Victoria Hospital, Ontario; Associate Professor, Faculty of Medicine, The University of Western Ontario, London, Ontario, Canada

O. Skalli PhD
Department of Cell, Molecular and Structural Biology, North Western University Medical and Dental School, Chicago, USA

J. D. Spencer MS MRCP FRCS
Senior Lecturer/Honorary Consultant, Orthopaedic Department, Guy's Hospital, London, UK

J. J. Tomasek MD
Assistant Professor, Department of Anatomy, New York Medical College, New York, USA

J. P. W. Varian MA FRCS FRACS(Orth)
Consultant Hand Surgeon, Blackrock Clinic, Dublin, Eire

K. I. Welsh PhD BSc
Senior Lecturer in Immunogenetics, Guy's Hospital, London, UK

L. Zachariae MD
Department of Hand Surgery, Kobenhavns, Amts Sygehus 1 Gentofte, Denmark

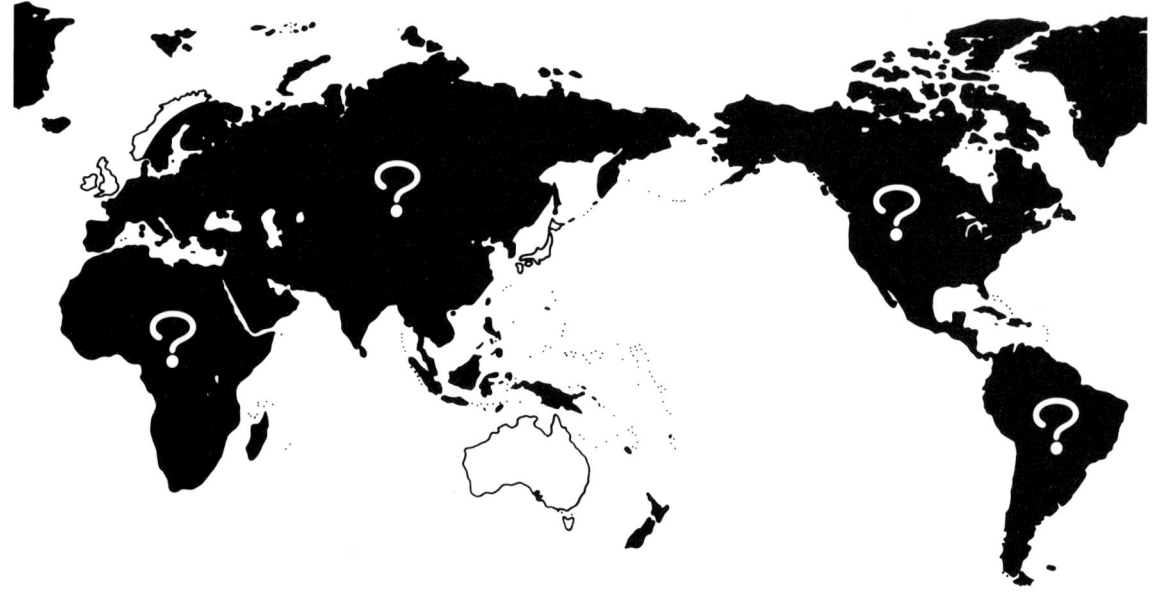

Dedication

Tsuneichi Egawa 1928–1987

This illustration of the known incidence of Dupuytren's Disease was submitted by Dr Tsuneichi Egawa with his manuscript that was completed just prior to his death. It graphically demonstrates the paucity of information about the epidemiology of Dupuytren's Disease and the need for further studies, such as those reported in this book by Dr Egawa and his co-workers.

Contents

1. The early history of contracture of the palmar fascia   1
   D. Elliot

SECTION 1 Biology   11

2. Connective tissue biology   13
   M. H. Flint

3. Histopathology   25
   D. T. Shum

4. Cellular biology   31
   W. Schürch, O. Skalli and G. Gabbiani

5. Proteoglycans and glycosominoglycans   48
   A. F. Delbrück and E. Gurr

6. Collagen   58
   A. J. Bailey

7. Collagen organization   72
   M. J. Glimcher and H. M. Peabody

8. Cellular structure and interconnections   86
   R. J. Schultz and J. J. Tomasek

9. Immunology and genetics   99
   K. I. Welsh and J. D. Spencer

10. Contraction and contracture   104
    M. H. Flint and C. A. Poole

SECTION 2 Normal and pathological anatomy   117

11. The development of the palmar fascia   119
    K. A. Caughell and R. M. McFarlane

12. The palm   127
    D. A. McGrouther

13. The genesis of the palmar lesion   136
    M. H. Flint

14. The finger   155
    R. M. McFarlane

15. The extensor mechanism and knuckle changes   172
    D. A. McGrouther

16. The radial side of the hand   168
    E. J. Hall-Findlay

17. The ulnar side of the hand   176
    N. J. Barton

SECTION 3 Epidemiology   185

18. The clinical diagnosis   187
    D. A. McGrouther

19. Epidemiology of a Norwegian population   191
    O. A. Mikkelsen

20. Epidemiology of surgical patients   201
    R. M. McFarlane, J. S. Botz and H. Cheung

21. Epidemiology of the oriental patient   239
    T. Egawa, H. Senrui, A. Horiki and M. Egawa

22. Dupuytren's diathesis   246
    J. T. Hueston

23. Associated diseases   253
    L. C. Hurst and M. Badalamente

24. Manual work and industrial injury: a personal commentary 261
    S. W. Meagher

25. A single injury to the hand 265
    R. M. McFarlane and D. T. Shum

SECTION 4 Aetiology and pathogenesis 275

26. An insight into the Italian literature on etiology and treatment 277
    V. Salvi

27. Is Dupuytren's disease an inherited disorder? 280
    D. A. McGrouther

28. Is Dupuytren's disease a connective tissue response? 282
    M. H. Flint and D. A. McGrouther

29. Is Dupuytren's disease a neoplasm? 288
    R. M. McFarlane

SECTION 5 Treatment 291

30. Assessment of the patient for operation 293
    R. M. McFarlane

31. An overview of operative treatment 295
    D. A. McGrouther

32. Various views and techniques 311
    P. Bedeschi   W. E. Burkhalter
    V. Salvi   R. I. Gonzalez   J. T. Hueston
    F. Iselin   J. Colville   B. Nagay
    J. Varian   L. Zachariae
    E. A. Rosenthal   J. P. Moermans
    D. A. McGrouther   R. M. McFarlane

33. Postoperative management 368
    E. J. Mackin and P. M. Byron

34. Complications and their management 377
    R. M. McFarlane and D. A. McGrouther

35. Recurrence and extension 383
    D. A. McGrouther

36. The results of treatment 387
    R. M. McFarlane and J. S. Botz

Bibliography of literature before 1900 413

References 420

Index 443

D. Elliot

1 The early history of contracture of the palmar fascia

The earliest reference in surgical history to the contracture of the palmar fascia which has become known as Dupuytren's disease (DD) is in the writings of Felix Plater of Basel in 1614 (Fig. 1.1). In the third volume of his observations, he described the case of a stonemason with this condition: the irrevocable drawing into the palm of the hand of the ring and little fingers and ridging of the palmar skin is pathognomonic. Plater's stonemason, like many patients since, associated the onset of the disease with a specific traumatic event, though the relative timing of this injury and the onset of the contracture are not recorded. Plater believed the tendons to have contracted and pulled out of their sheaths, so raising the palmar skin in ridges as they bow-stringed across the palm — an interpretative error which was to persist for 200 years.

Contractio digitorum sinistræ manus, in volam illius.

INsignis artifex lapicida quidam, saxum immensum voluens, adeò téndines in sinistræ manus vola ad digitos, annularem & minimum desinentes, ei attracti sunt, vt illi à vinculis quib. retinétur laxati, eleuatique, duas chordas sub cute tensas in altum referrent, contractique duo hi digiti & attracti, postea semper manserint.

Digiti

Fig. 1.1 Plater's description of Dupuytren's contracture, 1614. 'Contraction of the fingers of the left hand into the palm. A certain well-known master mason, on rolling a large stone, caused the tendons to the ring and little fingers in the palm of the left hand to cease to function. They contracted and in so doing were loosed from the bonds by which they are held and became raised up, as two cords forming a ridge under the skin. These two fingers will remain contracted and drawn in forever.'
'Translation by J. B. St. Clair, 1987.'
(Reproduced by kind permission of the Wellcome Institute for the History of Medicine.)

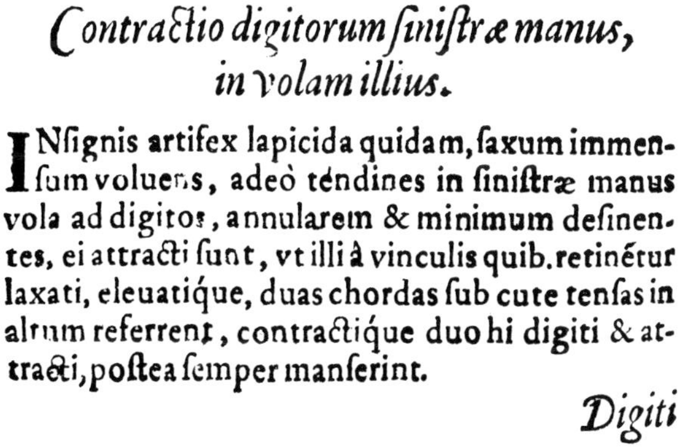

The advent in Europe of the anatomist surgeons of the late 18th century sparked a revolution in surgery. Foremost among these were the Hunter brothers; John Hunter is considered to be the father of British surgery. Surprisingly, the voluminous works of the Hunters contain few preparations of diseased hands and none of contraction of the palmar fascia. However, it was one of John Hunter's pupils, Henry Cline Senior, who first dissected a hand with this condition in 1777 (Fig. 1.2) and described its treatment, by palmar fasciotomy, soon after (Cline 1787) (Fig. 1.3).

Though little known today, Henry Cline was a

185
Contraction of the Fingers

The Contractions of the fingers which so frequently happens in laborious people arises from a thickening and shortening of the fascia in the palm of the hand, without any alteration in the muscles and tendons. This has been seen on dissecting two subjects, in one all the fingers were contracted, but upon cutting through the fascia they were immediately extended. In the other the ring finger only was contracted, which was found to arise from a thickening and shortening of that portion of ligament, which is inserted into that finger. It appeared from the last case, that the fascia is not blended with the theca of the fingers, but inserted into the phalanges distinctly by the side of it.

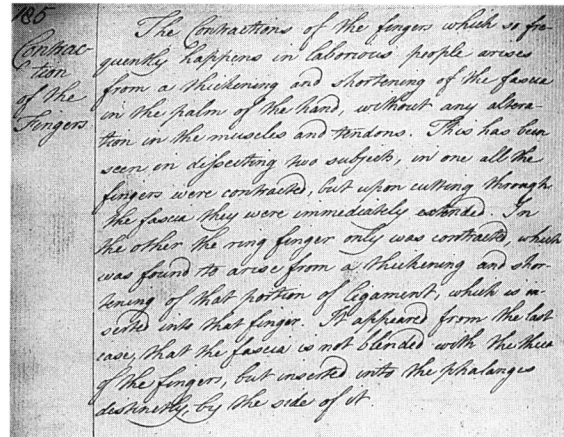

Fig. 1.2 Henry Cline's note-book, 1777, page 185.
(Reproduced by kind permission of the Library of St Thomas' Hospital Medical School, London.)

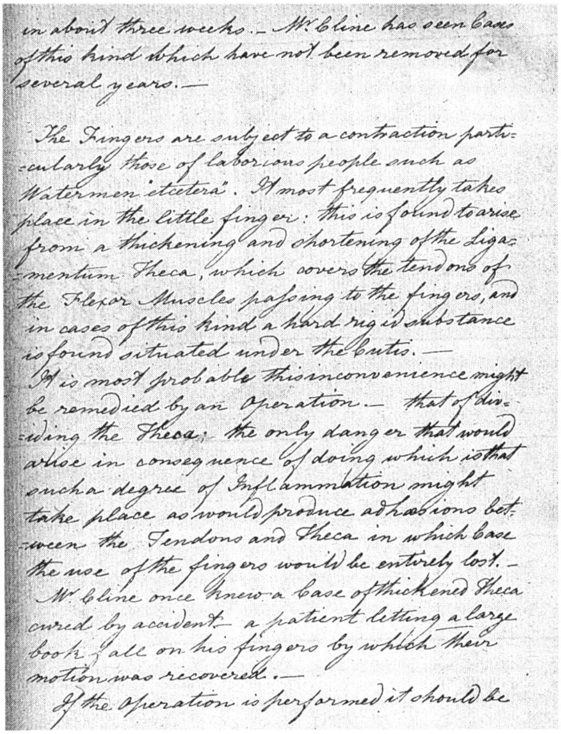

in about three weeks. — Mr Cline has seen Cases of this kind which have not been removed for several years.—

The Fingers are subject to a contraction particularly those of laborious people such as Watermen etcetera. It most frequently takes place in the little finger: this is found to arise from a thickening and shortening of the Ligamentum Theca, which covers the tendons of the Flexor Muscles passing to the fingers, and in cases of this kind a hard rigid substance is found situated under the Cutis.—

It is most probable this inconvenience might be remedied by an Operation — that of dividing the Theca; the only danger that would arise in consequence of doing which is that such a degree of Inflammation might take place as would produce adhesions between the Tendons and Theca in which case the use of the fingers would be entirely lost.— Mr Cline once knew a Case of thickened Theca cured by accident — a patient letting a large book fall on his fingers by which their motion was recovered.—

If the Operation is performed it should be

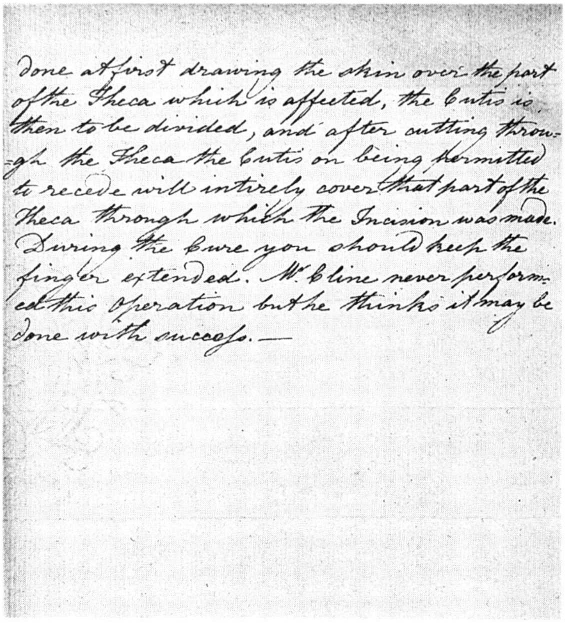

done at first drawing the skin over the part of the Theca which is affected, the Cutis is then to be divided, and after cutting through the Theca the Cutis on being permitted to recede will intirely cover that part of the Theca through which the Incision was made. During the Cure you should keep the finger extended. Mr Cline never performed this Operation but he thinks it may be done with success.—

Fig. 1.3 Notes of Thomas Smart, student, from a lecture by Henry Cline, 1787.
(Reproduced by kind permission of the Library of St Thomas' Hospital Medical School, London.)

prominent medical figure in London in his time. He was born in 1750 and was apprenticed at the age of 17 to Thomas Smith, surgeon to St Thomas's Hospital. On the death of Thomas Else, in 1781, Cline was appointed lecturer in anatomy and surgery to the hospital. Three years later, he succeeded Smith as consulting surgeon to St Thomas's. Cline dominated this hospital for 30 years, at a time when it was pre-eminent among the London hospitals, and his teaching played an important part in the spread of the new discipline of surgery throughout the UK. In 1811, at the age of 61, he retired from his teaching appointment and in the following year resigned his clinical post in favour of his son. Having been appointed to the Court of Assistants of the Surgical Company in1796, he continued to serve on the Court of the new College of Surgeons of England from its inception in 1800. He was a member of the Court of Examiners in 1810 and Master of the College in 1814. He served as President of the College in 1823 (the title of master having been changed to that of president in 1821). He delivered the Hunterian orations in 1816 and again in 1824. He died in 1826 at the age of 76. Though Cline's contribution to the expansion of surgery in his time was by no means modest, perhaps his most lasting influence on the development of the specialty in England was as a link between John Hunter and Astley Cooper. In 1789, after an apprenticeship of five years, Cooper was invited by Cline to share his lectures. This partnership dominated surgical teaching in London for 22 years and, on the retirement of Cline in 1811, Cooper continued to lecture with his son until the premature death of the latter in 1820.

Though Cooper was eventually to eclipse his mentor and Cline's name has submerged beneath those of Hunter and Cooper, nevertheless it was Cline who first recognized the true nature of the condition now known as Dupuytren's disease. In 1777 — by coincidence, the year of Dupuytren's birth — he dissected two cadaveric hands with this contracture of the fingers. The entry in his notebook records the involvement of the palmar fascia and the effect of dividing it (Fig. 1.2). He recognized the disease as one of 'laborious people'. In one of his dissections, the disease involved all of the fingers.

The record of his long career as a lecturer in

anatomy and surgery is fragmentary and the earliest indication that his observations were passed on to his students are the lecture notes of Thomas Smart in 1787 (Fig. 1.3): here, Cline proposed an operative cure (by palmar fasciotomy), though he had not performed the procedure at this time.

The lecture notes of John Windsor described the state of the art in 1808. After a brief description of the anatomy of the palmar fascia, the lecturer, Henry Cline Junior, comments:

One or more of these tendinous columns of the aponeurosis palmaris sometimes becomes contracted and thickened; most generally one only is affected, but sometimes more, and proportionably so many fingers are bent into the palm of the hand. The treatment is easy and efficacious; it consists in cutting through the aponeurosis with a common knife. In performing the operation, carefully dissect through, fibre by fibre, the aponeurosis palmaris, in order to avoid the blood-vessels and nerves beneath; the finger or fingers may be kept extended afterwards by a splint, for the flexor muscle has in some degree become shortened, and without this the disease might be reproduced.

There follows a brief discussion of the differential diagnosis from Volkmann's ischaemic contracture. Cline echoes Plater's description of the stonemason's hand, reiterating what is the clinical hallmark of Dupuytren's disease: 'the latter [aponeurosis palmaris] feels like a very hard cord raising the skin'. He then adds: 'but the flexors are too low to start thus, and are also bound down by the ligamentum annulare', so excluding the flexor tendons from further involvement in this disease in the UK.

Cooper, writing again of this condition in 1822, was equally brief, but perhaps considerably more astute than has been realized. He wrote:

The fingers are sometimes contracted in a similar manner [he had been discussing the treatment of hammer toes], by a chronic inflammation of the thecae (the flexor tendon sheaths), and aponeurosis of the palm of the hand, from excessive action of the hand, in the use of the hammer, the oar, ploughing, etc. etc. When the theca is contracted, nothing should be attempted for the patient's relief, as no operation or other means will succeed; but when the aponeurosis is the cause of the contraction, and the contracted band is narrow, it may be with advantage divided by a pointed bistoury, introduced through a very small wound in the integument. The finger is then extended, and a splint is applied to preserve it in the straight position.

Cooper's discussion of the treatment of Dupuytren's disease was to be misquoted again and again in the French literature, first by Dupuytren, then by those who followed him, as an absolute statement that the disease was incurable. In fact, Cooper had realized, presumably as a result of long clinical experience (this description of the management of the condition was written 14 years after the lecture recorded by John Windsor), that only disease of the palm was amenable to fasciotomy and then only if the bands were narrow.

Surgery of the hand featured in clinical practice at that time only in so far as injury and infection demanded attention. Without anaesthesia, and with death from sepsis a not infrequent sequel to surgery, there can have been few candidates for elective hand surgery and few surgeons willing to attempt more than the smallest of procedures. Thus might be explained the seeming lack of interest of the London surgeons in this condition, and the limitations which they set on the use of surgery for its cure.

It is of interest to speculate why Dupuytren was unaware of this work by the surgeons of the United Hospitals, when most of the surgeons in the UK had probably heard, directly or indirectly, of Cline's treatment of the condition, and when Astley Cooper and Dupuytren communicated and visited each other on several occasions during the period which preceded the latter's famous lecture of 5 December 1831 (Fig. 1.4). Whereas Dupuytren worked in an environment where the newly introduced medium of medical journalism had flourished to the extent that Paris had at least three weekly and two monthly medical journals, Cline belonged not only to a different generation but also to a less medically cosmopolitan city: even by 1830, London had a much smaller medical press. Cline's active surgical life largely predates medical journalism. He wrote virtually nothing: his medium was the lecture and it is only through the notes of his students and the writings of his younger contemporaries, particularly Cooper, that his work is known. It is likely that the only knowledge Dupuytren had of Cline was that gleaned in conversation with Cooper. In an era of great surgical discovery — with these two men pioneering the treatment of aneurysms: Dupuytren the first to resect the lower jaw and Cooper per-

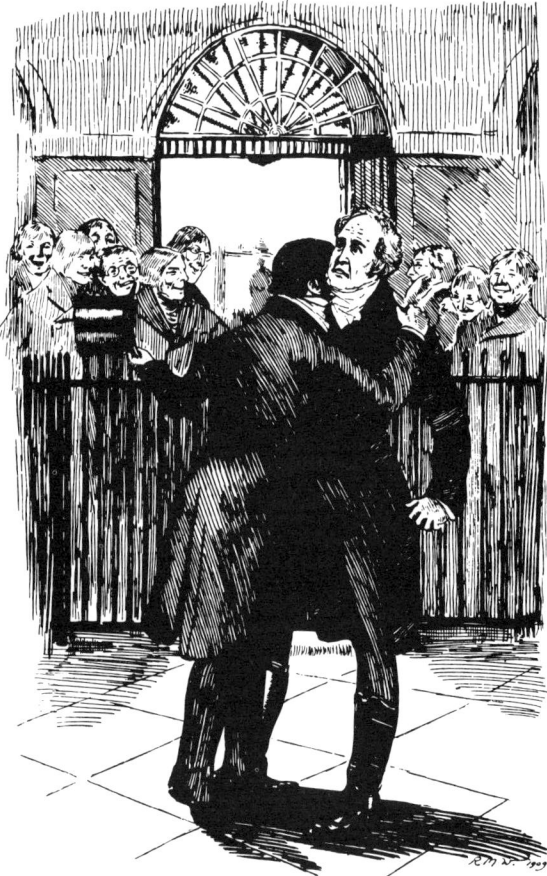

Fig. 1.4 Dupuytren's visit to Guy's Hospital, London, in 1826. **Episode for a Guy's Pageant:** 'Sir Astley's fame was European, so that distinguished foreign surgeons never failed to visit him at the Hospital. We read of Dupuytren going round the wards with him . . . . . When he took leave he saluted the worthy baronet on each cheek. The manner in which Sir Astley submitted to the ceremony afforded no small amusement to the pupils standing round.' — *Wilks and Bettany's History.*
(Reproduced by kind permission of the Editor of the Guy's Hospital Gazette.)

forming a hindquarter amputation (without anaesthesia) in 35 minutes — the two men must have had so much to discuss that Cooper may have forgotten even to mention this condition of the hand about which he was consulted little, on which he operated even less and for which the treatment was 'easy and efficacious'.

Although many of the surgical texts written in France during the 18th century discuss surgery of the hand — the bias being, as one would expect,

towards the emergency treatment of infection and trauma — I have found no reference to contracture of the palmar fascia. The condition began to appear in various guises in the writings of the new subspecialties of medicine developing in Paris at the beginning of the 19th century. In 1813, Chomel submitted an *Essai sur le Rheumatisme* as his graduation thesis, in which this flexion contracture of the fingers is considered to be a complaint associated with rheumatism or gout. In 1832, Baron Alibert, physician to Louis XVIII and the founder of dermatology in France, described what may have been Dupuytren's disease, in his classic *Monographie des Dermatoses*, under the name of *le paratrime palmaire*.

Recognizable in the latter part of Alibert's description of *le paratrime palmaire* is the condition which Boyer had described in 1826, using the name *crispatura tendinum*, by which it had been known to earlier surgeons. Boyer attributed the contracture of the fingers to a drying, hardening and stiffening of the flexor tendons and the overlying skin. It is clear from his description that the surgeons of Paris were aware of this disease before his time and he himself had sufficient experience of the disease to warn his readers strongly against dividing the flexor tendons, as this was 'probably never a practical proposition and a prudent surgeon would always refrain from it' — advice Dupuytren was to echo five years later. Dr Mailly, one of Boyer's pupils, was a wise surgeon or, at least, a diligent pupil: in 1831, he was consulted by a wine-merchant, M. L——, who lived at 25 quai de la Tournelle, about such a contracture of the fingers; remembering Boyer's advice, he was reluctant to advise surgery, as others had done. Instead, he referred the patient to Dupuytren, the senior surgeon of the neighbouring Hôtel-Dieu and, with the decline of Boyer, Larrey and Percy — the older generation of napoleonic surgeons — now considered the greatest surgeon in Paris. Dupuytren subsequently performed his first palmar fasciotomy on this patient.

On 5 December 1831, Dupuytren presented his findings on the contracture of the palmar fascia to the Hôtel-Dieu. This lecture was reported verbatim in the Journal Universel et Hebdomadaire de Médecine et de Chirurgie Pratiques et des Institutions Médicales — one of the Paris weekly journals — by his assistants Paillard and Marx. They wrote that they had attempted to report the exact words of the professor so that the readers might have an idea of his style of presentation — a unique account preserving a lecture by Dupuytren. This lecture was to be repeated in the following session, probably for the last time, as Dupuytren's illness at the end of November 1833 cut short his career. It was widely reported in the Paris medical press, where discussion began involving most of the surgeons of that city, continuing in a series of articles over several years. Reports appeared later in the British press; the first lecture was summarized in the London Medical and Surgical Journal of 1832 and the second, from the session of 1832–1833, appeared in the Lancet of 1834. It was in response to the latter that Windsor wrote to the Lancet, quoting Henry Cline Junior's lecture of 1808. The formal collection of Dupuytren's work and views in the *Leçons Orales de Clinique Chirurgicale faites à l'Hôtel-Dieu de Paris par M. le Baron Dupuytren* began in 1832 and a précis of the above lecture takes pride of place as the first article of the first volume.

Article XVII, later in the afore-mentioned book, is largely a summary of another lecture, which was first reported in the Journal Universal (Dupuytren 1832b), in which Dupuytren discussed the differential diagnosis of flexion contracture of the fingers. There is some elaboration of the original lecture, including an interesting demonstration on a cadaveric specimen of the critical role of the aponeurosis in *rétraction permanente*. Otherwise, both contain a fairly standard list of the various causes of flexion contracture of the fingers recognized at the time, which can be found in several of the French surgical texts of that period.

The differential diagnosis of conditions causing flexion contracture of the fingers also featured strongly in the discussion in the Paris press which followed publication of Dupuytren's first lecture. Nevertheless, the second lecture is interesting in that it was presented as a series of case histories, including a case of contraction of the palmar fascia which he related to a single traumatic event and a surgically induced bow-stringing of a flexor tendon (following overzealous treatment of an infection of the finger in which the whole length of the tendon sheath had been opened). Industrial injuries leading to flexion contracture of the fingers, as a result of joint damage from holding fixed positions of the fingers for extended periods of time, were also mentioned. Dupuytren cited the example of women knitting, adding: '*Cette dé formation était plus commune autrefois que de nos jours*' (This deformity was more common previously than it is nowadays): one wonders whether he was thinking of the notorious *tricoteuses* who knitted below the guillotines of the Revolution during his schooldays in Paris.

Another patient in this lecture, presented as an example of clawing secondarily to ulnar nerve division, met with his injury when shot by a thief caught in the act of stealing lead from the roofs of neighbouring houses. The lecture finished with a summary of the pertinent points of differential diagnosis.

The Paillard & Marx article of 1831 was reported with varying degrees of accuracy, with the second-hand descriptions becoming less precise with increasing time and distance from the event. Thus, Dupuytren's mention of Cooper's opinion began in 1831 as: '*Sir Astley Cooper, praticien non moins distingué, dans un pays voisin, donnât, ainsi que le rapporta M. Bennati, un conseil tout-à-fait semblable à M. Ferrari, maitre de piano*' (Sir Astley Cooper, a no less distinguished practitioner, in a neighbouring country, as M. Bennati has reported, gave quite similar advice to M. Ferrari, a piano teacher). In the *Leçons Orales* (Dupuytren 1832), this had become: '*M. le Docteur Bennati, consultant Astley Cooper pour un italien, nommé Ferrari*' (Dr Bennati, consulting Astley Cooper on behalf of an Italian called Ferrari) and was translated in the London Medical and Surgical Journal of 1832 as 'M. Bernali consulted Sir Astley Cooper for an Italian named Tersori'. The patient had acquired a nationality and lost the profession which probably explained his desperate search for a cure, at any cost, to a condition which was destroying his livelihood.

It seems appropriate to concentrate an analysis of Dupuytren's opinion of this disease on the 1831 account, though the Paris journals indicate that he added to his initial interpretation over the next two years. That Paillard & Marx were in a position to have reported the lecture as they claimed is substantiated by their close association with

Dupuytren — Marx was his personal secretary in all but name and the beneficiary in his will who received half of his books and observations and was instructed to publish any of them worthy of note.

In the manner of the day, the event of the 5 December was a lecture demonstration: the patient was brought from the adjoining Sainte-Marthe ward to be introduced to the audience, and used for clinical demonstration, before discussion of the pathology of his condition. The patient then underwent surgery and the lecture was concluded with a homily, stressing the pertinent facts.

Dupuytren introduced M. Demarteau, a 40-year-old coachman, who was to be the subject of his talk, with the dramatic words: '*Je ne vous parlerai aujourd'hui que d'un seul malade et d'une seule maladie*' (Today I am only going to speak to you of one patient and one illness). He discussed the history and relevant clinical signs shown by this patient, including a demonstration of the subcutaneous bands crossing the patient's palms and their exaggeration by extension of the fingers. After mentioning that he had seen 30–40 cases of this disease over the previous 20 years, he proceeded to consider the aetiology of the condition, dismissing any association with inflammatory conditions, with rheumatic or gouty disorders, or with trauma to the ligaments, joints or bones. He firmly associated the disease with chronic local trauma, indicating the patient's profession and his use of a heavy-handled whip, and citing other examples of professions where work involved pressure of a heavy object on the palm with resultant chronic damage, leading to development of this disease. He admitted, however, that not all cases could be explained in this way.

He emphasized the clinical course of the disease, including the predilection for the ring finger, the spread to adjacent fingers, especially the little finger, and the progressive lifting of the palmar skin into folds over the contracting subcutaneous bands as they pulled the fingers into the palm. He stressed the normality of the joints, none of which — with the exception of the proximal interphalangeal joint — showed evidence of ankylosis. He described having witnessed on several occasions futile attempts to rupture these bands by hanging weights of 100 and even 150 lb (45 and 67.5 kg) from the fingers. He passed on to the nature of the bands, mentioning previous theories, in particular that of chronic thickening of the flexor tendons with loosening from their sheaths — the so-called crispatura tendinum — which had been popular up to this time. He also dismissed the possibility that the condition was due to pathology of the joints. At this point, he digressed to discuss the lateral ligaments of the interphalangeal joints, citing his own work (his *Thèse pour le doctorat* of 1803). It was not, however, until 1836 that Dr John Reid of Edinburgh described secondary shortening of the ligaments of the joints in this condition.

Dupuytren then demonstrated his own opinion. He described in detail the morbid dissection of an affected hand, which he had had drawn at each stage of the dissection. At this point in the lecture, he passed round the audience a drawing of the dissected hand, which Paillard & Marx (1831) pointed out was similar in appearance to that of the coachman in the room. Essentially this presentation repeated Cline's observations of 1777. Though giving greater detail, Dupuytren's dissection was nevertheless restricted to the palm of the hand. The skin, tendons and joints were demonstrated to be normal and the retracting force on the fingers shown to be not the tendon but the palmar aponeurosis and its prolongations to the sides of the finger.

He then returned to what had gone before, listing a host of time-honoured remedies, all of which he had tried without success in the past. Even splinting had been of no avail; at this time, splinting was a popular treatment for many conditions of the limbs and contemporary surgical texts and journals often included diagrams of splints which were sophisticated in design and differ from those of today only in their construction from wood, iron and leather. By way of indicating that the splints which he had tried were of the best, Dupuytren mentioned that they had been made by the celebrated Lacroix, who was probably the most well known of the Parisian *mécanicien-bandagistes* of his day. This man's nephew was probably the Lacroix who wrote the single remaining admission book of Dupuytren's service at the Hôtel-Dieu, and who subsequently helped Denonvilliers compile the first catalogue of the Musée Dupuytren in 1842. Dupuytren then described two occasions when he had witnessed division of the flexor tendons: one operation had been ineffectual and the other ended in near fatal sepsis.

After citing Boyer and Astley Cooper as having pronounced the disease incurable, he introduced the audience to his thoughts of surgical treatment following the above cadaver dissection. He related his first opportunity to test the proposed operation of fasciotomy, reading the tale of M. L ——, the wine-merchant of 25 quai de la Tournelle, as it had been written by Dr Mailly, who had originally referred the case to him and who subsequently assisted at the operation on 12 June 1831. Fasciotomy through a transverse incision at the level of the distal palmar crease successfully released the ring finger but was only partially successful in releasing the little finger. This finger was only completely straightened after three fasciotomies, one at the distal palmar crease, one at the level of the mid proximal phalanx and one at the proximal interphalangeal joint. Postoperative extension splinting — probably rather too vigorously from the pain and inflammation which ensued — with an apparatus made by a trussmaker was started the following morning. The crudity of this splint was blamed for the pain and swelling and the ubiquitous Lacroix was called to provide a more serviceable splint. However, pain persisted and had to be relieved over the following week with soaks of lead acetate solution.

The skin incision had been left unsutured and healed by secondary intention in 20 days. Though stiff on removing the splint, the fingers soon regained full flexion. Night splinting was maintained for another month and an excellent result was achieved.

Dupuytren then analysed what had been seen at operation. He made the point that the skin was bound intimately to the palmar aponeurosis by dense fibrous tissue, in which there was little fat. As the aponeurosis contracted, the skin was thrown into folds. He described four bundles of aponeurotic tissue extending into the two involved fingers from where the prolongations of the aponeurosis to each finger forked to allow the passage of the flexor tendons. These bundles inserted into the proximal ends of the two proximal phalanges and into the deep transverse metacarpal ligament. He stressed the role of these bundles in causing the condition. These had to be cut, but warning was given that it was immediately below these bundles that the nerves and arteries entered the finger. Fortunately the retraction of the fingers lifted the bundles like a bridge, leaving enough room below to make the incisions without risk. He maintained that the normal function of the palmar aponeurosis was not only to contain the deeper structures, but also to brace the fingers in a state of flexion — a resting state seen in humans, certain animals and particularly in birds (in which the aponeurosis was of great elasticity to increase the flexion force and so assist perching). In humans this disease could, therefore, be considered as an exaggeration of the normal state.

The operation was then performed upon the right hand of Demarteau, the coachman. This proceeded much as on the previous occasion, except that only palmar fasciotomies were required. A Lacroix splint was applied, and the demonstration concluded with a further description of the true pathology and its correct treatment. Finally, Dupuytren warned that this operation was not a panacea for all flexion contractures of the fingers.

Dupuytren's final words on this occasion, and again, when he talked of the differential diagnosis of flexion contracture of the fingers, were that he would speak on another occasion of contracture of the plantar aponeurosis and the associated flexion contracture of the toes, which was much more common and no less important. Unfortunately, he does not appear to have done so. The association of this disease of the hand with hammer-toes — for it is more probably of this and not true plantar Dupuytren's disease that he spoke, since the latter does not usually affect the toes — is interesting. Cooper had already made the association and two of the prominent figures who wrote on both diseases later in the century — William Adams (1892) and William Anderson (1897) — independently included both conditions in single volumes.

In January 1832, Vidal de Cassis began a series of review articles of Dupuytren's clinics in the *Gazette Médicale de Paris*. He outlined his intention to explain briefly the doctrines developed by Dupuytren from his clinical observations and qualify these with his own comments and reflections. Again the contracture of the palmar aponeurosis was given pride of place: in his own words, he described the clinical features of the disease, making the observation that in the early stages, only the metacarpophalangeal joint is involved, the interphalangeal joints being straight and mobile. After describing Dupuytren's original contribution of the previous month, he posed the question of his professor — why, particularly, is the ring finger involved by this condition? He then advanced his own theory that the explanation may be that the ring finger has the least power of extension. He pointed out that this fact was well known to musicians, who recognize this finger as the most feeble and the most gauche. Having pointed out the importance of the extensors in the primary development of this deformity, he indicated his intention to write further on this subject. There were also several things he intended to discuss at a later date about the treatment; in particular, the conservative management of the condition.

Later in the same year, the *Gazette Médicale de Paris* reported again from Dupuytren on this subject: in July, he saw a 6-year-old child with flexion contractures of the ring and little fingers which had been present since birth. There was no evidence of burn or any other scars and extension of the fingers raised the characteristic cords under the palmar skin. The contracture was identical to that of the child's grandmother. Dupuytren concluded that one must add congenital and even hereditary causes to the list of aetiological factors of the disease and must, perhaps, consider a congenital predisposition in those who developed the condition as a result of chronic trauma of the palm. This confusion of camptodactyly with Dupuytren's disease was to persist and the term juvenile Dupuytren's disease remained in use until the end of the century (Hutchinson 1897).

Other causes of contracture of the fingers were then considered, including the case of a small girl who had developed tethering of the extensor tendon of the middle finger just proximal to the wrist as a result of an infection. This had caused hyperextension of the wrist and metacarpophalangeal joint. Dupuytren explained the secondary flexion of the interphalangeal joints by the wrist tenodesis effect, pointing out that it was impossible to extend the normal wrist beyond a certain point without the fingers flexing.

In 1833, Guérin wrote again from Dupuytren's clinic in the *Gazette Médicale de Paris*. In the description of the first case reported, we are reminded of the grim reality of surgery without anaesthesia: '*le malade avait commencé à crier avant le premier coup de bistouri*' (the patient had begun to shout before the bistoury had made its first incision). Guérin then described a much more severe case of Dupuytren's contracture than any that had gone before. This patient, a 22-year-old mason, had involvement of all five digits of the right hand. In this case, it was noted that the skin was so thickened that it appeared like burn-scarring in places and could not be separated from the subcutaneous bands; the interphalangeal joints were also involved. Four different bands to the thumb were described: one crossing the first web space from the index finger; one passing from the palmar disease in the line of the middle finger; another from the palmar disease in the line of the ring finger and a separate band commencing in the thenar eminence and passing to the radial border of the thumb. This hand was treated by what was becoming the routine operation, followed by prolonged postoperative extension splinting. Perhaps not surprisingly, this hand could not flex on removing the splint. With physiotherapy, the range of movement returned to almost normal.

Guérin pointed out that this was an atypical case. Nevertheless, he maintained that it was difficult to explain the involvement of the thumb on Dupuytren's theory that this was a disease of the aponeurosis alone, since there was no extension of the aponeurosis to this digit. In this case, the subcutaneous tissue of the thenar eminence was fibrous and very much involved in the retraction of the thumb. The skin was also involved in the fibrous change, and the natural planes deep to the skin had largely disappeared.

Though it could be argued that the operation had been successful because of the fasciotomy, incision of the apneurosis had only been achieved by first incising the cutaneous bands. Guérin doubted the lasting success of surgery in this case and was in complete agreement with Dupuytren that it would certainly recur if the patient did not continue to use the splint from time to time. By way

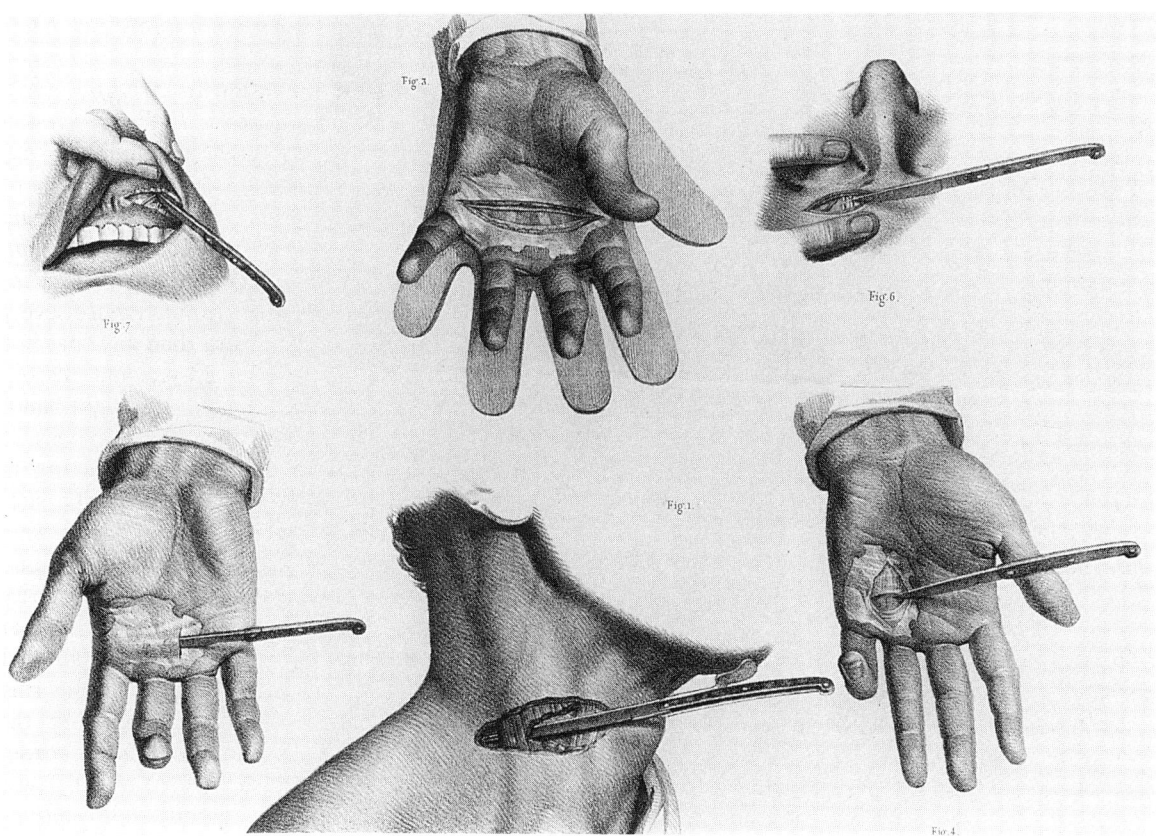

Fig. 1.5 Illustrations from a French Atlas of Surgery of 1839 showing the incisions of Cooper, Dupuytren and Goyrand. Top centre — Dupuytren's incision; Bottom right — Goyrand's incision; Bottom left — Cooper's incision. (Bougery and Jacob, 1839.)

of contrast with this case, he concluded by describing two dissections which he had recently performed in which the disease was exactly as Dupuytren had described, affecting only the ring and little fingers and without involvement of the skin.

Dupuytren's contribution to this disease, and to all surgery, had ended (Fig. 1.5). It is unfortunate that he was unable to answer in person the violent criticism of his contribution which followed in the Académie Royale de Médecine.

Bibliography — see pp. 413–419.

SECTION 1

Biology

M. H. Flint

2

Connective tissue biology

Much of the material that has been previously published on the subject of palmar nodular thickening and contraction has regarded the process as essentially pathological or diseased. This is reflected in its various eponyms — Dupuytren's disease, maladie de Dupuytren, morbus Dupuytrens, Dupuytren's contracture and even by the generic term, palmar fibromatosis. Some of the difficulties in characterization of the disease process as a pathological entity were stressed by Hueston (1977), who suggested; 'indeed there is much to indicate that we are dealing with an almost unique condition'. However, careful examination of histological, biochemical and metabolic features of the process indicates that many of these are non-specific biological responses common to a variety of mesenchymal connective tissue situations. For this and other reasons, I believe that a better understanding of the aetiology of the process and its progress through its various stages can be gained by viewing the process and its antecedents as a variety of biological phenomena occurring within the palmar connective tissues.

Connective tissues in general are characterized by the fact that their extracellular matrix forms the greater part of their bulk. This extracellular matrix is generally, if not always, functionally involved in the transmission or absorption of physical forces such as tension, compression and shear stress or in supporting or maintaining three-dimensional space, or the morphological interrelationship of one tissue with another (Flint 1981).

The general morphological features of connective tissues which govern their physical characteristics and their response to changing environmental loading will be briefly outlined later in this chapter and in greater detail in other chapters which specifically deal with the main structural elements of connective tissues, collagen and proteoglycans. However, as most readers of this book will probably be practising clinicians, it is important not to overemphasize either the biochemical or the biological minutiae of DD and its antecedents, but rather to try and present a readily comprehensible, holistic concept of its biological background and indicate how this might relate to changes in the connective tissue framework of the palm.

Although it has been known for 200 years or more that bones are remodelled during growth and development and after injury (Flint et al 1980), it is only comparatively recently that biologists and clinicians have come to realize that most, if not all connective tissues are, in more subtle ways, involved in continual remodelling and that there is no constancy of even apparently solid objects such as ligaments and tendons. Connective tissues are vital dynamic structures, ever changing and responding to the needs of their environment (Flint 1972, 1981; Reid & Flint 1974; Merrilees et al 1978; Gillard et al 1979). This applies not only to normal palmar connective tissues but also to the tissues of the Dupuytren's process itself.

It has been previously recognized (McFarlane 1974, 1985) that the Dupuytren's process does not develop or extend in haphazard or random manner but always begins in or extends along established anatomically identifiable connective tissue structures. However, the key to understanding its aetiology is the realization that these anatomically defined structures are subject to the various influences which constantly affect connective tissue organization and synthetic activity throughout the body. Consequently, it may be that the process known as DD arises not as a pathological disorder but rather as a consequence of morphological and metabolic changes, resulting from adaptive responses to applied stimuli in one or more of the anatomically defined constituents of the 'palmar connective tissue continuum'.

PALMAR CONNECTIVE TISSUE CONTINUUM

Over the past two decades there has been considerable debate between proponents of two opposing schools of thought about the site of development of the initial Dupuytren's lesion, due to different concepts of the distribution and extent of the palmar fascia. In other sections of the book it will be shown that the initial lesion of DD frequently occurs in fibres of the palmar fascia — not necessarily in the obvious thicker longitudinally running fibres of the triangular-shaped palmar aponeuroses of anatomical textbooks (Millesi 1985), but in the finer, almost microscopic fibres of the more superficial longitudinal fibre bundles coursing distally amongst the hypodermal fat pads to interact with fascial fibres of the dermis itself and the subjacent hypodermis. The connective tissues of the superficial palm from the underside of the epidermis to the deeper aspect of the deep longitudinally running fibres of the palmar fascia are really an integrated functional unit and should be regarded as a palmar connective tissue continuum. From this standpoint most would happily accept that the Dupuytren's process starts somewhere within this palmar connective tissue continuum — somewhere deep to the underside of the epidermis but superficial to the transverse fibres of the palmar aponeurosis which are apparently never primarily involved in the disease process (Skoog 1967).

The concept that the collagen fibres, the enclosed fibrofatty compartments and the other constituents of the extracellular connective tissue matrix of the superficial palm are a single unified structure allows us to examine the integrity and interdependence of these structures and to realize how changes in their biomechanical properties can drastically affect the functional capability of the palm leading to areas of biological reorganization which we recognize as DD. I would venture to suggest that, when viewed biomechanically or biologically in relation to the function of the hand, and particularly in relationship to the development of DD, the most important part of the palmar fascia lies superficial to the well defined layer of palmar aponeurosis.

CONNECTIVE TISSUE RESPONSIVENESS

Research over the last decade has demonstrated that connective tissues are remarkably constant in their response to physical and physicochemical changes in their environment, producing predictable changes in cellular synthetic activity and consequently in extracellular morphology in response to changing load (Flint 1972, 1983; Gillard et al 1979; Flint et al 1980). In fact, one can almost guarantee that if connective tissues are subjected to a change in environmental stimulus, say tension or pressure, an appropriate homeostatic response will be initiated in the cells leading to a synthetic or metabolic shift and a consequent reorganization of the cells' extracellular environment to deal more effectively with the changes in environmental load. Conversely, if certain applied forces are withdrawn, the cell will respond equally rapidly, and metabolic and matrix adjustments will inevitably follow (Flint 1972; Gillard et al 1979; Flint & Gillard 1980a; Flint et al 1980; Sharpe et al 1980). Experiments in our laboratories have demonstrated that quite profound metabolic shifts can occur within 24–48 hours of changes in the applied load to tissues and that profound matrix reorganization can occur within 10–14 days (Brown & Flint 1982, 1983). However, these changes are not spread uniformly throughout the whole of the connective tissue matrix; some constituents change much more rapidly than others.

Research in various parts of the world has demonstrated the essential similarities and differences in biochemical composition, cellular synthetic activity and extracellular organization of connective tissues in tensional, non-tensional, pressure-bearing and shear-resisting situations (Thaxter et al 1965; Akeson et al 1967; Hall 1970;

Telhag & Lindberg 1972; Flint 1972; Leung et al 1975; Caterson & Lowther 1978; Flint et al 1980). In essence, all connective tissues are basically composed of collagen, glycosaminoglycans, proteoglycans, water, salt and cells and associated extracellular glycoproteins such as fibronectin. In some situations, elastin is added to this basic framework to provide elastic recoil and sometimes hydroxyapatite is added to the collagen fibres to provide torsion-resisting strength and bony stability.

Collagen

The main constituent of connective tissues on a dry weight basis is the fibrous protein collagen. Until about 15 years ago it was thought that there was only one type of collagen, that collagen was the same anywhere in the body and even that collagens from different animals were more or less identical. However, more precise analytical methodologies have now shown that there is a considerable number of different collagen species (at the time of writing in 1989 at least 12 discretely different collagens have been identified). Although basically similar, in that they are extracellular proteins which contain three helical polypeptide chains possessing a similar repeating sequence of amino acids, each appears to have different biochemical composition, physicochemical structure and aggregation properties. For this reason it has been speculated that each has a particular specific biological function. The essential features of the different collagens found in skin, tendon, fascia and DD and their biophysical and biochemical interrelationships to other connective tissues are fully described in Chapter 6. For the purposes of understanding the concepts outlined in this chapter, it is sufficient to note that the major extracellular structural collagen of skin, tendon and fascia which largely subserves a tension-transmitting or resisting function is now known as type I collagen, whilst the more ephemeral collagen found in increased amounts in fetal and remodelling situations, such as wound healing, is known as type III collagen.

The presence of increased amounts of type III collagen in connective tissues generally indicates tissue immaturity or persistent connective tissue remodelling. For this reason it is quite common to see it in increased amounts in the early stages of wound healing, repair or hypertrophic scarring. Its persistence at a supranormal level in Dupuytren's nodular tissue is indicative of the immaturity of this tissue or of persistent active tissue remodelling process (Bailey et al 1977; Bailey & Duance 1980, Bazin et al 1980; Brickley-Parsons et al 1981). It is not, as some have suggested, a specific pathognomonic indicator of DD or an indicator of some genetic malfunction (Hueston 1975).

The increased amounts of type III collagen found in apparently clinically normal parts of the palmar aponeurosis well away from the areas of diseased fascia have aroused considerable interest; it has been suggested that collagen in apparently normal parts of the palm may be abnormal before there is any manifest evidence of DD (Bazin et al 1980; Brickley-Parsons et al 1981; Hueston 1985). However, there is now considerable histological and electron microscopical evidence indicating that the increased levels of type III collagen in apparently normal palmar aponeurosis arise as the result of active collagen remodelling in submicroscopic areas of damage in apparently clinically and visually normal palmar fascia (see Chapters 10 and 12).

PROTEOGLYCANS AND GLYCOSAMINOGLYCANS

Although collagen fibres provide the structural tensile elements of most connective tissues, their accretion, development and integration, and thereby the biophysical and biomechanical characteristics and properties of the tissue, are largely dependent upon the presence of a relatively small amount of large branching chains of disaccharide sugar units known as glycosaminoglycans (previously known as acid mucopolysaccharides; Serafini-Fracassini & Smith 1974). The glycosaminoglycan molecules which are often of very large molecular weight are generally, but not invariably, associated and integrated with specialized protein cores to form much larger functional units known as proteoglycans. The details of these proteoglycans and their constituent glycosaminoglycans are fully discussed in Chapter 5.

However, for the purposes of the present discussion of the biology of the connective tissue matrix in relationship to DD, it will suffice to confine consideration of the glycosaminoglycans to a simplistic understanding of their relationships to each other and to collagen and other extracellular matrix components (Flint 1981).

Essentially, there are five or six glycosaminoglycans found in connective tissues; only four of these are regularly found in normal palmar connective tissues or in Dupuytren's tissue (Flint et al 1982; Gurr et al 1984) or in cultures of cells grown from these tissues (Slack et al 1982; Delbruck & Schroder 1983). Hyaluronic acid (or sodium or calcium hyaluronate if it is compounded with its counterions) is a very large unsulphated polymer which has the property of enclosing vast amounts of water within its molecular domain. Consequently, this polymer is often found in situations requiring lubrication such as tendon sheaths and joint fluid; in situations where cell movement through a gel is required, such as the papillary layer of the skin or in embryonic tissue or wound repair and tissue remodelling. It also entangles water to act as a space-filler or as a means of disaggregating collagen fibres during tissue remodelling (Flint 1971, 1972). One of its great virtues as a biological material is the fact that it has a very short half-life and may only last in the tissues for a couple of days. For this reason I feel that it has a very important role in connective tissue homeostasis (Flint 1972). It is invariably associated with fine collagen fibril formation and appears to limit the size of collagen fibre aggregation (Parry et al 1982; Flint et al 1984).

The other glycosaminoglycans or proteoglycans found in connective tissue carry additional regularly spaced sulphate groups. These impart a higher negative charge and therefore a strong binding capacity to these materials; one of them, dermatan sulphate, is integrally associated with the collagen fibril structure (Toole & Lowther 1968; Scott et al 1981; Scott 1984). Collagen fibrils associated with dermatan sulphate tend to be thicker and have a higher tensile strength. For this reason, dermatan sulphate is found as the dominant polymer in tension-transmitting structures such as tendon (Parry et al 1982). In functionally active tendons, the total glycosaminoglycan content is very low, usually of the order of 0.2% of the dry weight (Gillard et al 1977). However, when the tendons are relieved of their tensional load, or if they are subjected to additional compressional loads, the amount of glycosaminoglycan may be markedly increased (Flint 1972, Reid & Flint 1974). In some specialized instances small intratendinous cartilagenous sesamoids may develop where the tendon is subjected to additional focal compressive loading. In these pressure-bearing regions the total glycosaminoglycan content may be 15–20 times as much as in the tension-transmitting parts of the tendon (Gillard et al 1979; Flint et al 1980).

In tissues which are subject to intermittent compressive loading, or even to less unidirectional tensional forces, chondroitin sulphate is found as the major glycosaminoglycan. Developing tissues such as in the embryo or in wound repair also contain relatively larger proportions of chondroitin sulphate than do their more mature counterparts. It is interesting in this regard that even cells from tensional situations, such as tendon, tend to synthesize chondroitin sulphate in preference to dermatan sulphate when grown in tissue culture, especially in non-confluent conditions (Mourao & Machado-Santelli 1978; Gallagher et al 1980).

Collagen fibres which are normally associated with higher levels of chondroitin sulphate are generally finer than those associated with dermatan sulphate but thicker than those associated with hyaluronate (Parry et al 1982; Flint et al 1984). In normal wound healing there is usually a relatively high concentration of both hyaluronate and chondroitin sulphate early in the phase of wound repair, but the level of chondroitin sulphate normally tails off and/gives way to a higher concentration of dermatan sulphate as the wound matures. It is noteworthy that in hypertrophic scarring and keloids the total concentration of glycosaminoglycans is much higher than normal and the concentration of chondroitin sulphate may be persistently greatly increased as compared with the situation in the well matured wound or scar (Bazin et al 1970; Kischer & Shetlar 1974; Shetlar & Shetlar 1977; Donoff & Burke 1978; Honda et al 1986).

PROTEOGLYCANS AND GLYCOSAMINOGLYCANS IN DD

Studies of glycosaminoglycan levels in palmar connective tissues and Dupuytren's material have been undertaken by various workers (Carr 1970; Hunter & Ogdon 1975; Bazin et al 1980). In our own work (Flint et al 1982) we studied the differences between different parts of the DD process and compared this with normal palmar fascial specimens, specimens of palmar skin and of the underlying digital flexor tendons. Whenever possible the excised specimens from Dupuytren's tissue were carefully dissected to identify and separate regions of nodular thickening from the thicker cellular bands and the denser fibrous cords. The results of this study, outlined in Tables 2.1 and 2.2, demonstrate that the overall levels of glycosaminoglycans in Dupuytren's tissue were significantly higher than those in normal palmar

Table 2.1 Glycosaminoglycan content (% dry weight) of Dupuytren's and control tissue

Tissue	n	Total glycosaminoglycans	Hyaluronic acid	Dermatan sulphate	Chondroitin sulphate
Dupuytren's					
Cellular bands	11	1.396 ± 0.054	0.121 ± 0.012	0.81 ± 0.056	0.454 ± 0.045
Nodules	15	1.172 ± 0.045	0.135 ± 0.010	0.680 ± 0.038	0.353 ± 0.031
Fibrous cords	18	0.704 ± 0.045	0.098 ± 0.011	0.431 ± 0.033	0.175 ± 0.017
Nodular bands	6	0.711 ± 0.081	0.106 ± 0.006	0.436 ± 0.047	0.17 ± 0.060
Uninvolved 'traction band'	1	0.228	0.08	0.07	0.06
Pooled nodules and bands	50	0.999 ± 0.045	0.120 ± 0.007	0.590 ± 0.029	0.283 ± 0.021
Pooled bands	29	0.957 ± 0.074	0.107 ± 0.009	0.572 ± 0.046	0.278 ± 0.032
Controls					
Palmar fascia (aponeurosis)	6	0.318 ± 0.028	0.111 ± 0.014	0.171 ± 0.020	0.035 ± 0.009
Palmar dermis	4	0.385 ± 0.030	0.17 ± 0.014	0.166 ± 0.020	0.043 ± 0.003
Pooled palmar connective tissue	10	0.351 ± 0.030	0.144 ± 0.020	0.168 ± 0.002	0.039 ± 0.006
Palmar segment of digital flexor tendons	4	0.221 ± 0.030	0.070 ± 0.010	0.090 ± 0.007	0.06 ± 0.020

Note
1. The chondroitin suphate content of nodules and cellular bands as compared with fibrous cords and bands, uninvolved fascia and underlying tendons.
2. The constancy of hyaluronic acid throughout all tissue.
3. The obvious activity of cellular bands as compared with the uninvolved traction band.

Table 2.2 Differential proportion of glycosaminoglycans in Dupuytren's nodules, bands and cords

Tissue	n	Glycosaminoglycans (% dry weight)	Hyaluronic acid (%)	Dermatan sulphate (%)	Chondroitin sulphate (%)
Cellular bands	11	1.396	9	58	33
Nodules	15	1.172	12	58	30
Fibrous cords	18	0.704	14	61	25
Palmar connectives tissue	10	0.351	41	48	11

connective tissue. However, this increased glycosaminoglycan concentration was not uniformly spread amongst the three main glycosaminoglycan fractions or the different manifestations of the disease process, i.e. nodules, cellular bands and fibrous cords. Cellular bands and nodules contained significantly greater amounts of glycosaminoglycans than did dense fibrous cords, which in turn contained significantly more glycosaminoglycans than palmar skin or fascia from the palms of age-matched controls.

The demonstration of an overall increase in glycosaminoglycans agreed with the findings of previous workers, but the differential proportional increases of chondroitin and dermatan sulphate and the concomitant reduction of hyaluronate observed in the study did not. Earlier investigators had suggested that only the dermatan sulphate levels were increased in the Dupuytren's process (Hunter & Ogdon 1975) whereas a more recent study had indicated that the increase was spread equally amongst the three main glycosaminoglycan fractions (Bazin et al 1980). The work of Flint et al (1982) demonstrated that whilst the dermatan sulphate level found in Dupuytren's tissue was four times greater than that of normal palmar connective tissues, the concentration of chondroitin sulphate was 11 times that of the control tissue.

In contrast, whilst the concentration of hyaluronate was similar in both diseased and normal tissues, there was a marked decrease in the relative proportion of hyaluronate in the diseased material (Tables 2.1–3; Figs 2.1 and 2.2). These variations in the tissue concentration of the three main glycosaminoglycan fractions indicated that there were differences in the rate of their synthesis or degradation, or that there was a differential retention of the synthesized products by the fibrous matrix of the Dupuytren's tissue.

The differences in the glycosaminoglycan content of the various manifestations of the DD process probably reflected differences in the de-

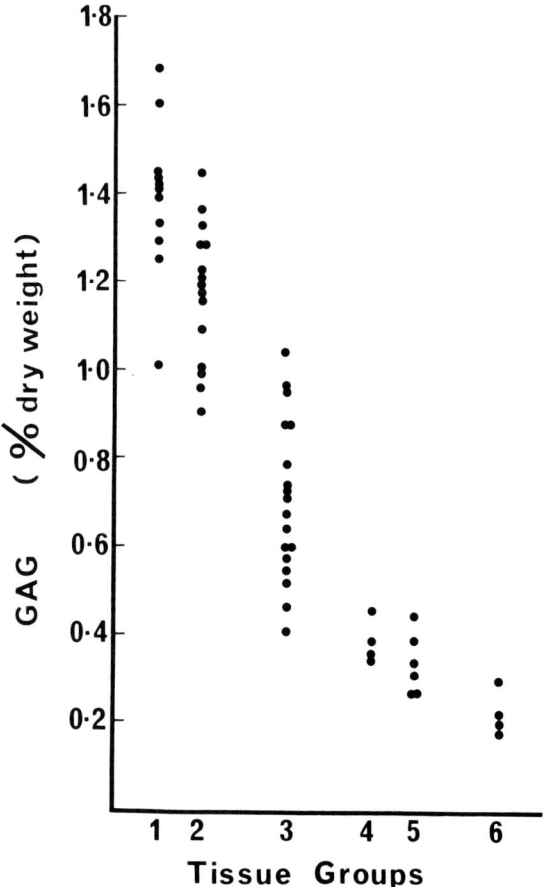

Fig. 2.1 Glycosaminoglycans (GAG) as % dry weight of **1** cellular bands; **2** nodules; **3** fibrous cords; **4** palmar dermis; **5** palmar fascia; **6** flexor tendons.

Table 2.3 Percentage change of glycosaminoglycans in different parts of Dupuytren's lesion as compared with normal fascia (100%)

Tissue	Total glycosaminoglycans	Hyaluronic acid	Dermatan sulphate	Chondroitin sulphate
Normal palmar	100	100	100	100
Cellular bands	398	84	482	1164
Nodule	334	93	404	905
Fibrous cords	200	68	257	449

Note the relative decrease of hyaluronic acid in all affected tissue.

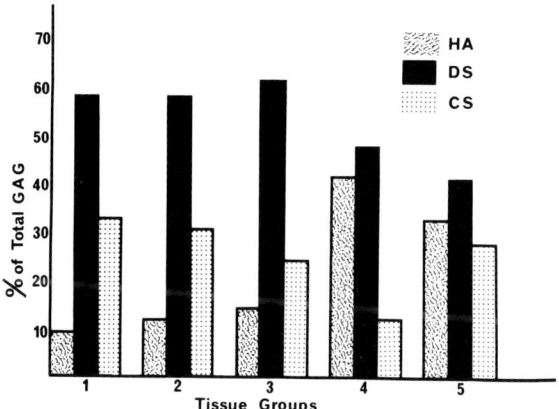

Fig. 2.2 Proportion of major glycosaminoglycan (GAG) fractions in Dupuytren's and normal tissues. 1 Cellular bands; 2 nodules; 3 fibrous cords; 4 normal palmar connective tissues; 5 digital flexor tendons.

gree of tissue maturation and the differences in the physical forces to which these tissues were subjected. The cellularity, glycosaminoglycan content and fraction profile of the cellular bands were surprisingly similar to those of the developing rabbit tendoachilles during the first week of postnatal development before it became subject to increased tensional forces from locomotory movement (Gillard & Flint 1981). On the other hand, the gross and microscopic morphological appearance of the fibrous bands and the associated reduction in total glycosaminoglycans particularly chondroitin sulphate, much more closely resembled a more mature — less cellular — tension-transmitting tendon.

The relatively high level of hyaluronate in normal palmar fascia could be related to the need for its free mobility and compliance. A decrease in hyaluronate levels in the fascia would markedly affect its gliding, sliding and compliance capability and might be a predisposing factor to the development of changes in palmar fascial compliance which have been implicated in the pathogenesis of DD (McGrouther 1982).

It is frequently suggested that the bands which extend into the fingers from the nodules arise in response to an increased tensional load resulting from cellular contraction within the nodule (Luck 1959). However the higher total glycosaminoglycans and particularly the increased chondroitin sulphate fraction found in the cellular bands strongly suggested that they are also part of the primary disease process. Certainly, histological examination of specimens shows that these bands are far more cellular than the mature dense fibrous bands. Whilst the cells of both the cellular and fibrous bands were more longitudinally orientated than those in the nodule, the former were plumper and more ovoid than those in the fibrous cords (see Fig. 2.3).

The total glycosaminoglycan levels and the relative proportional changes of their fractions in the nodules and cellular bands were surprisingly similar to those previously observed in hypertrophic scarring (Bazin et al 1970; Kischer & Shetlar 1974; Shetlar & Shetlar 1977; Donoff & Burke 1978; Honda et al 1986). The increased proportion of chondroitin sulphate in both hypertrophic scarring and Dupuytren's nodular tissue indicated that they were similar biological phenomena. The increased concentration of type III collagen which was found in both Dupuytren's nodules and hypertrophic scarring strengthened the impression that both processes reflected their prolonged tissue immaturity and perhaps the lack of appropriate cellular control mechanisms.

When the cells from the Dupuytren's nodules and bands were grown in tissue culture, the type and amount of synthesized glycosaminoglycans were almost identical to that produced by cells from normal fascial controls (Slack et al 1982). These findings strongly indicated that the cells were not, as some would believe, genetically abnormal or switched over to an abnormal synthetic pathway, but rather that the cells in the Dupuytren's nodules and cellular bands were synthesizing large quantities of chondroitin sulphate and type III collagen because of some local factor or factors within the palm.

What are these local factors and why should they lead to the development of the nodular bands and contractures recognized as DD? After looking at a vast amount of histological material from diseased and normal palms I have come to believe that the answer to these questions lies in the specialized microarchitecture of the palmar connective tissue continuum and the changes which take place in this in response to a variety of local and systemic environmental stimuli.

20 DUPUYTREN'S DISEASE

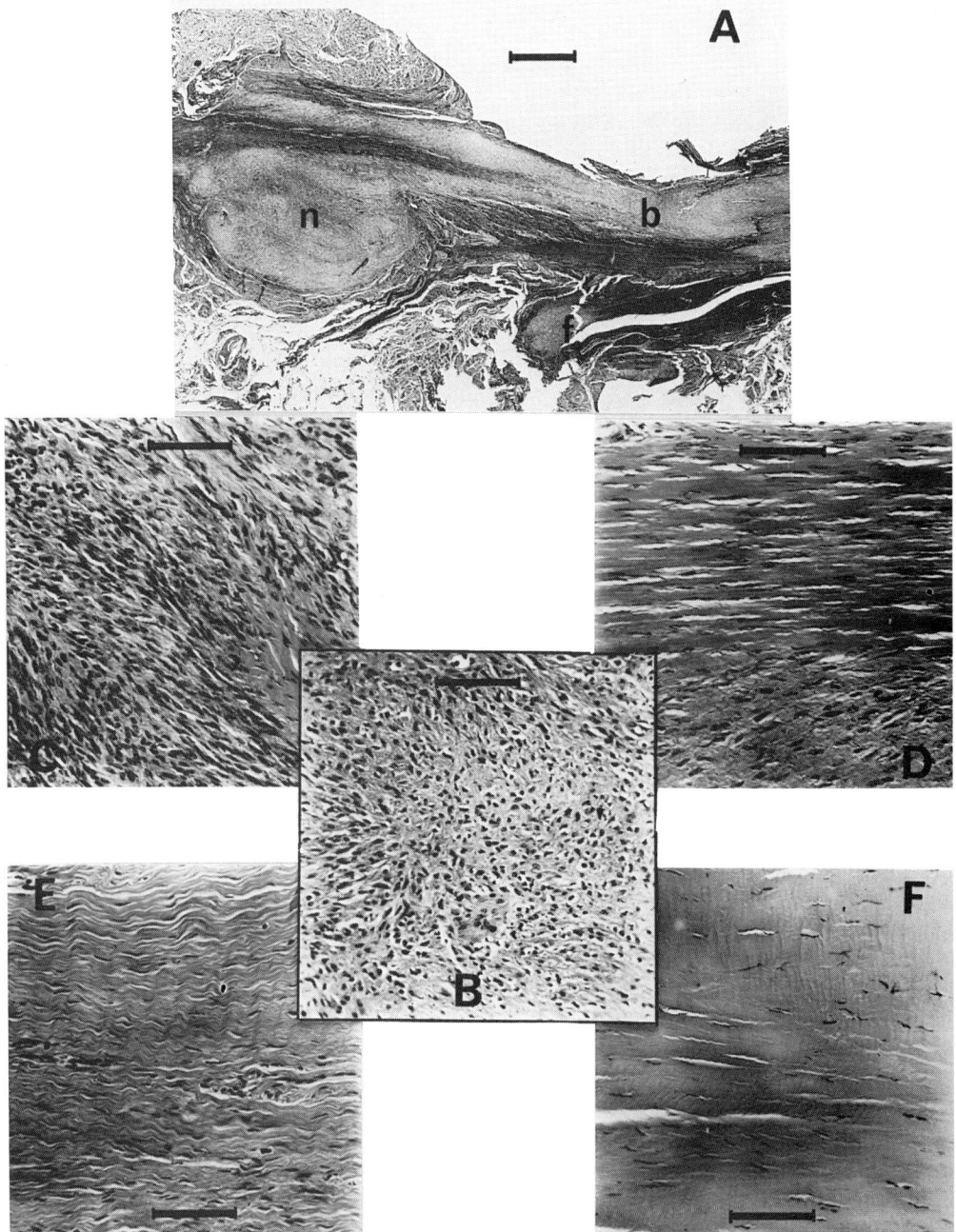

Fig. 2.3 Histological sections showing differences in cellular content in different parts of a Dupuytren's lesion. **A** Continuity of Dupuytren's nodule (n) with cellular band (b). Thicker, denser fibrous cord (f). Bar = 1 mm. **B** Section of nodule (n) showing ovoid and 'chondroid' cells. Bar = 100 μM. **C** Oriented plump cells of cellular part of band (b). Bar = 100 μm.
D Fibrous band with elongated cells (above) contiguous with more cellular area with more ovoid cells (below). Bar = 100 μm.
E Collagenous fibrous band with fibrocytic type cells. Bar = 100 μM. **F** Densely compacted, hyaline-type collagen fibres of mature fibrous cord and sparser distorted elongated fibrocytes.
Bar = 100 μm.

RELATIONSHIP OF BIOLOGY TO PATHOGENESIS

When viewed in isolation, DD appears to many to be a mysterious and almost inexplicable disease process. However, when the process and its antecedents are considered as a series of interrelated connective tissue biological events it is possible largely to demystify the enigma. One of the most fascinating aspects of connective tissue biology is the way in which it is possible to extrapolate information from one situation or tissue to another. This is made possible by the fact that the various connective tissues, even though apparently so dissimilar, are in reality variants on a theme. They share a common inheritance and a common cellular and metabolic response to any particular environmental stimulus, whether locally or systemically mediated. This constancy of responsiveness makes it possible to extrapolate information with amazing accuracy. For example, if a low level of proteoglycan is found in a tissue with a predominance of dermatan sulphate, it may be supposed fairly confidently that this tissue has been subjected to tensional forces and probably uniaxial tensional forces. It is then possible to predict that the collagen fibres will be longitudinally aligned and probably closely packed and that the contained fibroblasts will appear to be elongated with a length:breadth ratio of at least 4:1. Conversely, if microscopic examination of a tissue demonstrated these particular histological features, one could predict with a fair degree of certainty that the biochemical analysis will reveal a predominance of type I collagen, a relative paucity of proteoglycan or glycosaminoglycan on a dry weight basis, and a dominance of dermatan sulphate. However, if biochemical examination of a tissue sample demonstrated a greater amount of proteoglycan, and particularly a predominance of chondroitin sulphate, one could almost categorically assert, without examining the tissue, that it could not have been subject to uniaxial tensional forces. Furthermore, this single biochemical analysis permits the prediction that the collagen fibre pattern of this material shows signs of non-linearity and that the associated cells in consequence will also be non-aligned or randomly dispersed.

In essence, the Dupuytren's process can be regarded as a series of interrelated, and sometimes sequentially occurring, connective tissue responses:

1. Palmar fascial thickening.
2. Intrafascial nodule formation.
3. Cellular contraction.
4. Connective tissue remodelling and contracture.

In some cases of DD all these responses are evident; in others, only one or two may be apparent. However, each of these separate responses is explicable in terms of connective tissue biology.

The thickening and increased deposition of tendon collagen is well recognized as a response to increased loading (Craik & McNeil 1965, 1966; Tipton et al 1967; Viidik 1967, 1979; Rigby 1977; Woo et al 1980, 1982; Carlstedt 1987). The factors responsible for the thickening and coalescence of the fibres of the superficial longitudinal fascial bundles are fully discussed in Chapter 13.

Whilst some of the thickening of the longitudinal fibres undoubtedly occurs as a result of natural growth and homeostatic response, histological studies suggest that the thickening and coalescence of the superficial longitudinal fibre bundles may be exacerbated by alterations in the biomechanical and stress-absorptive properties of the palmar connective tissue continuum.

In some instances the longitudinal palmar fascial fibres are thickened without any evidence of intrafascial nodule formation, but in other cases, discrete intrafascial cellular thickenings or nodules are apparent (Fig. 2.4). These localized intrafascial cellular nodules are almost pathognomonic of DD. Whilst biochemical assays and histological studies indicate that they are zones of repair or connective tissue remodelling, there has as yet been no satisfactory explanation of their development or of their persistence.

Our histological and biochemical studies indicate that they may be analogous to similar intratendinous lesions seen in the tendoachilles or in the long head of biceps resulting from partial intratendinous rupture in which the overall continuity of the tendon is maintained.

In these various clinical situations, the intratendinous rupture or separation of fibres leads to the

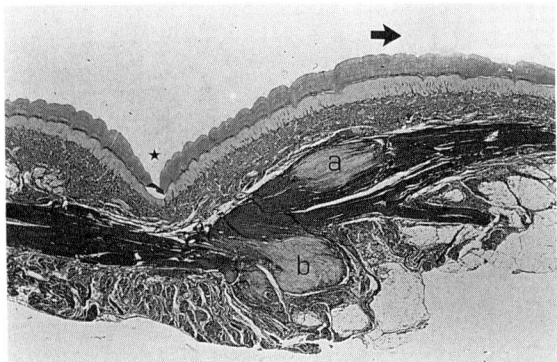

Fig. 2.4 Longitudinal section of palm taken along the fourth ray of the hand of an adult male shows thickening of superficial longitudinal fascial bundle. Proximal to the distal palmar crease (*) the bundle is thickened to approximately 3 mm. Distal to the crease intrafascial nodules are apparent in the superficial longitudinal bundle (a) and in an oblique band inferiorly (b). Arrow indicates distal part of section. Note the loss of subcutaneous fat proximal to and beneath the distal palmar crease.

development of localized nodular formation within the tendon. Histological examination demonstrates discontinuity of the collagen fibres, alteration in their staining pattern with the Masson trichrome procedure (Dreyer 1961; Craik & McNeil 1965, 1966; Flint 1972; Flint et al 1975), increased cellular reaction and changes in cellular morphology from elongated to round chondrocytic type of cells (Merrilees & Flint 1980). Histochemical and biochemical examination demonstrates a marked increase in glycosaminoglycan material, particularly chondroitin sulphate, within these nodular areas.

It has long been recognized amongst orthopaedic surgeons that these partial intratendinous ruptures are particularly refractory and slow to heal spontaneously. In normal circumstances, complete division of a tendon stimulates a wound-healing response with activation of paratenon and endotenon cells which come to be aligned across the gap between the divided ends of the tendon. Uniaxial tensional forces transmitted along the tendon and through the fibrin in the repair zone lead to the alignment of the primary biological scaffolding, the fibroblast ingrowth and the linear deposition of collagen fibres. Experimental wound-healing studies that I have undertaken on wounds made in various directions (Flint & Gillard 1980b) indicate that these uniaxial tensional forces appear to aid wound maturation, leading to a decrease of type III collagen and a gradual deposition of type I collagen. There is concurrently, a decrease in the initial post-traumatic accumulation of glycosaminoglycans, particularly chondroitin sulphate, so that eventually dermatan sulphate proteoglycan predominates, albeit at a very small level in relation to the total dry weight of the tissue.

However, it appears that if the fibril separation or division takes place within the substance of a tendon or fascial bundle with maintenance of fibre continuity around the periphery, a different set of physical forces, and consequently a different biological response, ensues (Fig. 2.5). Whilst division or tearing of central core fibres produces a discontinuity of fibrils, relaxation of collagen fibres and stimulation of an endotenon cellular response akin to that seen in complete division, the eventual cellular morphological and metabolic response appears to be quite different. There is less longitudinal directional organization of either fibrin or collagen fibres across the gap between the divided tendon ends; the post-mitotic reparative cells remain plump and round, are randomly arranged, and continue to produce significantly increased amounts of proteoglycan, particularly chondroitin sulphate. These features strongly indicate a lack of unidirectional tensional control. How does this occur in a longitudinally running structure like a tendon and how does it apply to the Dupuytren's nodule?

I suggest that in circumstances of central fibre rupture or dehiscence in either tendon or fascial fibres, the persistence of an outer rim of intact tension-transmitting fibres allows the transmission of tensional forces along the length of the fibre bundle (Fig. 2.6). The maintenance of intermittent tensional forces around the periphery of an internal zone of non-continuous collagen fibres and a wound-healing repair would exert intermittent compressive loading on the content of the internal healing zone, especially if it was swollen by inflammatory oedema (see Fig. 2.7). The biological effect of intermittent pressure on this central repair zone would be to encourage the further production of sulphated proteoglycan, particularly chondroitin sulphate, by the non-

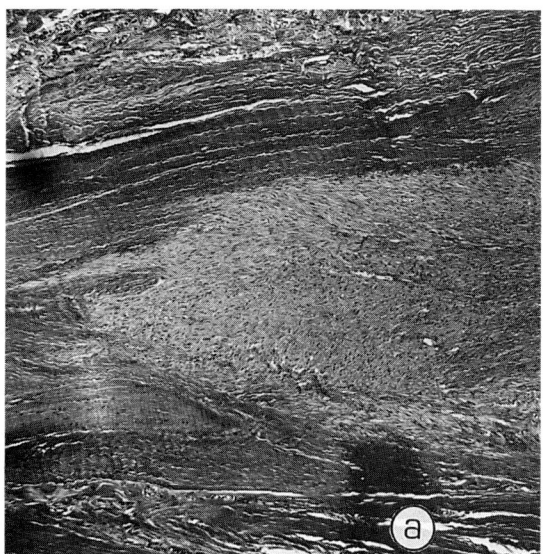
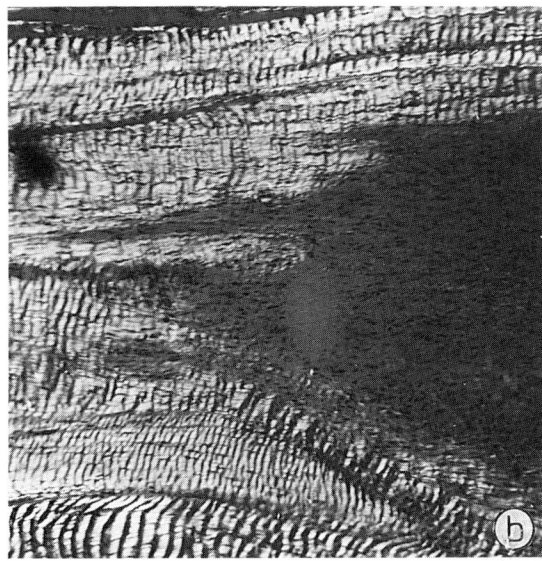

Fig. 2.5 (a) Intrafascial nodular lesion showing continuity of fibres around periphery of cellular nodule but discontinuity of fibres across the central reparative zone. (b) Proximal portion of section shown in (a) viewed through cross-polarized prisms, showing continuity of brightly refractile collagen fibres proximal to and around the periphery of the nodule, but absent across the central cellular zone.

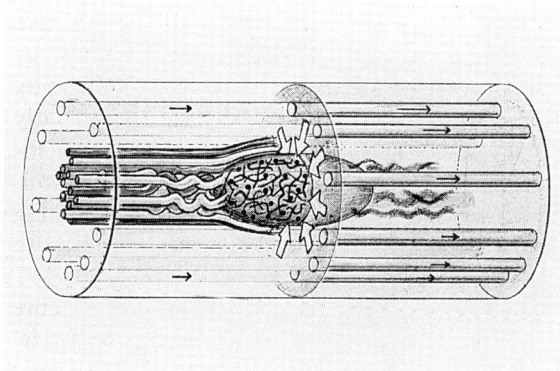

Fig. 2.6 Orientation of longitudinal fibre bundles in relationship to the development of an intrafascial nodular lesion. Note that the fibres are continuous proximal to and around the periphery of the lesion, but are discontinuous and disaggregated through the central core. Also note that the cells within the central zone are round or ovoid because of lack of longitudinal tensional forces.

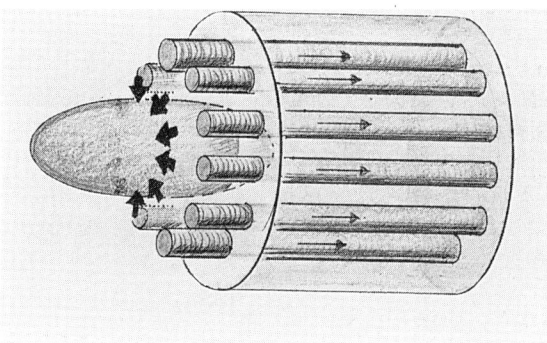

Fig. 2.7 Distribution of forces acting on an intrafascial nodular lesion; centripetal pressure forces act on the central core defect as a result of the maintenance of continuity of the peripheral tension-transmitting fibres.

aligned cells and discourage the longitudinal organization and alignment of collagen fibres (Gillard et al 1979; Flint et al 1980). The situation would be compounded by the fact that the lesions tend to be self-perpetuating, as the intermittent pressure causes a further synthesis and retention of chondroitin sulphate proteoglycan. This would lead to a further disaggregation of collagen fibres and a weakening of the fibre bundles, leading to further rupture.

I believe that this aberrant biological repair — or internal callus formation — is the basis of the intrafascial nodular thickening found in DD and that the longitudinal fibre aggregation of the palmar fascia favours the development of these intrafascial lesions once the optimal biomechanical properties of the palmar fascia have been disturbed. The data presented in Chapter 12 strongly indicates that the optimum biomechanical properties of the palmar connective tissue continuum may be lost at a surprisingly early age by replacement fibrosis of the subdermal fibrofatty oleoelastic suspension systems which, when intact, appear to protect the longitudinally running palmar fascial bands, particularly those of the superficial layer.

When viewed from a biological standpoint, it becomes possible to understand the predilection for fascial thickening to occur initially in the longitudinal fascial bands; the pathogenesis of the intrafascial nodule; the local differences in cellular morphology, proteoglycan content and collagen fibre morphology in various parts of the Dupuytren's process, and even the reasons for the recurrence of the disease.

In Chapter 10 an attempt has been made to apply the same connective tissue biological approach to the interrelated problems of contraction and contracture.

D. T. Shum

3

Histopathology

NORMAL PALMAR SKIN AND SUBCUTANEUM

Palmar skin (Fig. 3.1) is similar to the skin of the sole, but differs from skin covering the rest of the body. Skin of the palms and soles is non-hair-bearing and possesses the thickest horny and epidermal cell layers. The average thickness of the epidermis of palmar skin is 1.6 mm, as compared with 0.04 mm on the eyelids. The only adnexal structures present are the eccrine sweat glands and nerve end organs. Eccrine glands have basally located secretory lobules from which a duct emerges to conduct the secretion on to the surface of the epidermis. Special nerve end organs include the Meissner's corpuscles which are located in dermal papillae and the Vater–Pacinian corpuscles which are large nerve end organs located in the subcutis and which mediate a sense of pressure.

As in other parts of the body, the dermis of the palmar skin can be divided into the papillary dermis, which is the thin zone immediately beneath the epidermis and surrounding the epidermal rete ridges and, lying deeper, the thicker reticular dermis. Vital to the dermis are the fibroblasts, which have spindle-shaped cell bodies and nuclei. Three types of fibres can be recognized in the dermis by light microscopy; these fibres are all produced by the fibroblasts. Collagen represents by far the most abundant constituent of the filamentous components of the dermis. The diameter of collagen fibres on light microscopy ranges from 2 to 15 μm. Reticulum fibres are recognizable by impregnating sections of dermis with silver nitrate; they are also known as agyrophilic fibres. Reticulum fibres are first formed during embryonic life and appear

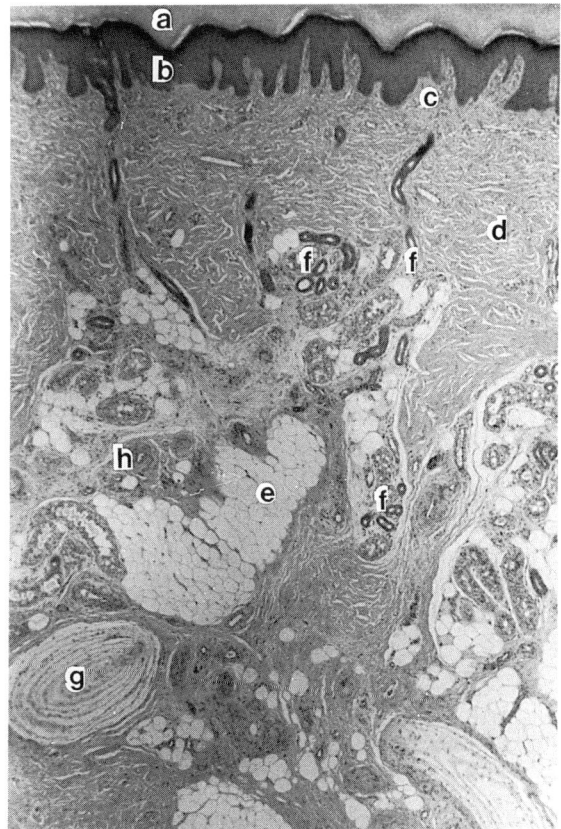

Fig. 3.1 Normal skin and subcutaneum of palm (haematoxylin & eosin; × 10 original). **a** stratum corneum; **b** epidermis; **c** papillary dermis; **d** reticular dermis; **e** subcutaneous fat; **f** eccrine sweat gland and duct; **g** Pacinian corpuscle; **h** artery.

around the third month of gestation. As these fibres increase in number and become thicker, they are organized into bundles, lose their agyrophilic properties and become collagen fibres.

The elastic fibres, the third type of filament, on the hematoxylin–eosin-stained sections appear as wavy, thin, 1–3 μm eosinophilic refractile fibres. They are especially highlighted by stains like orcein or Verhoeff–VanGieson. Under the electron microscope, elastic fibres lack periodicity, but are seen to consist of two components. Elastin is the amorphous protein occupying the centre of each fibre whereas the microfibrils — thread-like fibrillary protein — are embedded within the elastin and are numerous at the periphery of individual fibres, giving it a frayed appearance. While collagen is a structural protein and forms a fibrous network of support, elastic fibres provide the normal elasticity and resilient character of the skin. Unique to the palm is the palmar aponeurosis. This three-dimensional ligamentous system of the palm comprises three groups of collagenous fibres (Fig. 3.2), as described in Chapter 12.

HISTOPATHOLOGY

Even with the light and electron microscope techniques of the present day, there can be little improvement on Meyerding et al's (1941) paper: 'The Etiology and Pathology of Dupuytren's Contracture'. They wrote: 'other investigators have focused their attention on the palmar fascia to the exclusions of the surrounding tissue' and 'that Dupuytren's contracture is not merely a disease of the palmar fascia, but involves all structures from the skin down to the tendon sheaths'. As shown in Figure 3.3, we now know that this is certainly the case, and that the fibrosis, especially in more advanced cases, extends to the overlying dermis and surrounding subcutaneous tissue.

Meyerding et al described changes in the palmar fascia as well as in the adjacent tissues. In the former, they observed that: 'the characteristic change is the proliferation of fibroblasts in the nodules of the contracture'. More importantly, they noted the variable cellularity in lesions of Dupuytren's disease (DD) (Fig. 3.4). Meyerding was the first investigator to attempt a functional interpretation of the histopathological changes by assuming that the cellularity of the nodules was indicative of the activity of the disease. He suggested a gradation of one to four to reflect the activity of the proliferative process. With regard to the surrounding connective tissue changes, he noted that in advanced cases of DD 'evidence of subcutaneous adipose tissue is not revealed and sweat glands are rare or completely absent' (Meyerding et al 1941). This was the result of an increase in

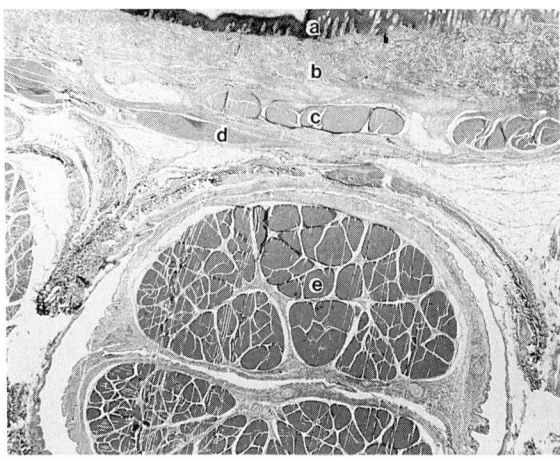

Fig. 3.2 a Transverse section of normal palmar skin through distal palmar crease (haematoxylyin & eosin; × 10 original). **a** Epidermis; **b** dermis; **c** longitudinal fibres; **d** deep transverse fibres; **e** flexor tendon.

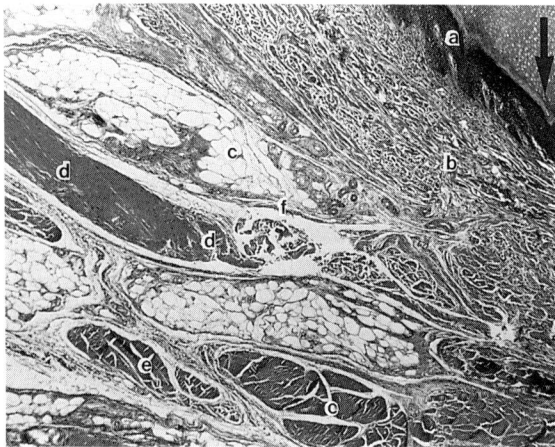

Fig. 3.2 b Longitudinal section of normal palmar skin just proximal to the proximal digital crease. Left: direction of proximal palm (haematoxlyin & eosin; × 25 original). Arrow = proximal digital crease. **a** Epidermis; **b** dermis; **c** subcutaneous fat; **d** longitudinal fibres merging with dermal collagen; **e** deep transverse fibres; **f** delicate vertical fibres.

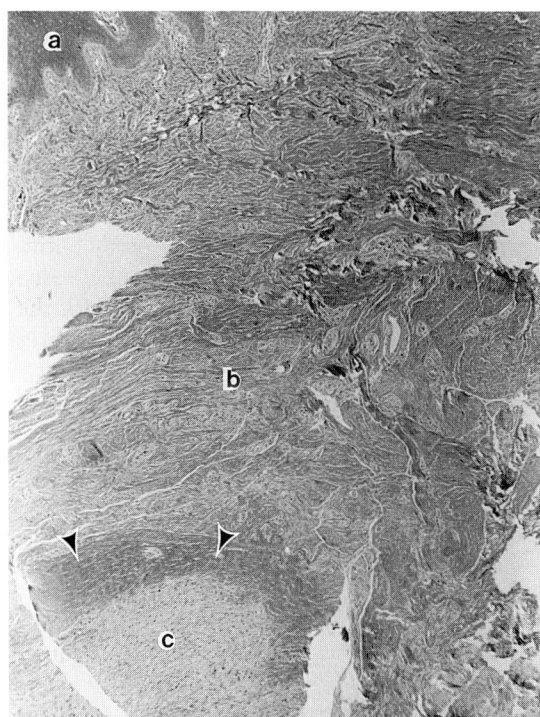

Fig. 3.3 Advanced lesion of DD. Note the nodular configuration and extension into dermis (haematoxylin & eosin; × 10 original). a epidermis; b dermis; c pale staining, cellular fibrous tissue of DD. Arrows = thick collagen fibres at periphery of lesion.

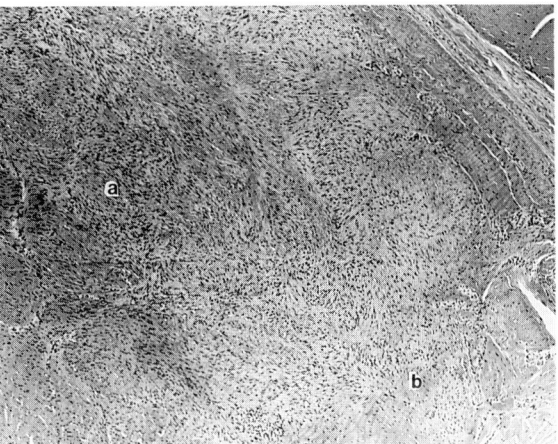

Fig. 3.4 Varying cell density within an active lesion of DD (haematoxylin & eosin; × 40 original). a cellular and dark staining area; b fibrous and less cellular area.

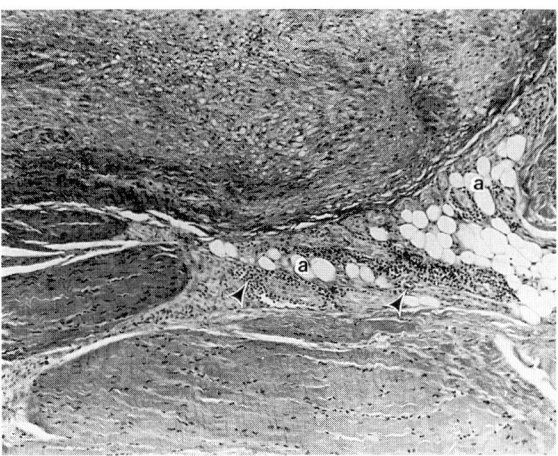

Fig. 3.5 Active lesion of DD resulting in loss of normal subcutis and adnexal structures (haematoxylin & eosin; × 40 original). a Encroachment of subcutaneous fat by DD. Arrows = perivascular lymphocytic infiltrate.

the size and number of connective tissue bands which normally separated the lobules of fat. There was also an increase in the number of capillaries in the interstitial connective tissue and the capillaries were infiltrated by lymphocytes (Fig. 3.5).

Such detailed and accurate accounts of the histopathological changes noting the involvement of not only the fascia, but the adjacent subcutaneous tissue and overlying skin, surpassed all previous descriptions.

Luck (1959) further classified the disease into three stages: proliferative, involutional and residual. He subdivided diseased tissue into essential fibrous nodules, reactive tissue and residual tissue. He defined the essential fibrous nodule as the initial lesion in the proliferative stage; he stated that histologically the nodule was a focus of proliferating fibroblasts that resembled a fibroma. He wrote: 'in this focal fibroplasia, the fibroblasts do not align themselves with lines of stress and have, in fact, no purposeful arrangement' (Fig. 3.6). The involutional stage was characterized by fibroblasts aligning themselves with major lines of stress that pass through the nodules (Fig. 3.7). Luck considered that the fibrous cords represented reactive functional hypertrophy in response to the repeated tension stresses on the hand of fascia from which the nodule took its origin, hence the term reactive tissue. Finally,

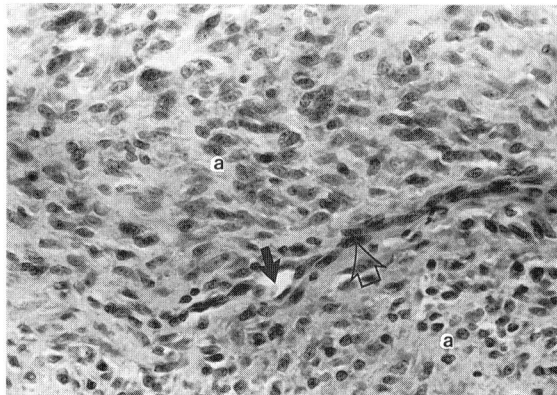

Fig. 3.6 Essential fibrous nodule as defined by Luck (1959) (haematoxylin & eosin; × 100 original). **a** Haphazardly arranged fibroblasts. Solid arrow = capillary lumen; hollow arrow = endothelial cells.

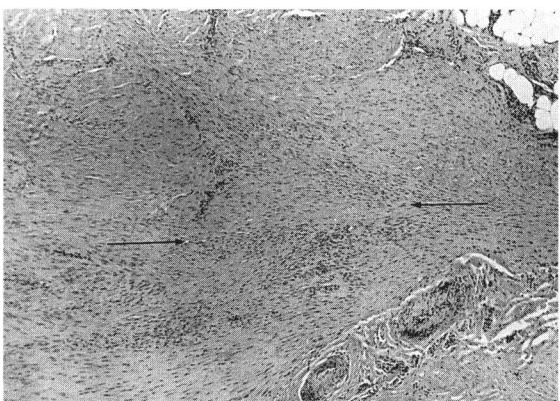

Fig. 3.7 Reactive tissue during the involutional stage of DD. The nodular configuration of the proliferative lesion is lost. (Haematoxylin & eosin; × 25 original). Arrows = alignment of fibroblasts along lines of stress with loss of the nodular configuration of initial lesion.

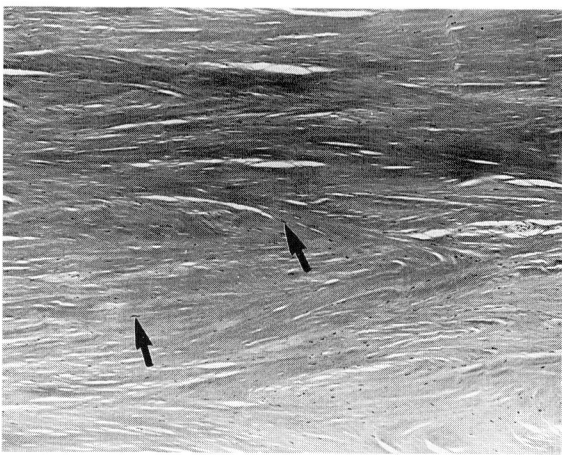

Fig. 3.8 Dense fibrous cord of residual stage (haematoxylin & eosin; × 25 original). Arrows = spindle-shaped nuclei of fibrocytes in between dense collagenous fibres.

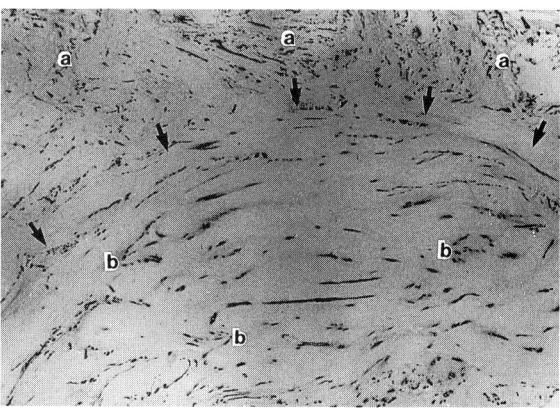

Fig. 3.9 A Dupuytrens nodule during the proliferative stage of the disease. The section was reacted with antibodies against factor VIII in order to demonstrate the endothelial cells of the capillaries (factor VIII antibodies peroxidase stain; × 10 original). **a** Normal vessels in surrounding subcutaneous tissue; **b** arborescent network of vessels in DD. Arrows = nodular boundary of Dupuytren's nodule.

with the complete involution of the nodule came the residual stage which he described as follows: 'the nodule disappears, leaving only a focus of dense adhesions and the reactive proximal fibrous cord which is almost acellular and tendon-like' (Fig. 3.8).

MacCallum & Hueston (1962) continued the investigation with their publication entitled 'The Pathology of Dupuytren's Contracture'. In their microscopic observations they recognized two rather than three phases of activity, and they correctly pointed out that the two phases may freely intermingle or be separated in a lesion. Their attention focused on the increased vascularity in the surrounding tissue and within the hyperplastic foci where they stated that: 'the new fibroblasts are arranged around sheets of branching blood vessels' (Fig. 3.9). They were first to suggest that: 'the sequence [of production of the Dupuytren's lesion] can be followed from vascular invasion and perivascular cellular proliferation to a maturing

HISTOPATHOLOGY

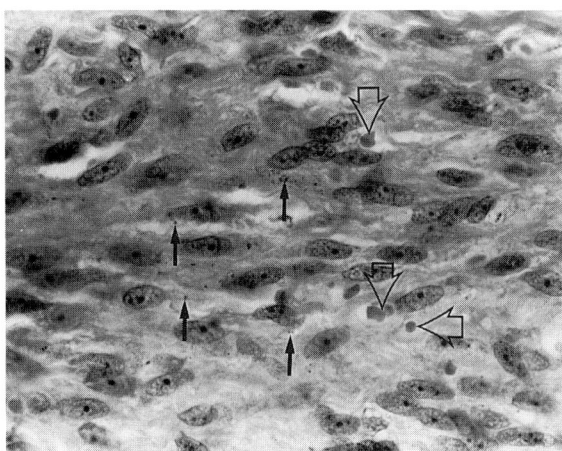

Fig. 3.10 Proliferative stage of Dupuytren's nodule. The haemosiderin pigment derived from breakdown of extravasated red cells is yellow-brown in colour (haematoxylin & eosin; × 1000). Solid arrows = yellow-brown haemosiderin pigment; hollow arrows = extravasated red blood cells.

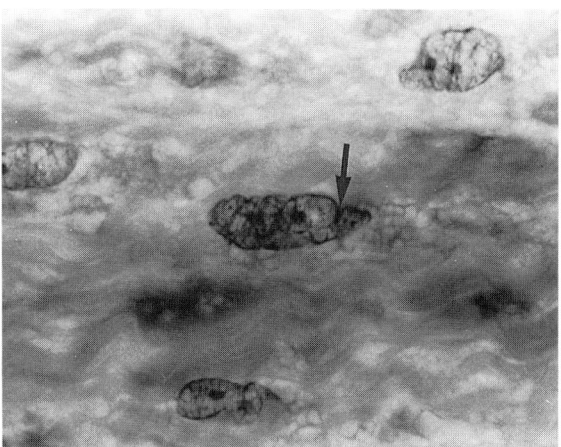

Fig. 3.11 Myofibroblasts in a Dupuytren's nodule (haematoxlyin & eosin × 1250 original). Arrow = myofibroblast with cross-banded nucleus.

nodule and finally to a relatively acellular dense atrophic tendinous band'. They also noted microhaemorrhages and deposits of haemosiderin pigment, in about one in ten specimens of DD usually in the hyperplastic foci (Fig. 3.10). This finding was interpreted as evidence of past interstitial haemorrhage from recently formed ingrowing capillaries.

Gabbiani et al (1971) used electron microscopy technique to study granulation tissue and discovered a special type of fibroblast that was capable of 'modulating' into cells very similar to smooth muscle cells. In 1972, Gabbiani & Majno reported on six cases of DD in which they specifically looked for these specialized or adapted fibroblasts, the so-called 'myofibroblasts' which they believed were the driving force behind the contraction of the palmar fascia and with it the overlying skin and digits. In this study, new features were reviewed both at the light and electron microscopic levels. With the light microscopy, they reported on the presence of intercellular fibrils which were visible as 'red streaks or filaments' with Masson's trichrome stain in cells of Dupuytren's nodules; these cells had 'crossbanded' nuclei (Fig. 3.11). Ultrastructurally, they reported that these cells had three distinctive features (Fig. 3.12). First, a complex system of

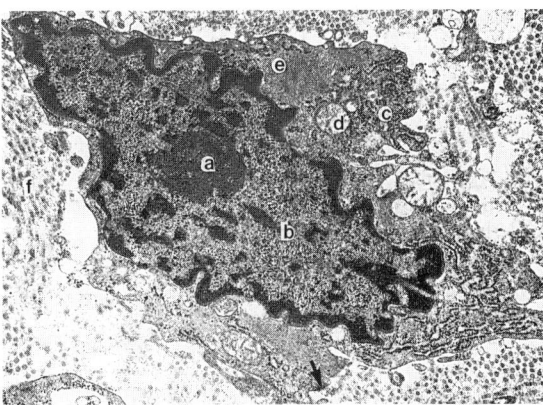

Fig. 3.12 Electron micrography of a myofibroblast from a Dupuytren's nodule (× 14 000 original). **a** nucleolus; **b** nucleus with irregular nuclear membrane; **c** cytoplasm; **d** mitochondria; **e** intracellular fibrils with electron densities; **f** collagen. Arrow = hemidesmosome.

intracellular fibrils with electron densities similar to the dense bodies in smooth muscle cells was present. Second, the nuclei contained frequent indentations and folds which the authors thought corresponded to the nuclear cross-banding seen under light microscopy. Third, they described the surface differentiations of these cells which consisted of basement membrane and hemidesmosomal structures. Indeed, ample ultrastructural morphological evidence was presented to support their hypothesis that these myofibroblasts possessed the essential intracellular bundles of fibrils, and cell surface adaptations for transmission of forces. The nuclear foldings were indirect evidence that these cells had been shortened during contraction. Their observations were later confirmed by Hueston et al (1976) and Chiu & McFarlane (1978) who reported that myofibroblasts were seen in the nodules.

Another innovative technique using fluorescent dye tagged on to antibodies was used by Hueston et al (1976) who demonstrated 'smooth muscle antigens' in 10 cases, thus confirming that cells akin to smooth muscle cells were present in lesions of DD.

Articles by Iwasaki et al (1984), Ushijma et al (1984) and Nezelof (1985) have further reviewed the histopathology of DD and a summary of pertinent changes at various stages of the disease is given in Table 3.1.

CONCLUSIONS

Histopathology is the basis of our knowledge. To date, however, it is probable that all significant histological features of DD have been recognized; it is unlikely that histological appearance alone could lead to any further breakthrough in our understanding of the disease.

The use of monoclonal antibody against desmin has demonstrated a subpopulation of desmin-positive cells in the proliferating lesion of DD which is undetectable with the haematoxylin & eosin stain (Shum & McFarlane 1988). Similar studies by Schürch et al, reported in the next chapter, using innovative techniques and multidisciplinary research in areas of molecular biology, biochemistry and cytogenetics, should provide more meaningful interpretation and new insight into the familiar morphological tissue changes in DD.

Table 3.1 Summary of histopathological changes*

Features of early lesions
1. Focal increase in vascularity with ingrowth of capillaries and proliferation of endothelial cells.
2. Proliferation of perivascular cells, many of which are desmin-positive and probably akin to perivascular smooth muscle cells.
3. Formation of angiocentric, nodular lesion by centrifugal spread of proliferating cells.
4. Extravasation of red cells focally from the newly formed capillaries.
5. Production of reticulum but not elastic fibres.

Features of intermediate lesions
1. Proliferating cells are undergoing morphosis from cells with round nuclei and scanty cytoplasm to spindle-shaped cells with indented, elongated nuclei and a moderate amount of cytoplasm. These are the morphological features of myofibroblasts.
2. Lesion becomes less cellular with increasing stromal collagen.
3. Alignment of cells along lines of stress.
4. Fibrous infiltration of adjacent skin and subcutaneous tissue.
5. Focal deposition of a haemosiderin pigment as a result of degeneration of extravasated red cells.
6. Lymphocytic infiltration.

Features of late lesions
1. Relatively acellular cords of densely packed and aligned collagen fibres.
2. Cells appear as typical fibrocytes with hyperchromatic, wavy and spindle-shaped nuclei between dense collagen bundles.
3. Few cells are positive for desmin-type intermediate filaments.

*As different stages of microscopic changes occur even within a small nodule, careful examination of all tissue removed is necessary. The activity or chronological age of a lesion is best indicated by the area with the highest cellularity. All of these features are seen in haematoxylin & eosin sections under light microscopy.

W. Schürch, O. Skalli and G. Gabbiani

4 Cellular biology

THE MYOFIBROBLAST

Definition, ultrastructural features and role in wound contraction

The progressive contraction of the palmar aponeurosis is considered to be responsible for the retraction of one or more digits. The fibroblasts of the Dupuytren's nodule have been shown to be ultrastructurally similar to myofibroblasts of granulation tissue (Gabbiani & Majno 1972). Since granulation tissue myofibroblasts were thought to be responsible for wound contraction (Gabbiani et al 1971; Majno et al 1971), the presence of this cell type in Dupuytren's disease (DD) nodules suggested that it could well be responsible for contractile events. Indeed, in addition to packed cisternae of endoplasmic reticulum typical of fibroblasts, myofibroblasts exhibit ultrastructural features reminiscent of smooth muscle cells. These consist of microfilament bundles usually arranged parallel to the long axis of the cell, amongst which are interspersed electron-opaque areas similar to the dense bodies of smooth muscle cells. Myofibroblasts are partly covered by a well defined layer of material having the structural features of a basal lamina and are interconnected by gap junctions (Gabbiani et al 1978). Myofibroblasts are connected to the extracellular matrix by fibronexus, which are transmembrane complexes of intracellular microfilaments in apparent continuity with extracellular fibronectin fibres (Singer 1979; Singer et al 1984). Finally, the nucleus of myofibroblasts consistently shows indentations or deep folds, an ultrastructural feature that has been correlated with cellular contraction in several systems (Lane 1965; Bloom & Cancilla 1969; Franke & Schinko 1969; Majno et al 1969).

The in vitro contraction of myofibroblast-containing tissues in response to various drugs known to act on smooth muscle contraction strongly suggested that myofibroblasts were responsible for the contractile events of wound healing (Gabbiani et al 1971; Majno et al 1971; Ryan et al 1974) and of liver (Irlé et al 1980) and lung (Evans et al 1982) contracture. The ability of myofibroblasts to produce forces strong enough to generate tissue contraction has also been deduced from experiments carried out on in vitro fibroblasts, which are structurally similar to in vivo myofibroblasts (see below). This was well shown in an in vitro model of wound contraction in which fibroblasts cast into a collagen lattice caused its contraction; the rate of this phenomenon was directly dependent on the number of cells seeded within the gel (Bell et al 1979). During the active phase of contraction fibroblasts exhibited numerous stress fibres and gap junctions, but when the gel was fully compacted, the number of microfilament bundles and gap junctions was decreased while the number of synthetic organelles was increased (Bellows et al 1982).

The forces generated by the cultured fibroblasts are traction rather than contraction forces, as shown by experiments in which fibroblasts distorted a sheet of silicon on which they were grown (Harris et al 1981). Several observations suggested that stress fibres are probably the force generating elements in wound contraction since:

1. They contract upon addition of adenosine triphosphate on glycerinated fibroblasts (Hoffman-Berling 1954; Isenberg et al 1976; Kreis & Birchmeier 1980).
2. Microinjection experiments showed that they

were functionally analogous to skeletal muscle fibrils (Kreis & Birchmeier 1980; Burridge 1981).

Fibronexus are probably the elements through which the forces generated by the actin filament bundles of myofibroblasts are transmitted to the extracellular matrix (Singer et al 1984) and the gap junctions found between these cells may synchronize their contractile action (Gabbiani et al 1978). To our knowledge the contractility of Dupuytren's nodules or of cells derived therefrom has not yet been examined; it remains to be shown whether the model of wound contraction by myofibroblasts also applies to Dupuytren's contracture.

THE MYOFIBROBLAST IN PATHOLOGICAL CONDITIONS

Following the recognition and characterization of the contractile myofibroblast in granulation tissue of healing wounds (Gabbiani et al 1971; Majno et al 1971), this cell was described in a wide assortment of normal and pathological conditions (for review on myofibroblasts in normal conditions see Skalli & Gabbiani 1988). Pathological settings in which myofibroblasts represent a principal cellular component fall into three groups (Seemayer et al 1980, 1981):

1. Response to injury and repair phenomena.
2. Quasineoplastic proliferative conditions.
3. Stromal response to neoplasia.

Response to injury and repair phenomena

These comprise the following:

1. Human and experimental liver cirrhosis (Bhatal 1972; Rudolph et al 1979; Irlé et al 1980).
2. Tenosynovitis (Madden 1973).
3. Radiation-induced pseudosarcoma of skin (Woyke et al 1974).
4. Burn contracture (Larson et al 1974).
5. Ischaemic contracture of intrinsic muscles of the hand (Madden et al 1975).
6. Renal interstitial fibrosis during obstructive nephropathy (Nagle et al 1973).
7. Pulmonary sarcoidosis (Judd et al 1975).
8. Giant cell granuloma of jaws (El-Labban & Lee 1983).
9. Schistosomal liver fibrosis (Grimaud & Borojevic 1977).
10. Regenerating tendon (Postacchini et al 1977).
11. Fibrous capsule around silicone mammary implants (Rudolph et al 1978; Zimman et al 1978).
12. Nodular hyperplasia of the liver (Callea et al 1982).
13. Ganglia of soft tissue (Ghadially & Mehta 1971).
14. Hypertrophic scars (Baur et al 1975).
15. Cataract (Novotny & Pau 1984).
16. Bleomycin-induced interstitial fibrosis of the lung in the rat (Woodcock-Mitchell et al 1984).

Quasineoplastic proliferative conditions

This group embodies the poorly understood, but very important and frequent fibrous tissue proliferations included under the broad heading of fibromatoses, as well as many other soft tissue proliferations, often mimicking sarcomas, which share their predominant myofibroblastic composition and which display a variable proliferative potential, yet do not disseminate or metastasize. (Seemayer et al 1980, 1981). Myofibroblasts constitute the principal cellular components of superficial and deep musculoaponeurotic fibromatoses (Enzinger & Weiss 1983). Superficial fibromatoses include palmar fibromatosis (Gabbiani & Majno 1972; Chiu & McFarlane 1978, Meister et al 1979; Navas-Palacios 1983; Ushijima et al 1984), plantar fibromatosis (Gabbiani & Majno 1972), penile fibromatosis (Ariyan et al 1978) and knuckle pads. Deep musculoaponeurotic fibromatoses comprise extra-abdominal, abdominal and intra-abdominal variants, collectively also called desmoid tumours. To this group also belong infantile fibromatoses, the childhood counterpart of adult musculoaponeurotic fibromatoses, infantile myofibromatosis (Chung & Enzinger 1981) and desmoplastic fibroma of bone (Lagacé et al 1979). Other soft tissue proliferations predominantly composed of myofibroblasts are:

1. Nodular fasciitis (Wirman 1976).
2. Proliferative fasciitis (Chung & Enzinger 1975).
3. Proliferative myositis (Povysil & Matejovsky 1979).
4. Giant cell fibroma of oral mucosa (Weathers & Campbell 1974).
5. Dermatofibroma (Stiller & Katenkamp 1975).
6. Elastofibroma (Ramos et al 1978).
7. Plasma cell granuloma of the lung (Buell et al 1976).
8. Juvenile nasal angiofibroma (Taxy 1977).

Myofibroblasts are also present, to a lesser extent, in the right heart plaque of carcinoid heart disease (Lagacé et al 1975), cardiac myxomas (Ferrans & Roberts 1973) and uterine plexiform tumours (Fisher et al 1978).

Stromal response to neoplasia

Many, invasive and metastatic carcinomas are characterized by hard consistency, retraction and are often fixed to adjacent tissues due to what is generally designated as a myofibroblastic stromal reaction. Myofibroblasts are particularly numerous within the stroma of desmoplastic carcinomas (Seemayer et al 1979a, 1979b; Tremblay 1979; Ohtani & Sasano 1980; Schürch et al 1981, 1982). The retraction phenomenon associated with such carcinomas is attributed to the contractile forces generated by stromal myofibroblasts. These stromal cells are not observed in in situ carcinomas (Seemayer et al 1980; Schürch et al 1982), suggesting that stromal invasion, beyond the epithelial basal lamina, is required to evoke a myofibroblastic stromal reaction. Myofibroblasts are notably absent or equivocally present within carcinomas lacking significant stromal desmoplasia (Schürch et al 1981). Myofibroblasts have been found in sarcomas where they generally constitute a small fraction of the cellular population (Gabbiani et al 1972, Lagacé et al 1980) and in nodular sclerosing Hodgkin's disease (Seemayer et al 1980).

Finally, a few reports describe myofibroblastic tumours, some considered as sarcomas (Churg & Kahn 1977; D'Andiran & Gabbiani 1980; Ghadially et al 1983), although the existence of such tumours as bona fide neoplasms has been questioned (Seemayer et al 1980).

CELLULAR AND EXTRACELLULAR COMPOSITION OF THE DIFFERENT STAGES OF DD

With the electron microscope, three main cell types are identified within the nodules of DD: — immature fibroblasts, myofibroblasts and mature fibroblasts or fibrocytes (Iwasaki et al 1984). Nodules of the proliferative phase (Luck 1959) are composed mainly of myofibroblasts admixed with a few immature fibroblasts (Gabbiani & Majno 1972; Enzinger & Weiss 1983; for review see Skalli & Gabbiani 1988). Lesions of the involutional phase consist of nodules and fibrous cords.

There is general agreement on the cell type composing nodules of DD in the involutional and residual phases (Meister et al 1979; Iwasaki et al 1984). However, according to Meister et al (1979), nodules of the proliferative phase are composed of cells displaying ultrastructural features of fibroblasts, thereby assigning a dominant cell to the proliferative, involutional and residual phases of Luck (1959), i.e. fibroblastic, myofibroblastic and fibrocytic, respectively.

Proliferative phase nodules

Ultrastructurally, the nodules are composed of large myofibroblasts with numerous long cytoplasmic extensions, joined by various gap junctions and relatively undifferentiated junctions (Fig. 4.1a-c). Their plasma membrane reveals focal deposition of basal lamina, some plasmalemmal attachment plaques and pinocytotic vesicles, as well as cell to stroma attachment sites in the form of fibronexus (Singer 1979; Fig. 4.1d). The cytoplasm reveals a well developed granular endoplasmic reticulum and Golgi apparatus and a number of bundles of microfilaments with dense bodies, often oriented parallel to the long axis of the cells. The nucleus is typically indented and often shows one or several nuclear bodies. Among these typical myofibroblasts, a few smaller cells are observed, corresponding to fibroblasts with a well developed granular endoplasmic reticulum and smooth contoured nucleus but lacking bundles of cytoplasmic microfilaments with dense bodies. The extracellular matrix in this phase contains a few mature collagen fibres (64 nm periodicity) ad-

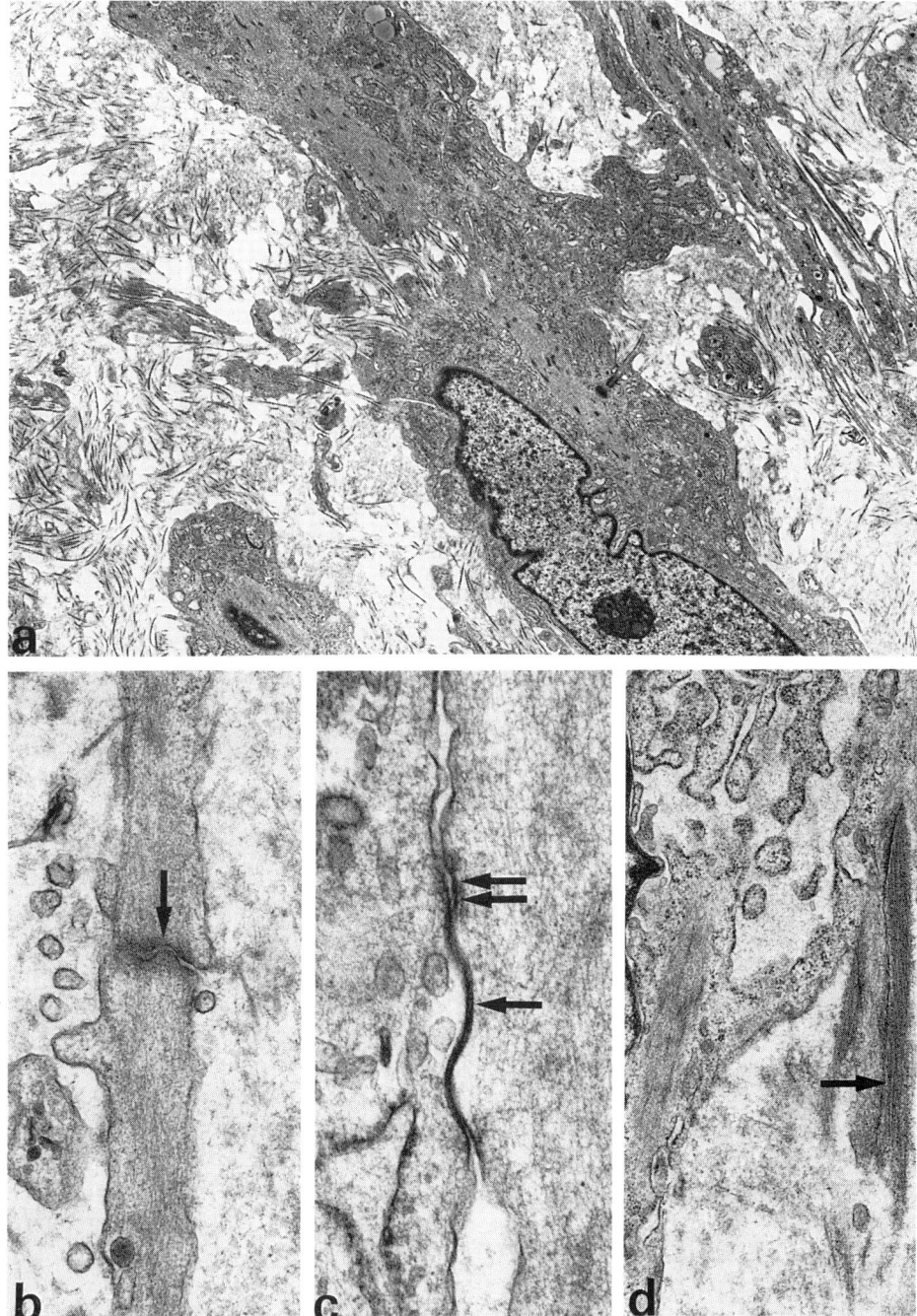

Fig. 4.1 Transmission electron micrographs of proliferative phase nodules. **a** Large typical myofibroblast with numerous cytoplasmic extensions, well developed granular endoplasmic reticulum, cytoplasmic bundles of microfilaments, oriented parallel to the long axis of the cell, cilium and indented nucleus. The extracellular matrix contains few mature collagen fibres. **b** Poorly differentiated junction between cytoplasmic extensions of two myofibroblasts (arrow). **c** Gap junction between two myofibroblasts (arrow) followed by poorly differentiated junction (double arrow). **d** Microtendon (fibronexus) establishing cell to stroma contact (arrow). Uranyl acetate and lead citrate (**a** × 4200; **b** × 30 000; **c** × 60 000; **d** × 20 000).

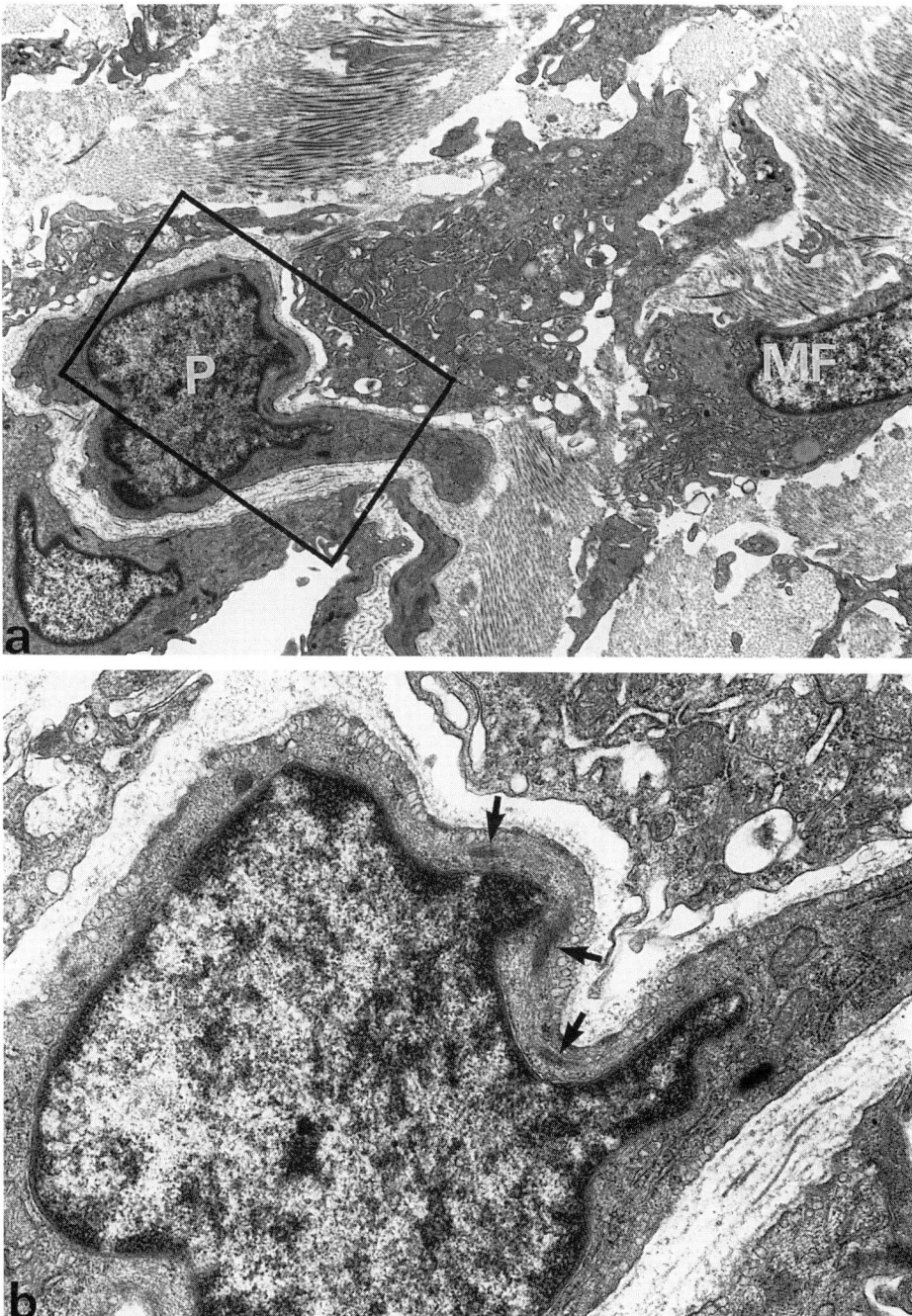

Fig. 4.2 a Transmission electron micrograph illustrating capillary of proliferative phase nodule with large pericyte (P) enveloped by a continuous basal lamina and in the close vicinity of a large myofibroblast (MF) revealing aggregate of microfilaments with dense bodies. **b** Detail of pericyte illustrated in **a** showing bundles of microfilaments with dense bodies (arrows).

mixed with granular, non-distinct fibrillar and basal lamina-like material (Fig. 4.1a). The capillaries reveal large prominent pericytes often displaying bundles or aggregates of cytoplasmic microfilaments with irregular densities. These large pericytes are often in the close vicinity of typical myofibroblasts (Fig. 4.2).

Involutional phase nodules

These regions also feature high cellularity but individual cells are smaller than in proliferative phase nodules and tend to be aligned in the same direction (Fig. 4.3). Ultrastructurally, these nodules are essentially composed of myofibroblasts which are also connected by gap junctions and poorly differentiated junctions. Intercellular junctions, however, seem to be less numerous than in proliferative phase nodules. The most striking difference compared to proliferative phase nodules is the amount of collagen. Individual myofibroblasts are enveloped by thick bundles of mature collagen fibres (Fig. 4.4). The myofibroblasts are somewhat smaller than in proliferative nodules and their cytoplasmic extensions are less numerous and appear shorter. Otherwise, the myofibroblasts composing involutional phase nodules are essentially similar to those observed in proliferative nodules and display indented nuclei (Fig. 4.4a). Capillaries are numerous and reveal prominent large pericytes.

Residual phase nodules

Such regions are hypocellular and the slender and aligned cells are surrounded by thick bands of collagen, giving them a tendon-like appearance on semi-thin sections (Fig. 4.3). Ultrastructurally, they are composed of mature fibroblasts (fibrocytes), some containing small aggregates of cytoplasmic microfilaments. The fibrocytes are connected by a few poorly differentiated junctions. Gap junctions, however, are no longer observed.

The slender fibrocytes also show smooth contoured nuclei and are embedded in a dense collagenous matrix formed by thick bands of mature collagen fibres (Fig. 4.5). The poorly vascularized nodules contain small pericytes with little cytoplasm devoid of a well developed microfilamentous apparatus with irregular densities, as observed in proliferative and involutional phase nodules (Fig. 4.6).

In summary, significant ultrastructural differences exist between proliferative, involutional and residual phase nodules in DD in relation to the cells, intercellular junctions, extracellular matrix and capillaries. In the proliferative phase, nodules are composed of typical large myofibroblasts connected by numerous poorly differentiated junctions as well as gap junctions, the latter considered as low resistance pathways for intercellular communication (Gabbiani et al 1978). The extracellular matrix is scant, but capillaries are numerous and feature large prominent pericytes displaying smooth muscle features. The involutional phase nodules, still composed of typical myofibroblasts, reveal fewer gap junctions and poorly differentiated junctions and the extracellular matrix is more abundant and composed of large amounts of mature collagen. Capillaries are numerous and reveal prominent large pericytes. In the residual phase, nodules are composed of slender fibrocytes embedded in a dense collagenous matrix. Gap junctions are not observed and fibrocytes are connected by occasional poorly differentiated junctions. Capillaries, few in number, show small inconspicuous pericytes devoid of a well developed microfilamentous apparatus.

CYTOSKELETAL COMPOSITION OF MYOFIBROBLASTS IN NON-TUMOURAL CONDITIONS

Intense efforts have been directed to establish whether myofibroblasts are derived from smooth muscle cells or fibroblasts. The resemblance in the organization of actin filament between myofibroblasts and smooth muscle cells obviously does not establish that myofibroblasts are of smooth muscle origin. Indeed, cultured fibroblasts acquire ultrastructural features which closely resemble that of myofibroblasts (Buckley & Porter 1967; Gabbiani et al 1973; Bellows et al 1982); moreover, other cell types, such as endothelial cells, develop under various circumstances bundles of actin filaments similar to those observed in

CELLULAR BIOLOGY 37

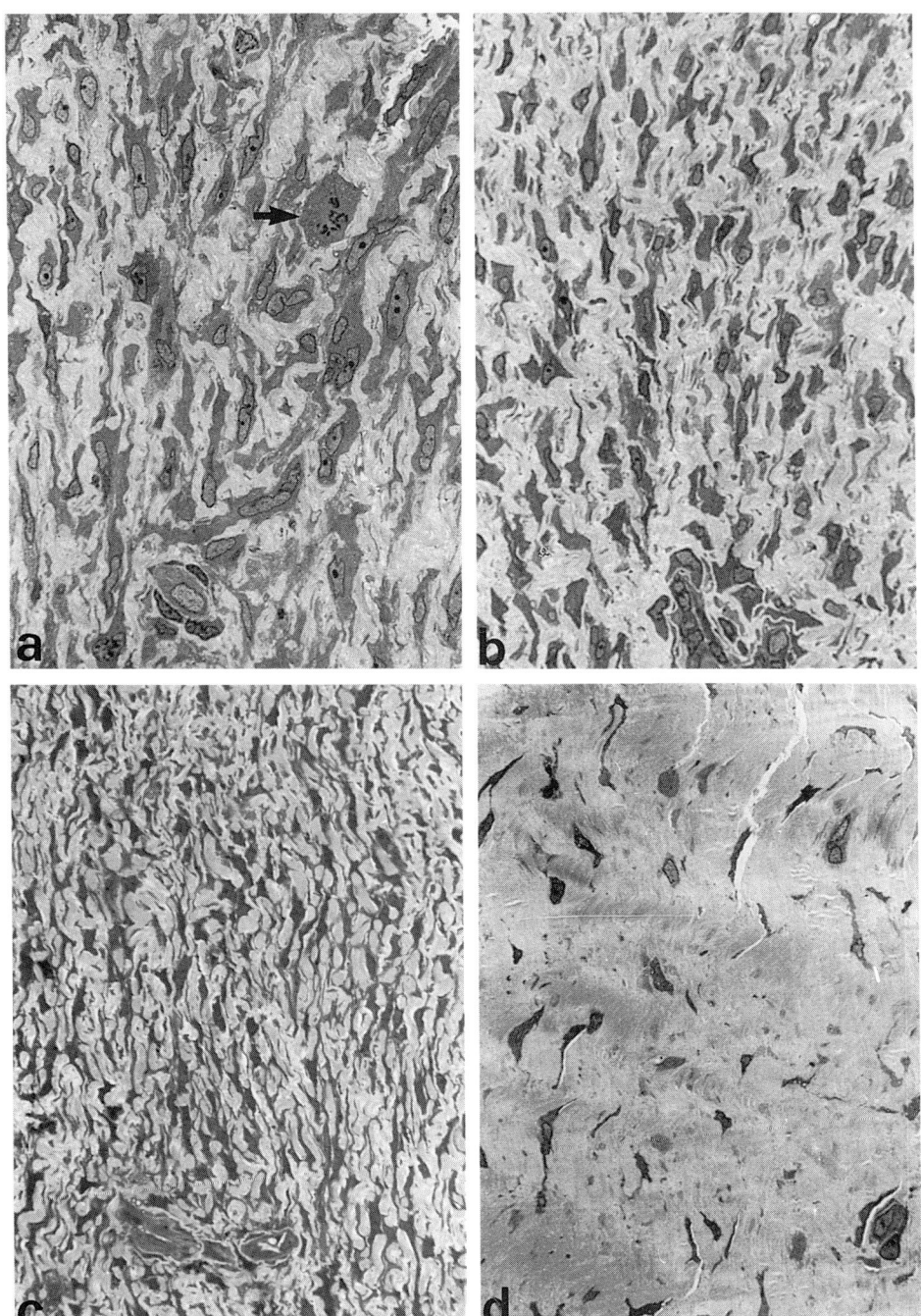

Fig. 4.3 Toluidine blue stained semi-thin sections. **a** Proliferative phase nodule illustrating large elongated cells with numerous cytoplasmic extensions and indented nuclei, some of them in division (arrow). **b** and **c** Involutional phase nodule composed of aligned spindle cells which display fewer and shorter cytoplasmic extensions than in **a** and which are also smaller in size. **d** Residual phase nodule showing slender spindle cells in a poorly vascularized and intensely collagenous matrix ($\times$ 500).

38 DUPUYTREN'S DISEASE

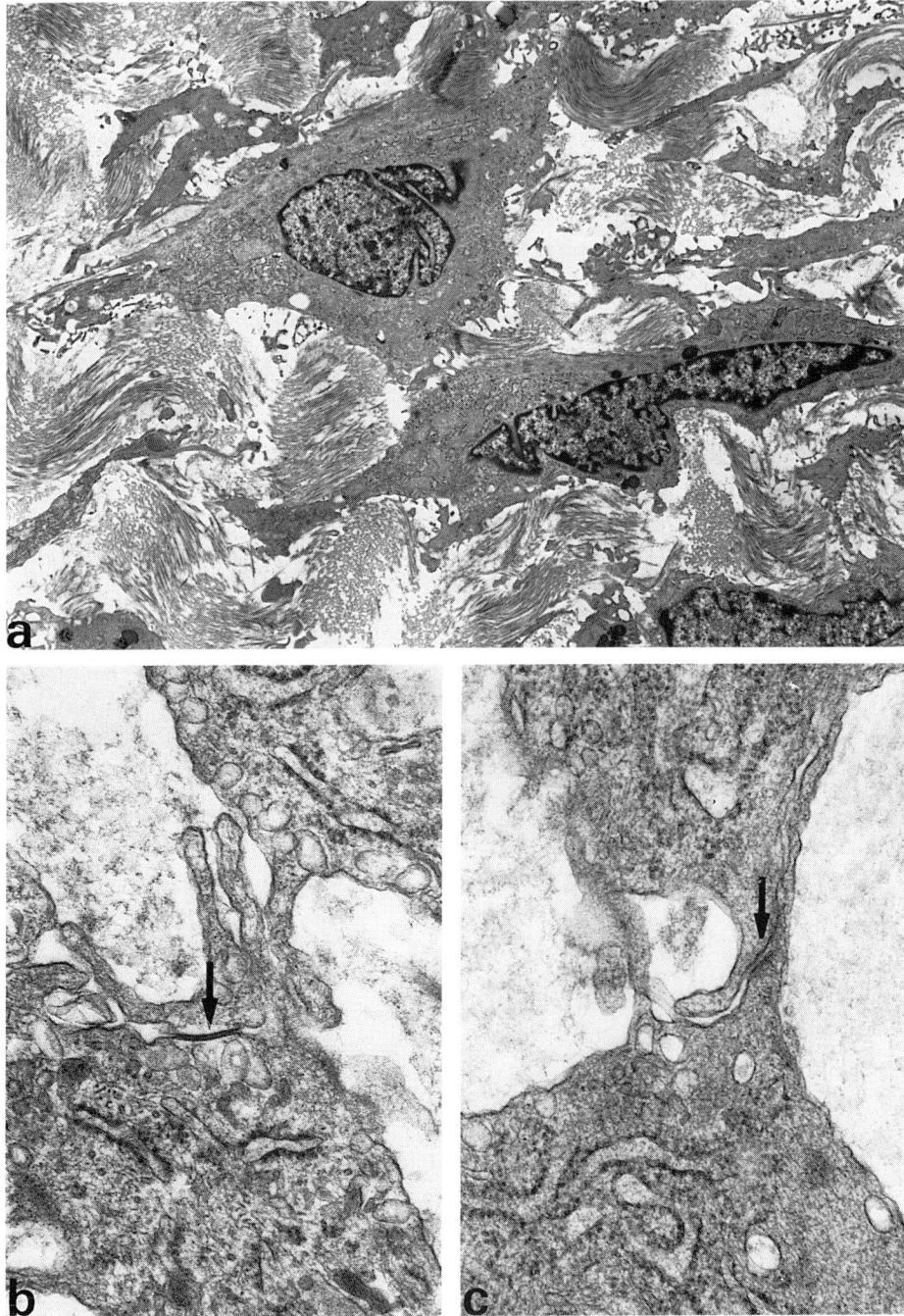

Fig. 4.4 Transmission electron micrographs from involutional phase nodule. **a** Two typical myofibroblasts with cytoplasmic extensions, bundles of cytoplasmic microfilaments, indented nuclei, surrounded by bands of mature collagen fibres. **b** Gap junction between two myofibroblasts (arrow). **c** Poorly differentiated junction connecting two myofibroblasts (arrow). Uranyl and lead citrate (**a** × 4200; **b** × 28 000; **c** × 42 000).

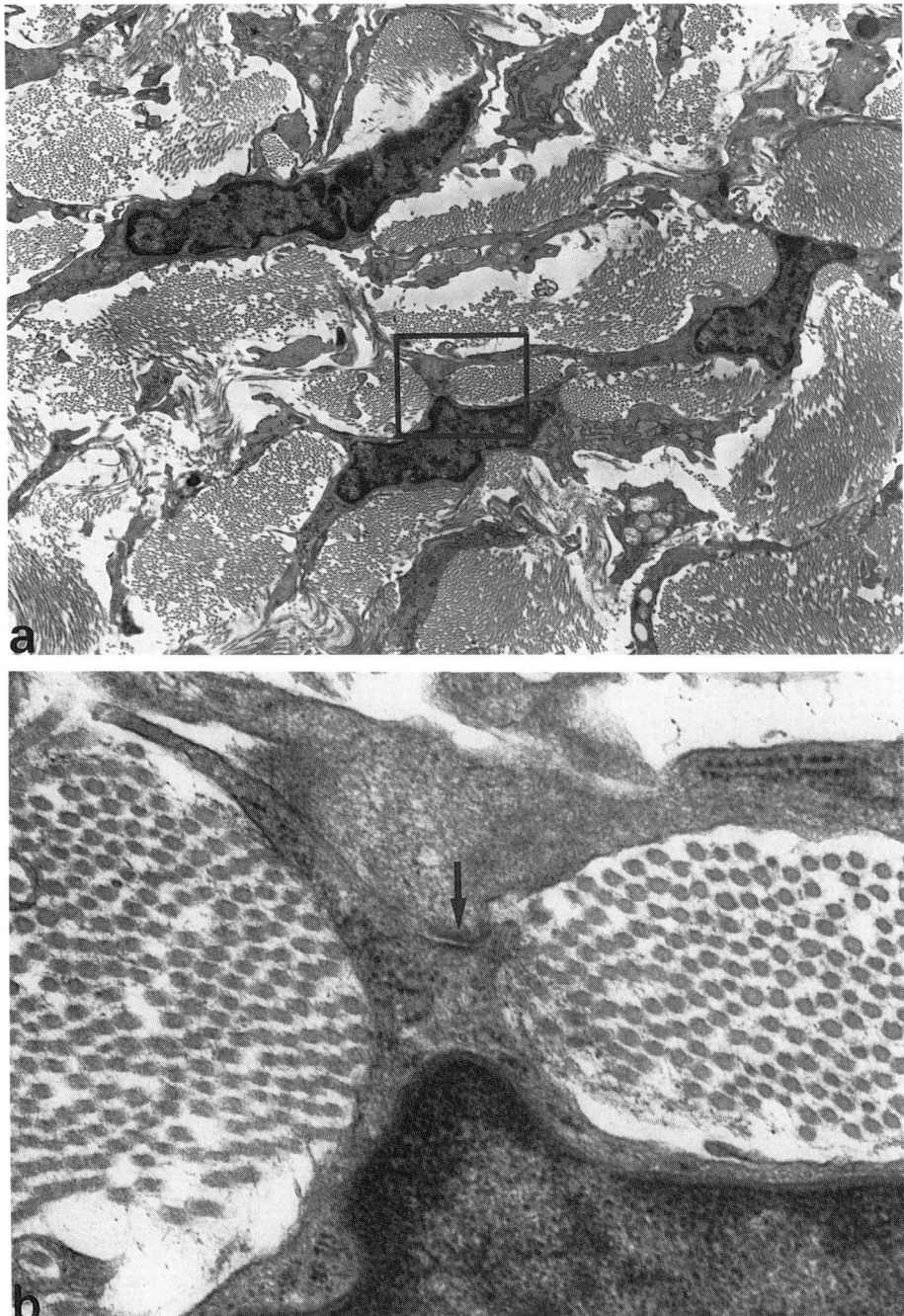

Fig. 4.5 Transmission electron micrographs from residual phase nodule illustrating a slender fibrocytes with smooth contoured nuclei embedded in a dense collageneous matrix, and b joined by few poorly differentiated junctions (arrow). Uranyl acetate and lead citrate (a × 6300; b × 48 000).

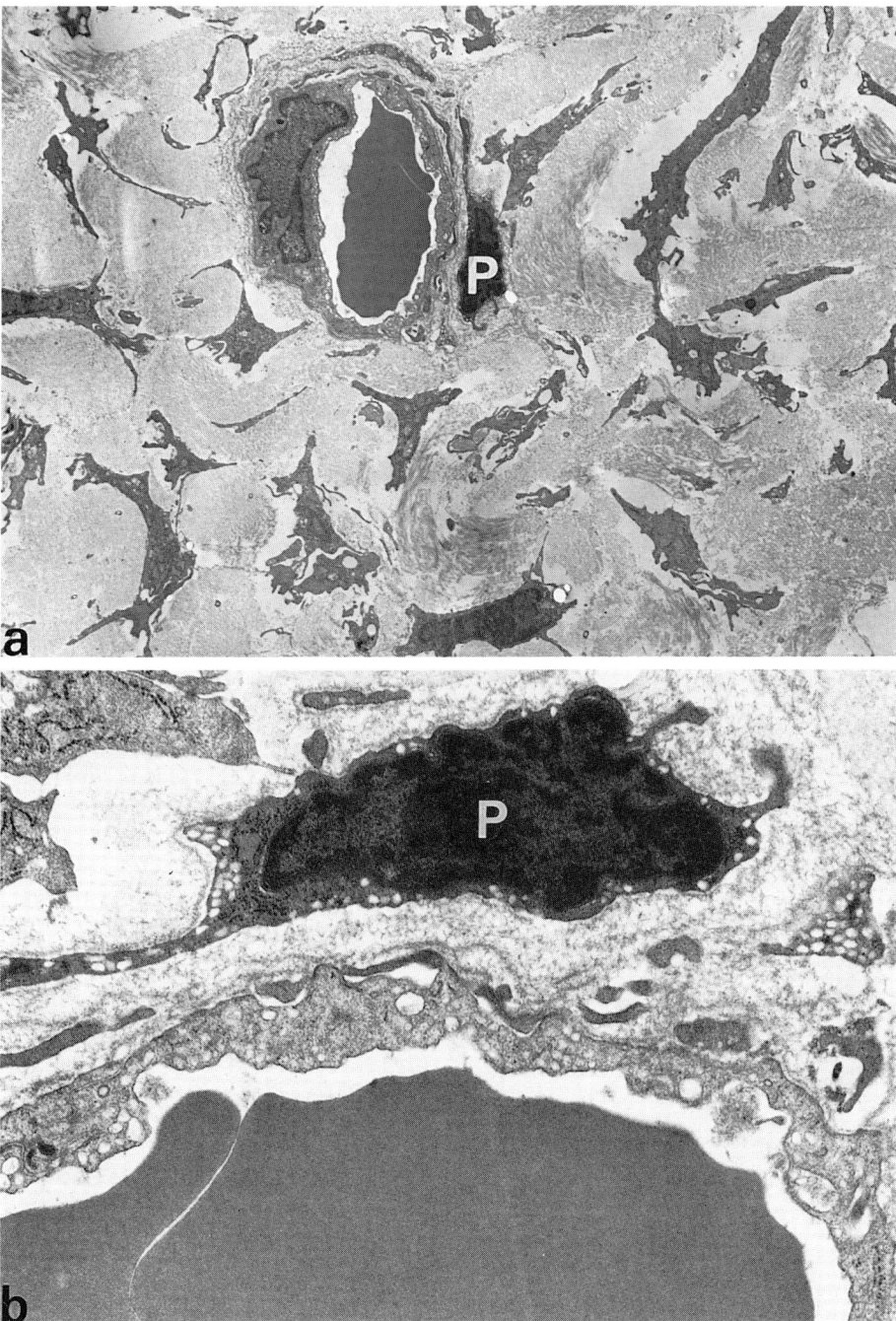

Fig. 4.6 Transmission electron micrographs from residual phase nodule illustrating: **a** small capillary with pericyte (P); **b** this pericyte is small with little cytoplasm and is devoid of bundles of microfilaments. For comparison, see Figure 4.2b. Uranyl acetate and lead citrate (**a** × 4200; **b** × 14 000).

myofibroblasts (Giacomelli et al 1970; Gabbiani et al 1979, 1983, White et al 1983; Wong et al 1983; Kocher et al 1985). On the other hand, proliferating smooth muscle cells from different pathological conditions and in vitro exhibit ultrastuctural features very similar to those of myofibroblasts (Poole et al 1971; Chamley-Campbell et al 1979; Olivetti et al 1980; Kocher et al 1984; 1985). From these considerations, it can be concluded that ultrastructural studies do not furnish any proof about the cellular derivation of myofibroblasts. Different authors have thus attempted to address this question by examining the cytoskeletal composition of myofibroblasts. Cytoskeletal proteins are of particular interest for this purpose since they display multiple variants that are encoded by multigene families or are the result of differential mRNA splicing (Caplan et al 1983). Intermediate filament proteins are good markers of cellular origin since they have a tissue-specific distribution which is retained during neoplastic conditions (Osborn & Weber 1983; Rungger-Brändle & Gabbiani 1983). Other cytoskeletal proteins, such as myosin isoforms also have a tissue-specific distribution but their expression changes promptly and reversibly in response to many physiological and pathological stimuli; such proteins are useful to evaluate the degree of cellular differentiation.

The determination of the intermediate filament protein content of myofibroblasts is of limited value for solving the riddle of their origin. Since myofibroblasts are of mesenchymal lineage (MacDonald 1959; Grillo 1963; Ross et al 1970) they may express vimentin and/or desmin. Vimentin is the unique protein subunit composing the intermediate filaments of most non-muscle mesenchymal cells such as fibroblasts, histiocytes, endothelial cells and white blood cells; desmin is the unique protein subunit composing the intermediate filaments of striated muscle cells and parenchymal smooth muscle cells. The two limitations for the use of these proteins as markers of myofibroblast origin are:

1. A large proportion of vascular smooth muscle cells express vimentin only, while others express vimentin and desmin (Berner et al 1981; Frank & Warren 1981; Gabbiani et al 1981; Schmid et al 1982).

2. Desmin has been increasingly found in an number of non-muscle mesenchymal cells such as endothelial cells (Fujimoto & Singer 1986; Toccanier-Pelte et al 1987), podocytes (Stamenkovic et al 1986) and stromal cells from various locations (Glasser & Julian 1986; Skalli et al 1986a; Franke & Moll 1987; Toccanier-Pelte et al 1987).

Other cytoskeletal proteins which may provide useful information about the histogenesis of myofibroblasts are actin isoforms, since the six actin isoforms expressed in mammals show a tissue-specific distribution (Vandekerckhove & Weber 1978a, 1978b, 1981). Thus, striated muscle cells coexpress various proportions of alpha-skeletal and alpha-cardiac actin, whereas smooth muscle cells coexpress various proportions of alpha- and gamma-smooth muscle actin. The two other actin isoforms are called beta- and gamma-cytoplasmic and are found in the cytoplasm of every cell. Alpha, beta and gamma refer to the electrophoretic mobility of these isoforms, when separated by isoelectric focusing or two-dimensional gel electrophoresis (Fig. 4.7). Further separation of the three isoforms with an alpha-electrophoretic mobility and of the two with a gamma-electrophoretic mobility requires electrophoretic analysis of the NH_2-terminal peptide (Vandekerckhove & Weber 1981). Two-dimensional gel electrophoresis of the actin isoform pattern of different mesenchymal tissues demonstrated that the presence of an alpha-actin spot allows the distinction between smooth muscle and fibroblastic tissues (Skalli et al 1987). This was confirmed at the histological level with a monoclonal antibody raised against the NH_2-terminal decapeptide of alpha-smooth muscle actin which recognizes exclusively this isoform (Skalli et al 1986a); this antibody did not stain normal fibroblasts but constantly decorated smooth muscle cells. Examination of actin isoform expression in various soft tissue tumours by means of immunofluorescence and two-dimensional gel electrophoresis showed that alpha-smooth muscle actin was present in well differentiated smooth muscle tumours, including leiomyomas and well differentiated leiomyosarcomas, but absent in poorly differentiated leiomyosarcomas (Schürch et

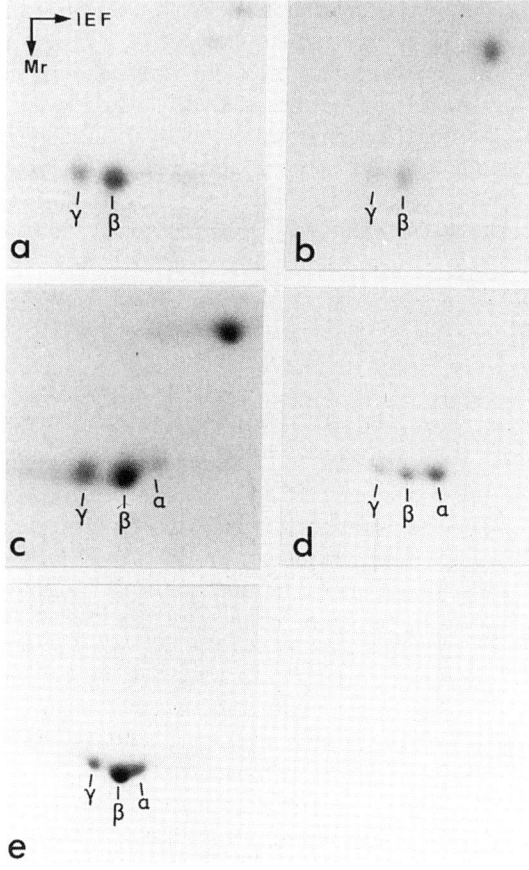

Fig. 4.7 Two-dimensional gel electrophoresis of actin isoforms in a dermis, b normal scar c, d hypertrophic scars and e palmar fibromatosis (e). Dermis and normal scar contain beta- and gamma-actins, whereas hypertrophic scars and palmar fibromatosis contain alpha-, beta- and gamma-actins. Note the alpha-spot is prominent in the hypertrophic scar occurring at the site of a smallpox vaccination (d). IEF, Mr, and the corresponding arrows indicate the direction of migration of isoelectric focusing and second dimension, respectively. Reproduced from Skalli et al (1989a), with permission.

al 1987). In benign smooth muscle proliferations alpha-smooth muscle actin was always present but at levels lower than in quiescent smooth muscle cells (Schürch et al 1987; Skalli et al 1987). This was also shown in human and experimental atheroma (Gabbiani et al 1984; Kocher et al 1984; Kocher & Gabbiani 1986) and for cultured aortic smooth muscle cells (Gabbiani et al 1984; Owens et al 1986; Skalli et al 1986b). Thus, the presence of alpha-smooth muscle actin in a cell can be taken as a good indication of a smooth muscle origin, as far as benign mesenchymal proliferations (such as those involving myofibroblasts) are concerned, and might indicate the state of differentiation in smooth muscle neoplasms.

Like actin, myosin is a ubiquitous cytoskeletal protein displaying a tissue-specific microheterogeneity (for review see Bandman 1985) which makes it potentially useful for the determination of myofibroblast origin. Smooth muscle cells express two myosin heavy chains, not normally found in other muscle or non-muscle cell types (Beckers-Bleukx & Maréchal 1985; Rovner et al 1986a; Kawamoto & Adelstein 1987). However, in proliferating smooth muscle cells the expression of smooth muscle myosin is replaced by that of non-muscle myosin, as has been established for benign and malignant smooth muscle proliferations (Donner et al 1983) and for cultured aortic smooth muscle cells (Chamley et al 1977; Larson et al 1984; Rovner et al 1986b; Kawamoto & Adelstein 1987; Benzonana et al 1988). Interestingly, in confluent aortic smooth muscle cell cultures, smooth muscle myosin is re-expressed (Chamley et al 1977, Larson et al 1984), indicating that the expression of myosin isoforms can be reversibly altered in these cells. Thus, myosin isoforms appear more useful for evaluating the degree of smooth muscle differentiation of cells or tissues than for determining their origin.

The determination of the cytoskeletal composition of myofibroblasts led some authors to postulate a fibroblastic origin whereas others favoured a smooth muscle derivation. Granulation tissue myofibroblasts were proposed to be of fibroblastic derivation since they are stained by vimentin and not by desmin antibodies (Skalli & Gabbiani 1988) and because two-dimensional gel electrophoresis failed to reveal the presence of an alpha-actin spot (Skalli et al 1987); (Fig. 4.7). A similar conclusion was reached for myofibroblasts from the stroma of invasive breast carcinoma (Shürch et al 1984) and pulmonary fibrosis (Woodcock-Mitchell et al 1984). However, myofibroblasts from these conditions reacted with a monoclonal antibody specific for alpha-smooth muscle actin, showing that they have smooth muscle cytoskeletal features (Skalli et al 1986a; Sappino et al 1988; Mitchell et al in press)

A positive reaction for desmin antibodies also suggested a smooth muscle origin for myofibroblasts of DD (Shum & McFarlane 1988) and infantile myofibromatosis (Fletcher et al 1987). Interestingly, desmin positivity was not found in all cases examined (Schürch et al 1984; Fletcher et al 1987). Staining with an antibody recognizing the four muscle actin isoforms further suggested a smooth muscle derivation for myofibroblasts from DD (Tsukuda et al 1987) and for inclusion body fibromatosis of adulthood (Viale et al 1988). Taken together, these studies suggested that myofibroblasts from different tissues disclose cytoskeletal heterogeneity. This point was systematically investigated by double immunofluorescence with antibodies against vimentin, desmin, alpha-smooth muscle and alpha-sarcomeric actin in diverse settings where myofibroblasts are present (Skalli et al 1989a). By this means it was possible to define four cytoskeletal phenotypes among myofibroblasts (Skalli et al 1989a):

1. Phenotype V, represented by myofibroblasts positive for vimentin only.
2. Phenotype VAD, represented by myofibroblasts positive for vimentin, alpha-smooth muscle actin and desmin.
3. Phenotype VA, represented by myofibroblasts positive for vimentin and alpha-smooth muscle actin.
4. Phenotype VD, represented by myofibroblasts positive for vimentin and desmin.

Myofibroblasts from all conditions examined were negative for alpha-sarcomeric actin. The recognition of these different cytoskeletal phenotypes allowed the distinction of two kinds of myofibroblastic proliferations: the first contains only V-cells and comprises normally healing granulation tissue, eschars and normally healed scars; the second embodies hypertrophic scars and fibromatoses, including Dupuytren's. In these settings V-cells were mixed with various proportions of cells expressing cytoskeletal markers of myogenic differentiation, i.e. VAD-, VA- and VD-cells. In most Dupuytren's nodules and other fibromatoses the number of VA-cells exceeded the number of VAD-cells (Fig. 4.8).

The tissue distribution of VA- and VAD-cells was homogeneous in some cases but in others it was focal. Whether these differences in the regional distribution of cells with various phenotypes affect the course of DD is unknown. Within the same nodule, cells with cytoskeletal smooth muscle features were present within the proliferative, cellular regions, and their number decreased progressively at the interface between these areas and sclerotic areas (Shum & McFarlane 1988; Skalli et al 1989a). The same observation was made for musculoaponeurotic fibromatoses (Skalli et al 1989a). Despite their heterogeneity in intermediate filament proteins and actin isoforms, myofibroblasts from different settings, including granulation tissue (Benzonana et al 1988; Eddy et al 1988), Dupuytren's nodules (Tomasek et al 1986; Benzonana et al 1986), and hypertrophic scars (Eddy et al 1988) express only non-muscle myosin. In these tissues, the extracellular matrix around myofibroblasts is strongly stained for anti-fibronectin but not for anti-laminin (Tomasek et al 1986; Eddy et al 1988).

The heterogeneous cytoskeletal composition of myofibroblasts raises questions as to their origin. Ultrastructural data provide evidence that during pathological and/or culture conditions fibroblasts and smooth muscle cells acquire morphological features similar to those of myofibroblasts (Moss & Benditt 1970; Poole et al 1971; Chamley-Campbell et al 1979, Olivetti et al 1980; Kocher et al 1984, 1985; Mosse et al 1985), thereby suggesting that both cell types may be the progenitor of myofibroblasts. The heterogeneous cytoskeletal composition of myofibroblasts may be in agreement with that theory since V-cells could be derived from fibroblasts, and VAD- and VA-cells could be derived from smooth muscle cells and/or pericytes, since these latter cells have cytoskeletal features similar to smooth muscle cells (Joyce et al 1984; Herman & D'Amore 1985; Fujimoto & Singer 1987, Toccanier-Pelte et al 1987; Skalli et al 1989b).

A vascular origin of myofibroblasts was also proposed on the basis of morphological observations, suggesting that desmin-positive cells were migrating from vessel walls to the tissue (Shum & McFarlane 1988); this suggestion is consistent with earlier studies showing an intimate relationship be-

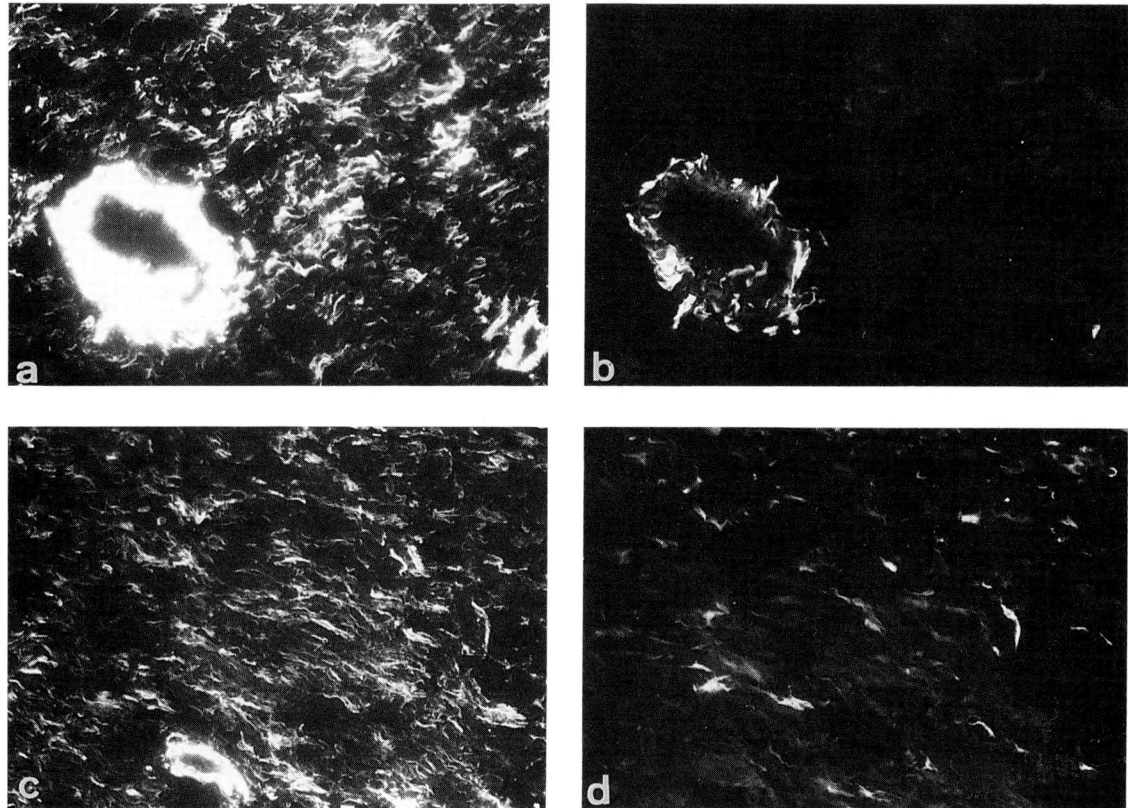

Fig. 4.8 Double immunofluorescent staining of a Dupuytren's nodule with anti-alpha-smooth muscle actin (**a,c**) and anti-desmin (**b,d**) disclosing areas of cells with different cytoskeletal phenotypes. **a** and **c**: area where many cells are positive for anti-alpha-smooth muscle actin and negative for anti-desmin; **c** and **d**: area where cells positive for anti-alpha-smooth muscle actin and anti-desmin are admixed with cells positive only for anti-alpha-smooth muscle actin ($\times$ 400).

tween proliferating cells of DD and blood vessels (Janssen 1902; Larsen & Posch 1958). One possible origin of VD-cells is the stromal cells positive for anti-desmin and negative for alpha-smooth muscle actin that are present in the stroma of various organs (Glasser & Julian 1986; Skalli et al 1986a; Franke & Moll 1987; Toccanier-Pelte et al 1987). The negative staining of DD myofibroblasts for a monoclonal antibody specific of alpha-sarcomeric actin (Skalli et al 1986a) strongly argues against an early theory which proposed that Dupuytren's nodules arise from residues of embryonic muscle in the palm (Krogius 1920; Stein et al 1960) or from local striated muscle (MacCallen & Hueston 1962).

In addition to an origin from different cell types, the cytoskeletal heterogeneity of myofibroblasts may also be accounted for by two alternative explanations. First, myofibroblasts may stem from fibroblasts which are induced to express smooth muscle cytoskeletal proteins upon some yet unknown stimuli. Secondly, myofibroblasts may originate from smooth muscle cells and/or pericytes, which in some instances, would 'switch off' the expression of alpha-smooth muscle actin and/or desmin. From these considerations it is clear that the data presently available on the cytoskeletal composition of myofibroblast do not allow a definitive conclusion of their cellular derivation; however, they demonstrate that subsets of myofibroblasts possess smooth muscle phenotypic features, as shown by their expression of alpha-smooth muscle and/or desmin. Interestingly, this smooth muscle differentiation is never fully expressed since smooth muscle myosin and laminin are not expressed by myofibroblasts from various tissues (Tomasek et al 1986; Benzonana et al 1988; Eddy et al 1988).

PATHOGENESIS OF DD

The pathogenesis of DD remains obscure. The finding that the major cellular component involved in this disease is also found in granulation tissue and tumour stroma is of interest for this issue. Indeed, at the cellular level, a number of similarities exists between the process of wound healing, certain quasineoplastic proliferative conditions, especially fibromatoses, and the desmoplastic stromal reaction to invasive carcinomas (Schürch et al 1981). In such a conceptualization, myofibroblast induction may be viewed as a fundamental pathobiological process which, at one end of the spectrum, effects the closure of wounds or, in a pathologically excessive reparative reaction, is responsible for the reaction of the palmar fascia in DD. At the other extreme it represents a cellular response to invasive neoplasia (Seemayer et al 1982). Myofibroblasts possess not only contractile forces, but also synthetic properties for type III collagen (Gabbiani et al 1976). In granulation tissue of healing wounds myofibroblasts are especially numerous and the collagen produced is principally type III. When granulation tissue is resorbed following wound closure, myofibroblasts disappear (Rudolph et al 1977) and the more rigid type I collagen is identified (Gabbiani et al 1976). In like fashion, the proliferative cellular phase of DD is characterized by numerous myofibroblasts and contains a predominance of type III collagen, whereas in the residual fibrocytic phase, type I collagen predominates (Meister et al 1979). Finally, types pro-III and III collagen are present in increased amounts in the 'young' oedematous mesenchyme (Lagacé et al 1985), areas laden with myofibroblasts, corresponding to zones of early stromal invasion of breast carcinomas (Schürch et al 1981, 1982); contrariwise, type I collagen is most prominent within the central sclerotic zone of breast carcinomas (Lagacé et al 1985), areas where myofibroblasts are replaced by fibroblasts (Schürch et al 1981, 1982).

Substantial evidence has been provided about analogies between wound healing and the generation of tumour stroma at the level of spillage of plasma proteins including fibrinogen, fibronectin and plasminogen (Dvorak 1986). These plasma proteins form an extravascular clot serving as provisional stroma which provides a matrix for the immigration of fibroblasts, macrophages and new capillaries, i.e. granulation tissue, which is eventually resorbed and undergoes retraction and scarring.

Some important topographical differences, however, exist between the desmoplastic stromal reaction in invasive carcinomas and the resorption of granulation tissue. The organization of granulation tissue during would healing is centripetal, whereas in carcinomatous invasion, the stroma is organized from within (point of departure of the carcinoma) outward and amidst the neoplastic elements. Organization in the desmoplastic stromal reaction of invasive carcinomas is therefore centrifugal and might limit (in theory) neoplastic extension and access of neoplastic cell to lymphatic and vascular channels, especially when the stromal reaction is precocious, that is, myofibroblasts precede the carcinoma cells by some distance into the adjacent tissue (Schürch et al 1982, Seemayer et al 1982).

The organization of granulation tissue and probably, Dupuytren's nodules is centripetal. The maturation of the principal cellular elements proceeds the opposite way, — blastic cells (myofibroblasts) are in the poorly collagenized centre and mature fibroblasts (fibrocytes) in the intensely collagenized periphery.

Although a number of similarities exists between the process of wound healing, quasineoplastic proliferative conditions and the desmoplastic stromal reaction of invasive carcinomas at the cellular and extracellular level, several fundamental differences exist concerning the maturation of the cellular elements. Myofibroblasts, during normal wound healing, disappear (Rudolph et al 1977), whereas in the stromal reaction to invasive carcinomas they persist. Thus, the stroma of invasive carcinomas resembles the non-healing wound (Dvorak 1986). In fibromatoses and also in DD myofibroblasts seem to persist more than in granulation tissue, therefore these quasineoplastic proliferations probably occupy a position intermediate between granulation tissue in normal wound healing and the desmoplastic stromal reaction of invasive carcinomas.

It has been suggested long ago that DD may be related to the repair of minor trauma of the palmar aponeurosis. This hypothesis has gained some support from experiments on monkeys showing that a pathological response similar to that of DD was induced by stretching the palmar fascia (Larsen et al 1960). Moreover, the proliferative nodule of DD often contains small foci of perivascular haemorrhage and haemosiderin deposition accompanied by the accumulation of macrophages and lymphocytes (Iwasaki et al 1984). Although these findings represent weak evidence for trauma as a cause of DD, in humans the presence of macrophages in this disease is of interest, in view of the central role played by these cells in wound healing and in the stimulation of fibroblast and smooth muscle cell proliferation (for review see Riches 1988).

Experimental evidence for DD as a benign tumour of mesenchymal origin (Enzinger et al 1970) has come from culture of cells derived from nodules and palmar aponeurosis of patients affected by DD (Azzarone et al 1983). The growth properties of Dupuytren's nodule myofibroblasts were intermediate between those of normal fibroblasts and embryonic or virus-transformed fibroblasts.

As with normal cells, Dupuytren's nodule myofibroblasts displayed contact inhibition at the plateau phase and had a limited life span. But, like transformed cells, Dupuytren's nodule myofibroblasts formed colonies in soft agar, grew in the presence of reduced amounts of fetal calf serum and secreted high levels of the urokinase-like species of plasminogen activator. Karyotypic abnormalities were also found in these cells (Bowser-Riley et al 1975; Azzarone et al 1983; Sergovich et al 1983). Interestingly, cultures derived from the apparently normal palmar aponeurosis of patients affected by DD showed some, but not all, of the abnormal properties of cells derived from nodules. In situ, myofibroblasts and type III collagen have been found in the 'normal' palmar aponeurosis of patients affected by DD (Bazin et al 1980), suggesting that the syndrome is not strictly focal. These findings may provide a possible explanation for the local recurrences observed in DD.

The concept of a neoplastic transformation of Dupuytren's myofibroblasts is not incompatible with trauma as an aetiological factor. It could be hypothesized that trauma occurring in the palmar aponeurosis will heal normally in most instances but that in some cases the myofibroblasts involved in repair become transformed. Diseases associated with DD and/or certain hereditary settings could explain why this transformation occurs only in certain cases.

CONCLUSIONS

Ultrastructural, immunohistochemical, biochemical and cell culture experiments have revealed important information about the cellular biology of DD. These studies have established that the main cell type present within Dupuytren's nodules has contractile and synthetic features similar to those of myofibroblasts present in granulation tissue, where they are thought to generate contractile forces responsible for wound closure. Thus, myofibroblasts present within Dupuytren's nodules might also be responsible for the contractile events observed in this disease.

These observations reveal a number of analogies between the process of wound healing, Dupuytren's nodules and the generation of tumour stroma. These analogies concern primarily the formation of a vascularized 'young' mesenchyme rich in type III collagen, in which the myofibroblast represents the predominant cell. The analogies and discrepancies between wound healing, DD and tumour stroma formation are to a large extent unexplored, but represent an attractive area of research. Their detailed analysis could well encourage the development of new therapeutic strategies, modulating stroma formation to limit neoplastic growth.

Immunohistochemical studies have shown that Dupuytren's nodules always contain a subset of myofibroblasts exhibiting smooth muscle cytoskeletal markers — alpha-smooth muscle actin and/or desmin. Moreover, within the same nodules, cells with cytoskeletal smooth muscle features revealed zonal differences. They were present within the cellular centre of proliferative nodules and decreased progressively at the interphase between these areas and the sclerotic zones. The presence of myofibroblasts in Dupuytren's nodules reinforces the notion that these cells are responsible for the contractile events in DD but does not provide any conclusive answer about their origin. Ultrastructural examination of Dupuytren's nodules reveals differences in proliferative, involutional and residual phase nodules concerning the cells, intercellular junctions, capillary pericytes and extracellular matrix. While myofibroblasts progressively disappear during evolution of the nodules, they are replaced by fibrocytes. The large and prominent pericytes of proliferative phase nodules, displaying smooth muscle features, are replaced by small inconspicuous pericytes in the poorly vascularized residual nodules. At the same time, gap junctions between myofibroblasts of proliferative and involutional phase nodules also disappear, and fibrocytes of residual nodules are connected by a few poorly differentiated junctions. Gap junctions are considered as low resistance pathways for intercellular communication. Parallel to these cellular events, a progressive collagenization takes place and the nodules are transformed into a scar-like tissue.

Ultrastructural examination of Dupuytren's nodules provides no information concerning the origin of myofibroblasts, even though morphological similarities exist between them and pericytes. Since Dupuytren's nodules are composed of cells with similar ultrastructural features but different cytoskeletal composition, the question has to be raised how these cells can be present within the same tissue. The phenotypic differences of myofibroblasts could be explained by the concept of isoformic transitions according to differences in cell function. For Caplan et al (1983), the concept of cellular isoforms is defined as 'the replacement of individual molecules and cells by molecular and cellular variants called isoforms because they are both similar and distinctly different and arise during embryonic development and later life'. According to this concept, the phenotypic modulation of myofibroblasts in DD might be viewed as isoformic transitions of a common ancestor cell which is still not defined. Future effort should be directed to determine which factors regulate the expression of smooth muscle proteins in myofibroblasts of DD and other pathological settings composed of myofibroblasts.

Acknowledgements

This work was supported by the Swiss National Science Foundation, grant no 3.108–0.88, by the Foundation de Recherches Médicales Carlos et Elsie de Reuter, and by the Cancer Research Society Inc., Montreal, Quebec, Canada.

We thank Mrs M.-M. Rossire for typing the manuscript.

A. F. Delbrück and E. Gurr

5

Proteoglycans and glycosaminoglycans

NORMAL PALMAR FASCIA

In the normal, healthy palmar fascia a network of specifically oriented connective tissue fibres consisting of collagen type I is embedded in a ground substance made up of proteoglycans, hyaluronate and proteins. Distributed throughout this substance are the cells that synthesize the macromolecular components of the palmar fascia and keep them functioning via a steady state of synthesis and degradation. The interactions of these macromolecules with each other and the effects of mechanical forces contribute to the formation of the architecture that is typical for this tissue, the basic characteristics of which are already evident in the morphological three-dimensional arrangement of the connective tissue cells at the embryonal stage (Chapter 11).

Proteoglycans are biological macromolecules with a protein core to which at least one glycosaminoglycan chain and oligosaccharides are covalently linked. The glycosaminoglycans are polyanionic chains of different lengths consisting of repeating series of disaccharide units. One component of these disaccharides is always an N-acetylated amino sugar, to which a sulphate group may be attached. The other component is a uronic acid. These macromolecules play an important role in the physical and functional characteristics of the connective tissue, e.g. molecular interactions, aggregation, viscosity, permeability, water-attracting capacity and swelling (Donoff & Schweidt 1982; Flint et al 1982).

The type and pattern of the glycosaminoglycans is specific for the individual types of connective tissue. Figure 5.1 shows the types and amounts of

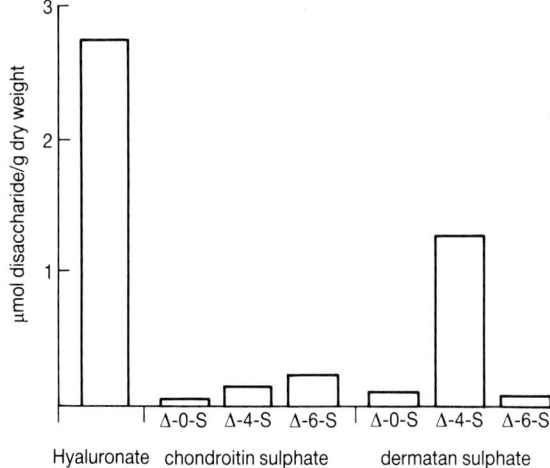

Fig. 5.1 Glycosaminoglycan pattern of human healthy palmar fascia. Combined enzymatic–high performance liquid chromatography analysis according to Gurr et al (1985). Biopsy.
Δ–0–S = non-sulphated disaccharide metabolite of glycosaminoglycan;
Δ–4–S = C–4–sulphated disaccharide metabolite of glycosaminoglycan;
Δ–6–S = C–6–sulphated disaccharide metabolite of glycosaminoglycan.
Total glycosaminoglycans = 4.45 μmol/g dry weight.

the different sulphated and non-sulphated glycosaminoglycans in healthy human palmar fascia (Tunn et al 1988). Characteristically there is a high percentage of the non-sulphated hyaluronate, and among the sulphated glycosaminoglycans dermatan sulphate predominates, as also shown by Flint et al (1982). Heparan sulphate occurs in trace amounts and is probably a component of the cell surface structure.

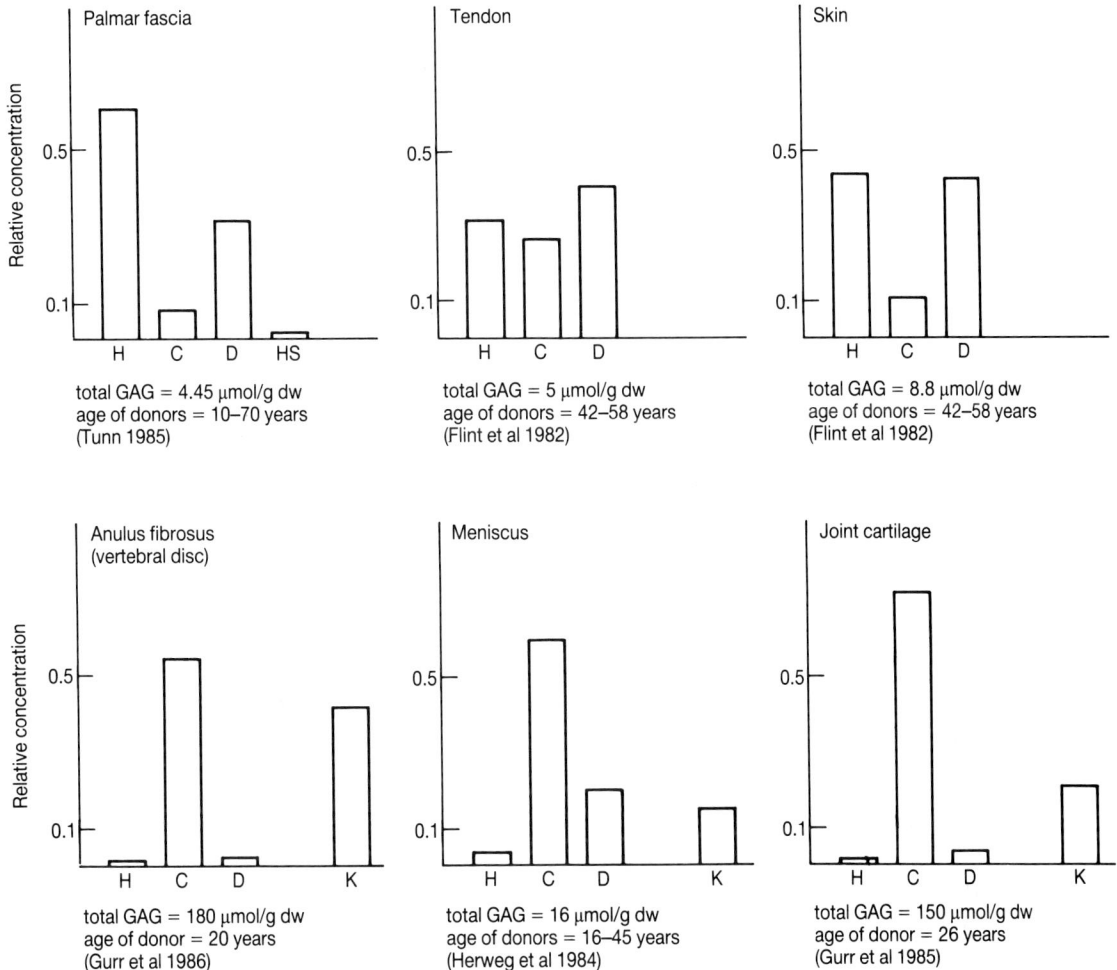

Fig. 5.2 Glycosaminoglycan (GAG) pattern from healthy human palmar fascia in comparison with other human connective tissues in relative concentrations. H = hyaluronate; C = chondroitin sulphate; D = dermatan sulphate; HS = heparan sulphate; K = keratan sulphate. dw = Dry weight.

Figure 5.2 shows that in spite of limitations in comparability related to methodology, the profiles for other types of connective tissue are clearly different from that found in the palmar fascia. Skin and tendon tissue also have relatively large proportions of dermatan sulphate, whereas anulus fibrosus, meniscus and joint cartilage all contain very small proportions of hyaluronate and large amounts of chondroitin sulphate and keratan sulphate. The large amount of hyaluronate in the palmar fascia cannot be explained solely by the formation of complexes with proteoglycans such as occurs in cartilage. Rather, we must assume that the physical and chemical properties of hyaluronate are of importance for the function of the tissue as such, as for example Viidik et al (1982) have discussed regarding the function of the tendons. The characteristic glycosaminoglycan content is paralleled by an equally typical collagen profile consisting almost exclusively of collagen type I; there is less than 5% collagen type III in healthy palmar fascia (Menzel et al 1979).

The structures of the proteoglycans from palmar fascia have not yet been studied. The best we can do is to make assumptions on the basis of our knowledge about proteoglycans isolated from tissues related to palmar fascia. Proteoglycans extracted from tendon consist of two different subpopulations (Vogel & Heinegard 1985). One of these, which contains about 12% of the total proteoglycan content, has a high molecular weight and chondroitin sulphate side chains. In areas where the tendons are subject to relatively high compressive loads, the percentage of large proteoglycans containing chondroitin sulphate increases to about 50%, and this difference is maintained when the tendinocytes are placed in cell cultures and synthesize proteoglycans under culture conditions (Vogel et al 1986).

In contrast to the small proteoglycans containing dermatan sulphate, the large proteoglycans from tendon containing chondroitin sulphate bind to hyaluronate in the same way as the proteoglycans in cartilage. In contrast, Scott (1984) found that the low molecular weight dermatan sulphate proteoglycan of tendon binds specifically to the surface of the collagen type I fibrils. Vogel et al (1984) showed that it binds via the protein core. From skin it was possible to isolate a subpopulation of the proteoglycans containing chondroitin sulphate with a high molecular weight and another subpopulation containing dermatan sulphate with a lower molecular weight.

In contrast to tendon and cartilage, the proteoglycans in the skin that contain chondroitin sulphate do not bind to hyaluronate. Moreover, the proportions of the two types of proteoglycans in the skin are age-dependent; the percentage of proteoglycans containing dermatan sulphate increases with age (Habuchi et al 1986). Studies on human rectus sheath revealed the presence of three types of proteoglycans. In addition to a high molecular weight fraction, two low-molecular weight proteoglycans are present, distinguished by a difference in their electrophoretic mobility (Gurr et al, unpublished observations). If hypotheses about the structure of the extracellular matrix of the palmar fascia are based on these findings, one would expect to find (at least) two different types of proteoglycans. The glycosaminoglycan pattern of healthy palmar fascia suggests that the main portion of proteoglycans in this tissue belongs to the dermatan sulphate-containing fraction of low molecular weight.

The steady state of the extracellular matrix of healthy palmar fascia is maintained by the metabolism of the fascia cells. Specific enzymes catalyse the different steps in the synthesis and degradation of the matrix components and the intermediary and energy metabolism. The extracellular matrix provides a pathway for the metabolic exchange with the vascular system, and therefore factors affecting metabolism produced in specific organs or tissues also reach the cells of the palmar fascia. Information on the activity of the enzymes involved in the intermediary and energy metabolism of the palmar fascia can be found in Hoopes et al (1977) and Delbrück et al (1981). Although differences in the methods employed make it difficult to compare the findings, the two studies are in agreement that fascia cells, which synthesize the specific components of the palmar fascia matrix from basic components such as glucose and amino acids and make available the necessary energy (Delbrück et al 1981), have a high metabolic potential. Energy production is mainly via glycolysis, as is evident from the activity of lactate dehydrogenase (EC no. 1.1.1.27) and glucose-6-phosphate dehydrogenase (EC no. 1.1.1.49) in the enzyme profile (Delbrück et al 1959). An enzyme profile which is almost identical to that of the palmar fascia in vivo can be found in fibroblast cultures of cells from human palmar fascia (Delbrück et al 1981). The authors could also show that the activity of lysosomal enzymes in vivo behaved in the same manner as in fibroblast cultures of cells from the palmar fascia.

Studies on the synthesis of extracellular matrix components in which [^{35}S]-sulphate and [^{3}H]-proline were incorporated into glycosaminoglycans and collagen respectively have shown the ability of these cells to synthesize the specific matrix components of the palmar fascia in a defined in vitro system (Fig. 5.3). The fact that the rates of synthesis depend on the cell density in the cultures indicates that the interaction of the cells with each other and/or with the surrounding matrix has a regulatory influence on cell metabolism (Delbrück & Schröder 1982). Handley et al (1985) hypothesized a feedback regulation of the synthesis of the proteoglycans for cartilage, and this would appear to hold for the palmar fascia, too. Although there is no evidence so far that any hormones play a role in the regulation of metabolism

THE PALMAR FASCIA IN DD

Under pathological conditions, various factors can have inhibitory or activating effects on the complex metabolic processes that take place in the cells of the palmar fascia, resulting in an imbalance, with consequences for the structure and function of this tissue. To do justice to the dynamics of the pathological process in DD, a careful treatment is required of the individual stages seen in the development of the disorder. In agreement with Flint et al (1982), a classification according to macroscopic appearance is recommended: apparently normal fascia; fascia adjacent to bands or nodules (termed fibrous bands by Flint et al); bands (called fleshy bands by Flint et al) and nodules.

Assessed in terms of DNA concentration, fascia tissue affected by Dupuytren's process has a much larger cellular component than normal fascia (Hoopes et al 1977; Delbrück et al 1981, Tunn 1985; Fig. 5.4). Morphologically, cell proliferation begins in the perivascular space (Millesi 1981). Mohr & Vossbeck (1985) found an increase in [^{3}H]-thymidin uptake by the cells which Kischer & Speer (1984) have termed pericytes and that they consider to be the initial manifestation and

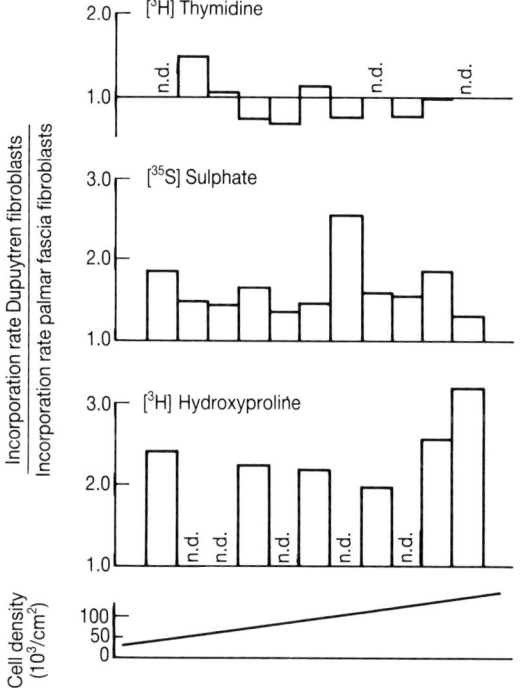

Fig. 5.3 Incorporation of labelled precursors into DNA, glycosaminoglycans and collagen by cultured fibroblasts from DD and normal human palmar fascia. Determinations in quadruplicate cultures, Dupuytren and palmar fascia lines are matched according to the cell density. The incorporation rates of palmar fascia are set at 1.0
n.d. = not determined.

in the cells of the palmar fascia, within the framework of the overall control of metabolism in the human body such influences must be assumed to exist. Another factor involved in the regulation of the metabolic equilibrium and the types and amounts of the extracellular matrix components was identified by Gillard et al (1979), Merrilees & Flint (1980), and Gurr et al (1985a), namely the mechanical forces which act on tissues and cells, which can, among other things, lead to a change in the glycosaminoglycan content of rabbit tendon.

Although there are many gaps in our knowledge about the biochemistry of the palmar fascia, it is evident that complex metabolic processes produce and maintain the biochemical and morphological structure of healthy palmar fascia, enabling the mechanics of hand movements to function smoothly.

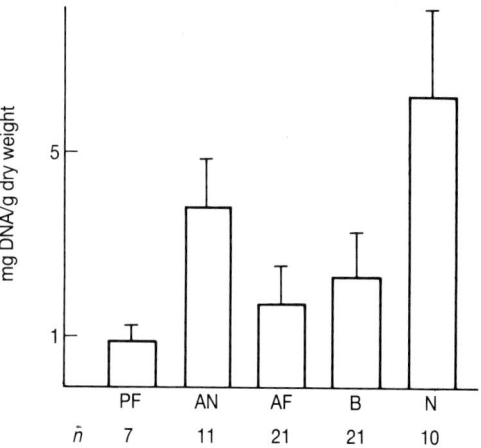

Fig. 5.4 DNA content in specimens of DD in comparison with normal palmar fascia (PF). AN = Apparently normal fascia; AF = fascia adjacent to bands or nodules; B = bands; N = nodules. n = number of biopsies (patients). Bars indicate standard deviation. From Tunn (1985).

starting point of the pathogenetic chain. In DD these authors found perivascular cell proliferation even in palmar fascia tissue which had not yet shown any macroscopic changes. This morphological picture is consistent with the finding that the increase in DNA concentration as a measure of the cell count is particularly marked in specimens of diseased fascia that have been classified as 'apparently normal' (Fig. 5.4).

No differences were observed in the growth rates of isolated cells from healthy palmar fascia and DD tissue in cell culture (Delbrück & Schröder 1982), however. Furthermore, there was no activation of [^{3}H]-thymidin incorporation into the cells from DD tissue.

Azzarone et al (1983) also found identical cell growth kinetics for cells from tissue of DD and healthy palmar fascia. The number of DNA-synthesizing cells was unaltered in the plateau phase of growth. However, the authors were able to show that in contrast to skin fibroblasts, the cells from DD tissue grow and form colonies in an agar culture medium. In monolayer cultures they reach a higher final cell density than healthy skin fibroblasts.

The findings were similar in a study by Rüssel & Witt (1976) on cell cultures of human fibroblasts from keloid and scar tissue. As in DD tissue in vivo, the cells in these tissues are apparently stimulated to proliferate by factors outside the cells such as connective tissue-activating peptide (Castor et al 1979) and growth factors from platelets (Dresow et al 1986) which stimulate cell proliferation in vivo and, after substitution, also in vitro. In addition to cell proliferation, the rates of synthesis of the glycosaminoglycans and collagens can be increased in vitro by the action of the growth factor from platelets on cells of healthy palmar fascia (Dresow et al 1986).

In tissue of DD the total glycosaminoglycan content and the proportions of the different glycosaminoglycans are different from those in healthy palmar fascia. In the papers published on this subject over the last 15 years there has been general agreement about the increase in the total glycosaminoglycans and the shifts in proportions of different glycosaminoglycans, as Table 5.1 shows. The few contradictory findings (Hunter et al 1975) are probably due to methodological problems, which in the past have severely limited the usefulness of the experimental findings. Characteristic differences in the total and fractional content at different stages of DD have been identified, and they suggest associated structural and quantitative changes in the proteoglycans.

Figure 5.5 shows the glycosaminoglycan profile in the palmar fascia at different stages of the disease (Tunn 1985). There is a decrease in the concentration of hyaluronate, with a 50% reduc-

Table 5.1 Biochemical characteristics in specimens from Dupuytren's contracture

Component	Concentration in Dupuytren's contracture	References
Glycosaminoglycans	Exceeding normal tendon Exceeding normal palmar fascia (autopsy) Exceeding normal skin (autopsy) Exceeding palmar fascia (biopsy carpal tunnel syndrome)	Viljanto et al (1971) Flint et al (1982) Bazin et al (1980) Carr et al (1970)
Total collagen	Exceeding normal tendon Exceeding normal palmar fascia (biopsy)	Bazin et al (1980); Gelbermann et al (1980) Brickley-Parson et al (1981)
DNA	Exceeding normal palmar fascia (autopsy)	Delbrück et al (1981)
Water	Exceeding normal tendon	Bazin et al (1980)
Hyaluronate	Lower than normal palmar fascia and tendon (autopsy)	Flint et al (1982)
Dermatan sulphate	Exceeding normal palmar fascia and tendon (autopsy)	Flint et al (1982)
Chondroitin sulphate	Exceeding normal palmar fascia and tendon (autopsy)	Flint et al (1982) Bazin et al (1980)

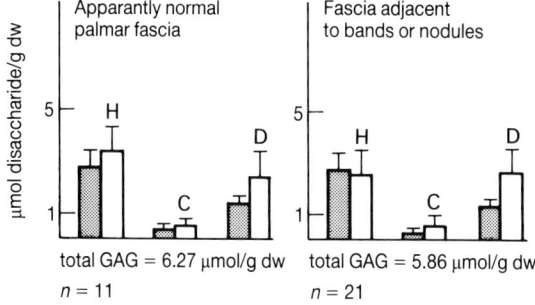

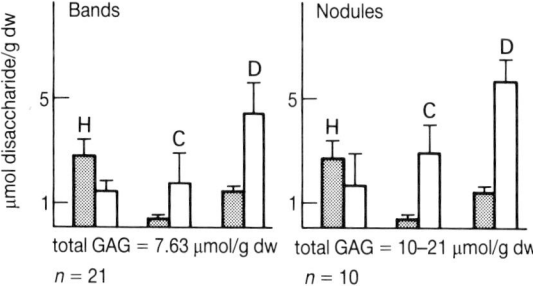

Fig. 5.5 Glycosaminoglycan (GAG) concentrations in different stages of DD. Specimens are grouped according to macroscopic appearances. H = hyaluronate; C = chondroitin sulphate; D = dermatan sulphate. Shaded boxes indicate the respective reference values from healthy palmar fascia biopsies ($n = 7$; 4.45 μmol/g dry weight total GAG; see Fig. 5.1). Bars indicate standard deviation; dw = dry weight. From Tunn et al (1988).

tion in bands and nodules compared with healthy palmar fascia after a slight initial increase in apparently normal fascia material. Parallel to these changes there is an increase in the proportions of chondroitin sulphate and dermatan sulphate, reaching a concentration three times the normal level. As in healthy palmar fascia, the concentration of dermatan sulphate exceeds that of chondroin sulphate. There is thus an overall shift from the non-sulphated to the sulphated glycosaminoglycans; the quotient of non-sulphated divided by sulphated glycosaminoglycans drops from 1.62 to 0.20.

The findings of Flint et al (1982) on the total and fractional glycosaminoglycan content of these three components are generally consistent with those of Tunn (1985) and Tunn et al (1988), in spite of differences attributable to different methods. Tunn et al used a method that enables differentiation of the individual sulphated subfraction (Gurr et al 1985b). As Figure 5.6 shows, they found the greatest relative increase in the chondroitin sulphate fractions, and within that fraction a substantial increase in chondroitin-6-sulphate. The overall concentration of the dermatan sulphate fraction increased by a factor of five compared with normal fascia, but there was no change in the proportions of the various subfractions.

Characteristic changes in the composition of glycosaminoglycans and their subfractions (see above) in specimens from diseased portions of palmar fascia allow classification of the biopsy material according to the stage of the disease. With multivariate analysis (Schneider 1970) it was possible to group exactly the bands and nodules and the normal palmar fascia. As expected, apparently normal tissue and fascia adjacent to bands and nodules were not significantly different from each other but were significantly different from the other groups (Fig. 5.7). Microscopic examinations using the Millesi (1981) classification yielded poorer agreement, however. The discrepancies between morphological (microscopical) and biochemical classifications resulted from the morphological inhomogeneity of the diseased tissue examined and the consequent effect of sample selection on the classification.

The distinct glycosaminoglycan patterns in the various stages of DD lead us to expect similar findings for the proteoglycans in the afflicted tissue portions. However, no data have been published so far on the types and amounts of proteoglycans in DD tissue. Gurr & Borchert (1988) were able to isolate proteoglycans from DD. Gel permeation chromatography and electrophoresis in agarose or polyacrylamidegel enabled identification of at least two proteoglycan subpopulations differing in size and electrophoretic mobility. Based on the proportion of chondroitin sulphate and dermatan sulphate in DD, one can assume that in the course of this disease the high molecular weight proteoglycans increase to 30–40% while the low molecular weight proteoglycans decrease to about 60% of the total proteoglycans (Table 5.2). The low molecular weight proteoglycan population seems to be com-

54 DUPUYTREN'S DISEASE

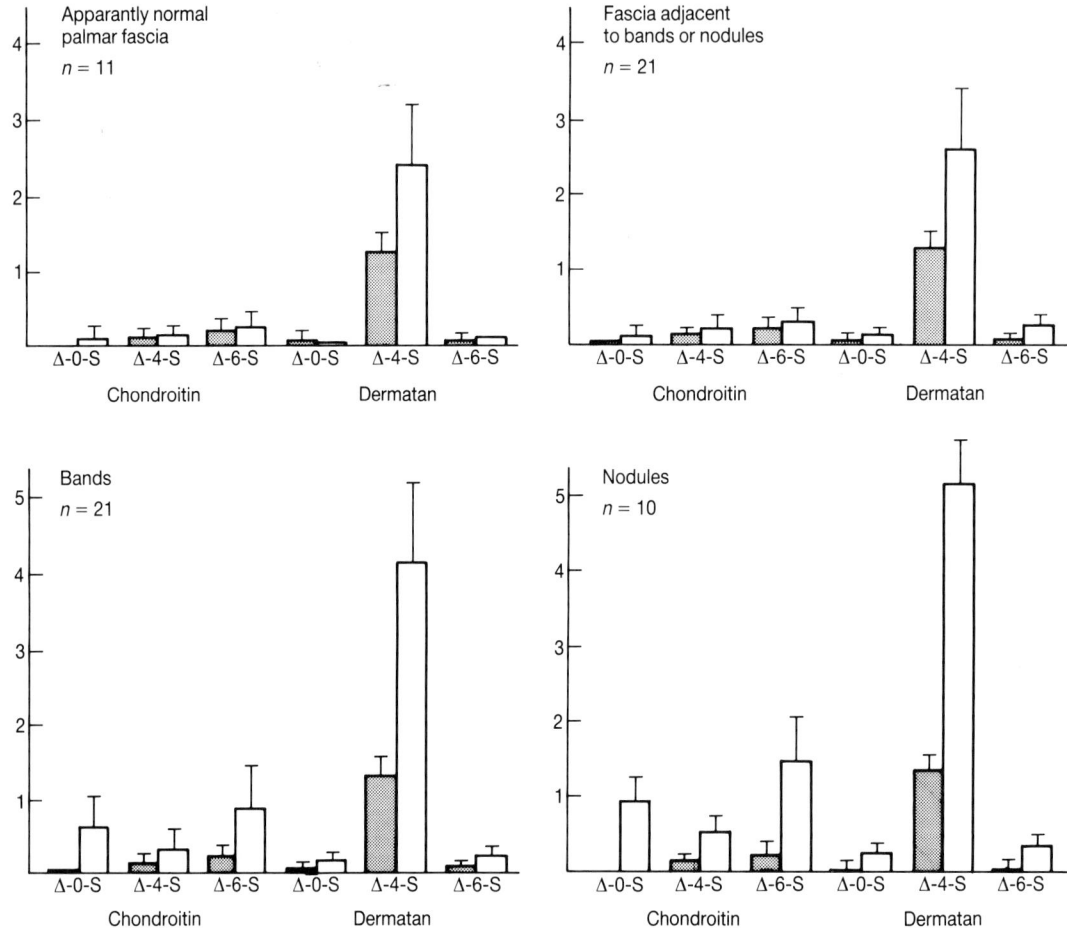

Fig. 5.6 Glycosaminoglycan patterns in Dupuytren's contracture specimens, grouped according to macroscopic appearance. Shaded boxes indicate the pattern of healthy palmar fascia biopsies for reference ($n = 7$). Bars indicate standard deviation. From Tunn et al (1988).

Table 5.2 High and low molecular weight (HMW, LMW) proteoglycans in palmar fascia and DD calculated on the basis of the proportion of chondroitin sulphate or dermatan sulphate

Proteoglycan	Normal palmar fascia	Dupuytren's disease
HMW proteoglycan (chondroitin sulphate)	19.4%	31.6%
LMW proteoglycans (dermatan sulphate)	80.6%	68.4%

posed of two subpopulations. The importance of these changes in the proteoglycan pattern for the fibrillogenesis and the collagen or dermatan sulphate proteoglycan interaction (Scott & Hughes 1986) is still unknown.

The altered steady state of matrix components in DD tissue makes it likely that there are metabolic aberrations in the cells of the palmar fascia or in those cells invaded from foreign tissues. In a study of the types and amounts of main metabolic pathway enzymes it was found that the increases in enzyme activity correlated with the increase in the amount of DNA in specimens of healthy palmar fascia and DD tissue (Delbrück et al 1981). Furthermore, when the activity of glycerinaldehyde-phosphate dehydrogenase (EC no. 1.2.1.12), one of the key enzymes of the

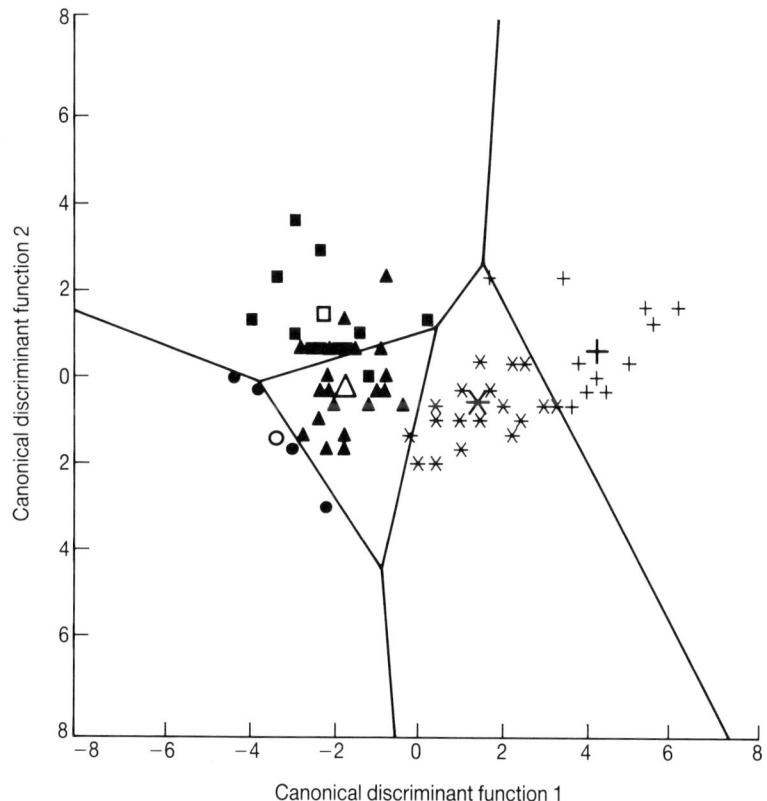

Fig. 5.7 Classification of specimens from healthy palmar fascia and DD by multivariate statistical evaluation (18) of the glycosaminoglycan patterns: nine variables (hyaluronate, total chondroitin sulphate, total dermatan sulphate, and the respective unsulphated, C4 and C6-sulphated isomers). Open symbols indicate group centres. ● = Healthy controls; ■ = apparently normal fascia; ▲ = fascia adjacent to strands and nodules; ★ = strands; ◆ = nodules. From Tunn et al (1988).

Embden–Meyerhof pathway, was used as a point of reference (Delbrück et al 1959), no changes were found in the relative amounts of activity of the different enzymes in fascia tissue at different stages of DD (Delbrück et al 1981). Moreover, even in isolated cultured cells from healthy and pathological palmar fascia tissue there were no changes in the proportions or in the overall activity of the enzymes. The contradictory findings of Hoopes et al (1977) can be explained by methodological differences, which have been discussed elsewhere (Delbrück et al 1981).

In contrast to the main metabolic pathway enzymes, the activities of those enzymes involved in the synthesis of the specific extracellular matrix components show a marked increase in the cells of DD tissue, as could be demonstrated in a study on the incorporation rates of marked precursors of glycosaminoglycan and collagen synthesis in isolated cells in vitro (Delbrück & Schröder 1982; Fig. 5.3). It must be assumed that there has been a modulation of synthesis metabolism and that it has been transferred to the culture.

The findings have been similar in studies on isolated cells from other fibromatous tissues such as keloid tissue (Diegelmann et al 1977), cirrhotic liver (Galambos et al 1977) and arteriosclerotic vessel wall (Mey et al 1980). On the other hand, there are no changes in the types and amounts of lysosomal enzymes involved in the degradation of the matrix components in the cells of DD tissue as compared with healthy palmar fascia (Delbrück et al 1981). This is true for the hexosaminidases, glucuronidases and sulphatases just as it is for the collagen peptidases. No data are available on the collagenases. For fibroblasts from normal palmar fascia and DD tissue there are no differences in vitro in the activity levels of the lysosomal enzymes (Delbrück et al 1981). The differences between these findings and those of Hoopes et al (1977) are probably of a methodological nature (see above).

The site of action of these enzymes is sometimes extracellular, and intracellularly the lysosomes are only required to the extent that pieces of the extracellular matrix components are internalized. Therefore, the enzymes involved in degradation are probably subject to regulatory mechanisms which activate only a portion of the enzyme activity available from a constant pool of lysosomal total enzyme activity. In the case of cartilage, for example, it is known that interleukin I, as the mediator of cartilage degradation, acts by stimulating the release of proteinases, proteoglycanases and other lysosomal enzymes from the chondrocytes (Tyler 1985). Another possibility is that lysosomal enzymes of different origins, e.g. from macrophages or granulocytes that have migrated into the matrix, may initiate the degradation of the matrix outside the cell. Similar mechanisms need to be discussed with reference to the pathogenesis of DD; as yet, no experimental data are available to support this hypothesis.

On balance, the metabolic rates of the synthesis and degradation of the extracellular matrix components in Dupuytren's disease tissue are shifted toward synthesis. Therefore, an accumulation of both proteoglycans and collagen would be expected; in fact this does occur. In addition to this increase in collagen in DD tissue there is also an enormous increase in the collagen type III fraction, which is extremely small in the healthy palmar fascia (Menzel et al 1979; Bazin et al 1980; Gelbermann et al 1980; Brickley-Parson et al 1981).

Although a good number of detailed studies have been conducted on biochemical changes in DD, the causes of the disease are still unknown. Furthermore, the pathogenesis of the disorder is still only poorly understood. The heterogenous morphological picture of the disease at different stages (Mohr & Vosbeck 1985), which leads to a much wider range of findings than in healthy palmar fascia, is a complicating factor in the interpretation of findings obtained in biochemical studies. However, biochemical and microscopic investigations have clearly demonstrated that the onset of the pathological changes in the palmar fascia occurs before the afflicted tissue is diseased by clinical observation. The cell population in the diseased palmar fascia is not uniform. Mohr & Vosbeck (1985) differentiate between the tendinocytes, i.e. the cells of the healthy palmar fascia, and the proliferating endothelial cells and pericytes as well as the macrophages and lymphocytes that have migrated into the fascia. All types of cells found in a tissue sample can contribute in differing degrees to the metabolism of the diseased palmar fascia. Therefore, it is not surprising that in DD the composition of the proteoglycans indicated by their glycosaminoglycan patterns does not resemble any known pattern for other types of connective tissue (Fig. 5.8). The same holds for a calculated pattern of glycosaminoglycans produced by a mixed tendinocyte and pericyte population present in an assumed ratio of 1:4 (see Fig. 5.8). The most likely explanation for this aberration is atypical synthesis of matrix components caused by a modulated or uncontrolled metabolism in the cells of the DD tissue. In this case there may be a lack of differentiation of cells of the palmar fascia or of those cells which invaded the fascia from other tissue sources.

In as much as no changes of any consequence are apparent in the activity levels of the enzymes involved in the energy and intermediary metabolism in the direction of what is found in malignant tumours, from a biochemical perspective the presence of a malignant process is rather unlikely. This view is supported by the studies of Azzarone et al (1983), in which Dupuytren cells were compared with healthy skin fibroblasts and the tumour cell lines for a number of cell physiology criteria. From the criteria selected the authors found that the Dupuytren's cells were in a middle position between the healthy fibroblasts and the tumour cells. It is interesting to note that these phenomena of modulation of cell behaviour could be observed even in cells isolated from macroscopically normal fascia tissue taken from an individual with DD. The aetiology of this modulation of metabolism and of the proliferation

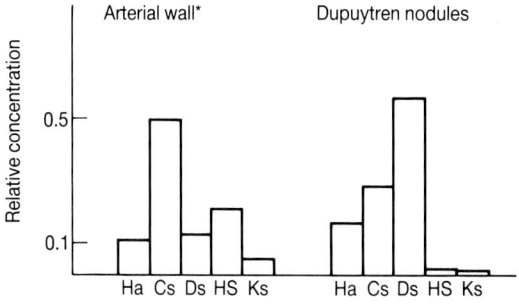

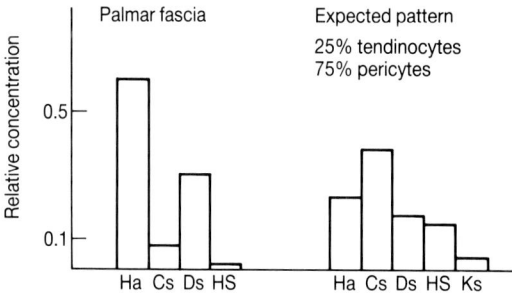

Fig. 5.8 Glycosaminoglycan patterns of arterial wall, Dupuytren's contracture (nodules) and palmar fascia in relative concentrations. Calculated pattern of a diseased palmar fascia containing 25% normal tendinocytes and 75% pericytes. H = Hyaluronate; C = chondroitin sulphate; DS = dermatan sulphate; HS = heparan sulphate; K = keratan sulphate. ★ = Stuhlsatz et al (1980).

behaviour of the cells in the diseased palmar fascia is still unclear. The explanation will probably be found on the level of the genome, the translation or the post-translational modifications of the synthesis of the matrix components. On all three levels exogenous, still unknown factors could be the precipitating factors. If there is an alteration in the genetic code or if exogenous factors affect metabolism constantly, then the modulation is perpetuated, and it can be increased through feedback mechanisms in the production of atypical matrix components. The latter also alter the characteristics of the pathway for the metabolites of the cells in DD tissue, thus contributing to the vicious circle. The result is the predominant symptom of DD — the contracture with thickening and shrinking of the palmar fascia.

In spite of marked progress, our understanding of the pathobiochemistry of DD is still limited, and this prevents a detailed characterization of the factors directly responsible for the development of the contracture. It is conceivable that in addition to the altered physical chemistry, i.e. the pathological content of the extracellular matrix, external mechanical forces or the contractile elements of atypical cells (tractofibroblasts; Tomasek et al 1986) may be involved.

A. J. Bailey

Collagen

Whatever the aetiology, the cellular biology and the overall biochemical changes, the proliferation of fibrous collagen is the major biochemical characteristic of Dupuytren's disease (DD). The excess collagen impairs normal function and also provides the disease with its clinical feature, the contracture of the fingers.

Considerable progress has been made in detailing the biochemical changes of collagen in DD but we still are not certain of the stimuli which actuate the process, or the mechanism by which the tissue contracts. In contrast to most fibrotic situations, in DD it is possible to distinguish the early and late stages of the disease. It is therefore possible to follow, at least in part, its course; from the early stages it should be possible to distinguish the stimulating factors, and hence the means to devise rational treatment. This chapter will seek to describe briefly the currently perceived role of collagen in DD.

DEPOSITION OF COLLAGEN

The lesion primarily involves the palmar fascia. In the early stages of DD discrete highly cellular nodules form, but in the later stages the characteristic feature is of dense fibrotic bands or cords in the palmar fascia. Biochemical investigations have therefore concentrated on comparing normal fascia with nodules and bands.

The nodules of DD are highly cellular, comparable to granulation tissue formed during wound healing. Amongst the collections of cell types present in the nodules are the fibroblasts, the major synthesizer of collagen. The excess collagen produced could result from an increasing fibroblast population, increased synthesis or by transformation of the fibroblasts. In the majority of fibrotic situations, it appears that a select number of fibroblasts synthesize more collagen per cell than the other fibroblasts in the tissue. Whether this is through stimulation via mediators or there is an inherent defect through transformation in these fibroblasts has not yet been established, and indeed the situation may be different in different fibrotic situations.

The disease often progresses to the irreversible deposition of thick fibrous collagen bands. Changes in the physical appearance of the fibres, their composition in terms of genetic type of collagen, changes in post-translational modification, extracellular cross-linking and changes in the organization of the tissues have been reported. An understanding of the mechanisms leading to these changes and their significance on the functional properties of the collagenous tissues requires some appreciation of the structure of collagen and details of its biosynthetic and degradative processes.

THE METABOLISM OF COLLAGEN

As a number of reviews adequately cover the genetics, structure, biosynthesis and degradation of collagen (see, for example Bailey & Etherington 1980; Piez & Reddi 1984; Fleischmajer et al 1985; Martin et al 1985 and its role in fibrosis (Evered & Whelan 1985), only the salient features of these properties in the metabolism of collagen need be outlined here.

Structure

It is now apparent that there is a large family of collagens, which are for the most part tissue-specific (Martin et al 1985). At the time of writing 12 genetically distinct types of collagen have been identified. These molecules are basically similar in that they contain three helical polypeptide chains possessing the repeating sequence $(Gly-X-Y)_n$; wound into a stable triple helix to produce a thin rod-like molecule. The genetic differences lie in the small variations in primary structure, and in the size and composition of the globular domains at the N and C termini of the molecule. In addition, each of the molecular types undergoes different degrees of post-translational modification. These variations result in dramatic differences in the self-assembly of the molecules, thus providing a wide range of supramolecular structures. The identification of these distinct collagens over the last decade has provided some of the answers to the question of the biological diversity of the simple collagen molecule. This diversity is expressed in the rope-like fibres of skin and tendon, the transparent amorphous membrane of the lens capsule and glomeruli, and the filamentous collagen surrounding some cells.

Fibrous collagens

Collagen types I, II and III are the major fibrous collagens (Fig. 6.1). Self-assembly occurs through lateral association of the molecules in a quarter-stagger and end-overlap fashion (Hulmes et al 1973, Fraser et al 1987). This relative displacement of the molecules leads to the characteristic cross-striations observed in the electron microscope (Fig. 6.1).

Type I collagen is the most abundant structural component of skin, tendon and bone, generally comprising 90% of the collagen. Type II confers the structural framework on cartilage and the intervertebral disc. Type III occurs in many tissues,

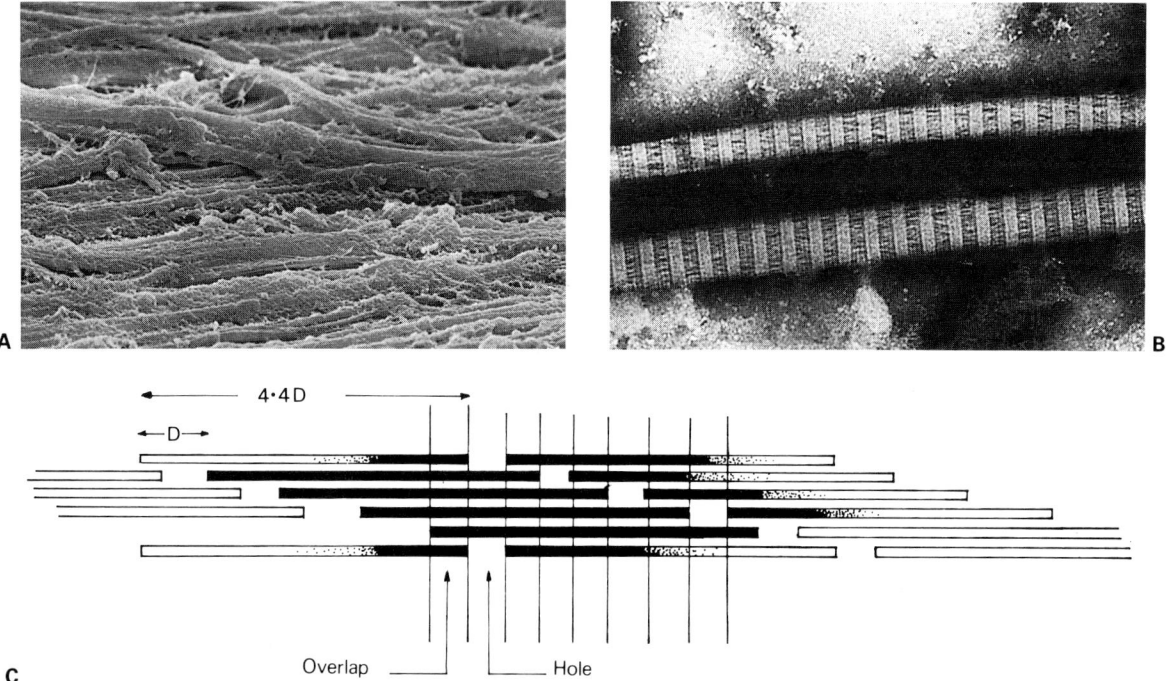

Fig. 6.1 **A** Scanning electron micrograph of fibrous collagen (magnification × 960); **B** Transmission electron micrograph of collagen fibres showing regular axial periodicity of 70 nm (magnification × 56 000); **C** Representation of the end-overlap and quarter-stagger alignment of molecules in collagen fibres responsible for the axial repeat observed in the electron microscope. The electron dense stain preferentially fills the whole region.

as a minor component in tendon (1–2%), a significant component in skin (10%) and a major component in the vascular system (40–50%). It forms fine fibres and occurs mainly in distensible tissues, although its function in relation to the other collagens has not been established. Similarly, type V collagen is a minor component (5–10%) and forms fine fibres in many tissues. The typical striations are not observed. The proportion of type V is generally higher in embryonic tissue. Like type III, the functional role of type V has not been identified.

Non-fibrous collagens

Type IV collagen provides the structural framework of the non-fibrous basement membranes which act as an underlying support for epithelial and endothelial cells, a protective sheath for myofibrils and the filtration membrane of the glomeruli. The type IV molecule possesses a longer triple helix than types I–III and, following secretion, the terminal globular domains are retained. This, together with differences in the primary sequence of the helix, causes a unique charge profile and a more flexible rod-like molecule which results in the self-assembly of an open network rather than the laterally associated fibril (Timpl et al 1981). The type IV molecules aggregate via their N-terminal ends in an anti-parallel fashion, and the tetramer formed acts as the unit 'monomer' to produce an open network

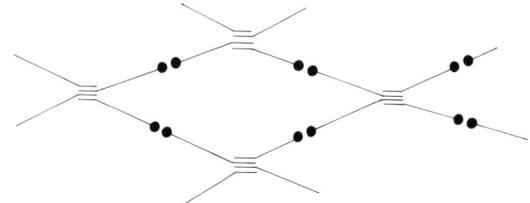

Fig. 6.2 Proposed 'chicken wire' net for the organization of type IV collagen molecules in basement membrane. The N-terminal regions are aligned in an anti-parallel fashion and the 'tetramers' so formed are organized into a network by the linking of the globular C-terminal regions.

through interaction of the C-terminal globular domains (Fig. 6.2). Our own recent evidence suggests that there may be some lateral aggregation of the type IV molecules, at least in lens capsule basement membrane (Barnard et al 1987a).

Filamentous collagens

Types VI and IX form loose assemblies of microfibrils rather than a tightly packed striated fibre (Fig. 6.3). Type IX appears to be associated with cartilagenous tissues (Duance et al 1982), whilst type VI seems to have a wide distribution (Hessle & Engvall 1984). It has been identified in cornea, skin and tendon, but its functional role has not been established. The type VI molecule is small — 100 nm compared to the fibrous (300 nm) and non-fibrous collagen (400 nm) — but

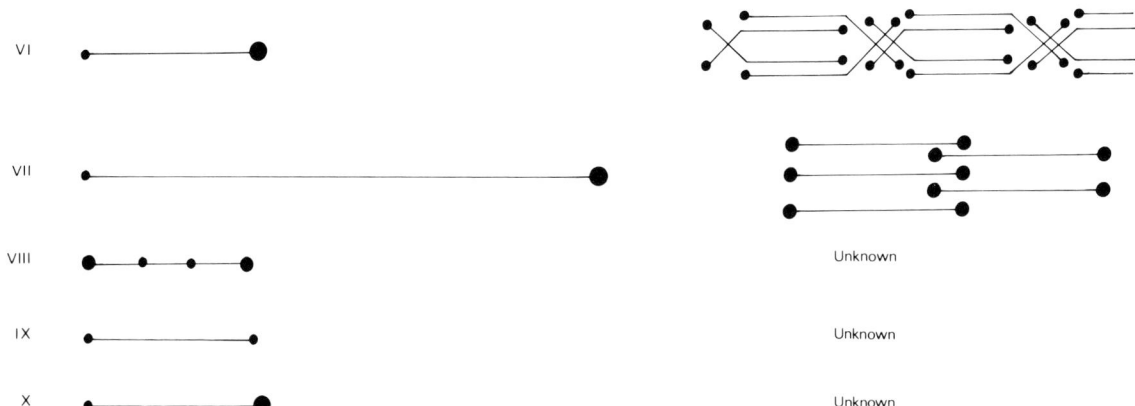

Fig. 6.3 Left: Diagrammatic comparison of the molecular length of the minor collagens types VI–X. Circles represent the globular regions at the ends of the triple helix. **Right:** The proposed macromolecular structures for types VI and VII.

self-assembles to a fibril by a complex series of anti-parallel and parallel interactions (Engel et al 1985 see; Fig. 6.3).

Biosynthesis

Collagen is synthesized as polypeptide chains by the same mechanism of mRNA and ribosomes as other proteins. The major difference is the number of post-translational modifications that take place in the nascent polypeptide chains (for reviews, see Bailey & Etherington 1980, Kivirikko & Myllylä 1984). These modifications require a complex series of enzymes and cofactors (Fig. 6.4). The prolyl residues in the Y position of the repeating sequence $(Gly-X-Y)_n$ are converted to hydroxyproline by prolyl hydroxylase; some of the lysine residues in the Y position are converted to hydroxylysine by lysyl hydroxylase; the hydroxylysine residues are 0-glycosylated with galactose or glucosyl-galactose by the relevant hexosyl transferases; a mannose-rich oligosaccharide is added to the carboxy terminal globular region by other transferases. Assembly of the triple helix is initiated by registration of the C-terminal globular region. The helical procollagen molecule is secreted from the cell and then undergoes further processing. The N- and C-terminal propeptides are, when necessary, selectively removed by N- and C-peptidases. In the case of the fibrous collagens this then permits self-assembly of the molecules in fibres. In contrast, the propeptides are retained in type IV and the molecules self-assemble in the extracellular milieu to form the network structure. These supramolecular structures are then stabilized by modification of specific lysine residues by lysyl oxidase which then spontaneously form intermolecular cross-links. Without the formation of covalent intermolecular cross-links, none of the collagenous assemblies described can function as a structural framework for body tissues.

Cross-linking

The cross-linking enzyme acts on the fibrillar form of collagen binding to a specific region of the triple helix, the sequence Hyl-Gly-His-Arg, and oxidizes a lysine or hydroxylysine in the vestigial propeptide region at the N and C termini. The lysyl-aldehyde produced then reacts with the Hyl in the enzyme-binding site sequence (Bailey et al 1974; Eyre et al 1984). This reaction results in a covalent intermolecular cross-link of the aldimine bond type (Fig. 6.5). If the residue in the N- or C-terminal telopeptide region is hydroxylysine then hydroxylysine aldehyde reacts with the hydroxylysine to form an oxo-imine bond (Fig. 6.5). The relative proportion of these two cross-links varies with the tissue and with age. The aldimine is the predominant cross-link in skin collagen, and the oxo-imine in cartilage and bone, whilst Achilles tendon contains equal proportions of both cross-links.

During maturation of the tissue these cross-links are believed to be transformed into stable multivalent cross-links (Bailey et al 1980; Light & Bailey 1980). The stabilization of collagen through the formation of intermolecular cross-links appears to be a two-stage process. Initially cross-linking occurs through head-to-tail cross-linking of the end-overlap region, i.e. at 4D stagger, to form longitudinal cross-linked filaments (see Fig. 6.5). In the second stage these intermediate divalent cross-links react with cross-links in other filaments, i.e. with molecules in register at 0D stagger, to form transverse multivalent cross-links (Light & Bailey 1980). These longitudinal and transverse cross-links build up a three-dimensional network of cross-links (Fig. 6.6), and can therefore account for the increasing tensile strength of collagen as the tissue ages.

The nature of these multivalent cross-links has not been completely established. One trivalent compound, 3-hydroxy-pyridinoline (Fujimoto et al 1977), has been identified and a derivation from two oxo-imine cross-links has been proposed (Eyre & Oguchi 1980). The location of this cross-link has not been confirmed. An alternative cross-link, hydroxyaldolhistidine (Housley et al 1975) has been proposed as the mature cross-link of tissues that do not possess the precursor oxo-imine cross-link, for example, skin. More recently, the structure of this cross-link has been reassessed (Yamauchi et al 1987). On the other hand, one as yet uncharacterized mature cross-link has been identified in all mature tissues (Barnard et al 1987b). Confirmation of this compound as a cross-

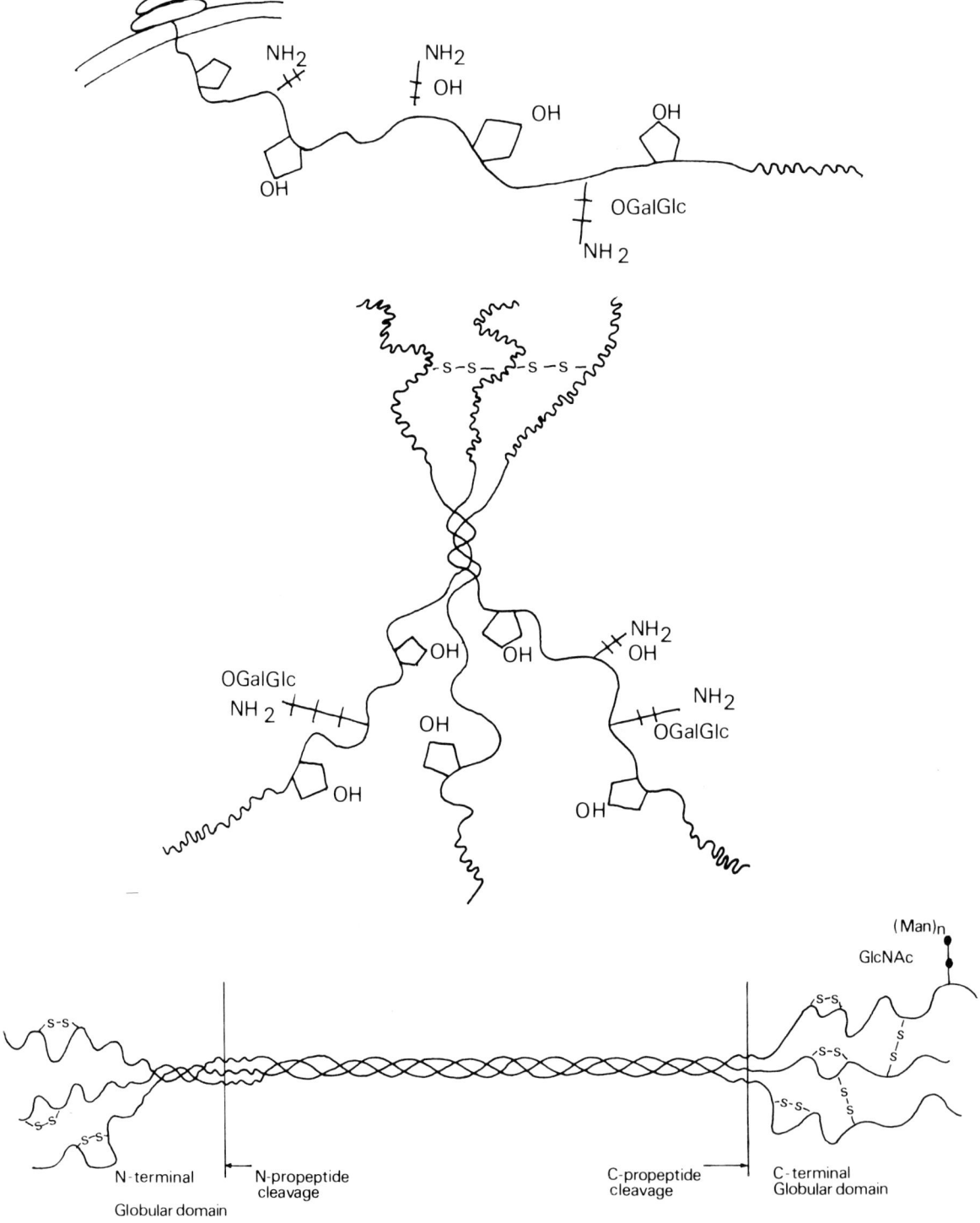

Fig. 6.4 Diagrammatic representation of the synthesis of procollagen (**top**) on the ribosome; (**middle**) during triple helix formation following aggregation of the C-terminal propeptides and (**bottom**) the procollagen molecule possessing a stable triple helix and globular domains at the N- and C-termini.

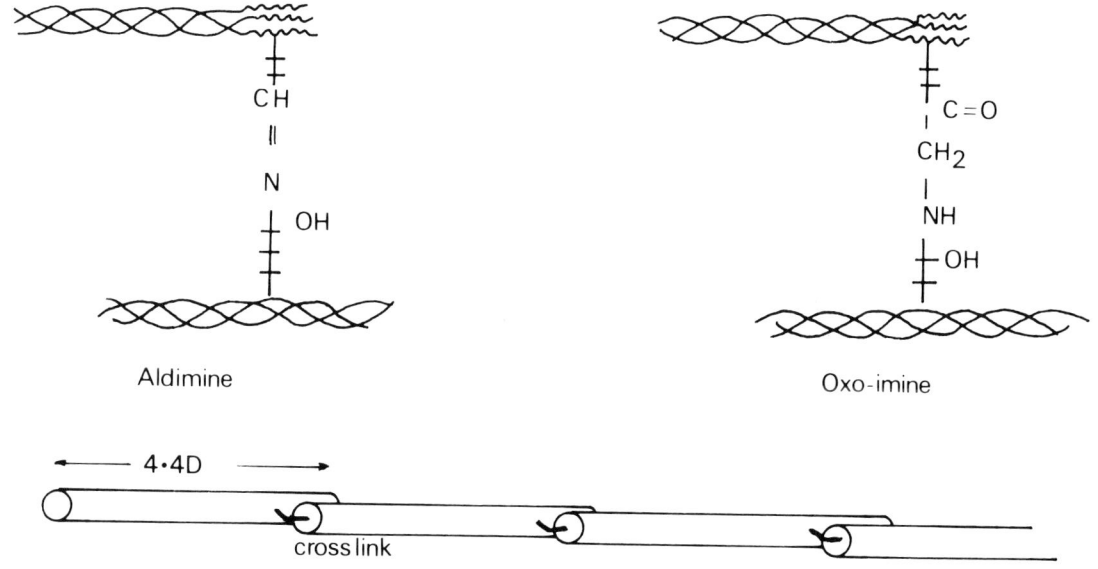

Fig. 6.5 Initial cross-linking of collagen molecules. The structure of the two major cross-links, the labile aldimine and the stable oxo-imine, is shown. The head-to-tail location, including the end-overlap of these cross-links in the microfibril, is also depicted.

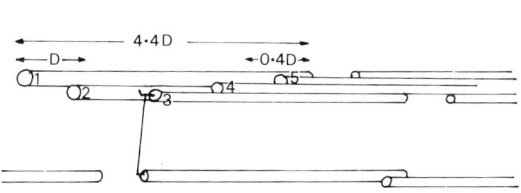

Fig. 6.6 The mature cross-linking of collagen fibres. The diagram illustrates the further reaction of the head-to-tail lateral cross-links within a microfibril to form interfibrillar transverse cross-links. These mature cross-links would form a three-dimensional network, thereby stabilizing the collagen fibre and providing the structure with a high mechanical strength.

link would suggest that there is a common mechanism for the maturation of collagen rather than different mature cross-links for different tissues.

Despite the unique network organization of type IV collagen in basement membranes, the molecules are intermolecularly cross-linked by the same mechanism (Bailey et al 1984). The divalent oxo-imine cross-link has been identified and localized in the N-terminal assembly of the tetramers. Although this cross-link must be present in cross-linking of the tetramers to form the larger network structure, its location has not been established but clearly must involve interaction of the C-terminal region. Basement membrane collagen also matures in the same way as the fibrillar collagen. However, analysis failed to reveal the presence of pyridinoline or hydroxyaldolhistidine. The unknown compound M was, however, found to be present (Barnard et al 1987b). To achieve the same maturation reaction through reaction of the divalent cross-links or their precursors necessitates the molecules of the network structure to be in register. This can be achieved if the type IV networks are overlaid in sheets.

The nature of the cross-links affects the properties of the collagen fibre by providing it with tensile strength. Although the two intermediate divalent cross-links present in mature tissue are chemically different, the physiological difference in terms of function, if any, has not been established. Certainly the oxo-imine bond is chemically more stable than the aldimine bond and this may be reflected in mechanical properties. For example, tissues under stress may contain a higher proportion of the stable oxo-imine cross-link. In this context we have noted that the extensor tendon and the flexor tendon of the rabbit foot are cross-linked by the oxo-imine and the aldimine bonds respectively (Bailey, unpublished observations).

The presence of these cross-links affects the extractability of the collagen. Tissues containing the aldimine, e.g. skin, are readily extracted in dilute acidic solution, whilst those containing the oxo-imine, e.g. bone, are insoluble. As the tissue matures all the cross-links are stable and the collagen is virtually insoluble under these conditions, and can only be solubilized by degradative methods. These age-related changes in the collagen ensure that collagen is resistant to endogenous proteolytic enzymes, less susceptible to changes in pH and ionic concentrations, and that through the three-dimensional network of intermolecular cross-links it acquires its optimal functioning capacity.

Degradation

The degradation of collagen involves a complex and highly orchestrated series of enzymes (Murphy & Reynolds 1985). The connective tissue cells secrete a group of proteinases that are capable of acting on collagen under physiological conditions. A specific metallo-endopeptidase, generally referred to as mammalian collagenase, has been shown to cleave the three polypeptide chains of collagen at a single site along the helix (Woolley & Evanson 1980). These fragments of the helix are unstable at body temperature, hence are rapidly denatured, in which state they are then digested by many proteolytic enzymes (Fig. 6.7). The enzyme is synthesized as an active zymogen, and activation of the procollagenase is achieved by enzymes such as trypsin and plasmin.

The mammalian collagenase acts on mature fibrous collagen but release of the fragments is inhibited by the intermolecular cross-links. Release of these fragments can be achieved by the neutral cysteine or serine proteases (Burleigh 1977), by acting on the non-triple helical telopeptide ends of the molecule. Cleavage of peptide bonds on the helix side of the cross-links effectively depolymerizes the fibre (see Fig. 6.7).

Both types of enzyme are necessary for degradation of the fibre but the relative importance of each has not yet been established. The fragments are phagocytosed and degraded intracellularly by the lysosomal system of enzymes, primarily the cathepsins (Etherington 1980).

Metabolism

The biosynthesis and degradation has been shown to be a complex series of enzymic and non-enzymic reactions, the basic essentials of which are now understood. The rates of metabolism of collagens are less well known and collagen is generally thought to be metabolically inert. As a generalization, there is a high rate of turnover during early growth but this falls to a low level at maturity (Kivirikko 1970). The level of turnover in mature animals varies considerably with the particular tissue. In the majority of tissues — for instance, skin and tendon — the turnover is slow to non-existent whilst there is a slow but significant turnover in bone. In contrast some tissue, e.g. periodontal ligament, turns over in 2–3 days and therefore never matures (Sodek 1976).

STRUCTURAL CHANGES IN THE COLLAGENOUS TISSUE

Histological changes in DD have been well described in the literature (Larson et al 1960; Hueston 1963; Millesi 1966, 1974; Tubiana 1967), revealing two components — initially a highly cellular nodule and finally a virtually acellular fibrous cord. The nodules are characterized by a network of thin collagen fibres (reticulin) and proteoglycans staining metachromatically with toluidine blue. The collagen of the fibrous bands takes up the typical collagen stains, but the silver staining for reticulin is confined to fine fibres in the centre of

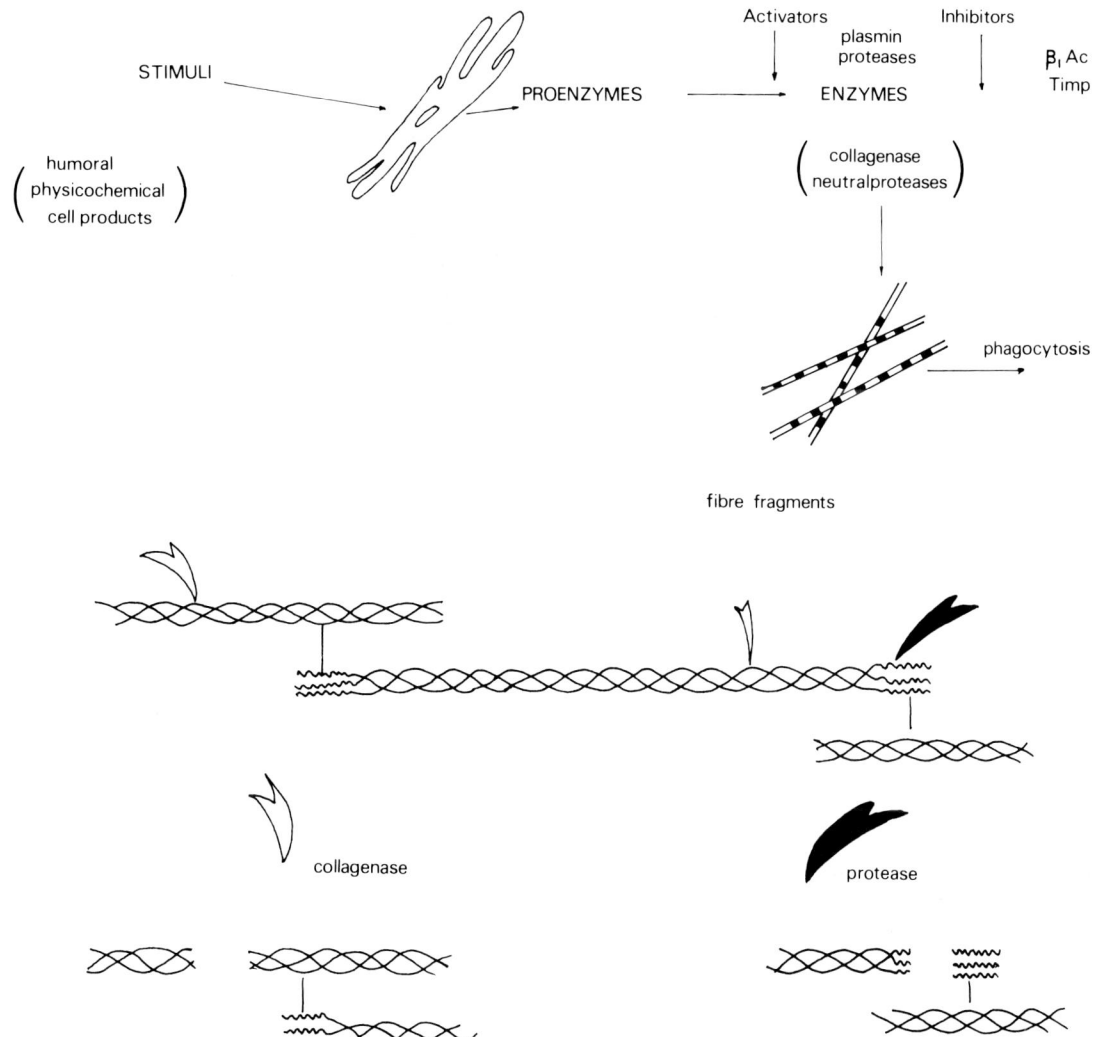

Fig. 6.7 Proposed degradative pathway of collagen fibres. **Top:** Cells are stimulated to synthesize proenzymes (procollagenase and other proteinases) which are then activated to digest intact collagen fibres. Control is believed to be exercised by the presence in the tissue of inhibitors (Timp). **Bottom:** The mechanism of two types of proteinase is illustrated. Collagenase acts at a highly specific location within the triple helix, whilst the other neutral proteinases act on the non-triple helical N- and C-terminal domains.

the band. Like the normal aponeurosis, metachromatic staining of the bands is minimal. The fibres are more highly oriented in a preferred direction in the band compared to the normal aponeurosis. At intermediate stages the collagen fibres appear to be degraded whilst others fuse together to form thicker fibres, and it would appear that the bundle structure breaks down. The elastic fibres are no longer evenly distributed but are reduced in number and located in the periphery of the fibre bundles. The sub-aponeurotic fat usually remains free of fibrotic infiltration.

Examination of the organization of the fibre bundles by the scanning electron microscope has revealed significant changes (Hunter & Ogdon 1975; Legge et al 1981). The normal parts of the palmar fascia consist of flat interweaving fibres.

Nodules are characterized by a meshwork of fine fibrils which appeared to be incompletely formed. In the bands the fibres are more compact and tended to be oriented in a specific direction. The fibres possess a wavy appearance indistinguishable from normal tendon. Legge et al (1981) also observed tighter bundles which had a shorter wave pattern than the normal fibres. The waves were frequently seen in the form of a helix that was never observed in normal tissue.

In cells in the proliferative stage, Gokel & Hübner (1977) observed intracellular structures surrounded by trilaminar membranes continuous with the endoplasmic reticulum containing banded structures with a periodicity of about 100 nm. These workers concluded the material was intracellular 'fibrous long-spacing' (FLS) collagen, based on comparison with in vitro reprecipitated FLS collagen fibres, but subsequent studies indicate that these FLS fibres were probably type VI collagen.

At high magnification using transmission electron microscopy the individual collagen fibres were seen to possess the normal structure and typical axial banding pattern of 67 nm. Similarly, analysis of the fibres by X-ray diffraction, both wide and low angle, showed no detectable difference between the normal tissue and that from DD patients (Brickley-Parsons et al 1981). It appears from these results that the structure of the individual collagen fibres in DD is indistinguishable from normal collagen fibres. However, at a higher level of order the histological evidence suggests that the structure of the fibre bundles appears to have broken down.

BIOCHEMICAL CHANGES IN THE COLLAGENOUS TISSUE

Recent studies in DD have attempted to identify and separate for analysis at least three regions of the aponeurosis:

1. The highly cellular nodules.
2. The fibrous bands.
3. The apparently unaffected regions, in terms of macroscopic appearance.

There is a progressive increase in the proportion of collagen in the aponeurosis from the control at about 60%, to the bands at about 90% and even higher in the nodules (Bazin et al 1980; Brinkley-Parsons et al 1981; Hamamoto et al 1982). The water content of this collagen increased from 55% in the controls to 62% in the nodules. The proportion of neutral salt-soluble and acid-soluble collagen was very small, about 0.2%, from the diseased tissue compared to virtually nothing from the control. Similarly, the amount of collagen digestible by pepsin treatment increased from 80% in the controls to almost complete solubilization for the diseased tissue. The latter tissues were also solubilized more rapidly by the pepsin than were the controls, as would be expected for immature collagen.

Amino acid compositional analysis of the collagen extracted revealed a higher level of hydroxylation, increasing from 5 to 13 residues of hydroxylysine per 1000 residues (Brickley-Parsons et al 1981). This increase was accompanied by a parallel increase in the number of glycosylated hydroxylysines so that the relative proportion of glycosylated hydroxylysine remained constant. However, it has not been established whether the increased glycosylation occurs predominantly in the type I or type III collagen.

All these changes in chemical and physical properties are consistent with the presence of increased quantities of newly synthesized collagen in the diseased tissue. Similar changes occur in the granulation tissue of healing wounds. Unfortunately no studies have been carried out on the time-related changes analogous to those in the healing wound.

Collagen types

The major collagen of normal aponeurosis is type I, although using the sensitive immunofluorescence technique (Fig. 6.8) it is possible to detect a small amount of type III collagen (Bazin et al 1980). This is similar to the situation in normal tendon where the type III can be located in the endotendinium surrounding the bundles of collagen fibres within the tendon (Duance et al 1977). This hierarchy of fascicles bound together by a collagenous sheath is presumably a requirement for mechanical integrity and normal function of

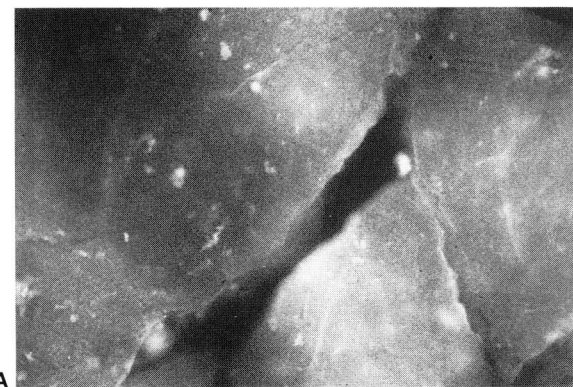

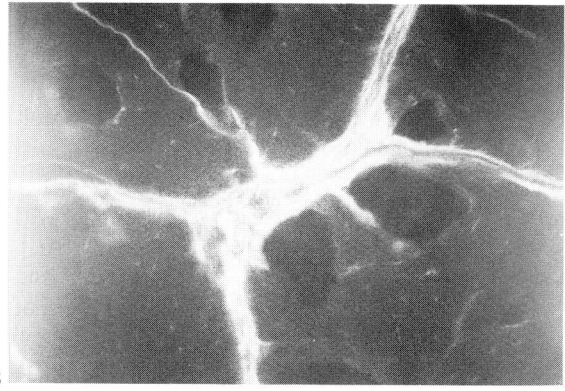

Fig. 6.8 Immunofluorescence location of type I and type III collagen in tendon fibres. **A** Overall staining of fascicles by type I collagen antibody; **B** Preferential staining of endotendinium by anti-type III collagen

Table 6.1 Analysis of normal and Dupuytren's aponeurosis

	Total Collagen (%)	Solubility (%)		Type III (%)	Type V (%)
		Acid	Pepsin		
Normal aponeurosis	65	0	80	<5	<2
Dupuytren nodules	100	0.2	97	30–40	10
Dupuytren bands	90	0.3	95	20–30	
Apparently unaffected Dupuytren	70	0	90	10–15	

tendons. Immunofluorescence studies also indicate the presence of types IV and V as part of the endotendinium sheath (Duance et al 1977) but these have not been confirmed biochemically. The presence of type IV and V in the interfascicular connective tissue has not been described, but is probably analogous to the endotendinium.

Using either pepsin digestion, which in this case solubilized over 90% of the collagen and therefore gave a representative sample (Bailey et al 1977; Bazin et al 1980; Gelberman et al 1980), or the complete dissolution of the sample by cyanogen bromide in formic acid (Brickley-Parsons et al 1981), similar results were obtained for ratios of types I to III (Table 6.1). Basically there was an increase from 1–2% type III in the normal aponeurosis to 10–15% in the apparently uninvolved, 10–20% in the nodules, and 30–40% in the fibrous bands (Fig. 6.9). The more accurate technique of cyanogen bromide peptide mapping indicated the nodule possessed a higher (28%) type III content than the bands (25%). These small differences between the bands and nodules may be due to differences in experimental techniques or in the duration of the disease in the tissue from which samples were taken.

These changes in collagen type are analogous to those occurring in the granulation tissue of dermal wounds (Bailey et al 1975a) and in hypertrophic scars (Bailey et al 1975b). As in the case of physicochemical properties, the time-related changes in the ratio of types I:III have not been investigated. One would expect a greater amount of type III in the nodules where there is a rapid proliferation of collagen and decreasing amounts in the bands as they mature if the Dupuytren's contracture follows the pattern of normal wounds and fibrotic lesions. On the other hand, a high type III would be retained over a long time period if the bands followed a similar course to the hypertrophic scar.

Other collagen types have been detected, as in granulation tissue, but in much smaller amounts. Type V collagen has been reported to be increased (Ehrlich et al 1982) and this may be associated with increased vascularity since it is a component of basal lamina; type IV of the capillary basement membrane has not been studied. The relative proportions of both type I trimer and type V were found to double from 2 to 5% and from 5 to 9% respectively and these increases are again similar to those found in hypertrophic scars (Ehrlich et al 1982).

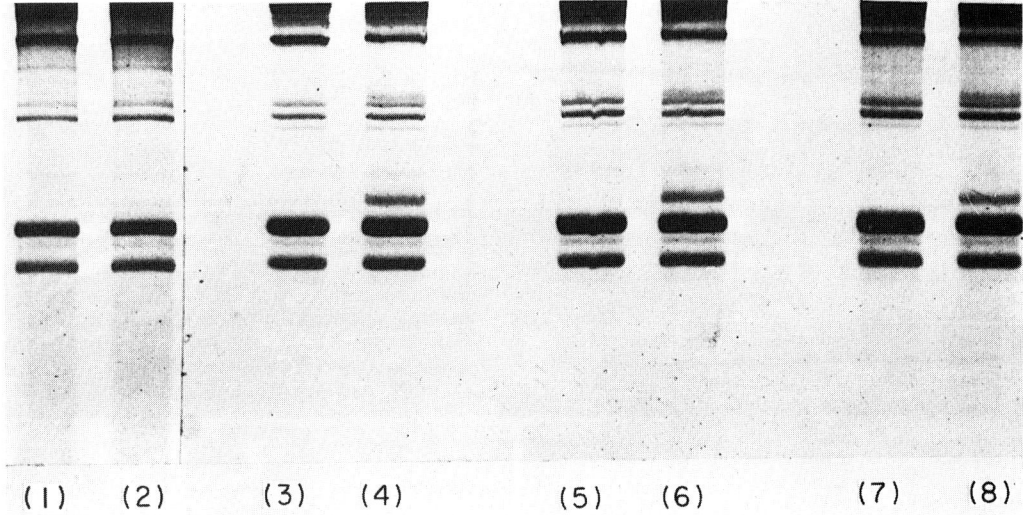

Fig. 6.9 SDS gel electrophoresis of pepsin-solubilized collagen from the aponeurosis of normal and Dupuytren's subjects. 1 and 2: normal type I collagen without and with mercaptoethanol; 3 and 4: collagen from the nodules; 5 and 6: collagen from the bands; 7 and 8: collagen from the apparently uninvolved aponeurosis. Tracks 3, 5 and 7 show the presence of type I collagen, and tracks 4, 5 and 8 type I and type III after treatment with mercaptoethanol.

Recently type VI collagen has been identified in a number of tissues (Hessle & Engvall 1984). This unusual collagen is not detected in normal tendon but can be readily observed in the electron microscope following in vitro incubation (Bruns et al 1986). Similarly, examination of the fibrotic bands in the aponeurosis of DD reveals the 100 nm banded filaments of type VI collagen (unpublished results). These fibres are probably the 'fibrous long spacing' with a banding periodicity of 100 nm, previously reported by Gokel & Hübner (1977). The suggestion is supported by the immunohistochemical studies on DD tissue using antibodies to type VI collagen (Bailey et al, unpublished results).

Cross-linking

Distinct differences in the cross-link pattern were reported by Bailey and co-workers (Bailey et al 1977; Bazin et al 1980) and have been confirmed by others (Gelberman et al 1980; Brickley-Parsons et al 1981; Hanyu et al 1984). The control tissue, as expected from previous studies of mature tissue, revealed the hexosyl-lysines as the major reducible components; the divalent reducible cross-links were barely detectable. In contrast, the major reducible components of the nodules and the bands were the two reducible cross-links dehydro-dihydroxylysinonorleucine and dehydrohydroxylysinonorleucine (Fig. 6.10). The reported increased levels of lysyl oxidase (Hamamoto et al 1982) is consistent with the high levels of these reducible cross-links. Surprisingly, the apparently unaffected parts of the aponeurosis also showed increased amounts of the reducible cross-links although a significant level of hexosyl-lysines was still present. It should be remembered that the hexosyl-lysines are not cross-links, but may be considered a good indicator of maturity (Robins & Bailey 1972).

As discussed earlier, the reducible cross-links are only present in immature, and the hexosyl-lysine in mature tissue. The gradual change of pattern shown by the different parts of the diseased aponeurosis indicates an increasing activity of the cells in synthesizing collagen. The apparently unaffected aponeurosis shows clear signs of some newly synthesized collagen, whilst the highly active nodules contain completely new collagen. The bands are mainly newly synthesized collagen, but contain some mature features similar to the control, clearly indicating that some maturation of the tissue has occurred. Surprisingly, Hanyu et al

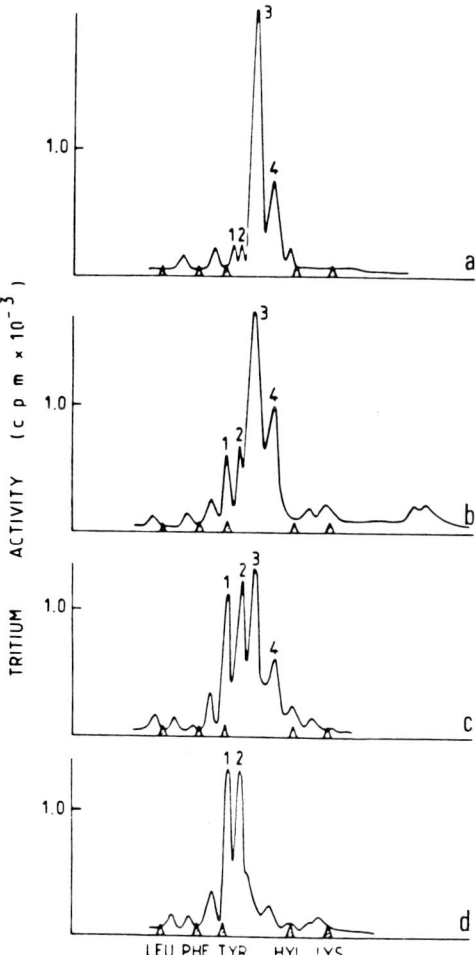

Fig. 6.10 Chromatographic profiles of the reducible cross-links present in control and Dupuytren aponeurosis. a nodules; b bands; c apparently uninvolved; d control. Peaks 1 and 2 represent hexosyl-lysines, 3 dihydroxylysinonorleucine, and 4 hydroxylysinonorleucine.

(1984) reported equal amounts of pyridinoline in the normal and affected aponeurosis and concluded the cross-link was not involved in the pathogenesis of the disease. The presence of the mature cross-link in the bands has not been reported. However, to be of value it would be crucial to know the physiological 'age' of the band in order to correlate this with the amount of pyridinoline and compound M.

The changes detailed above are characteristic of those occurring in hypertrophic scars (Bailey et al 1975b) which, in contrast to normal wounds, fail to mature and retain some of the characteristics of embryonic collagen. These studies indicated a continuing rapid turnover of the collagen even in hypertrophic scars that are many years old.

However, in contrast to this analogy with scar tissue, we observed that the disease is not strictly focal and limited to the nodules, but is clearly evident in the apparently unaffected parts of the aponeurosis (Bailey et al 1977; Brickley-Parsons et al 1981). This is consistent with the well accepted clinical observation that Dupuytren's disease can recur within the same aponeurosis, presumably due to the failure to eliminate the disease by excision only of the grossly affected tissue. We have suggested (Bazin et al 1980) that the disease is initiated and/or propagated by the cells migrating along the collagen bundles. The pathway would presumably be equivalent in the aponeurosis of the endotendinium. The presence of myofibroblasts in the apparently unaffected aponeurosis (Bazin et al 1980) supports the proposal, but this latter finding was not supported by Brickley-Parsons et al (1981). On the other hand, Gelberman et al (1980) have correlated recurrence of DD with those patients in whom myofibroblasts were detected.

Immunolocalization

Using the indirect immunofluorescence technique it is possible to determine the distribution of the various collagen types in tissues (von der Mark 1982). Few studies of the aponeurosis have been carried out. When stained with antibodies to type I collagen, uniform staining occurred as expected; with types III and V, however, the staining was limited to the periphery of the regularly arranged bundles (Bazin et al 1980). This can be compared to the staining of Achilles tendon where the fibre bundles of type I were surrounded by fibres of type III as a peritenon and, closer to the bundles, by a sheath of types IV and V collagen (Duance et al 1977; Fig. 6.11). A similar analysis of the diseased aponeurosis provided a different picture (Bazin et al 1980). The nodules were intensively stained with antibodies to type III and type V within the major bundles, and the bundles appeared to be dissociated into finer fibres (Fig. 6.11). Staining of the apparently unaffected areas revealed much the same picture as for the normal aponeurosis, but in some areas the staining was more intense and the distribution was similar

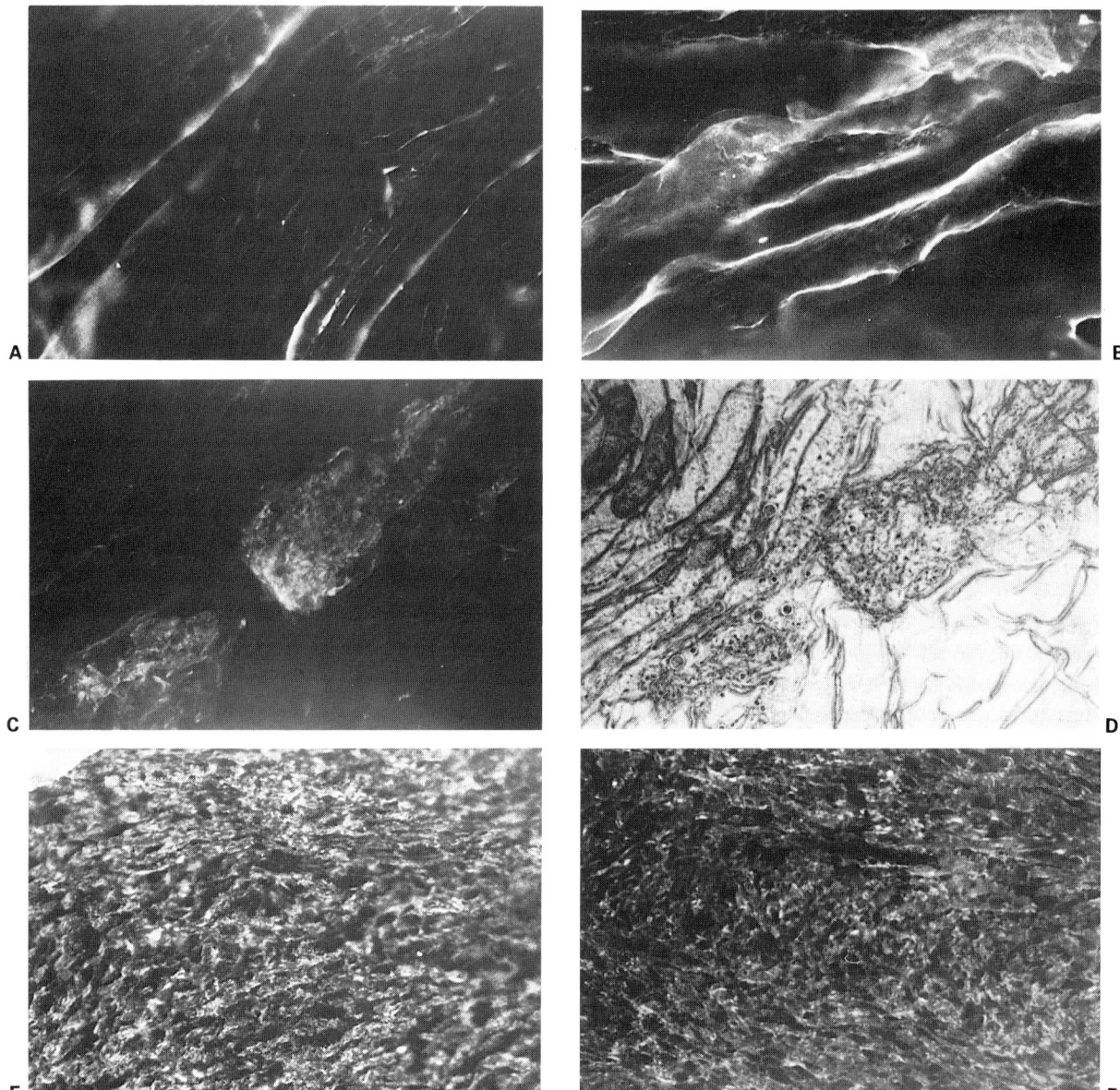

Fig. 6.11 A, Immunofluorescent staining of a longitudinal section from a normal human aponeurosis using anti-type III collagen, showing the type III collagen sheath surrounding the packed type I fibres (as in Fig. 6.8) (magnification × 160). **B,** Longitudinal sections from the apparently uninvolved region of the aponeurosis from a Dupuytren's subject demonstrating the large early increase in type III collagen (magnification × 160). **C,** Aponeurosis staining with anti-type III collagen showing the early stage of disorganization (magnification × 60). **D,** Phase contrast picture of similar field to Fig. 6.2c (magnification × 60). **E,** Late stage highly disorganized area of the aponeurosis from a Dupuytren's subject stained with anti-type I collagen (magnification × 160). **F,** Similar field to Fig. 6.2e but stained with anti-type III collagen, again demonstrating the random distribution and high proportion of type III collagen (magnification × 160).

to that in the nodules, although not as extensively dissociated into microfibrils. Unfortunately, no detailed immunohistochemical examination of the 'band' regions has been reported.

These observations certainly support the proposal that the initiating site is within the aponeurosis. However, more detailed studies on the changing location of the different collagen types using these techniques and following a time sequence in the disease would provide valuable information on the development of DD. In addition, the thin argyrophilic fibrils reported to be present by a number of workers are almost certainly type III collagen but this needs confirming both in the nodules and the bands. The presence of type V indicates vascularization but this requires confirmation using type V antibodies, since Type V may also exist as fibrils in the extracellular matrix. Similarly, the 100 nm banded fibrils seen in the electron microscope need to be confirmed as type VI using antibodies.

CONCLUSIONS

Although much has been learnt about the changes of the collagen in DD this knowledge has not as yet helped our understanding of the nature of the stimulating factors or the mechanism of contraction. Whilst the disease is initiated in the palmar connective tissues, it seems likely that these changes are not unique, but follow the same pattern as those occurring in wound granulation tissue and hypertrophic scar. However, there appears to be a significant difference in that DD does not remain localized but progresses along the tissue.

Collagen does not always respond the same way even to the same stimulus, and the nature of the tissue could alter the response. It is therefore conceivable that the collagen of DD patients is defective and responds in an abnormal way to stimuli that do not affect the majority of individuals. If indeed the collagen of DD patients is genetically abnormal, the change must be subtle since no major biochemical difference has been reported to date. A more detailed analysis of the collagen should be undertaken. Furthermore, the aberration is likely to show up as connective tissue defects in other tissues. The genetic background to DD is well known and the recent typing of patients using collagen antibodies suggests that it may be an inherited collagen disorder.

The ultimate solution to the disease may be to search for and identify the stimulating factor: an exogenous mediator or transformed cell which, based on the recurrence — albeit slow — of the disease appears to be retained in the tissue. A genetically defective collagen could produce an abnormal response to the trauma. Unfortunately, in DD fibrosis usually develops before clinical presentation and knowledge of the stimulating factor is unlikely to help clinically at this stage. However, based on our understanding of the fundamentals of the synthesis and degradation of collagen, several approaches may result in regression of the fibrosis:

1. Control of the production of mRNA at the transcriptional level. New techniques in molecular biology are becoming available to provide an understanding of collagen synthesis at the gene level. For example, dexamethasone and gamma-interferon decrease levels of type I mRNA in chick fibroblasts, and in the future it may be possible to regulate gene expression through the promoter regions of the gene.
2. Control of the post-translational modification. Specific inhibitors of prolyl hydroxylase are known to be effective in reducing synthesis. These act by sufficiently reducing the level of hydroxyproline to destabilize the triple helix at body temperature, and consequently leading to rapid degradation. Inhibition of secretion by colchicine and the use of a feedback mechanism utilizing the C-propeptide are feasible alternatives.
3. Controlled degradation of the collagen. The selective use of collagenases and neutral proteases, or in the future a genetically engineered collagenase, could be effective in removing the excess collagen.

Unfortunately, at the present time inhibiting synthesis and removing excess collagen present formidable difficulties in targeting the therapeutic agents to the specific tissues involved.

The increased understanding of the nature of collagen, its complex biosynthetic and degradative pathways, together with a more detailed biochemical analysis of the progression of the disease will surely provide not only a better explanation of the mechanism of contracture but at the same time may be an alternative treatment to surgery.

7

Collagen organization

The principal clinical deformity observed in Dupuytren's disease (DD) is a slowly progressive and irreversible flexion of the fingers as a result of decreased distance between the origin and insertion of the palmar fascia. This slowly progressive shortening of the longitudinal distance is termed a *contracture* (see Chapter 10). This term must be distinguished from the term *contraction*, which is usually used to describe the very rapid shortening of skeletal or smooth muscle cells. This rapid contraction results in the immediate shortening of the muscle cells, which in turn leads, in the case of skeletal muscle, to flexion or extension of a joint, and in the case of smooth muscle cells, to a decrease in the diameter of the lumen of an organ such as the bowel or a blood vessel. The contraction which can move a limb or diminish the diameter of the lumen of a bowel or blood vessel, occurs relatively quickly and is reversible when the muscle cells relax or when an antagonist groups of muscle cells contract. It does not produce a progressive, irreversible shortening of the muscle cells or of the surrounding connective tissues (*contracture*). However, contracture of the connective tissues about a joint can be induced experimentally by passively placing the joint in some desired position without any help from muscle contraction and fixing the joint externally or internally in the desired position for a long period of time.

The distinction between contracture and contraction is emphasized here because of reports demonstrating an abundance of cells (myofibroblasts) in the nodules of the palmar fascia of patients with DD which have the cellular components associated with cell contraction. Since these cells have the potential for contracting and shortening it is tempting directly to equate the presence of myofibroblasts and their putative contraction with palmar fascia contracture. It is important to recognize that the contraction of cells (muscle or otherwise) in a tissue is not the same as a contracture and indeed does not necessarily result in a contracture. The smooth muscle cells in the gut lumen, for example, contract and relax continuously for years in the life of the organism without any permanent contracture of the lumen occurring. Consequently, because a tissue like the palmar fascia contains cells which have the potential to contract or even those which definitely do contract, one cannot necessarily conclude that these cells produce a contracture. This point will be discussed further below.

CHANGES IN COLLAGEN STRUCTURE IN DD

There are a number of potential explanations as to just what the contracture of the palmar fascia represents physically and biologically (Brickley-Parsons et al 1981). The simplest situation that could explain the gross longitudinal shortening of the distance between the origin and insertion of the palmar fascia in DD would be one where the gross overall length of the palmar fascia is preserved, pleated or folded instead of being longitudinally stretched out (relatively) straight (Fig. 7.1). This results in significant shortening of the distance with no change in its 'running length' — external shortening. Both wide angle and low angle X-ray diffraction studies of palmar fascia in DD patients (Brickley-Parsons et al 1981) which

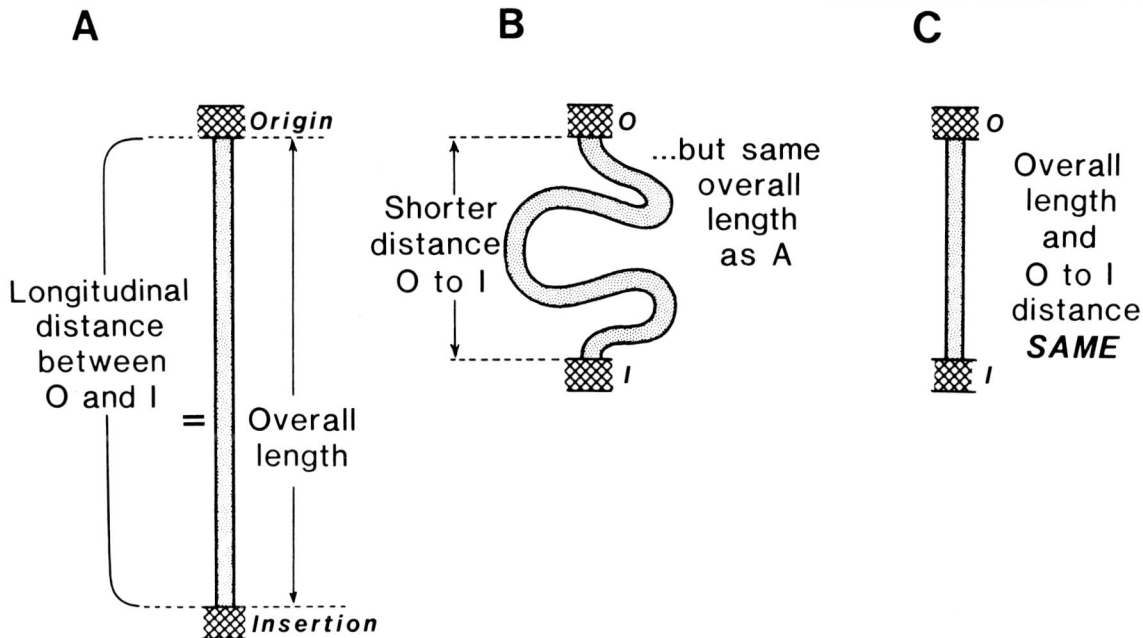

Fig. 7.1 How the palmar fascia (**A**) can be shortened; (**B**) physical folding or pleating, in which case the overall length of the palmar fascia remains the same while the longitudinal length is significantly decreased; (**C**) internal shortening where both the overall length and the longitudinal length are shortened.

are capable of detecting any change in the orientation of the collagen fibrils and fibres fail to show any evidence that the collagen has been reordered and redirected, as would have had to occur if the collagen was pleated or folded as depicted in Figure 7.1B. In other words, there is no evidence of pleating or plicating. Indeed, the longitudinal orientation and ordering of the collagen was considerably better in the DD tissue than in the normal palmar fascia (Brickley-Parsons et al 1981).

Scanning electron microscopy has also shown better alignment of the collagen fibrils in the palmar fascia of patients with DD than in patients with normal fascia, and there was no evidence of folding or plication in sufficient amount to account for significant gross longitudinal shortening of the tissue (Hunter & Ogdon 1975; Finlay & McFarlane 1981). Although there was a shorter wavelength and a helical form to the fibrils, these changes could not have accounted for the gross shortening seen in this condition.

These studies are consistent with clinical observations that there is no bunching of the palmar fascia in the palm, which would have to happen if there was shortening because the same initial length (and amount or volume) of the palmar fascia is simply folded into a space of less volume (Figs 7.1B and 7.2C).

Another possible explanation for the gross longitudinal shortening is that the collagen macromolecules, fibrils and fibres are internally shortened as a result of denaturation of the collagen (Figs 7.1C and 7.2B). Denaturation of collagen macromolecules results in the loss of the triple helical configuration of the alpha-chains which assume a random order, resulting in a marked shortening in their overall length without pleating or folding. This macromolecular shortening, together with the concomitant disruption of the ordered macromolecular aggregation state of the collagen macromolecules in the collagen fibrils and fibres, could theoretically account for the amount of gross clinical shortening observed in DD whilst maintaining the relatively straight longitudinal character of the tissue without folding (Fig. 7.1C). However, experimental examination of the collagen in the palmar fascia of patients with DD showed no evidence of denaturation of the collagen triple helix (wide angle X-ray diffraction) or loss of the highly ordered aggregation of the

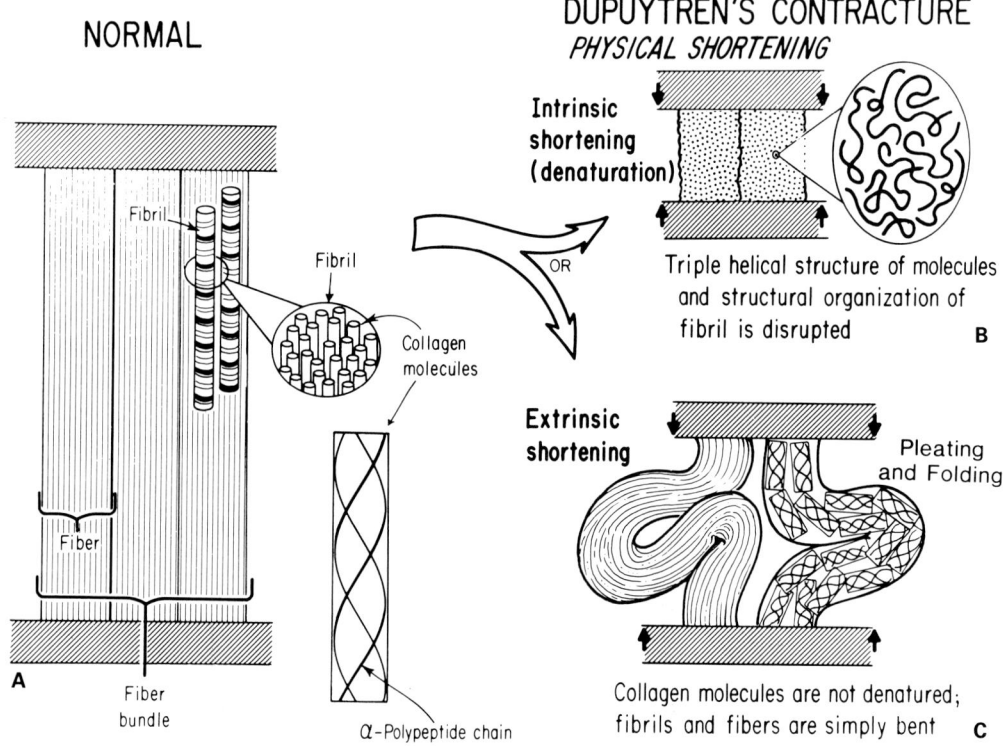

Fig. 7.2 Two possible ways that physical shortening of collagen may occur, accounting for the shortening of the palmar tissue fabric in DD by intrinsic changes within the collagen: (**B**) denaturation or (**C**) plication or folding of the fibrils, fibres, fibre bundles and higher ordered structural elements. Neither of these explanations accounts satisfactorily for the gross shortening or contracture of the palmar fascia in DD. Adapted from Brickley-Parsons et al (1981).

collagen molecules in the collagen fibril as studied by electron microscopy, low angle X-ray diffraction (approximately 70 nm axial periodicity characteristic of collagen; Brickley-Parsons et al 1981), and shrinkage temperature. Thus, neither of the two possible proposals, external or internal shortening of the collagen can account for the major clinical finding in DD the gross macroscopic shortening of the palmar fascia which is its hallmark (Jahnke 1960; Patel 1961; Dahmen 1968; Weiss et al 1976, Brickley-Parsons et al 1981; Finlay & McFarlane 1981).

CHANGES IN PALMAR FASCIA IN DUPUYTREN'S DISEASE

When tissues were sampled from patients with Dupuytren's disease they were categorized as being from specific regions, including the nodules (most severely involved tissue), longitudinal bands (next most seriously involved), mildly involved (sometimes not obtained) and most importantly, tissues from as far from the site of involvement in the palmar fascia as it was possible to obtain, and which the surgeon felt were clinically normal (Brickley-Parsons et al 1981). Samples of this latter tissue, referred to as apparently uninvolved palmar fascia, when examined by light microscopy were consistently considered normal. Some samples, however, when examined by electron microscopy did contain myofibroblasts, fibroblasts apparently in transition, fibroblasts showing evidence of increased protein synthesis, and normal fibroblasts. Biochemical analyses and structural characteristics of collagens in DD were presented in 1975, the data being derived from the tissues of approximately 150 patients (Albin et al 1975). The results were not significantly changed when the study was extended to more than 400 patients with DD and 100 control patients (Brickley-Parsons et al 1981); this study has now been extended to encompass approximately 500 patients. Similar results have been obtained by other investigators (Bailey et al 1977; Bazin et al 1980; Gelberman et al 1980) including studies which localized the increases in the genetic type III collagen in DD discussed in detail below. These results may be summarized as follows (Bailey et al 1977; Bazin et al 1980; Gelberman et al 1980; Brickley-Parsons et al 1981).

Composition of the palmar fascia

The collagen content of the palmar fascia is considerably increased in DD compared with that of normal controls; the increase is in parallel with the degree of severity. For example, in the Dupuytren's nodules of the palmar fascia, the collagen content is raised approximately 75% or more. However, it is important to note that it is also increased 20–25% in the apparently uninvolved tissue from patients with DD. Similar but considerably smaller increases were noted in the hexosamine content of the clinically involved tissues of the palmar fascia in DD compared with normal controls. There has been a significant change in the overall composition of the palmar fascia tissues in DD compared with normal palmar fascia.

CHEMICAL COMPOSITION OF COLLAGEN IN DD

Hydroxylysine content

One of the most striking changes in the biochemical composition of the collagens of the palmar fascia in DD is the marked increase in the content of hydroxylysine; values (like the content of collagen and hexosamine) parallel the severity of the disease. For example, there is a 300% or more increase in the hydroxylysine content in the Dupuytren's nodules in the palmar fascia with correspondingly smaller increases in longitudinal bands and in the apparently uninvolved fascia. The percentage of hydroxylysine residues which are glycosylated is unchanged from the values found in normal palmar fascia — the new lysyl hydroxylated residues (hydroxylysine) do not become more glycosylated than they do in normal type I collagen. Thus, the collagens in the palmar fascia of DD do not resemble the type II collagens of cartilage which likewise contain a high concentration of hyl but, in contrast to the collagen type I in DD have a high percentage of hyl residues which are glycosylated. The maintenance of the normal percentage of the hydroxylysine residues in collagen which are glycosylated in DD is typical of newly synthesized embryonic soft tissue and bone type I collagens (Miller et al 1967; Barnes et al 1971a, 1974; Royce & Barnes 1977; Strawich & Glimcher 1983) as well as the newly synthesized soft tissue collagens in healing wounds (Barnes et al 1971b, 1974; Bailey et al 1975a) and bone defects in post-natal animals (Bailey et al 1975a, b; Miller 1976; Glimcher et al 1980). A typical analysis from a large series of patients is shown in Table 7.1.

Reducible collagen crosslinks

The total number of reducible crosslinks in the collagen of the palmar fascia of tissues of patients with DD is significantly increased approximately three fold in the nodules and 40–50% in the apparently uninvolved portions of the fascia. However, even more striking than the overall marked increase in the total number of reducible crosslinks (Table 7.2; Brickley-Parsons et al 1981) is the finding that there is a complete reversal in the biochemical nature of the major reducible aldimine intermolecular cross-links in the palmar fascia in patients with DD compared with normal palmar fascia. Thus the predominant intermolecular reducible cross-link of normal type I collagen in human palmar fascia is hydroxylysinonorleucine. There is none or at best a trace of the cross-link hydroxylysinohydroxynorleucine in normal adult type I collagen. In contrast to the normal palmar fascia, the major reducible aldimine cross-links of the palmar fascia in DD is hydroxylysinohydroxynorleucine (Fig. 7.3; Table 7.3; Brickley-Parsons et al 1981). The cross-link profile shown in Figure 7.3 and the data from Table 7.3 make it clear that while the concentration of hydroxylysinonorleucine of the collagen remains relatively constant in various degrees of

76 DUPUYTREN'S DISEASE

Table 7.1 Hydroxylysine and glycosylated hydroxylysine Contents in normal and Dupuytren's fascia

Fascia	Hydroxylysine residues 100 hydroxyproline residues	Glycosylated hydroxylysine residues (%)	Glucosylgalactosyl hydroxylysine galactosylhydroxylysin ratio
Normal	5.3 ± 0.7	34.9 ± 1.7	1.53
Dupuytren's disease			
Apparently uninvolved	8.3 ± 1.1 (155)	34.6 ± 1.3 (42)	1.55
Mildly involved	10.3 ± 1.8 (200)	35.4 ± 1.9 (81)	1.57
Longitudinal bands	11.5 ± 1.7 (137)	34.8 ± 1.4 (80)	1.54
Nodules	13.9 ± 1.5 (107)	35.5 ± 1.8 (64)	1.55

Mean ± standard deviation; number of samples tested is in parentheses. From Brickley-Parsons et al (1981).

Table 7.2 Relative contents of reducible intermolecular cross-links in collagen after reduction with tritiated sodium borohydride

Fascia	Total of reducible intermolecular cross-links (cpm/mg)
Normal	575 ± 104
Dupuytren's disease	
Apparently uninvolved	810 ± 115
Mildly involved	945 ± 85
Longitudinal bands	1172 ± 106
Nodules	1588 ± 105

Mean ± standard deviation of 75 samples. Values expressed as counts per minute per milligram of hydroxyproline recovered in hydroxylysinohydroxyorleucine, hydroxylysinonorleucine, and hydroxymerodesmosine.

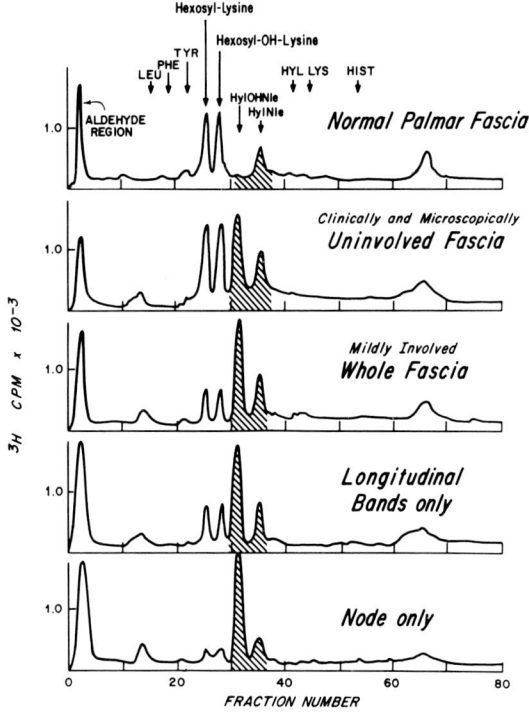

Fig. 7.3 Typical chromatographic profiles of reducible cross-links from normal palmar fascia and from palmar fascia of patients with Dupuytren's disease. Note the virtual absence of hydroxylysinohydroxynorleucine in the normal palmar fascia and its presence as the major reducible intermolecular cross-link in the palmar fascia of patients with DD including the tissue that was considered grossly and histologically normal. Adapted from Brickley-Parsons et al (1981).

severity the amount of hydroxylysinohydroxynorleucine in the collagen of the palmar fascia in DD rises from zero to such a concentration that it becomes the major intermolecular reducible aldimine cross-link. As with the other changes in the collagen of the palmar fascia in DD the absolute amount of this cross-link increases with the severity of the disease.

In contrast to the increase in the intermolecular aldimine cross-link hydroxylysinohydroxynorleucine, there is a decrease in the concentration of hexosylysine and hexosylhydroxylysine in the palmar fascia of DD. Similar findings with reference

Table 7.3 Reducible cross-link in collagen after reduction with tritiated sodium borohydride II

Fascia	No. of samples	Hydroxylysino-hydroxynorleucine	Hydroxylysino-norleucine	Hydroxymero-demosine	Hydroxylysino-hydroxynorleucine hydroxylysino-norleucine ratio
Normal	36	0	28.0 ± 1.6	72.0 ± 3.5	
Dupuytren's disease					
Apparently uninvolved	44	33.1 ± 1.8	22.1 ± 1.3	44.7 ± 3.3	1.5
Mildly involved	83	41.8 ± 1.6	24.5 ± 1.5	33.6 ± 3.9	1.7
Longitudinal bands	87	44.0 ± 1.5	21.2 ± 1.7	34.7 ± 3.1	2.1
Nodules	94	64.7 ± 1.2	21.0 ± 1.5	14.0 ± 2.2	3.1

Values expressed as percentage of counts per minute per milligram of hydroxyproline recovered.

to the reducible aldimine cross-links have also been reported by others (Bazin et al 1980).

Non-reducible stable cross-links

Hanya et al (1984) have reported that they find no significant differences in the concentration of the pyrolidine non-reducible cross-links in the palmar fascia of DD compared with normal controls. More recently, we have examined the concentration of pyrolidine cross-links in the palmar fascia, skin of the palm over the diseased area, skin of the palm from control patients and skin used for palmar grafts from normal regions of the upper arm in DD patients. Insufficient numbers of patients were examined to be statistically valid, but in several DD patients there appeared to be an increase in the level of the pyrolidines in the skin of the palm over the diseased area compared with normal palmar skin. Careful histological and ultrastructural examination of the skin biopsies will be necessary to rule out the possibility that the skin samples were contaminated with affected palmar fascia, but this seems unlikely to be the whole answer, since in several instances the palmar skin samples in DD had higher concentrations of the pyrolidines than did the pure Dupuytren's palmar fascia. These findings may reflect preliminary electron microscopic observations of palmar skin from regions involved in DD which have demonstrated some cellular abnormalities in the epidermis of the skin. These data raise the question once again of whether DD first arises in, or at least involves, the palmar skin as well as the palmar fascia.

In addition to the non-reducible pyrolidine cross-links, the formations of stable non-reducible bonds by reduction of the reducible bonds has been postulated as a mechanism for the development of stable covalent cross-links from reducible cross-links. Using very large quantities of tissue and preparative amino acid chromotography (Brickley-Parsons et al 1977), the various reduced forms of the putatively in vivo reduced cross-links were searched for unsuccessfully; no reduced forms of any of the reducible cross-links were detected in the palmar fascia of patients with DD. Similar results have been obtained from other soft tissues (Brickley-Parsons et al 1977).

Collagen polymorphism (Albin et al 1975; Bazin et al 1980; Gelbernab et al 1980; Brickley-Parsons et al 1981; Parsons et al 1985)

Type I collagen is the major collagen component of most soft tissues and bone, including palmar fascia. Normal palmar fascia, however, differs from most of the other soft tissue collagens in that it contains little or no detectable type III collagen in addition to type I collagen. Recent work using large amounts of collagen has detected a small amount of type III collagen in normal palmar fascia (less than 3%; Parsons et al 1985). In any event, under ordinary circumstances and using normal size samples, no type III is detectable in normal palmar fascia.

In sharp contrast to these findings in normal palmar fascia, a considerable amount of type III collagen is found in the palmar fascia of patients with DD: approximately 30% of the collagen is type III in Dupuytren's nodules, and this value decreases with decreasing severity of the diseased tissue. Once again, 10–15% of all of the collagen in the apparently uninvolved regions of the palmar fascia consists of type III collagen.

In addition to this major alteration in the types of collagen which must be synthesized during the development and pathogenesis of the diseased tissue, Ehrlich et al (1982) have also found that the palmar fascia in DD contains a slight increase in the amounts of type V and type I trimer.

DISTRIBUTION OF ADDITIONAL RESIDUE OF HYDROXYLYSINE

Hydroxylysine is an important functional amino acid residue of collagen. For example, some of its residues participate in the reducible intermolecular aldimine cross-links and eventually in non-reducible cross-links which provide much of the mechanical properties and solubility characteristic of the collagen and also provide sites for glycosylation. In addition, recent experiments have shown that some of the lysine residues in type I collagen are phosphorylated, an event which may be important in the intracellular metabolism and processing of the collagen chains (Urushizaki & Seifter 1985). It is therefore important not only to determine how many extra lysine residues do become hydroxylated, but also where the lysine residues are located along the alpha-chains which are hydroxylated. Tables 7.4–7.6 are a summary of results presented at the meeting of the Orthopaedic Research Society in 1985 by Brickley-Parsons et al (unpublished data). As with the other chemical abnormalities (Table 7.5), the degree to which lysine is hydroxylated is, for the most part, dependent on the severity, acuteness or activity of the condition, so the collagen in the Dupuytren's nodules show the most marked changes. Once again, the apparently normal fascia from patients with DD shows significant changes from the normal.

In type III collagen obtained from the fascia of patients with DD (Table 7.6) values for the percentage of lysine residues hydroxylated are compared with similar values obtained from type III collagen from normal skin and placental

Table 7.4 Concentration of hydroxylysine of highly purified α_1 (I) and α_1 (III) chains

	Residue/1000 residues	
	α_1 (I)	α_1 (III)
Normal	7	*
Dupuytren's disease		
Apparently uninvolved tissue	10	13
Minimally involved tissue	11	15
Longitudinal bands	13	17
Nodules	14	18

*Insufficient amount available. From Brickley-Parsons et al, unpublished data.

Table 7.5 Percentage hydroxylation of lysine residues in the CNBr peptides of α_1 (I) derived from normal patients and patients with DD

CNBr Peptide	Normal	Dupuytren's disease			
		AU	MI	LB	N
CB 3	6.3	8.2	16.0	17.0	18.0
CB 7	6.8	9.8	11.0	17.0	19.0
CB 8	12.0	12	13.0	29.0	18.0

AU = Apparently uninvolved tissue; MI = minimally involved tissue; LB = longitudinal bands; N = nodules. From Brickley-Parsons et al, unpublished data.

Table 7.6 Hydroxylation of lysine residues in peptides of α_1 (III) collagen of Dupuytren's fascia (% lysine hydroxylation)

Peptide	Apparently uninvolved tissue	Minimally involved tissue	Longitudinal bands	Nodule	Skin	Placental membrane
3	33	42	55	59	29	33
4	20	23	46	47	9	22
5	36	46	54	55	9	37
6	57	63	76	75	21	60
7	64	67	65	70	70	65
8	41	44	52	54	14	27
9	31	33	39	40	23	34

Peptides 1 and 2 contained no hydroxylysine. From Brickley-Parsons et al, unpublished data.

membrane. Except for peptide 7 and possibly peptide 9, all of the CNBr peptides in every stage of DD show a higher degree of lysyl hydroxylation than the corresponding peptide derived from normal skin and placental membrane, both of which are considered to have collagens characterized by particularly high hydroxylysine concentrations.

It is interesting to note that we have observed all the same significant changes seen in the collagen of the palmar fascia of patients with DD, in the plantar fascia of patients with plantar fibrosis and in the penile fascia of patients with Peyronie's disease.

Tissue culture experiments

Palmar fascia tissues from control patients and from the four sites of palmar fascia tissues involved in DD were cultured in vitro with ^{3}H-proline in the tissue culture medium (Brickley-Parsons et al 1977, unpublished data). After incubation, the amount of ^{3}H-proline remaining in the media, the amount of ^{3}H-hydroxyproline incorporated in the tissue and the amount of hydroxyproline and ^{3}H-hydroxyproline in the tissue culture media were measured. From these data, the rate of collagen synthesis and a good indication of the rate at which collagen was resorbed were computed (Stern et al 1963; Sakamoto et al 1979). These data showed that there were very marked increases in the rate of both collagen resorption and synthesis in the tissues of patients with DD as compared with the fascial tissues from normal subjects.

In addition to the study of collagen synthesis and degradation, investigations were carried out using ^{14}C-lysine and ^{3}H-NaBH$_4$ in the tissue culture medium to determine the post-translational modifications which occurred in the formation of the cross-links found in the collagen synthesized in organ culture. In normal palmar fascial tissues, collagen, newly synthesized in tissue culture in vitro, contained no excess hydroxylysine and the major intermolecular cross-link was found to be hydroxylysinonorleucine, as it is in normal palmar fascia in vivo. In contrast, the cells in the palmar fascia from patients with DD synthesized a collagen rich in hydroxylysine and containing hydroxylsinohydroxynorleucine as its major intermolecular reducible cross-link (Brickley-Parsons

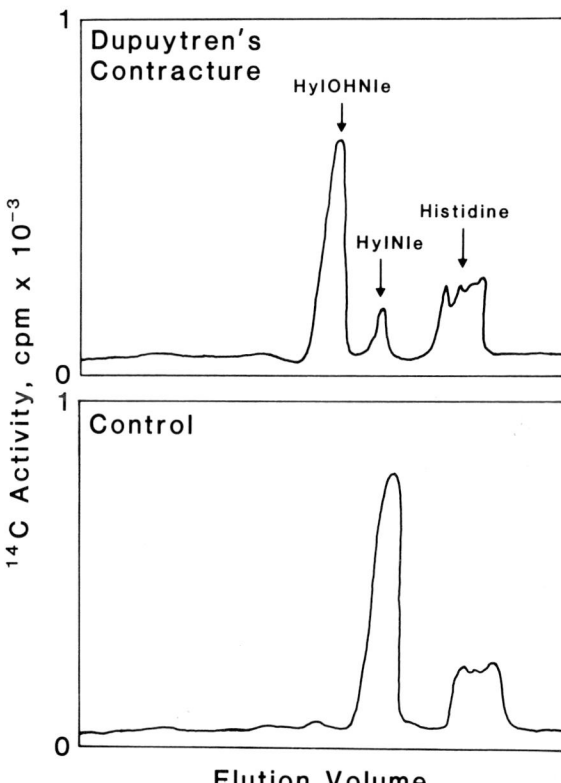

Fig. 7.4 Incorporation of ^{14}C lysine into reducible cross-links of collagen in *in vitro* tissue cultures of patients with DD (**top**) and controls (**bottom**). Adapted from Brickley-Parsons et al (1977).

et al 1977). Indeed, tissues from all four sites of the palmar fascia from patients with DD and most importantly, from tissue which was clinically and histologically normal, contained newly synthesized collagen having hydroxylysinohydroxynorleucine as essentially the only intermolecular reducible cross-link (Fig. 7.4).

BIOLOGICAL AND CLINICAL IMPLICATIONS

The changes in the biochemical characteristics of the collagen in the palmar fascia of patients with DD.

1. Increase in the content of hydroxylysine.
2. Emergence of hydroxylysinohydroxy-

norleucine, a minor reducible intermolecular cross-link in normal palmar fascia, as the major reducible intermolecular cross-link;
3. Marked increase in the amount of type III collagen of up to 25% of the total tissue collagen compared with an almost undetectable amount of type III in normal palmar fascia, and small increases in the amount of type V and type I-trimer collagens.

These are all characteristic of newly and rapidly synthesized collagen in newly synthesized collagen in embryos, of wounds and granulation tissue (Miller et al 1967; Barnes et al 1971a, 1974; Bailey et al 1975a, b, 1977; Royce & Barnes 1977; Bazin et al 1980; Strawich & Glimcher 1983) and of the collagens of healing bone tissue defects in postnatal animals (Glimcher et al 1980). However, it is important to note that in the late healing stages of wounds and healing tissue defects, and in chronic fibrosis such as occurs in cirrhosis of the liver or chronic pulmonary fibrosis, the biochemical changes in the collagen gradually return to normal or near normal.

In sharp contrast however, the biochemical changes of the collagen in DD remain significantly altered over long periods of time as measured either by site (chronic longitudinal bands) and/or with respect to the length of time the disease has been present. For example, tissues obtained from patients who have had DD for 20 years and longer still show the same biochemical lesions, although to a lesser extent. Thus, whatever the fundamental aetiological agent provoking the Dupuytren's response by the connective tissue cells (fibroblasts and possibly the myofibroblasts) which are similar to an acutely healing wound, it continues to be active for long periods after the initial episode. The synthesized collagen continues to show the same biochemical post-translational changes in vivo and in vitro. Chronic DD is biologically, cellularly and biochemically an ongoing disease with all of the characteristics of a healing and repairing injured connective tissue wound.

Another clinically important finding is that the palmar fascial tissue deliberately taken by the surgeon at the farthest distances from the clearly involved Dupuytren's tissue, and representing specimens believed to be indistinguishable clinically and later histologically from normal palmar fascial tissue, in all cases showed all the biochemical changes seen in Dupuytren's collagen. Even at the ultrastructural level (electron microscope), in a large number of cases there was no discernible pathology in the collagen or changes in the morphology of the cells. In other instances, myofibroblasts or fibroblasts in apparent transition to myofibroblasts were observed. Since the chemical changes were always present in such tissue whether or not the myofibroblasts were present, it appears that the biochemical clinical changes in the collagen occur before the fibroblasts are morphologically modified or replaced by myofibroblasts. Thus the aetiological agent of DD appears to stimulate and cause morphologically normal fibroblasts to synthesize collagen which can undergo the altered post-translational modifications of the collagen. From the surgeon's standpoint, it is clear from the biochemical studies that only in unusual cases is it possible surgically to remove anything like all of the involved palmar fascia. Thus, it seems that this is one of the major underlying reasons for the high recurrence rate reported after surgical excision of the palmar fascia in DD.

The palmar fascia in DD

What changes in the internal or external physical configurations of the collagen can account for the gross macroscopic decrease in the overall longitudinal length of the palmar fascia? We have concluded on the basis of a number of experiments already cited that it is *not*:

1. A simple folding or plication of the tissue (see Fig. 7.1B).
2. A denaturation of the collagen to gelatin resulting in the shortening of the polypeptide chains and molecules (see Fig. 7.2B; Brickley-Parsons et al 1981).

That leaves precious few rational explanations based on either external or internal shortening since even in the most active stage of the disease, the macromolecules of collagen are not denatured, and there is no disorder of the macromolecular aggregation of the fibrils (see Fig. 7.2B). We believe that the overall longitudinal length of the palmar fasica is shortened **because some of the palmar fascial tissue has been removed** — there is left a shorter piece of palmar fascial tissue which has replaced an originally longer piece and in which the normal orientation of undenatured normal collagen macromolecules, fibrils and fibres is maintained. This is accomplished by the resorption of some of the palmar fascial tissue and its replacement by newly synthesized collagen while the origin and insertion of the tissue are moved closer together by some external force (Figs. 7.5 and 7.6; see Chapters 12 and 26). This explanation is consistent with the observed increased resorption of old collagen and the simultaneous synthesis of and replacement by new collagen having the previously described biochemical modifications of DD.

Physical mechanism of shortening

The rapid turnover of the palmar fascia collagen, and the fact that the new collagen, synthesized partly to replace the old collagen, is biochemically different from the old collagen, due to post-translational changes, does not explain either why the tissue is resorbed and partly replaced with collagen having the post-translational modifications of collagen synthesized in healing wounds, or why the tissue slowly shortens irreversibly. Clearly some force external to the collagen fibrils and fibres is necessary to bring the ends of the palmar fascia tissue closer together. This must act at a rate similar to the rate of tissue resorption and its replacement with new, post-translationally modified collagen to ensure that the overall longitudinal length of the collagenous **tissue** (not the molecules or fibrils) of the palmar fascia is shorter than normal.

The critical question is what generates the external tensile force on the collagenous matrix necessary to pull the origin and insertion of the palmar fascial tissue closer together? The early ob-

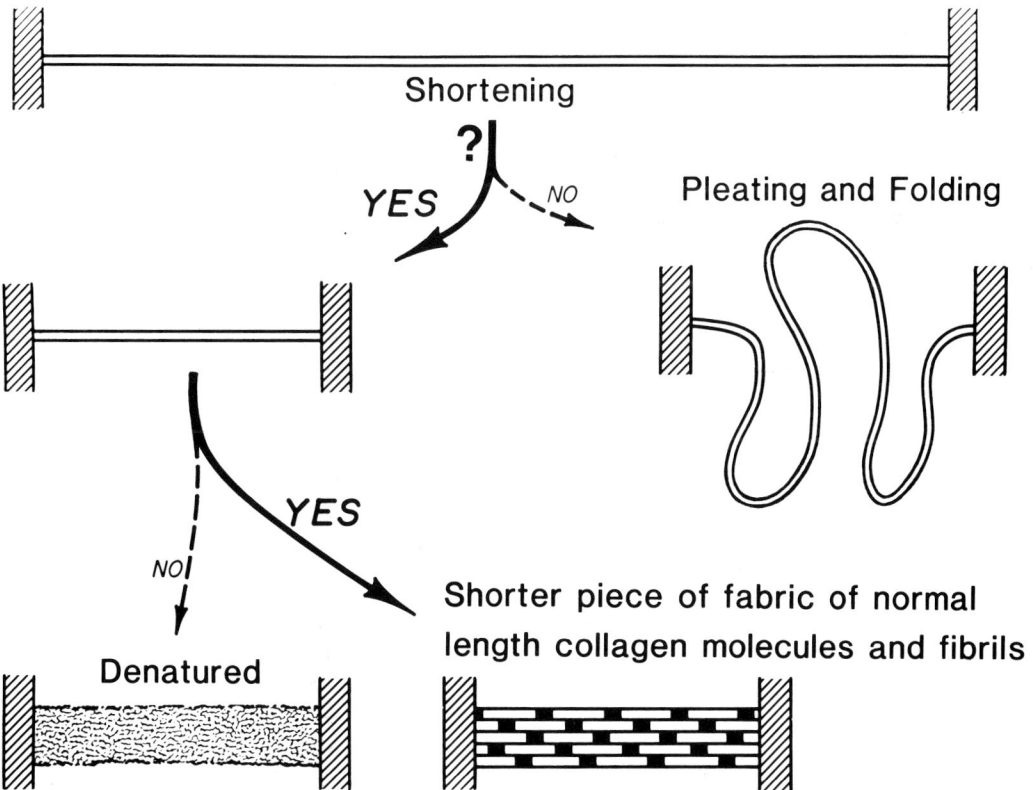

Fig. 7.5 How the palmar fascia can be shortened; authors' proposed solution.

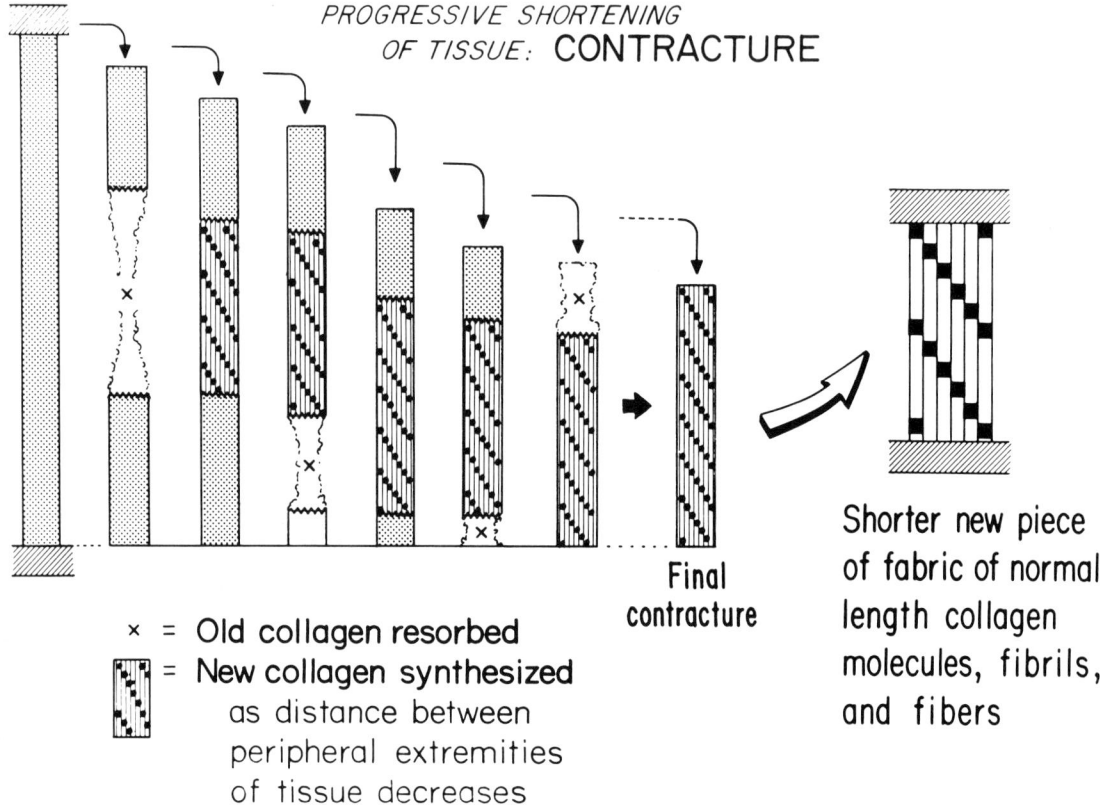

Fig. 7.6 Proposal that the gross shortening of the palmar fascia tissue fabric (the contracture per se) in DD represents a newly synthesized, shorter piece of palmar fascia containing structurally normal collagen that has replaced the original palmar fascia. In brief, as the distal ends of the palmar fascia are brought closer together (possibly the role of the myofibroblasts), the old collagen is resorbed and replaced by progressively less collagen; that is, by a smaller, shorter, new piece of tissue fabric. The configuration of the collagen molecules and their macromolecular organization in the fibrils are normal. There is no gross pleating or crimping of the higher ordered fibres in this new tissue fabric. From Brickley-Parsons et al (1981).

servation of Gabbiani and Majno (1971, 1972) that wound contracture tissue in general — including the palmar fascia in DD, contains cells with many of the ultrastructural characteristics of smooth muscle cells, has now been confirmed by a large number of independent workers (Badalamente et al 1983; Hurst et al 1986; Tomasek et al 1986). These cells (which Gabbiani & Majno named myofibroblasts) contain myosin and are therefore potentially capable of contraction, and, with the proper extracellular surface protein components, of generating a tensile force from these contractions on the extracellular matrix.

Recent immunofluorescence studies of myofibroblasts from Dupuytren's nodules have established that the myofibroblasts are probably modified or specialized fibroblasts rather than cells similar to smooth muscle cells (Tomasek et al 1986). (Because of the widespread use of the term myofibroblast and its general acceptance, this terminology will continue to be used in this chapter to avoid confusion.) This conclusion was reached as a result of immunocytochemical experiments which demonstrated that they possess a cytoplasmic contractile apparatus containing non-muscle myosin rather than smooth muscle myosin (Tomasek et al 1986). Furthermore, the extracellular matrix immediately surrounding the myofibroblasts does not stain for laminin as is the case of smooth muscle cells, but rather stains positively for fibronectin (Tomasek et al 1986). Significantly, the fibronectin staining is much more intense for the matrix surrounding the myofibroblasts than it is for that surrounding the fibroblasts present in normal palmar fascia (for further details see Chapter 8).

Several studies have shown that in vitro granulation tissue containing similar myofibroblastic cells contracts after it is subjected to a variety of specific substances used to cause contraction of smooth muscle cells (Gabbiani et al 1972, McFarlane 1982; Badalamente et al 1983; VandeBerg et al 1984). Further work needs to be done to characterize the physiology of the contractile mechanisms of the myofibroblasts, including determining which stimuli they respond to by contraction.

It has been postulated that contraction of these cells results from an interaction between the intracellular actin microfilaments and the non-muscle myosin as a result of as yet unknown stimuli. The intracellular force is thought to be transmitted extracellularly through the interaction of the actin cytoskeleton with transmembrane protein which interacts via specific receptors with the contractile actin–myosin cytoskeleton on the one hand, and fibronectin on the surface of the cell extracellularly on the other hand. The fibronectin transmits the tensile force to the extracellular matrix proper by virtue of its strong and specific interaction with collagen fibres, which in turn results in the pleating and folding of the collagen fibres. This tends to move the origin and insertion of the palmar fascia towards each other, thus shortening the distance between them. However, even if one accepts the proposition that the myofibroblasts not only have the potential to contract but actually do contract as a result of unknown stimuli, and also that the extracellular fibronectin layer is bound tightly enough to the actin microfilaments by the membrane protein and to the collagen to transmit the intracellular force to the extracellular collagen network, there still remain a number of other physical, biological and biochemical conditions which must be satisfied if the contraction of these cells is to lead to a gross longitudinal shortening of the palmar fascia, not just a simple pleating of the tissue (Brickley-Parsons et al 1981).

In the first place, the cells must be geographically ordered with respect to one another so that the simultaneous contraction of large groups of cells is transmitted in roughly the same correct linear direction. The resultant force from the contraction of all of the cells must have an overall vector in the proper direction to shorten the tissue in the appropriate direction, so that the origin and insertion approach one another. We have already detailed the experimental evidence that the shortening of the linear distance between the origin and insertion of the fascia is not solely the result of gross folding or pleating. Resorption and remodelling of the collagen and other macromolecular components of the tissue must also occur. The myofibroblasts may be involved in both synthesis and resorption of collagen in addition to contributing to the development of a tensile force on collagen fibres by virtue of their cellular contractions. While the contraction of myofibroblasts may be a critical phenomenon in shortening the longitudinal distance between the origin and insertion while the tissue is being replaced and remodelled, cell contraction alone does not explain the pathogenesis of the specific kind of physical shortening of the palmar fascia which occurs, or the biochemical changes which occur in the collagen and other components simultaneously with the shortening, and probably before it begins.

It has already been observed (Gelberman et al 1980) that a significant number of Dupuytren's nodules either do not contain any myofibroblasts or only a scattered few. This seems to rule out an obligatory role for the myofibroblasts either as the source of the external tensile forces tending to shorten the palmar fascia or as the cell-synthesizing collagen with the post-transitional changes observed in DD. Similarly, the complete or near complete absence of myofibroblasts in what appears to be clinically, morphologically and cellularly normal palmar fascia tissue in DD which already shows the biochemical abnormalities of composition and of the collagen components, effectively rules them out as the only cells involved in the remodelling of the palmar fascia collagen.

When fibroblasts (as opposed to myofibroblasts) are grown in culture, large net contractile forces are generated by the traction forces the cells exert by virtue of their *motility* (James & Taylor 1969; Bell et al 1979; Harris et al 1981; see Chapter 10).

Since the traction forces generated by the fibroblasts were found to be capable of rearranging collagen into ordered patterns when cultured on collagen gels, it was postulated that such forces are the basis of the contractures of the collagen network in healing wounds, burns and surgically implanted prostheses (Harris et al 1981). The movement of fibroblasts and the forces generated by the motility of fibroblasts and other cells cannot therefore be ruled out as a potential mechanism responsible for the generation of traction forces on the collagen which would tend to shorten the palmar fascia while it was being resorbed and partially replaced with the new, post-translationally modified collagen (Brickley-Parsons et al 1981; See Chapter 10).

While the electron microscopic morphological and immunofluorescence data indicate that myofibroblast contraction may account for traction forces which tend to shorten the palmar fascia in DD (Tomasek et al 1987), there is still little or no direct physical or chemical evidence that these chemical interactions between the intracellular and extracellular proteins occurs or that the ordered, geometrically organized contraction of those cells and this whole sequence of events occurs. There still remains the task of chemically establishing the links between the various intracellular and extracellular protein elements and establishing that they are strong enough to resist the mechanical forces generated by the cells.

On the other hand, movement of cells travelling away from a fixed point, and with sufficient bonding strength to the extracellular collagen and other constituents, could displace the tissue and, if the displacement was in the proper direction, shorten the tissue. During this shortening, these and other cells in the tissue might then resorb some of the collagen so that pleating and bunching did not occur. Additionally, some of the resorbed collagen could be replaced by collagen synthesis, and this collagen would be different from the normal mature collagen of the palmar fascia due to the post-translational changes observed analytically and described in detail in this chapter. For the authors and their colleagues collaborating in the research programme on DD, this seems to be a more likely scenario (see Chapters 2, 10, 13 and 28).

Further insight into the possible role of the myofibroblasts, the development of flexion contractures and the interrelationship between the two can be derived from the clinical observation that a number of patients with well developed nodules — and in some cases longitudinal bands — have no contractures and do not develop them for long periods of time, while nodules and in some cases longitudinal bands continue to be present. Tissues from nodules and bands removed at surgery from several of these patients were sent to us by several surgeons. Many samples, especially the nodules, were found to contain a high density of myofibroblasts. The collagen showed changes typical of DD. Thus, it is clear that there is a stage or phase of DD when cellular and biochemical changes may be present for a significant time without any evidence of a contracture. That is, the cellular changes and synthesis of new collagen in DD can be separated from the physical shortening and contracture of the palmar fascia.

A careful search of the literature reveals that there is essentially no concrete scientific evidence as to the basic underlying aetiology of DD; why the myofibroblasts form; what causes them to contract; if they do, what the cellular basis is for the resorption of collagen or of new collagen synthesis, and the stimuli which lead the cells significantly to alter the post-translational biochemical reactions in the collagen of the palmar fascia in DD. We do know that an aetiological agent has either directly or indirectly caused the cells in the palmar fascia to behave like those in an acute wound or in the reparative tissue synthesized during the healing of an open wound. In many respects these effects closely resemble the behaviour of cells in rapidly growing (and remodelling) embryonic tissue.

A significant difference between DD and these other conditions, however, is the fact that in the non-DD situations the cells' resorptive, synthetic and post-translational functions eventually return to normal (in skin wounds, for example), whereas in DD the increased turnover of collagen continues, as do the post-translational modifications of the collagen. Indeed even fibroblasts removed from the affected palmar fascia many years after the onset of the disease still show the same modified synthetic and post-translational changes when cultured in vitro (Brickley-Parsons et al 1977).

In reading much of the literature on DD, we

have been struck by the fact that supposed aetiologies are proposed which do not even address the question correctly, mixing pathogenesis, pathological anatomy and clinical appearance with aetiology. Aetiology must specifically address 'what' and 'how' an aetiological agent causes the biochemical and cell biological changes discussed here. The cause of the disease is the key question which needs to be answered in specific scientific terms based on clear-cut experimental data, demonstrating conclusively that the proposed aetiological agent can experimentally induce the cellular and biochemical changes characteristic of DD. Broad, general statements and terms like 'trauma', 'tissue composition and distribution of tissue components', 'metabolic changes', 'anatomical variations' and 'biomechanics' are of little use in this regard. Attempts to form causal relationships between Dupuytren's and other diseases which may occur in an increased percentage of patients with DD are interesting, but in no way do such data indicate causality. Similarly, general or specific anatomical/or biomechanical theories of aetiology — unless they can be shown experimentally to cause the disordered cell biology and biochemistry which occurs in DD — offer little to our understanding of the underlying cause of the disease.

Acknowledgements

This work was funded in part by grants from the National Institutes of Health (AM34078), the Peabody Foundation Inc., and a Faculty Scholar Award to M. J. Glimcher from the Josiah Macy Jr Foundation, Inc. The studies of the pyrolidine cross-links were a collaborative effort between Drs David Eyre, Rauol Tubiana, Caroline Leclercq, the late Richard Smith, and the authors, and currently also include Dr Richard Gelberman.

8 Cellular structure and interconnections

INTRODUCTION

Dupuytren's disease (DD) is characterized by the presence of a nodule and/or fibrous band which may ultimately produce a flexion deformity of the fingers. A specialized cell present in the diseased palmar fascia has been termed the 'myofibroblast' by Gabbiani & Majno in 1972 because of its morphological similarities to fibroblastic and smooth muscle cells. The structural similarities of this cell to the smooth muscle cell in its contractile apparatus and its presence in the clinical nodule during the active stage of contraction have led to the proposal that the myofibroblast is responsible for the digital contracture (Chiu & McFarlane 1978).

The cellular mechanisms underlying the digital flexion characteristic of Dupuytren's disease are still unclear. Studies by Brickley-Parsons and co-workers (1981) have suggested that the contracture of the palmar fascia is due to an active cellular process that progressively draws the extremities of the affected tissue together and at the same time replaces the original tissue. The result of these two processes is a shorter, smaller piece of tissue fabric. In order for a cell to be the active agent responsible for bringing together the extremities of affected tissue it must be able to generate an intracellular contractile force and secondly, it must be able to transmit this intracellular force to the surrounding tissue.

The generation of intracellular contractile force requires a specialized cytoskeleton, whereas the transmission of this contractile force to the surrounding tissues demands an adherent link between adjacent cells as well as other surrounding tissues. To understand these mechanisms one must have a knowledge of the intracellular contractile elements, namely the proteins present in the cytoskeleton of the cell, and the adhesion glycoproteins found at the cell's surface.

The structural similarities of the myofibroblast to smooth muscle cells and fibroblasts have stimulated research to determine which of these two cell types the myofibroblast more closely resembles and from which it is derived. As illustrated by Gabbiani & Majno (1972) and Chiu & McFarlane (1978), myofibroblasts contain numerous mitochondria and large amounts of rough endoplasmic reticulum typical of fibroblasts. They also contain large bundles of actin microfilaments, which are similar in appearance to the myofibrils of smooth muscle. Furthermore, myofibroblasts have an interrupted, amorphous extracellular layer at their surface, which resembles the basement membrane around smooth muscle cells.

Fibroblasts and smooth muscle cells can be more accurately distinguished by the proteins present in their cytoskeleton and extracellular matrix than by their appearance. Smooth muscle cells contain smooth muscle myosin and are associated with the extracellular glycoprotein, laminin (Burridge 1974; Foidart et al 1980). On the other hand, fibroblasts also contain an intracellular myosin — non-muscle myosin — and are associated with fibronectin in their extracellular matrix. Recent immunocytochemical studies, discussed below, indicate that Dupuytren's myofibroblasts are more akin to fibroblasts than smooth muscle cells. They were found to contain non-muscle myosin but no smooth muscle myosin or laminin and thus no muscle elements (Tomasek et al 1986). Immunocytochemical studies by Schürch and co-workers (1984) demonstrated that the cytoskeleton of myofibroblasts contains the intermediate filament protein vimentin and lacks desmin, further indicating that these cells are distinct from smooth muscle cells.

These studies indicate that Dupuytren's myofibroblasts closely resemble fibroblasts. In addition to the fact that they contain non-muscle myosin, the large bundles of actin microfilaments present in these cells are similar to stress fibres seen in cultured fibroblasts. Furthermore, the presence of fibronectin at the surfaces of Dupuytren's myofibroblasts and the transmembrane association between actin microfilaments and extracellular fibrils are also similar to observations in cultured fibroblasts. These findings further indicate that the Dupuytren's myofibroblast is a modified fibroblast with a specially organized cytoskeleton with large amounts of fibronectin accumulated at its surface. In view of this we feel that the term myofibroblast is rather misleading and prefer to call this cell a Dupuytren's specialized contractile fibroblast, or more descriptively a 'tractofibroblast', from the Latin *tractare* — to pull. In this chapter we have occasionally interchanged the terms myofibroblast and tractofibroblast, depending on the circumstances.

Cytoskeleton of the myofibroblast

The myofibroblast, felt to be the basic cell of DD, structurally resembles both fibroblasts and smooth muscle cells and thus derives its name. The most prominent feature of the myofibroblast is the fibrillar system present within its cytoplasm. Unlike the meshwork organization of actin microfilaments seen at the periphery of normal fibroblasts in vivo, myofibroblasts contain large bundles of actin microfilaments (Fig. 8.1). These bundles parallel the long axis of the myofibroblast and terminate at the cell surface in a specialized association with extracellular fibrils (see section on interconnecting bonds, below). This ultrastructure is similar to either that of myofibrils in smooth

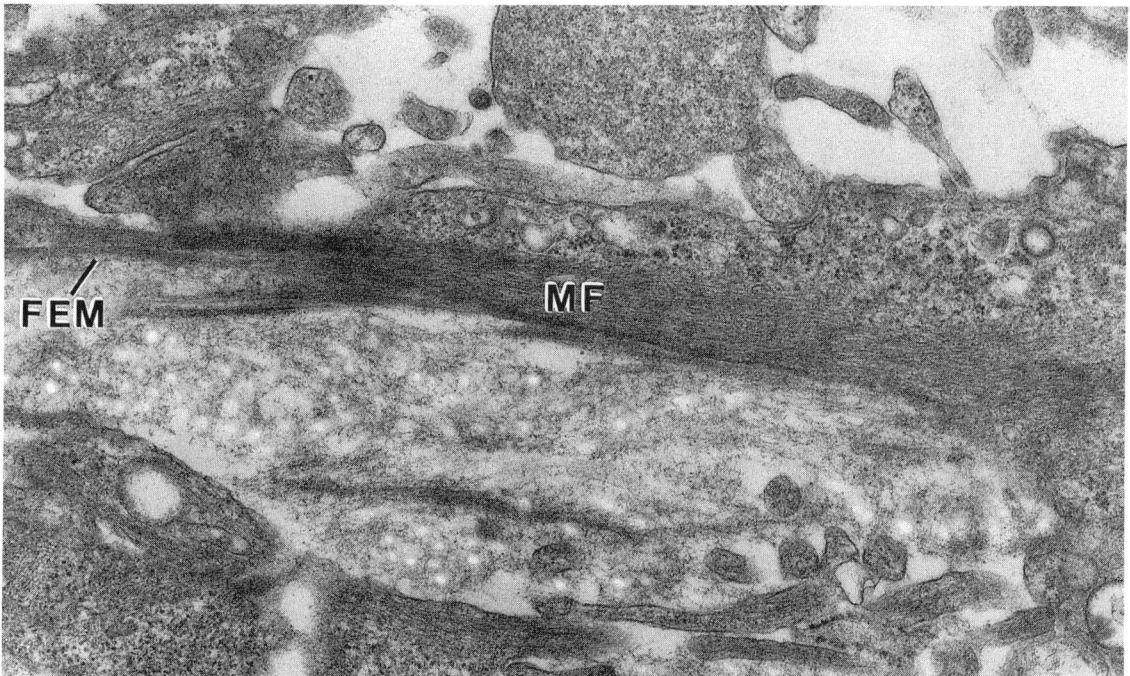

Fig. 8.1 Electron micrograph of a Dupuytren's myofibroblast. A large bundle of actin microfilaments (MF) with electron-dense regions along its length is present. This bundle terminates at the cell membrane in a well defined end-to-end transmembrane association with filamentous extracellular material (FEM). Magnification × 21 000.

muscle or stress fibres which form in fibroblasts under culture conditions (Fig. 8.2). To understand the cellular mechanism of force generation in the myofibroblast one must consider whether the large bundles of actin microfilaments within myofibroblasts more closely resemble myofibrils or stress fibres.

In 1986 we demonstrated by immunocytochemistry that Dupuytren's myofibroblasts stain intensely with a monoclonal anti-actin antibody (Fig. 8.3a; Tomasek et al 1986). It should be stressed that this antibody recognizes both non-muscle and smooth muscle actin. The fibroblasts in normal palmar fascia and in the surrounding band tissue show little if any staining with this anti-actin antibody (Fig. 8.3b). The intense staining pattern in Dupuytren's myofibroblasts and smooth muscle cells exists since the actin in both these cells is organized into bundles of microfilaments. The actin in fibroblasts is organized into a filamentous meshwork which stains only faintly.

Another important protein in DD is myosin. Myosin is a cytoskeletal protein that interacts with actin to generate contractile force in either muscle or non-muscle cells. The presence of myosin in Dupuytren's myofibroblasts was first demonstrated by Meister and co-workers in 1979; utilizing immunocytochemistry, these authors found that myosin was present in substantial

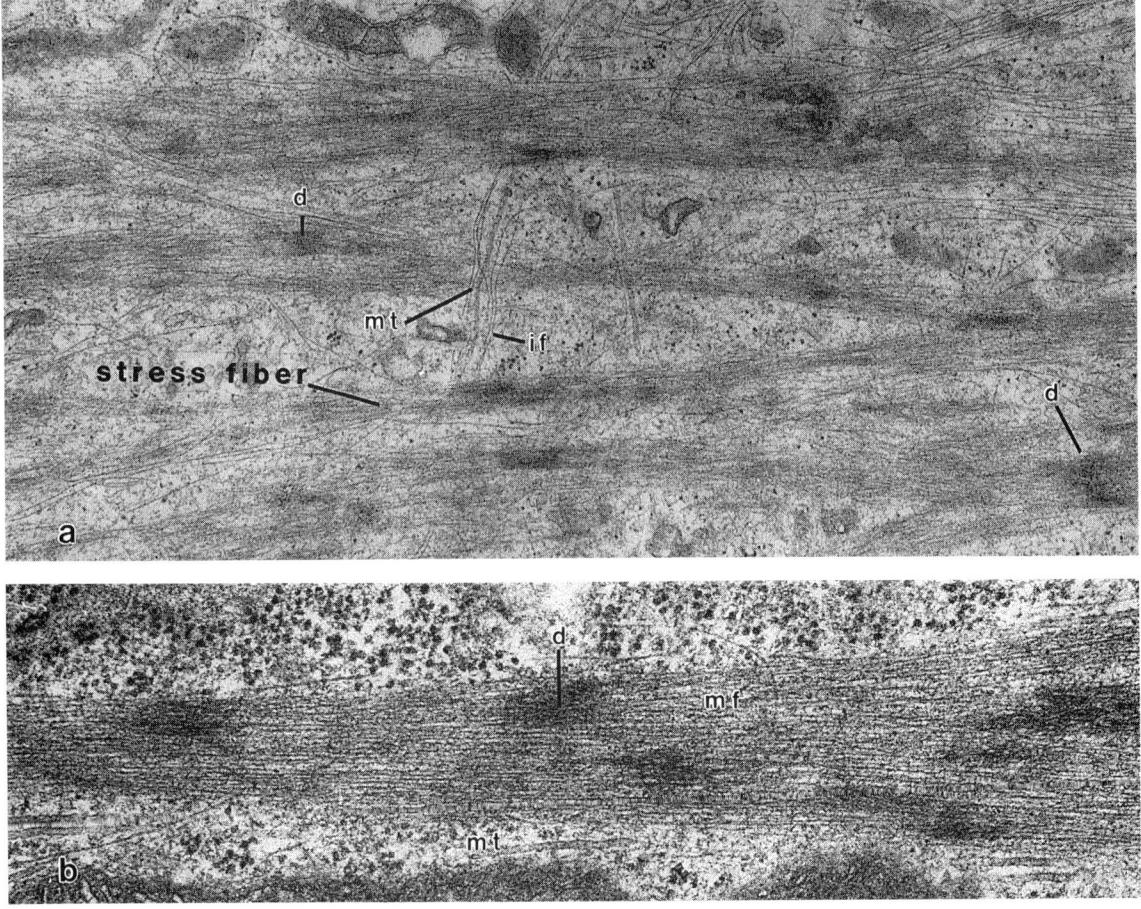

Fig. 8.2 Electron micrographs of fibroblasts cultured on coverslips a Bundles of actin microfilaments (stress fibres) with periodic densities (d) along their length are present throughout the cytoplasm near the substratum. Intermediate filaments (if) and microtubules (mt) are present. b High magnification electron micrograph of stress fibre. Periodic densities (d) are present. Magnification A × 24 000; B × 55 000.

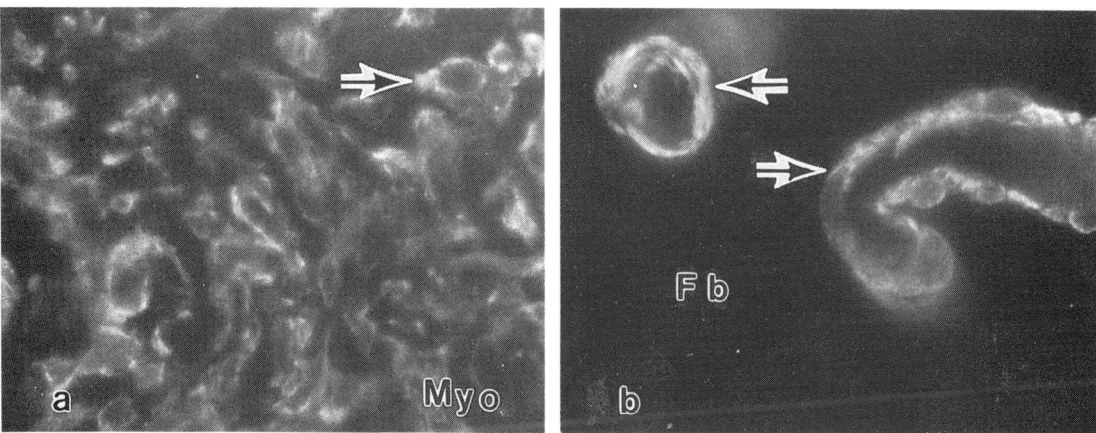

Fig. 8.3 Fluorescent micrographs of cryosections of (**a**) Dupuytren's nodular tissue and (**b**) normal palmar fascia stained with anti-actin antibody. **a** Bright staining for actin is seen in the cytoplasm of the cells in the stroma (arrow), showing the presence of a large population of myofibroblasts (Myo). **b** The fibroblasts (Fb) in the normal palmar fascia do not stain for actin. Vascular smooth muscle cells around blood vessels stain intensely for actin (arrows). Magnification × 800.

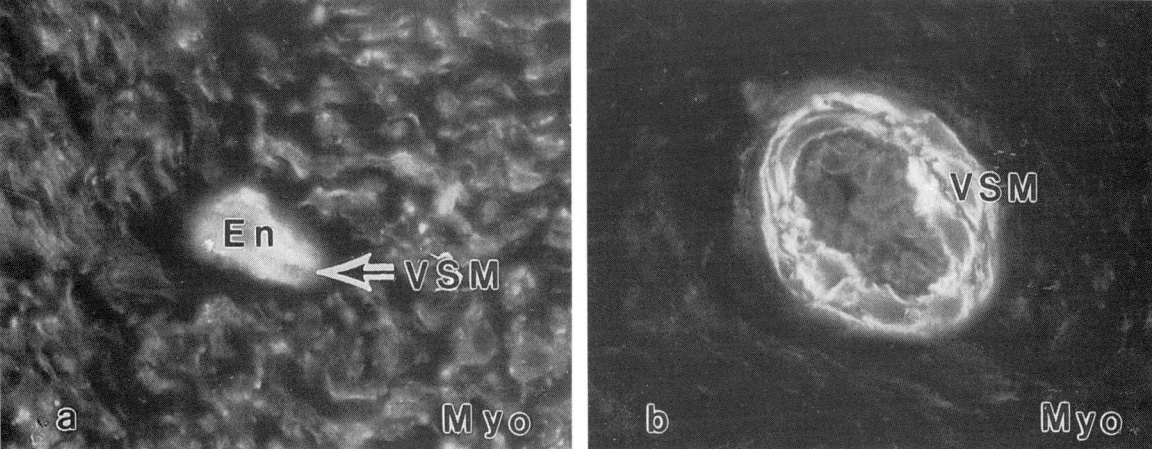

Fig. 8.4 Fluorescent micrographs of cryosections of Dupuytren's nodular tissue stained with either (**a**) anti-non-muscle myosin antibody or (**b**) anti-smooth muscle myosin antibody. **a** The myofibroblasts (Myo) in the stroma of the nodule stain heavily for non-muscle myosin. Vascular smooth muscle (VSM) does not stain with anti-non-muscle myosin antibody, but vascular endothelium (En) does. Myofibroblasts (Myo) present in the stroma of the Dupuytren's nodule do not stain with anti-smooth muscle myosin antibody. As expected, vascular smooth muscle (VSM) stains intensely with this antibody. Magnification × 800.

quantities in Dupuytren's myofibroblasts during the involutional phase of the disease. It should be emphasized that the myosin found in smooth muscle cells is distinct from that found in non-muscle cells. Although most anti-myosin antibodies do not distinguish between these two types of myosin, it is possible to prepare antibodies specific for the myosin in smooth muscle and non-muscle cells. These antibodies can identify these two distinct types of myosin in a variety of mammalian tissues examined by immunofluorescence microscopy. The anti-non-muscle myosin antibodies specifically stain non-muscle cell types, while anti-smooth muscle myosin antibodies stain only smooth muscle cells (Larson et al 1984).

Utilizing these specific antibodies in our 1986 study we found that Dupuytren's myofibroblasts-contain non-muscle myosin and do not contain smooth muscle myosin (Fig. 8.4). In these preparations only the vascular smooth muscle cells stained with anti-smooth muscle myosin antibodies (Fig. 8.4b). These results demonstrated that the Dupuytren's myofibroblast, with regard to its myosin, is a fibroblastic-type cell and not a smooth muscle-like cell; its cytoskeleton is that of an altered fibroblast.

STRESS FIBRES

If fibroblasts are cultured on a planar substratum such as plastic they can develop large bundles of actin microfilaments within their cytoplasm (Fig. 8.2). These intracellular bundles have been termed stress fibres and are found running parallel to the long axis of the cell (for review see Byers et al 1984). The distinguishing features of stress fibres are the organization of actin microfilaments into bundles, and the presence of various cytoplasmic proteins in an alternating pattern along their length. These proteins include non-muscle myosin, α-actinin, and tropomyosin. When examined by electron microscopy, stress fibres have electron-dense regions separated by an electron-translucent region along their length. Stress fibres terminate at the cell membrane, forming a specialized contact with the underlying substratum.

In DD the large actin bundles of microfilaments present in myofibroblasts appear similar to the stress fibres that form in cultured fibroblasts. These bundles of actin microfilaments parallel the long axis of the myofibroblast, have alternating electron-dense and electron-translucent regions along their length and terminate at the cell surface in specialized adhesion sites (see Figs 8.1, 8.9, 8.12 and 8.13). In addition our immunocytochemical studies demonstrated that myofibroblasts in Dupuytren's nodules contain large amounts of actin and non-muscle myosin but no smooth muscle myosin, similar to stress fibres.

The presence of stress fibres in myofibroblasts leads one to believe that this fibrillar system is contractile. The non-muscle myosin in stress fibres of cultured fibroblasts is organized in the form of bipolar filaments (Langanger et al 1986). In this configuration the myosin has the potential to mediate a sliding actomyosin movement. The addition of Mg^{2+}-ATP to isolated stress fibres causes these fibrils to contract (Isenberg et al 1976). Whether this will occur in cells is still unclear, although studies have suggested that stress fibres in cells can contract and exert tension upon the substratum (Harris et al 1980). Once formed, the contraction can be held for long periods of time.

This ability of stress fibres to contract and maintain tension is consistent with their proposed role in DD. It has been suggested that the active cellular process in DD involves contraction of the affected tissue and replacement of the contractile tissue with a new shorter tissue structure. The contraction of stress fibres in Dupuytren's myofibroblasts would bring together the tissue extremities.

The conditions leading to the development or visualization of stress fibres within Dupuytren's myofibroblasts are unknown. Fibroblasts will form stress fibres when cultured on a rigid planar substratum. The formation of stress fibres is dependent upon the adhesion of the cultured fibroblast to the underlying substratum. It has been demonstrated by Ali et al (1977) and Willingham et al (1977) that cells which adhere weakly to the substratum will not form stress fibres; however, when adhesion is increased by the addition of the extracellular glycoprotein fibronectin, stress fibres develop. Burridge (1981) proposed an explanation as to why tight adhesion to a substratum might induce the formation of stress fibres. Stress fibres may arise within a cell because it attempts to pull against a point of tight adhesion. If the substratum is resistant to deformation and the adhesion is strong enough so as not to break, tension will develop. Microfilaments would tend to line up along the line of force, forming large bundles of actin microfilaments. Thus strong adhesion to a substratum resistent to deformation would impose isometric conditions on a contraction, resulting in the formation of stress fibres. Once formed, stress fibres have the potential to contract and maintain tension upon the substratum. Dupuytren's myofibroblasts appear to be strongly adherent to the surrounding tissue, as demonstrated by the presence of fibronectin at their surfaces and filamentous extracellular material connecting them to adjacent myofibroblasts and surrounding collagen fibres (see below). Whether the stress fibres present in these cells form in response to isometric tension remains to be determined.

THE EXTRACELLULAR MATRIX

To produce clinical contraction the myofibroblast of DD, in addition to being inherently contractile, must also be able to transmit its intracellular force to the surrounding cells and extracellular matrix. In order for myofibroblasts to produce pathological effects they must be attached strongly to one another, and also to the surrounding collagen.

There are a group of adhesive glycoproteins that link cells to one another and to the surrounding extracellular matrix; these glycoproteins could fulfil the role of transmitting the necessary contractile force. The best understood of these anchoring molecules are the proteins known as fibronectins or, collectively, as fibronectin (*fibre* and *nectere* — to bind, tie; for review see Hynes 1986). The major function of fibronectin is as an adhesive protein. Fibronectin acts as a ligand attaching cells to various biological substrata including collagen and fibrin. The ability of fibronectin to link collagen and fibrin with the cell surface is related to its structure. The molecule is subdivided into functional domains that bind to collagen, fibrin and the cell surface (for review see Yamada 1983).

Laminin is another adhesion glycoprotein (for review see Kleinman et al 1984). Similar to fibronectin, laminin binds cells to surrounding collagen. Laminin however is specific in terms of its location and function, being found in basement membranes at the basal surface of epithelial cells and surrounding muscle cells.

We have demonstrated by immunocytochemistry the presence of increased amounts of fibronectin and the absence of laminin in Dupuytren's diseased palmar fascia. Cryosections of palmar nodules, which contained myofibroblasts as screened by anti-actin immunostaining and electron microscopy, were stained with anti-fibronectin antibody and anti-laminin antibody. These tissue cryosections demonstrated intense staining with anti-fibronectin antibody, whereas no staining was observed with anti-laminin antibody in the extracellular matrix surrounding myofibroblasts (Figs 8.5 and 8.6). Laminin was localized only in the basement membranes surrounding endothelial cells and smooth muscle cells in blood vessels (Fig. 8.6).

Fibronectin is present in increased amounts in diseased tissue but only in association with the presence of myofibroblasts (Fig. 8.7a). Little if any fibronectin is present around fibroblasts in the

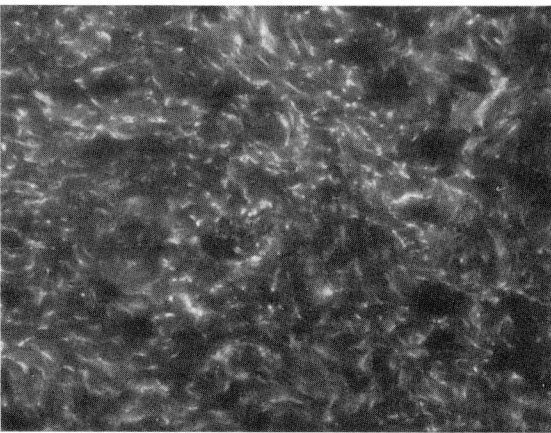

Fig. 8.5 Fluorescent micrograph of a cryosection of Dupuytren's nodular tissue stained with anti-fibronectin antibody. Bright fibrillar staining for fibronectin can be seen in the extracellular matrix around myofibroblasts. Magnification × 800.

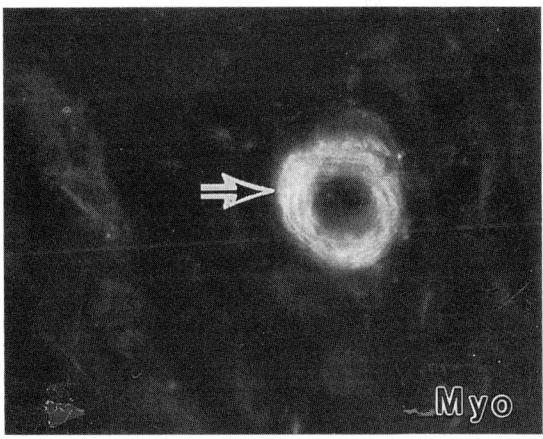

Fig. 8.6 Fluorescent micrograph of a cryosection of Dupuytren's nodular tissue stained with anti-laminin antibody. The basement membranes surrounding blood vessels and vascular smooth muscle stain brightly for laminin (arrow). No staining for laminin is observed around myofibroblasts (Myo) present in the stroma of the nodule. Magnification × 800.

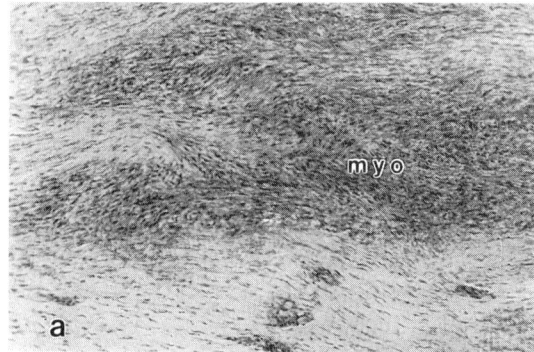

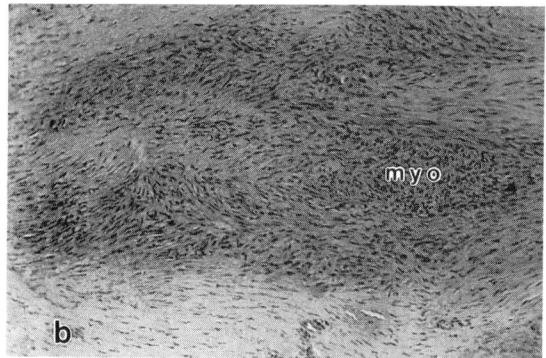

Fig. 8.7 Light micrographs of adjacent cryosections of Dupuytren's diseased palmar fascia stained by immunoperoxidase with either (**a**) anti-actin antibody or (**b**) anti-fibronection antibody followed by staining with haematoxylin & eosin. **a** The myofibroblasts (myo) organized into a nodule stain intensely with anti-actin antibody. The fibroblasts in the surrounding band tissue do not stain. Vascular smooth muscle cells around blood vessels in the surrounding band tissue also stain. **b** The extracellular matrix around myofibroblasts stains intensely with anti-fibronectin antibody. The extracellular matrix around fibroblasts in the surrounding band tissue does not stain. Magnification × 80.

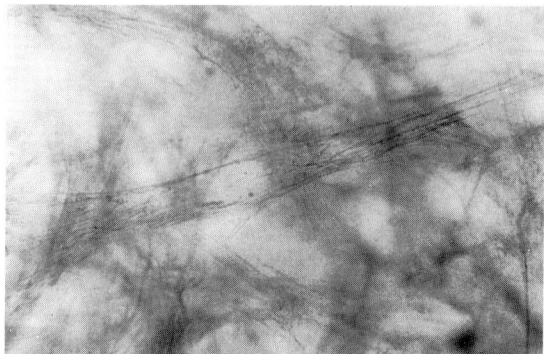

Fig. 8.8 Light micrograph of a Dupuytren's tractofibroblast cultured within a hydrated collagen lattice and stained by immunoperoxidase with anti-human fibronectin antibody. Fibrillar staining for fibronectin is present at the surface of tractofibroblasts. Since this antibody only recognizes human fibronectin, these fibronectin fibrils must have been produced by the cultured tractofibroblasts. Magnification × 400.

surrounding band tissue (Fig. 8.7b). Similarly, little if any fibronectin is present around fibroblasts in normal palmar fascia.

The fact that laminin does not appear to be present in DD, and therefore does not play a role in linking Dupuytren's myofibroblasts to the surrounding tissue, further demonstrates that the myofibroblast is not a smooth muscle cell.

For this reason we feel that the term myofibroblast may be misleading, and prefer to regard this cell as a 'specialized contractile fibroblast'. In view of this for the rest of the chapter we will refer to this cell as a 'tractofibroblast'.

As yet we have not determined whether the fibronectin present at the surfaces of Dupuytren's tractofibroblasts is synthesized by these cells. However, utilizing a monoclonal antibody specific for human fibronectin we have found that Dupuytren's tractofibroblasts cultured within hydrated collagen lattices can synthesize and accumulate fibronectin fibrils at their surfaces (Fig. 8.8). This suggests that they may be able to do the same in vivo.

Fibronectin probably plays a similar role in granulation tissue and hypertrophic scars. It has been localized by immunocytochemistry in the extracellular matrix surrounding myofibroblasts in granulation tissue and hypertrophic scars (Grinnell et al 1981; Kischer & Hendrix 1983). In addition, an immunocytochemical study from our laboratory has demonstrated the presence of fibronectin and the lack of laminin around myofibroblasts in these tissues (Eddy et al 1987), similar to our observations in DD.

THE INTERCONNECTING BONDS

Two features must be present to produce contracture: a contractile cell and the presence of an interconnecting link for the contracting cell to pull on. Ultrastructural studies by Gabbiani & Majno (1972), Chiu & McFarlane (1978) and Tomasek et al (1987) have demonstrated that there are physical connections between individual tractofibroblasts and collagen fibres in Dupuytren's nodules. By electron microscopy we have been able to identify further the nature of these physical connections.

Structure of filamentous extracellular material

Our ultrastructural studies have demonstrated that the extracellular connections are composed of two types of fibrils — fine fibrils with a diameter of 3–5 nm and, of lesser frequency, large fibrils, 10–13 nm in diameter (Fig. 8.9). These fibrils, found only associated with tractofibroblasts, intermingle with each other, making a complex which we refer to as filamentous extracellular material.

This extracellular material at the surfaces of Dupuytren's tractofibroblasts has been described by numerous investigators as basal lamina-like or basement membrane-like (Gabbiani & Majno 1972; Chiu & McFarlane 1978; Meister et al 1979; Gelbermann et al 1980). Although in some ways this filamentous extracellular material does resemble a basal lamina and therefore appears basal lamina-like, it is however ultrastructurally and biochemically (see above) distinct from other basal laminae located at the basal surfaces of epithelia, endothelia, and surrounding skeletal and smooth muscle cells.

The filamentous extracellular material at the surface of Dupuytren's tractofibroblasts is probably in part fibronectin. Preliminary results from our laboratory have demonstrated that Dupuytren's tractofibroblasts cultured in hydrated collagen lattices will form large bundles of actin microfilaments and associated filamentous extracellular material, identical to tractofibroblasts in vivo (Fig. 8.10). Immunoelectron microscopy has demonstrated that this filamentous extracellular material will stain with anti-fibronectin antibody (Fig. 8.11).

Location of filamentous extracellular material

The filamentous extracellular material associated with tractofibroblasts is present only in close transmembrane apposition to intracellular bundles of 5 nm actin microfilaments at the tractofibroblast's

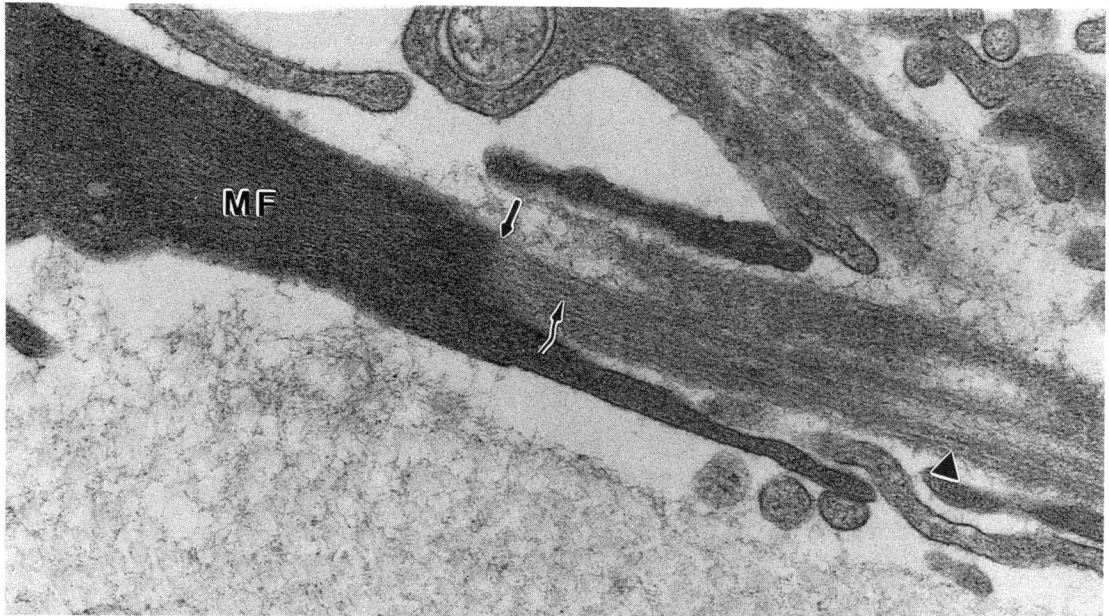

Fig. 8.9 Electron micrograph of a Dupuytren's tractofibroblast. Filamentous extracellular material is composed of fine filaments (curved arrow), 3–5 nm in diameter, and larger filaments (arrowhead) 10–13 nm in diameter. Intracellular actin microfilaments (MF) and extracellular filaments appear to be colinear at the cell surface in an end-to-end association (arrow). Note the absence of a morphologically distinct cell membrane in the region of this transmembrane association. Magnification × 35 000.

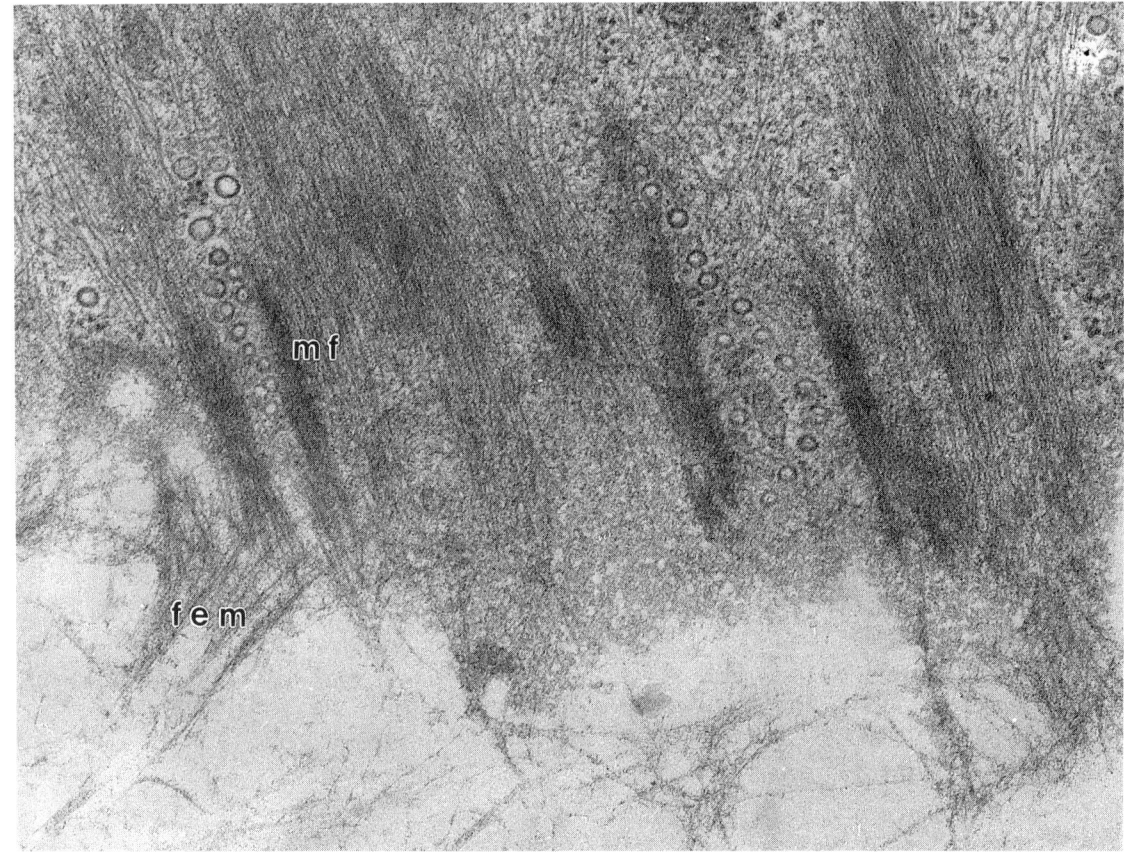

Fig. 8.10 Electron micrograph of a Dupuytren's tractofibroblast cultured within a hydrated collagen lattice. These cultured cells form large bundles of actin microfilaments (mf) and closely associated filamentous extracellular material (fem). Magnification × 38 000.

surface. Here there are two types of transmembrane relations between actin microfilaments and filamentous extracellular material: end-to-end and lateral associations. End-to-end associations consist of 5 nm actin microfilaments and filamentous extracellular material which appear to be colinear across the cell membrane (see Figs 8.1, 8.9, 8.12 and 8.13). Lateral associations are composed of bundles of 5 nm actin filaments and filamentous extracellular material which parallel the intervening cell membrane (Figs 8.12 and 8.13).

The filamentous extracellular material may extend from transmembrane associations at the tractofibroblast's surface to transmembrane associations at the surface of adjacent tractofibroblasts (Fig. 8.14), or to terminate in the surrounding extracellular matrix (Fig. 8.15). Thus filamentous extracellular material participating in transmembrane associations can link the actin cytoskeleton of one tractofibroblast with that of surrounding tractofibroblasts and also with the extracellular matrix.

Although at the time of writing, the exact function of the filamentous extracellular material is unclear, it is possible to speculate on its role in producing flexion deformity in DD. In its specific location the filamentous extracellular material is in a key position to transmit the contractile force generated by the tractofibroblast from cell to cell and to the surrounding tissue. The glycoprotein fibronectin is ideally suited for being the connecting macromolecule since it can bind to the surfaces of cells and collagen fibres and in addition, will form fibrils at the surface of cells. Thus we feel that this filamentous extracellular material is the

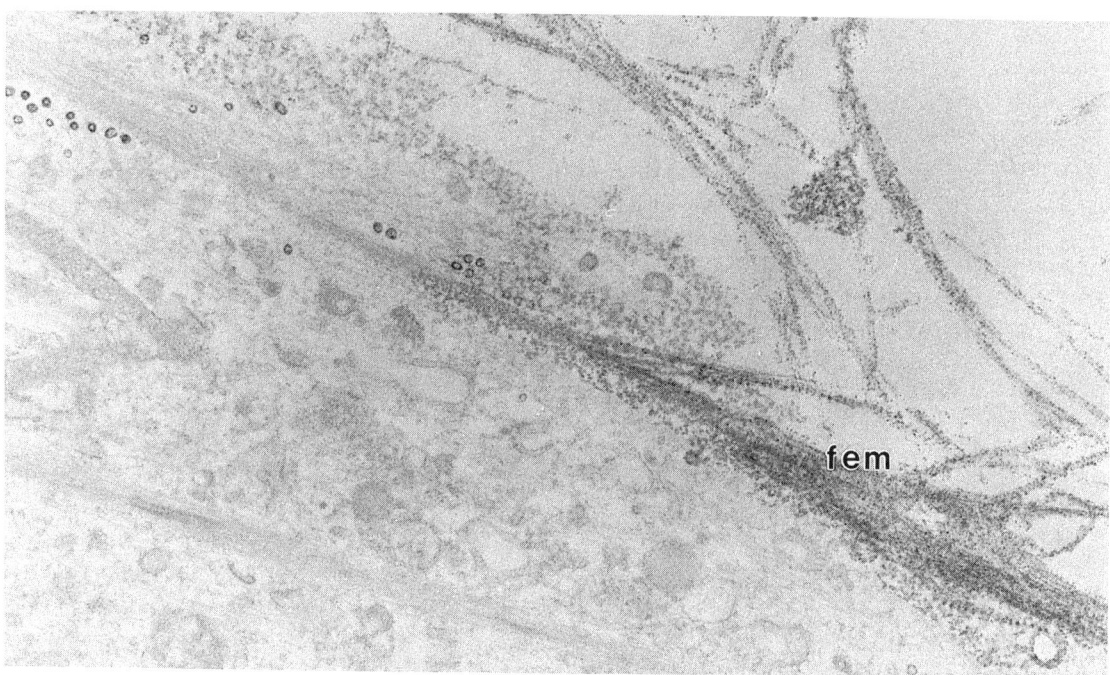

Fig. 8.11 Electron micrograph of a Dupuytren's tractofibroblast cultured within a hydrated collagen lattice and stained by immunoperoxidase with anti-fibronectin antibody. The filamentous extracellular material (fem) present at the surface of the tractofibroblast stains intensely for fibronectin. Magnification × 17 000.

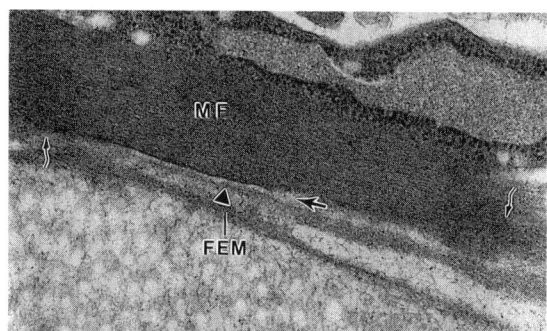

Fig. 8.12 Electron micrograph of a Dupuytren's tractofibroblast. Filamentous extracellular material (FEM) associated with this tractofibroblast is composed only of fine filaments 3–5 nm in diameter. Both end-to-end (curved arrows) and lateral (arrowhead) associations between actin microfilaments (MF) and filamentous extracellular material are present at the surface of this tractofibroblast. An electron translucent space (arrow) separates the cell membrane and filamentous extracellular material in the lateral association. Magnification × 24 000.

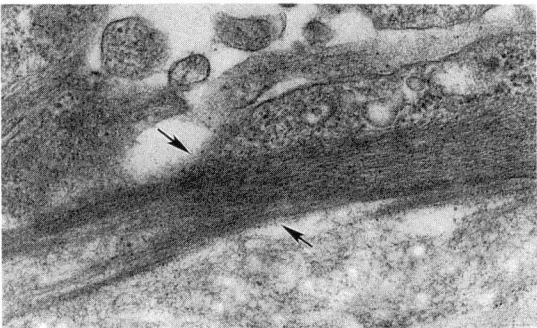

Fig. 8.13 Electron micrograph of a Dupuytren's tractofibroblast. A well defined end-to-end transmembrane association of a bundle of actin microfilaments (MF) and filamentous extracellular material (FEM) is present at the surface of this tractofibroblast. The cell membrane in the region of the end-to-end transmembrane association is not distinct (arrows). Actin microfilaments and filamentous extracellular material appear to be colinear across this transmembrane association. Magnification × 21 000.

key link in attaching tractofibroblasts in Dupuytren's diseased tissue to surrounding tractofibroblasts and collagen fibres.

Connections between bundles of actin microfilaments and filamentous extracellular material are not restricted to Dupuytren's diseased tissue. Fibronectin-rich filamentous extracellular material with the same ultrastructure and similar end-to-

96 DUPUYTREN'S DISEASE

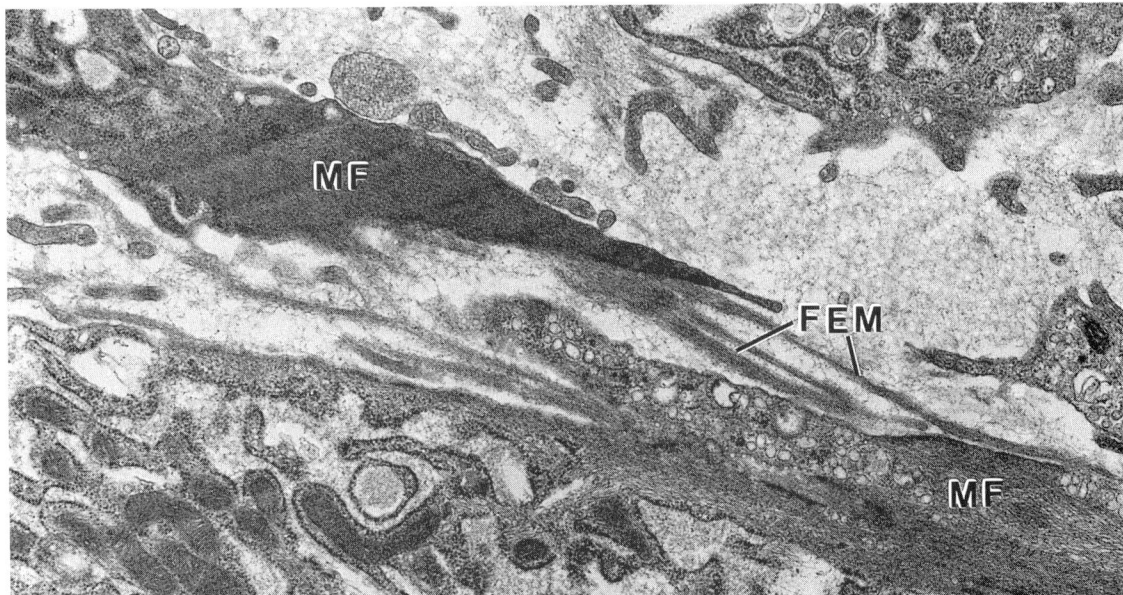

Fig. 8.14 Electron micrograph of a Dupuytren's tractofibroblast. Bundles of filamentous extracellular material (FEM) traverse the surrounding extracellular matrix connecting adjacent tractofibroblasts. Bundles of actin microfilaments (MF) are present within tractofibroblasts. Magnification × 14 000.

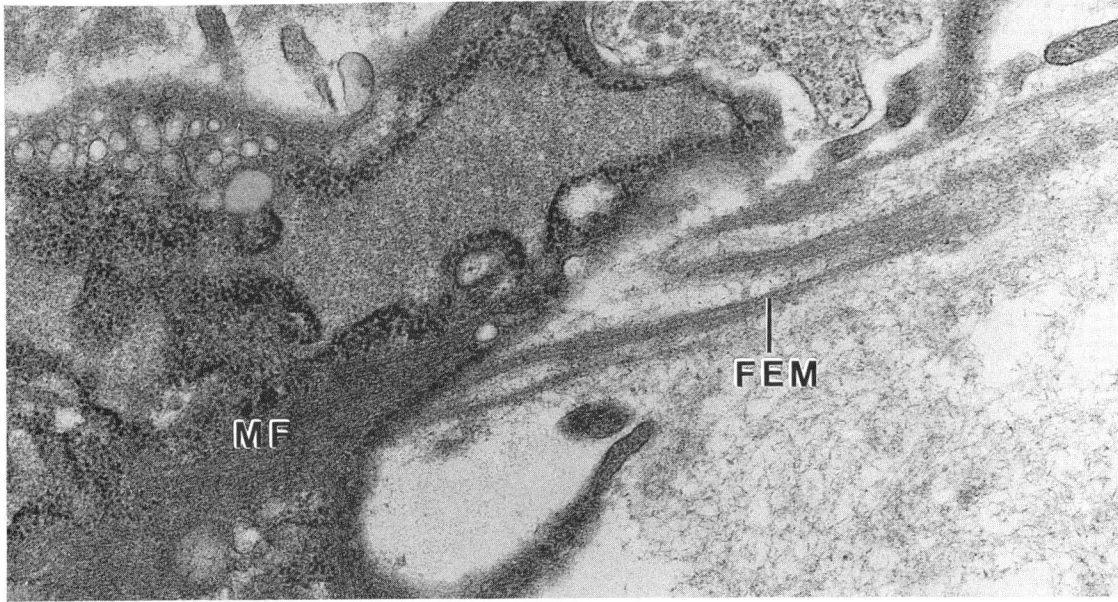

Fig. 8.15 Electron micrograph of a Dupuytren's tractofibroblast. Bundles of filamentous extracellular material (FEM) extend from the surface of a Dupuytren's tractofibroblast into the surrounding extracellular matrix. The filaments composing these bundles appear to disperse and interdigitate with the fibrous matrix surrounding these cells. This filamentous extracellular material is closely associated with an intracellular bundle of actin microfilaments (MF). Magnification × 21 000.

end transmembrane associations with actin microfilaments have been described at the surfaces of cultured fibroblasts by Singer (1979). This transmembrane association between extracellular fibronectin and intracellular actin has been termed the 'fibronexus'. The formation of fibronexus was suggested to occur as a result of attachment by fibronectin to the underlying substratum.

Fibronexus have been described at the surface of myofibroblasts in granulation tissue (Singer et al 1984). The presence of fibronexus in granulation tissue strongly suggests that they are an important in vivo cell surface adhesion site functioning in wound repair. The ultrastructural similarity between the fibronexus seen at the surfaces of myofibroblasts in granulation tissue and the transmembrane associations described at the surfaces of tractofibroblasts in DD suggest they may be the same structure.

TRANSMEMBRANE LINKAGE

The intimate relationship of filamentous extracellular material and intracellular actin microfilaments at the surfaces of tractofibroblasts in Dupuytren's diseased tissue suggests they are physically connected. Since the cell membrane is interposed between them they cannot be in direct contact. If they are to be physically joined there must be a transmembrane linkage connecting them.

This transmembrane linkage may be formed in part by integrin, a complex of cell surface receptors that connect the extracellular matrix and the cell's cytoskeleton (for review see Hynes 1987). This complex spans the cell membrane and contains an extracellular domain, a transmembrane segment and a cytoplasmic domain (Tamkun et al 1986). The extracellular domain can bind directly to fibronectin. The intracellular domain can bind to talin, a cytoskeletal protein that can bind indirectly to actin (Horwitz et al 1986). In addition, integrin has been localized at the surface of cultured cells where extracellular fibrils containing fibronectin and intracellular bundles of actin are closely associated (Chen et al 1985).

It would seem that integrin is a crucial component of the transmembrane linkage between fibronectin-rich extracellular matrices and the cytoskeleton. It is possible to speculate as to the role of such a linkage in the adhesion of Dupuytren's tractofibroblasts to the surrounding tissue. A simplified model of the connection of bundles of actin microfilaments within a Dupuytren's tractofibroblast to the surrounding tractofibroblasts and collagen fibres via such a transmembrane linkage and extracellular fibronectin fibrils is illustrated in Figure 8.16. As indicated in the diagram, actin microfilaments and associated non-muscle myosin could bind either directly or indirectly through actin-binding proteins to the transmembrane linkage. A transmembrane linkage such as integrin could span the cell membrane coupling intracellular actin microfilaments with extracellular fibronectin fibrils. Extracellular fibrils could extend from these surface associations attaching tractofibroblasts to either adjacent tractofibroblasts or surrounding collagen fibres. That the bundles of actin microfilaments in Dupuytren's tractofibroblasts are connected to surrounding tractofibroblasts and collagen fibres is clear; whether this connection involves integrin as the transmembrane linkage and fibronectin as the filamentous extracellular material remains to be determined.

CONCLUSIONS

The myofibroblast described so well by Gabbiani & Majno (1972) has the morphological appearance of both smooth muscle cells and fibroblasts. Analysis of proteins of the intracellular cytoskeleton and extracellular matrix by immunocytochemistry failed to demonstrate any muscle elements; only proteins characteristic of a fibroblastic type cell were observed. Thus the specialized contractile cell in DD appears to be a fibroblast which has altered its cytoskeleton and surrounding extracellular matrix. Based upon these results we suggest that the term 'myofibroblast' may be misleading for this specialized contractile fibroblast and prefer to call this cell a 'tractofibroblast' from the Latin *tractare* — to pull.

The altered cytoskeleton of the tractofibroblast

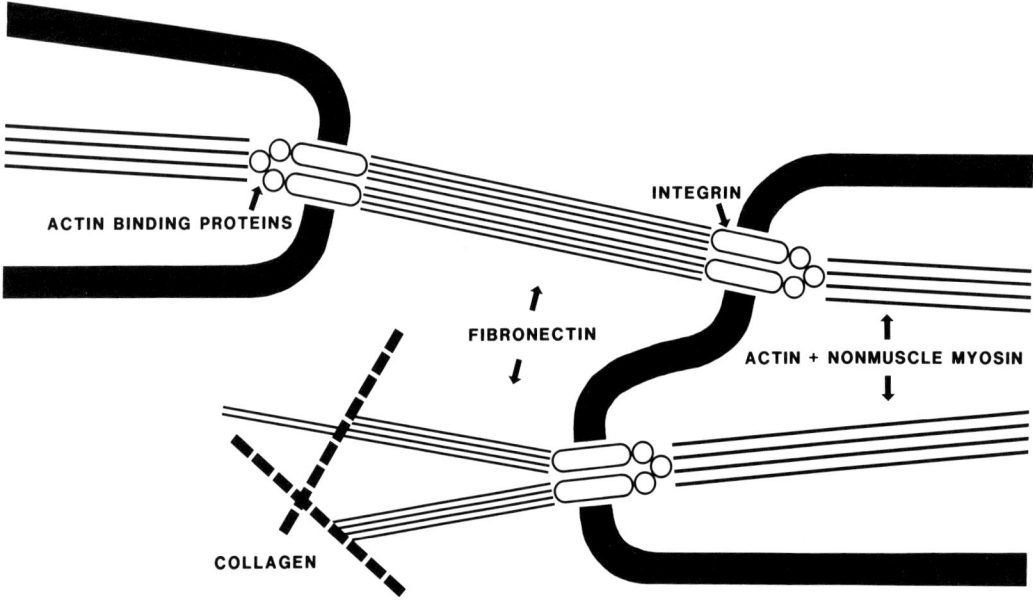

Fig. 8.16 The interconnection of tractofibroblasts with each other and the surrounding collagen fibres. See text for description.

is composed of large bundles of actin microfilaments with associated non-muscle myosin. These bundles of microfilaments resemble stress fibres in cultured fibroblasts. The generation of intracellular contractile force by the tractofibroblast could come about by an interaction of the actin and non-muscle myosin organized into these bundles.

Alterations in the extracellular matrix of tractofibroblasts occur in the form of increased amounts of fibronectin, along with the presence of filamentous extracellular material. Bundles of actin microfilaments terminate at specific locations at the tractofibroblast's surface in close association with filamentous extracellular material. At these specific locations the intracellular bundles of actin microfilaments are connected to filamentous extracellular material through a transmembrane linkage. Extracellular filamentous material extends from these transmembrane linkages on adjacent tractofibroblasts, connecting the contractile cytoskeletons of these cells to each other. In addition, filamentous extracellular material extends from these transmembrane linkages into the surrounding extracellular matrix, connecting the cytoskeleton with surrounding collagen fibres. This filamentous extracellular material, composed of fibronectin, forms a physical connection that could transmit intracellular contractile force to the surrounding tissue.

Acknowledgements

We thank Carol Haaksma and Charles Episalla for their excellent technical assistance in the experiments described in this chapter. We also thank the members of the New York Society for Surgery of the Hand for their contributions of Dupuytren's tissue. The original research reported in this chapter was supported by a grant from the Orthopedic Research and Education Foundation.

K. I. Welsh and J. D. Spencer

9

Immunology and genetics

Dupuytren's disease (DD) is common, with a high level of genetic predisposition. Indeed, there are arguments that it is inherited in a dominant fashion with high penetrance; if this is so then it is far and away the commonest of such diseases and warrants very much more attention by research workers and others. Immunological and genetic investigations into DD have not had a high priority as regards basic research, but tremendous strides have been made in the last few years towards understanding both the immunology and the molecular genetics of other collagen related disorders. In this chapter, our aim is to clarify the present position as regards the immunology and genetics of DD and to relate it at each stage to observations which have been made for related disorders. Hopefully this will enable us to produce evidence sufficient to justify a combined attack on the disease by surgeons and the relevant researchers.

AETIOLOGICAL QUESTIONS

Hueston (1963, 1974) considered that the continuing search for the nature of DD could be most conveniently directed by asking the following questions;

1. Who gets it?
2. What course does it run?
3. What therapy influences it?
4. What is its mechanism of production?
5. How can it be prevented?

We will reconsider Hueston's first question in this chapter.

Who gets it?

The simplified answer is mainly older white males especially if they have epilepsy and are from an affected family. Is it then a clear cut sex-linked disorder, restricted to a single ethnic group and can we explain its genetics by analogy with such a disorder? For example, could DD be a classic genetic disorder of the sickle cell disease type, but one in which the abnormal DNA sequence occurs in genes related to collagen as opposed to those which code for haemoglobin sequences?

In order to answer this question we need to review the evidence for the various parts of our simplified statement on who gets it.

Age and sex

Dupuytren's disease was reported to occur six to ten times more frequently in males than females (Mumenthaler 1961). The possibility existed, however, that as the disease's main economic import was on manual workers, the incidence in females may have been underestimated. Early (1962) tackled this problem by looking at the incidence of palmar contracture in 5000 clerical and manual workers at the Crewe locomotive works in England. Further, since the majority of the workers were male, he also undertook a similar study on the residents of a home for old people and on a random sample of the population of the town of Leigh. Early was able to confirm the work of Herzog (1951) and Hueston (1960) that, in general DD occurred with almost equal frequencies in manual and non-manual workers. However, he observed that although the male to

Table 9.1 Incidence of DD men and women in the Lancashire area (after Early 1962)

Age (years)	15–24	25–34	35–44	45–54	55–64	65–74	>74*
Men							
Number in survey	993	1089	1091	1145	1026	170	138
% with DD	0.1	0.2	1.2	4.4	10.0	15.0	18.1
Women							
Number in survey	264	180	180	212	141	129	221
% with DD	0.0	0.0	0.0	0.5	1.4	6.2	9.0

*Early puts the figure for the incidence of DD in men over the age of 85 at 30.8% but gives no figures for females in this age group.

female ratio was around 8:1 in the 15–64 age groups it fell to around 2:1 in the over 75's. Table 9.1 summarizes the relevant section of Early's data to illustrate this point. It is apparent therefore that the disease develops earlier in males than females but is by no means a specific disease of males.

Dupuytren's disease in non-white races

The prevelance of DD in Negroes, Chinese and Asiatic Indians is reportedly so small that James (1985) concluded that it probably does not occur among pure stock within these racial groups. A similar conclusion was also reached by Hueston (1974). However, such statements, even if they turn out to be incorrect, are a useful focus of attention, and since 1974 several case reports describing DD in the non-white races have specifically checked for gene admixture by careful questioning and by genetic tests. Mennen and Grabe (1979) described a case of DD of both feet and hands in a pure Negro patient with epilepsy. Red cell typing and enzyme polymorphisms strongly supported that the patient was of pure stock. Zaworski and Mann (1979) also reported DD in a black American patient and the letters to the editor following this publication as well as the editorial comment are of interest. Plasse (1979) wrote of a classic case in which the patient could trace his family lineage back three generations, into the time of slavery, and was unaware of any inter-racial marriages. Furnas (1979) reported DD in a 65 year old black tribesman in Southern Tanzania. There was no evidence of white settlements in the area of his home at any time prior to his birth. Maes (1979) described a case of unilateral DD in a Vietnamese patient but did not describe any geneological data.

These sporadic reports give us cause to doubt the conclusions reached by James and by Hueston and Tubiana, but do not justify a definitive statement that DD can occur in pure non-white groups. The blood group and enzyme tests are not conclusive, non-awareness of inter-racial marriages is not proof against gene admixture, and although the Tanzanian case looks convincing it is only a single incidence and lack of permanent settlement is insufficient evidence on which to prove non-exposure to white genes. It is apparent therefore that DD does occur in non-white races but with orders of magnitude of less frequency. It most probably can occur, at least in Negroes, even if the stock is pure but the new and very much more sophisticated genetic fingerprinting techniques would be necessary finally to prove this point.

Dupuytren's disease and diabetes mellitus

Dupuytren's disease has been shown to be associated with diabetes mellitus in several studies (Schneider 1971, Gunther & Miosga 1972, Ravid et al 1977, Heathcote et al (1981) although this has been disputed (Krall & Zorilla 1963). In the study of Heathcote et al, for example, DD was observed in 42% of 273 diabetic patients and 13% of age and sex matched controls. Two other points of note about this study are firstly that the predominant form of DD in diabetic patients (especially in females) is mild and occurs mainly in the middle and ring finger rays as opposed to the ring and little finger rays. Secondly, 57% of the patients with DD had had overt diabetes for less than ten years and characteristic lesions could be found in 16% of newly diagnosed diabetic patients. The authors conclude, and we would agree, that the fascial abnormality cannot be considered to be a late complication (as has been suggested by Gunther and Miosga (1972)) and may be considered as an early warning sign (as has been suggested by Schneider (1971) and by Spring et al (1970)). However, there are two forms of diabetes, one of which is most definitely immunological and has a primary genetic association in the MHC region of chromosome 6 whereas the other is not thought to be immunological and has no MHC association. Unfortunately none of the publications have indicated if diabetes per se or one of the two forms is linked to DD. Renal nephropathy for example is probably almost equally associated with insulin-dependent diabetes mellitus (IDDM) and non-insulin-dependent diabetes mellitus (NIDDM) although it is more often treated in the former. Nephropathy is thought to occur because of a glucose interaction with free amino groups on renal collagen which prevents natural collagen breakdown. Heathcote et al (1981) suggested that glucose intolerance might disturb fibroblast function and cited evidence that cultured skin fibroblasts from diabetic patients display abnormal patterns of growth and protein biosynthesis. However such mechanisms would seem unlikely if DD is associated with only one form of diabetes especially if that form was IDDM. Unfortunately, as we have already said, the question of whether or not diabetes in general or a subset of the disease is linked to DD has not been specifically addressed and may, by analogy of the experience in relating which form is associated with renal failure, actually prove quite difficult to answer. From our own experience DD is nearly always associated with NIDDM. This may be because of local patient handling and all we can say in summary is the rather unsatisfactory statement that DD is associated with NIDDM but may also be associated with IDDM.

Diabetes has two forms, does DD? It has been noted in diabetic patients, that DD is milder and affects preferentially the middle and ring finger rays. It has been shown very clearly that for certain collagen disorders such as Ehlers-Danlos syndrome that each case may have a slightly different genetic abnormality and, even more significantly, that many apparently normal individuals have slight differences in collagen gene areas. The enormous task of defining which modifications in which genetic area are pathogenic and which are not, is already underway and it seems extremely unlikely from the data so far that the same genetic abnormality would cause abnormalities either in the ring and middle finger rays or the ring and little finger rays. We believe therefore that DD will prove to be genetically as well as clinically two or more distinct but closely related disorders.

Dupuytren's disease and other diseases

The primary cause of the contracture has been related to many factors including a high alcohol intake with liver disease (Wolfe et al 1956), tuberculosis and more recently with Peyronie's disease (Billig et al 1975).

There appears to be only one report of a condition in which DD is less common than in the normal population, although it is possible that there may be more instances because negative associations are more difficult to recognize. Arafa et al (1984) observed a significant negative association between rheumatoid arthritis and DD in a study of 292 patients and 555 controls. The patients chosen were all suffering from rheumatoid arthritis and had a female:male ratio of 2:1; the controls were matched for age according to decade and comprised 254 males and 301 females. The results clearly showed the incidence of DD to be less in both male and female rheumatoid patients than in controls. Protective effects of the drugs, especially steroids, given to control the rheumatoid arthritis were considered a possible explanation. Rheumatoid arthritis is linked to the presence of genes in the HLA region on the short arm of chromosome 6 and of genes in the immunoglobulin region on the long arm of chromosome 14 (Sakkas et al 1987). Histocompatibility antigens are discussed in relation to DD below, and it is sufficient to say here that the antigen found raised in rheumatoid arthritis is not of lowered frequency in DD. Immunoglobulin region genes have not been studied in DD but it seems most likely that whatever the reason for the negative association between DD and rheumatoid arthritis, it is not genetic.

Family studies

Proof that DD is a collection, in genetic terms, of several disorders might be forthcoming by comparing inheritance patterns in large multicase families and by careful questioning and assessment of the apparent sporadic cases.

Twin studies would also be a useful adjunct but, considering the relatively high incidence of the disease, reports of cases in twins are small. Couch (1938) reported cases of identical DD in identical twins and as has been reviewed by Ling (1963), there are a few additional early reports but no recent ones. Whether or not this is due to a declining interest in the disease or a genuine lack of cases is unclear. The family studies indicate that DD or a form of the disease is transmitted as an autosomal dominant trait with variable penetrance (Ling 1963). Ling studied 50 probands and then examined all available relatives of each. On preliminary questioning 8/50 patients stated a positive family history. Clinical assessment of 832 relatives revealed that in actual fact 34/50 patients had a proven positive family history and that a further 3 probably had, although examination of the supposedly affected family members was impossible. Other interesting points in the Ling study are the suggestion that the expression of the disease gene is almost complete in males over the age of 75, but is of much lower penetrance in females unless it arises from both parents. Homozygosity for a pathogenic gene might also be expected to lead to an earlier age of disease expression in men and a more aggressive form of the disease. Unfortunately there is no conclusive evidence on these points although there are reports of more rapid recurrences of symptoms after surgery if both parents of male patients were also sufferers.

At this stage we can make several comments. Even if the higher estimates of positive family histories are correct around 30% of cases of DD are sporadic. We have no indication of whether children of sporadic cases will be affected. In the pedigrees published the earliest case can be considered sporadic if neither parent was affected. However, there appear to be no such instances in the literature. This may mean that the children of sporadic cases are not at risk or simply that authors have not included non-affected members of previous generations in their papers. Ling's data, for example (Ling 1963), shows that 8/11 fathers and 7/13 mothers of propositi had DD and one presumes, although the data is not given, that the number of propositi having both parents unaffected is quite small.

Histocompatibility antigens in DD

Tait and MacKay (1982) and Hunter et al (1981) were unable to find a significant association between DD and HLA-A, B or C locus products but Tait did find an increase of HLA-B12 in the patient group. We studied HLA-A, B, C and DR antigen frequencies in 37 consecutive patients attending the Guy's and Lewisham Hospital clinics (Spencer and Welsh 1984) and found an increase of HLA-DR4 (an antigen in linkage disequilibrium with B12), but again the association did not reach significance. We also observed a slight increase in the frequency of the A1, B8, DR3 haplotype, a haplotype common in patients with a range of autoimmune disorders. We also looked for any association between alcoholism-induced DD, familial DD or sporadic DD with HLA antigens but found none.

Collagen antibodies in DD

The suggestion that DD might be associated with an autoimmune response to collagen was made by Gay & Gay (1972) but it was not until 1979 (Menzel et al 1979) that serum antibodies to collagen were detected in a proportion of patients. The abnormal palmar fascia of the hand which characterizes the disease contains increased amounts of type III collagen (Bailey et al 1977, Bazin et al 1980) but the major collagen antibody observed by Menzel was directed against type I. Pereira et al (1986) showed 11/16 patients and 27/96 normal blood donor controls had antibodies to at least one collagen type. Patients had more antibodies to native collagen types III and V and more antibodies to denatured collagen types II and IV than controls. In addition, the antibodies to denatured collagen type II were restricted to those patients having HLA-DR4. These results are on a relatively small number of patients and no account has been taken of the length of disease duration.

In rheumatoid arthritis, for example, it is during early disease that collagen antibodies are most prevalent and it is again those who are HLA-DR4 who have highest incidence of antibodies. We feel that there is insufficient evidence to connect anticollagen antibodies with the pathogenesis of DD at this time. A sequential study on serum samples from non-affected members of multicase families would be all that is necessary to determine if anticollagen antibodies appear before or after the clinical manifestations of the disease. Such a study need not take more than a few years if selected individuals from a large number of families could be chosen for study.

Conclusion

We conclude from the last two sections that DD is not an HLA linked disease and that it is unlikely to have any autoimmune input into its pathogenesis. In addition, we can draw several conclusions from the studies presented in this chapter:

1. There appears to be a form of DD the primary cause of which is the presence of an abnormal gene. This gene is not on the X or the Y chromosome and is most likely to be one of those associated with collagen production.
2. This disease gene is dominant but homozygous expression may give a more aggressive disease.
3. Males or females carrying this gene will probably all develop DD if they live long enough.
4. A separate factor related to sex influences the age at which the disease manifests itself. This factor is not related to occupation, but may still be related to an environmental difference between the sexes, although it is more likely to be itself genetically controlled.
5. Sporadic cases of DD do occur but there is no evidence to show whether or not children of such cases will be susceptible. Neither is there any suggestion that the disease is clinically different or occurs at different ages in sporadic as opposed to familial cases. We cannot say therefore that the sporadic cases involve a different genetic lesion.
6. Cases of DD do occur in the non-white races and most probably in pure black genetic stock although reported cases in other ethnic groups could still be due to gene admixture. Such cases are sporadic and occur with much lower frequency than sporadic cases in whites.
7. DD apparently occurs more often with epilepsy and with diabetes mellitus than would be expected by chance but the majority of the disease which occurs in conjunction with diabetes mellitus may be of a different form.
8. It is not apparent if sporadic and/or familial DD is associated with epilepsy and yet the co-occurrence of the diseases in the same family members would provide solid evidence for a genetic link.
9. If drugs given for epilepsy do induce DD it is likely that they only do so in those who have the DD genetic susceptibility gene.

by authors*M. H. Flint and C. A. Poole*

10 Contraction and contracture

Although Dupuytren's disease (DD) may sometimes be restricted to a relatively asymptomatic thickening of the palm, patients' complaints of inconvenience, incapacity or frank disability generally relate to the contracture or flexion deformity of the fingers or the adduction contractures of the web spaces.

Whilst contracture may not be the primary event in the disease process, there would probably be general agreement that it is the most troublesome. The fact that the disease process is frequently referred to as Dupuytren's disease tends to give the impression that it is a unique or special type of contracture which is somehow different from other post-traumatic or postoperative contractures encountered in plastic or orthopaedic practice. To some extent this is true, but we feel that it is likely that the biological basis of the contractual process in DD is probably identical with, or at least similar to, other clinically observed contractural or remodelling processes. We believe that the special, and at times apparently unrelenting, aspects of the Dupuytren's contractual process relate more to the unique microarchitectural and anatomical features of the palmar skin and aponeurosis — especially the distribution and orientation of the longitudinal fibre fascial bundles — than to any unique cellular or extracellular contractural or remodelling process.

The palmar surface of fingers and palm, in common with the front of the neck, the antecubital fossa and the popliteal aspect of the knee, are all potentially concave surfaces, the longitudinal traverse of which is only maintained by active extension. This, and the fact that the fingers are frequently held in a semi-flexed position for long periods of the day and night, increases the likelihood that any contraction or connective tissue remodelling which may occur could produce a decrease in the available length or extensibility of the palmar connective tissue fabric. This would as a consequence lead to its further contraction, remodelling and shortening.

We believe that one of the basic reasons for the development of Dupuytren's disease on the palmar surface of the hands and fingers is the fact that the volar surface of the fingers and palm are anatomically and posturally poorly equipped to resist any active contractural process. In this chapter we will try to examine the biological mechanisms which give rise to the connective tissue fabric shortening which is clinically manifest as contracture.

The semantic confusion which has arisen over the usage of words such as 'contraction' and 'contracture' has tended to obscure the true biological basis of the process. Some writers have, for instance, indicated that the word 'contraction' should be limited to the active and reversible shortening associated with *muscular* activity (see Chapter 7), whilst others have dismissed the idea of the contractile potentiality of fibroblasts because they consider that there are not enough cells to pull the collagen fibres in such a manner as to 'contract' the tissue.

We feel that it is also useful to use the term 'contraction' to describe tissue fabric shortening attributable to cellular activity. This allows us to group together the contraction of granulation tissue in wound healing with the contraction of a collagen gel in tissue culture, or the contraction of a blood clot by platelets (Budtz-Olsen 1951, Gabbiani & Majno 1972; Bell et al 1979; Grinnell & Lamke 1984). As we shall see, this cellularly motivated change is brought about by active reorganization or realignment of the cell, its intracellular microfilaments and cytoskeleton and its relationship with the extracellular matrix (Gabbiani & Majno 1972; Gabbiani et al 1976). Until the resultant shortening of the extracellular fabric has been irreversibly locked in place by collagen reorganization and further collagen deposition, this process is partially or completely reversible (Guidry & Grinnell 1986). It is prevented or inhibited by drugs which affect the contraction of the cytoplasmic microfilaments, or which block or disaggregate the microtubular system and can be reversed by removal of the cells from the system, either by detergent or enzymic treatment (Gabbiani et al 1973; Butler et al 1977; van Bockxmeer et al 1985).

However, after a varying period of time this dynamic cell-dependent process of fabric shortening (contraction) is followed by physicochemical changes in the extracellular matrix which, as it were, lock the dynamic process of contraction into a more static, and progressively more irreversible state of 'contracture' (Guidry & Grinnell 1986). Initially, and for a short period of time, this contracture can be overcome by the application of an external distractive force of sufficient magnitude to return to the status quo ante. Until the new extracellular framework becomes sufficiently reorganized and remodelled to overcome this, the irreversibility of the contractual process is only relative. With the passage of time, and especially if the tissue is constantly relaxed by posturing, the process of shortening may become progressively irreversible.

The changes which lead to the contractural shortening — and often thickening — of the connective tissue fabric involve the active remodelling and recycling of the extracellular matrix. Collagen and the other constituents of the extracellular matrix are broken down by physicochemical and enzymatic degradation both within and outside the cell (Weber 1967; Woessner 1968; de Campos Vidal 1972; Slack et al 1986). Concurrently or sequentially, new collagen is synthesized by the cell and secreted into the extracellular matrix (Birk & Trelstad 1985). The newly formed tissue is generally shorter than that which was there prior to the contraction so the available and potential extensibility of the tissue is gradually reduced (Brickley-Parsons et al 1981). When this dense, irreversible fibrosis decreases the available tissue fabric length and extensibility and particularly when it limits joint movement, it is generally regarded as 'contracture'.

CONTRACTION AND TRACTION

Until the work of Abercrombie et al (1954, 1956) it had generally been considered that the shrinkage or contraction of wounds or scars was due to the physical shortening of the collagen fibres themselves, particularly the condensation of fine argyrophylic reticulin fibres into thicker collagen fibres. However, those studies on the contraction of wounds in rats and scorbutic guinea pigs some 30 years ago conclusively established that the contraction process was independent of the collagen content of the wounds and that cells were responsible for providing the motive force for contraction.

Subsequently James's group (Abercrombie et al 1960; James & Newcombe 1961; Highton & James 1964) were able to show, in a series of elegant experiments, that the stored energy of the cellular contraction process could be held in abeyance by splinting the periphery of the wound. Removal of the splints was followed by immediate contraction of the wound to the size that it would have been if contraction had been allowed to proceed uninhibited throughout the contraction phase. The studies also demonstrated that the force generated either by a sheet of fibroblasts in culture or by the granulating wound in vivo could be directly measured by strain gauges and were found to be of a similar order of magnitude (Highton & James 1964; James & Taylor 1969).

It is somewhat surprising that the matter is still currently being questioned and debated, notwithstanding the fact that Gabianni et al in a series of demonstrations of the contractile properties of the myofibroblasts (Gabbiani & Majno 1972; Gabbiani et al 1976; Gabbiani & Montandon 1985) confirmed these initial results and ideas. In experimental demonstrations of granulation tissue and myofibroblast contractility, Gabianni made it undeniably apparent that the myofibroblast, as he and his associates called the contractile fibroblast, was the prime candidate for the initiation of contraction.

It is, however, important to stress that the isolated myofibroblast is itself unable to induce the extracellular contractural process. The attachment of its contractural elements to the extracellular matrix and ultimately the collagen fibres is a prerequisite for the translation of the energy of cellular contraction into extracellular fabric shortening (Brickley-Parsons et al 1981; Grinnell & Lamke 1984; Gillery et al 1986; Guidry & Grinnell 1986). However, the necessary connections to facilitate the contractural process have now been demonstrated in various contractile situations linking the microfilamentous intracellular motor through the fibronexus on the cell membrane to the extracellular fibronectin and thence to the collagen fibrils themselves (Fig. 10.1; Singer et al 1985, 1987; Tomasek et al 1987). These matters are discussed in detail in Chapter 8.

Whilst, nowadays, few would deny the possibility of the generation of contractile forces by 'myofibroblasts', there is still some concern with this terminology, indicating as it does that the cell is a type of muscle cell. This point of view is

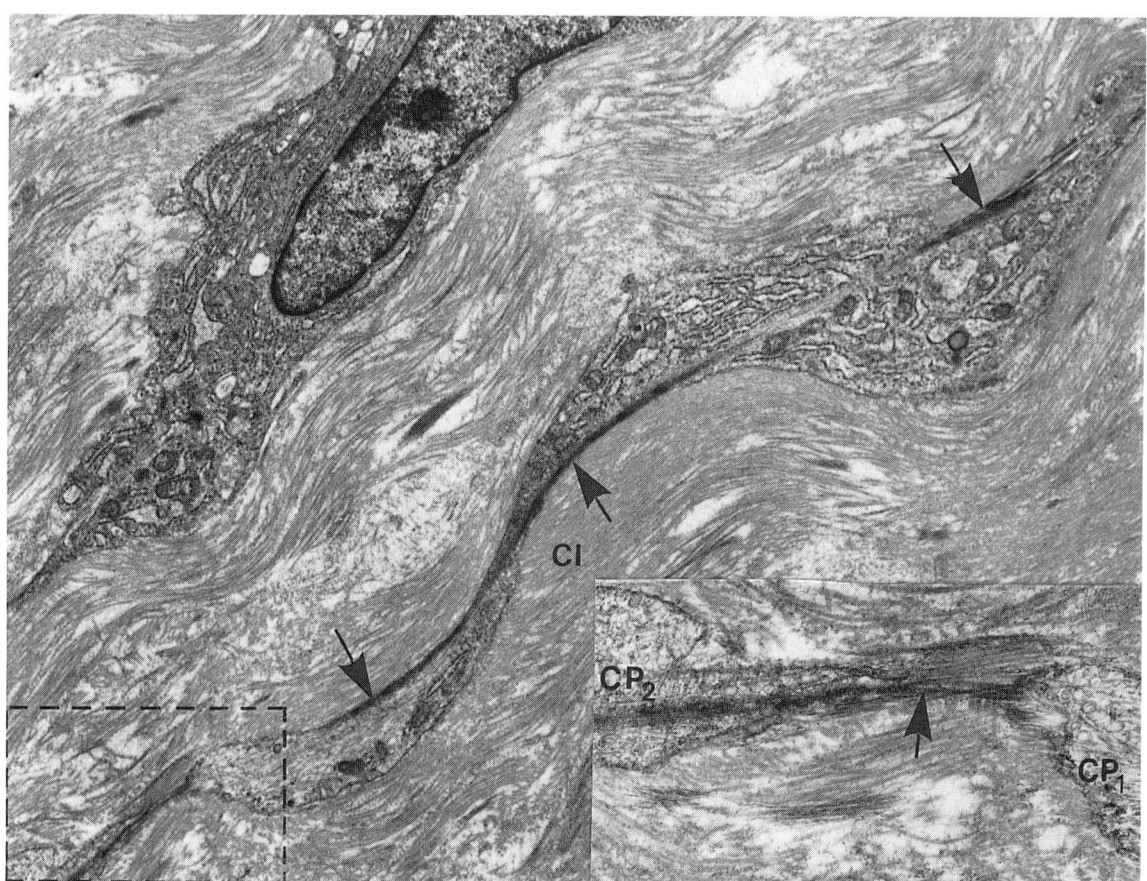

Fig. 10.1 Portion of an undulating myofibroblast from Dupuytren's band showing a dominant stress fibre running the length of the cell process with alternating attachments to the cell membrane on either side of the process (arrows). Retraction of the stress fibre is thought to cause ruffling of the cell process and results in the undulation of the surrounding collagen bundles (CP) during the contraction process. Magnification × 7120. **Inset** Detail of the myofibroblast at bottom left, showing a tandem fibronexus where stress fibres at the terminal end of the process (CP_1) form a continuum with extracellular microfilaments (arrow) and the stress fibres of an adjacent cell process (CP_2). Magnification × 15 000.

discussed in Chapter 8; the name tractofibroblast is suggested as being more suitable to express the function of these contractile cells without implying any connection with smooth muscle cells. The term tractofibroblast has much to commend it, for recent studies on the mechanism of the deformation (or contraction) of silastic substrates by fibroblasts grown upon them in culture indicate that the fibroblasts actually shorten (or contract) the underlying silastic sheet *by elongating* their own cytoplasmic pseudopodial extensions and rippling the underlying substrate beneath their cytoplasm (Harris et al 1980, 1981). Whilst these observations confirmed that fibroblasts and other similar cells can produce a reduction in fabric length by direct physical pull, Harris et al (1980, 1981) elegantly demonstrated that the resultant change was not produced by a simple contraction of the cells or their surface protrusions. They demonstrated that fibroblasts did not produce the contraction effect by simply shortening in length like contracting muscle cells but rather shortened the underlying substrate by exerting a shearing force tangential to their surface. This shearing force seemed to be similar to the mechanism which has been observed by which fibroblasts spread or propelled themselves on glass or polystyrene substrates.

Stopak & Harris (1982) used the term 'traction' to describe this force as being analogous to the traction exerted by an automobile wheel on the underlying highway. They distinguished it from 'contraction' which would necessitate a shortening of the cell itself. Although recognizing that cellular traction was caused by cytoplasmic contraction, they felt that it was very important to distinguish between the process of cell contraction as observed in muscle shortening, and cell traction as seen in the spreading or elongation of fibroblasts.

These and other workers, particularly Melcher and his colleagues in Toronto, have studied the forces generated by fibroblast traction and been able to observe the morphological consequences of the intense stress fields which develop in organ cultures of explants and which are of such importance in normal growth, development and repair (Bellows et al 1981, 1982). There is now no doubt that fibroblasts are capable of generating forces far in excess of those required for simple locomotion (Harris et al 1980, 1981; Bellows et al 1982).

Recent studies by Guidry & Grinnell (1986) conclusively demonstrated that the initial process of gel or wound contraction is cell dependent and that during this stage the collagen fibres are mechanically held in place by the cells. Subsequently, however, after about 2 hours, it appears that the collagen fibrils become stabilized by non-covalent chemical interactions independently of the cell, which will persist even when the cells are removed by either enzymatic or detergent extraction.

The cellular basis of contraction

Even though the investigative methods have become more refined since Abercrombie et al (1954, 1956) demonstrated that viable cells were necessary for wound contraction, the exact mechanism by which this contractile force is transmitted to the extracellular environment is, at the time of writing, still uncertain. However, during the last few years, high resolution electron microscopic studies have demonstrated connections between the cytoplasmic actin microfilaments — generally regarded as the intracellular 'motors' — and the cell membrane, and in some instances passing through the cell membrane to connect with extracellular fibrils (Fig. 10.2). In many instances there appeared to be dense plaques, either on the bundles of microfilaments, or on the inner surface of the cell membrane in close proximity to the bundles. The nature of these dense plaques is at the moment uncertain, but we wonder whether they are formed by localized zones of a cytoskeletal protein which may act as co-ordinator of the actin microfilamentous bundles (Small & Sabieszek 1980; Weeds 1982; Bray & White 1988). Brett & Godman (1986) indicate that fodrin (fibroblast spectrin) and ankyrin may also be important in linking the plasma membrane to the microfilaments whereas the substrate adhesion plaques appear to contain vinculin and talin.

In our studies of remodelling in a variety of connective tissues, we have frequently seen these dense plaques straddling and apparently binding the actin bundles (Fig. 10.3) and wonder whether they play a part in providing a registration for the

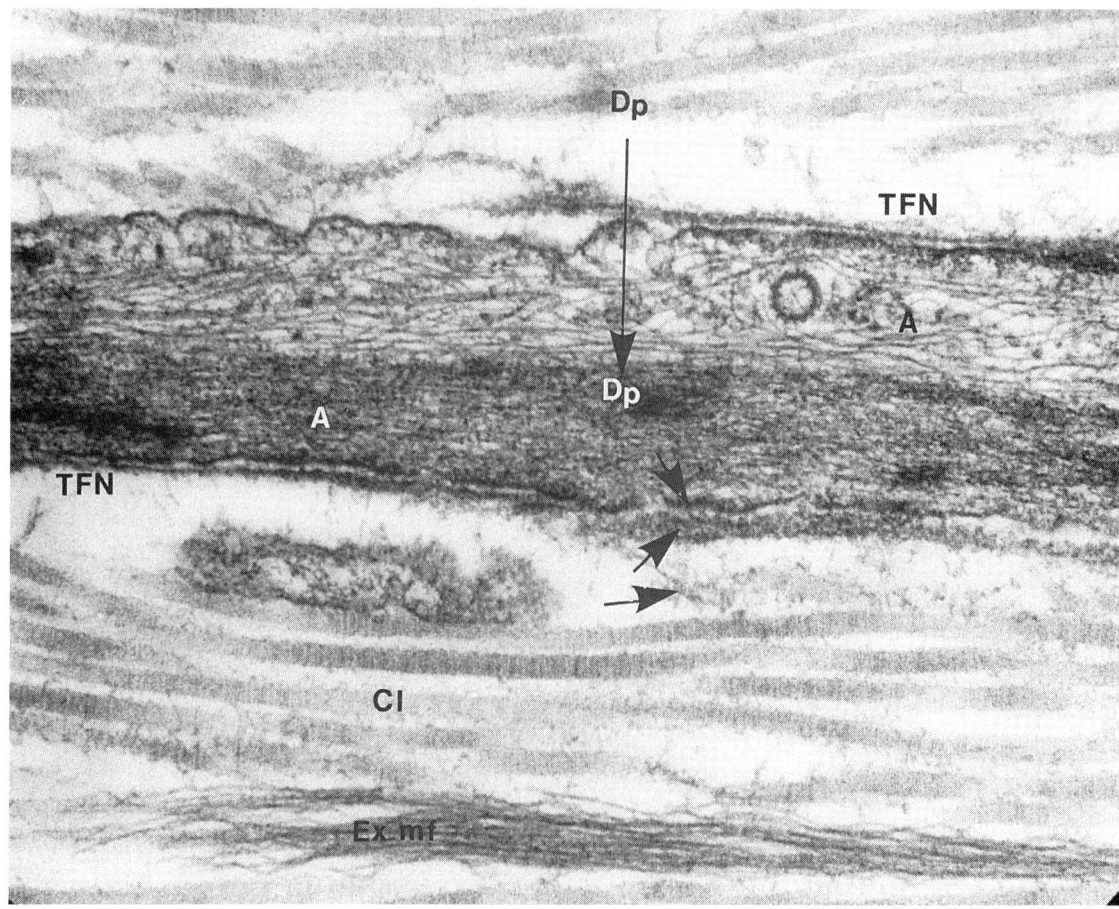

Fig. 10.2 Portion of the myofibroblast cell process showing details of actin filaments (A) organized into discrete bundles characterized by dense plaques (Dp), and their association with tract fibronexus (TFN) on the upper and lower surface of the process. Each fibronexus is characterized by an increased density at the point where actin filaments attach to the inner surface of the membrane (arrows), transmembrane attachment sites to extracellular fibronectin microfilaments (arrows) and the interaction between fibronectin filaments and adjacent collagen fibres (Cl). Magnification × 50 000.

actin microfilaments to act in concert. In non-contractile fibroblasts, actin microfilaments are present and identifiable, but are not so densely aggregated as they are in the active myofibroblasts (Gabianni & Rungger-Brondle 1981; Doillon et al 1987). The non-contractile cells also appear to have fewer dense plaques. We wonder whether one of the essential differences between an actively contractile and non-contractile fibroblast is the presence or absence of these dense plaques which might be involved in the registration and aggregation of the actin into contractile bundles. It may be that the actin microfilaments are normally present in similar numbers in contractile and non-contractile cells but are only placed in contractile readiness by the deposition of plaques of 'register protein'.

As yet, we do not know the exact mechanism or the ultrastructure of the actin–fibronexus–fibronectin–collagen interconnection, but evidence is gradually accumulating that there are indeed microfilamentous or intermediate filament connections capable of transmitting the forces from the motor to the extracellular matrix across the cell membrane (Gold & Pearlstein 1980; Hay 1981; Hynes 1981; Singer et al 1983, 1985; Bereiter-

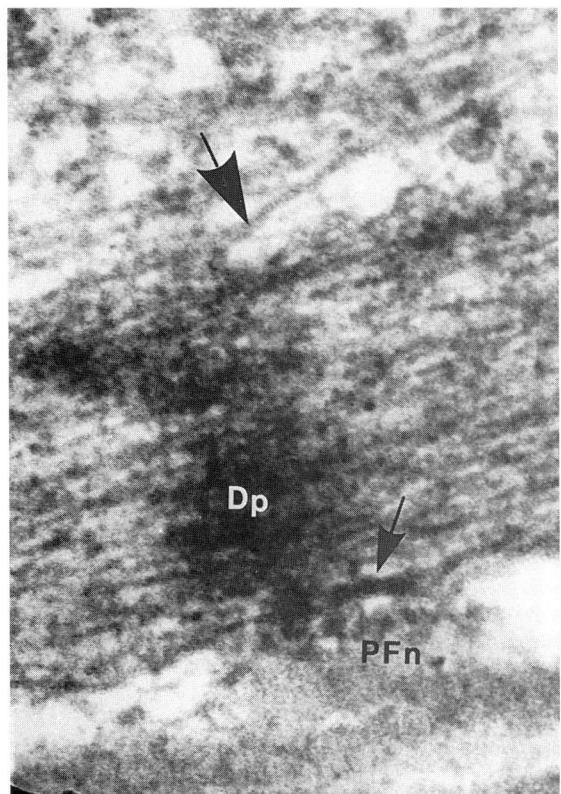

Fig. 10.3 Detail of a dense plaque (Dp) illustrating the incorporation of actin filaments (large arrow) into compacted organized stress fibres. The dense plaque also forms a dense attachment to the inner cell membrane (small arrow) which in turn is connected to a plaque fibronexus (PFn) in the extracellular space. Magnification × 109 000.

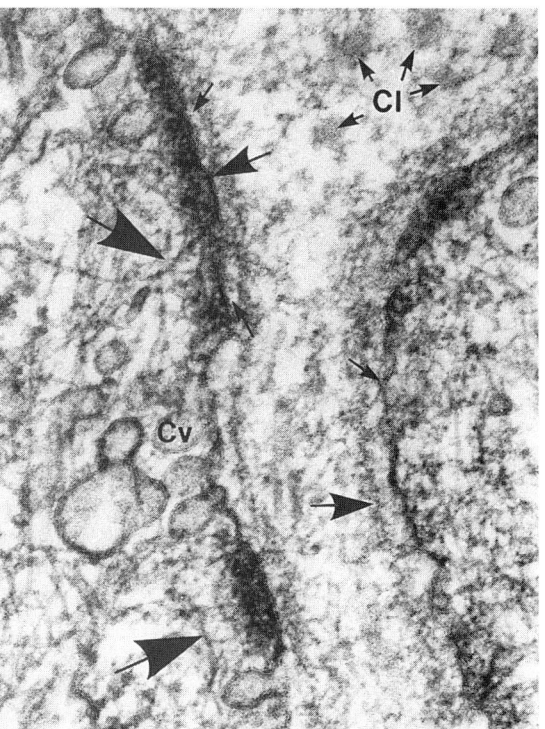

Fig. 10.4 Proliferating cells in the nodule are at first closely packed as they commence synthesis of new extracellular matrix. These round immature cells are seen to form the rudiments of a fibronexus at this early stage. Intracellular actin filaments are not yet combined into stress fibres and form individual attachments with the dense inner margin of the membrane (large arrows). Fibronectin in the extracellular space (intermediate sized arrows) is attached to the outer cell membrane by fine filamentous threads (small arrows). Cl = newly formed colagen fibres. Cv = caveolae. Magnification × 60 000.

Hahn 1985; Tomasek et al 1987; Figs 10.2 and 10.4). Recent evidence indicates that heparan sulphate and cell surface glycoproteins may be involved in this (Hedman 1982; Singer et al 1987).

Our own electron microscopic observations on remodelling tissues demonstrate that on occasions loops of collagen fibres may be entrapped within deep cytoplasmic invaginations as though the fibre has been dragged into the cell so that the cell could obtain a better purchase on the fibre (Fig. 10.5). Furthermore, we have observed active collagen remodelling occurring within these deep invaginations (Slack et al 1986). It appears that on occasions (at least) the entrapment and shortening of collagen fibrils proceeds directly to collagen remodelling to produce a definitive shorter fabric.

CONTRACTURE: ITS DEVELOPMENT AND CORRECTION

The production of a definitive shorter fabric by connective tissue cellular remodelling is an essential feature of all connective tissue contracture, and Dupuytren's disease is no exception. Unfortunately, this concept is not generally recognized and as a result, considerable debate has centred around the difficulties of appreciating what happens to the excess extracellular fabric, particularly the collagen fibres which have been rendered surplus to requirement following the fabric

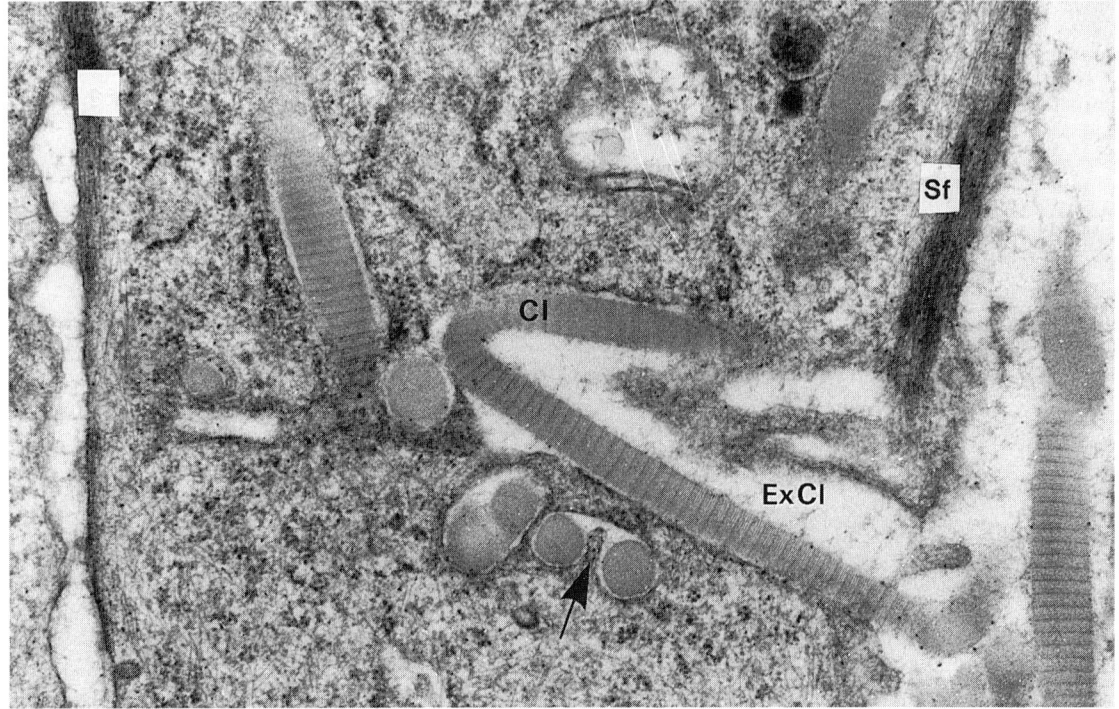

Fig. 10.5 Internalized collagen fibres (Cl) formed into a U-shaped loop within an extracellular cleft (ExCl). The regular appearance in our experimental remodelling studies of two collagen fibres within a common cleft (arrow) indicates that the collagen fibres are not necessarily phagocytosed from a divided end, but may be picked up along their length and internalized as a loop. These appearances are particularly common in experiments where the fibres are completely free of attachment. Sf = stress fibres. Magnification × 30 000.

shortening by cellular contraction (Brickley-Parsons et al 1981). Some writers appear to have difficulty in accepting the cellular basis of contraction because there does not appear to be any evidence of loose or pleated collagen fibres after the tissue has become shortened by the contraction process.

For almost 20 years the Connective Tissue Research Group in the Department of Surgery at Auckland, New Zealand has been involved in a study of connective tissue remodelling. In essence we have shown that connective tissues, whether fibrous or cartilagenous, are essentially plastic, ephemeral and ever-changing (Flint et al 1980; Merrilees & Flint 1980; Flint 1981). We have demonstrated changes occurring remarkably rapidly in connective tissues relieved of their normal loading or which have been subjected to additional load of the same or different mode (Gillard et al 1977, 1979; Slack et al 1983, 1986). All these rapid changes involved an active remodelling of the tissue with a concomitant collagenolysis or collagen degradation and collagen formation, often occurring within the same cell. Usually there is a concomitant and often marked change in the type and amount of proteoglycan or glycosaminoglycan synthesized by the cells and in proteoglycan turnover which is reflected in marked changes in the biochemical analysis of the tissues. These metabolic shifts occurring at the same time as, or following, activation of the plasminogen activator degradative cascade (Brown & Flint 1982, 1983), can produce massive changes in a whole tissue, such as a tendon, or alternatively may lead to localized contained changes, if they alone are sufficient for the remodelling needs of the tissue.

The concept of the potential dynamic nature of connective tissues of even the most inert and solid-looking structures such as tendon and cartilage makes it necessary to appreciate that the connective tissue fabric which was there yesterday or last week will not necessarily be there tomorrow or next week. Some evidence of the accretion of new material or the loss of old material is discernible on ordinary light microscopy with routine histological staining, but at the ultrastructural level the effects are magnified into a seemingly frenetic or sometimes apparently chaotic reorganization of the tissue fabric (Fig. 10.6) with collagen fibres being broken down, fragmented and disaggregated at the same time as fine new collagen fibrils are being formed and integrated into larger fibres and bundles. In fact it is frequently possible to see collagenolysis and collagen synthesis taking place within the same cell at the same time (Birk & Trelstad 1985; Slack et al 1986). This remodelling process may occur very rapidly, but certainly within 7–10 days after the appropriate stimulus has been applied by injury or release or application of load, major extracellular reorganization can be detected. In fact, in some of our work we found that there were profound metabolic changes in glycosaminoglycan synthesis and degradation within 48 hours of releasing fibrocartilage from load bearing (Brown & Flint 1982, 1983).

In recent studies undertaken in our department, individual fibre bundles of the rat tail tendon have been exposed, isolated and transected under the dissecting microscope and left to heal, remodel or realign for periods of up to 9 weeks. The effect of releasing these fibre bundles from their normal tonic load was observed by transmission electron microscopy using whole fibre preparations to avoid artefactual bias or error. These studies demonstrated the marked effect of connective tissue remodelling in the fibre bundles released from their normal tensional force transmission. Active collagen breakdown (collagenolysis), connective

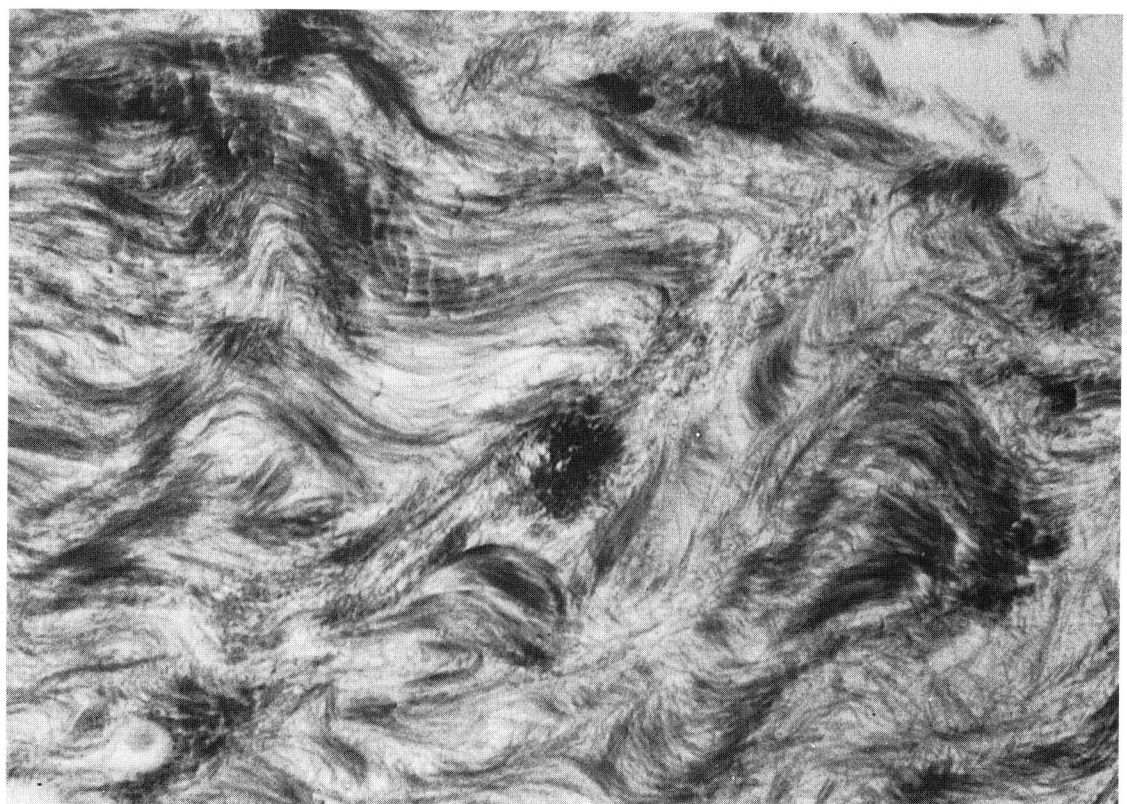

Fig. 10.6 Connective tissue remodelling in apparently uninvolved normally glistening longitudinal fascial bundle from the palm of a 28-year-old woman killed in a car accident. Magnification × 2000.

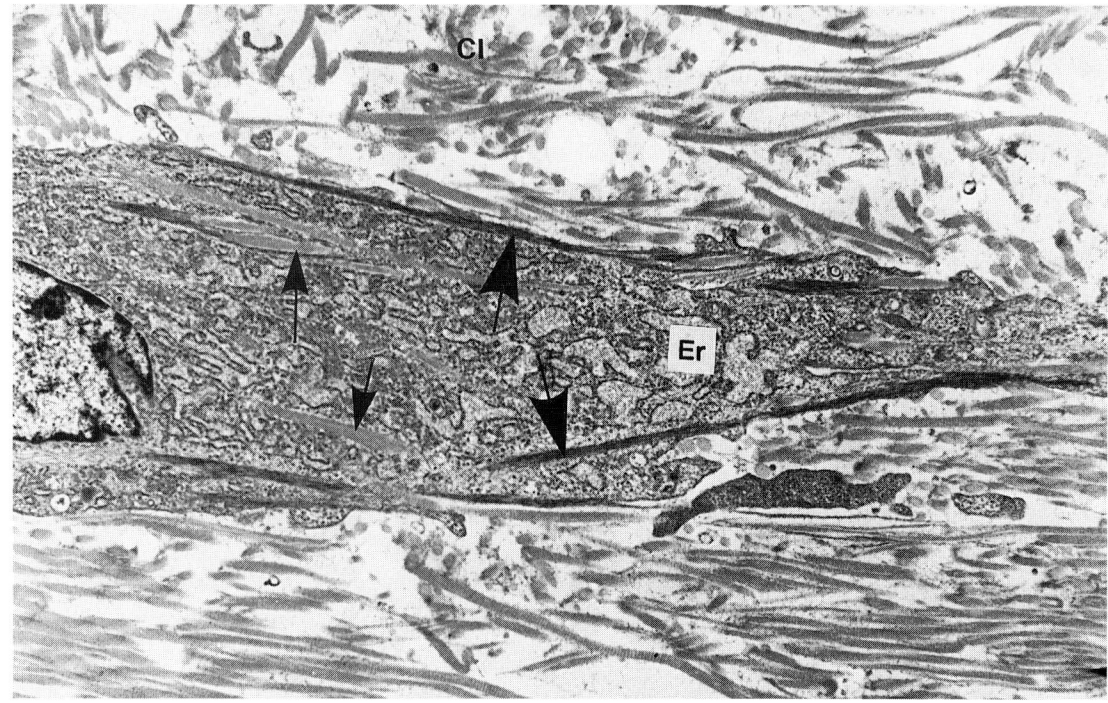

Fig. 10.7 Rat tail tendon resected 7 days in situ. Low power plan of remodelling fibroblast in a matrix of disaggregated collagen fibres (Cl). Dense stress fibres are common at the periphery of the cytoplasm (large arrows), with internalized collagen fibres deeper in the cytoplasm (small arrows) and an active and swollen endoplasmic reticulum in the central cytoplasm (Er). Magnification × 6500.

tissue remodelling, and collagen synthesis occurred concurrently within the same cells (Fig. 10.7; Birk & Trelstad 1985). Tendon bundles dissected free from the tail tendon, and transferred to and maintained in organ culture, also showed similar remodelling and shortening (contracture) within a 10-day period; (Slack et al 1986).

These and other electron microscopic studies of connective tissue remodelling which we have undertaken indicate that the cellular phagocytosis of extracellular collagen is often triphasic.

In phase one there is a cellular extension along and attachment to the collagen fibres via transmembrane linkages connecting the intracellular stress fibre and the fibronexus. Some collagen fibres appear to be drawn into extracellular clefts invaginated deep into the cellular cytoplasm. On longitudinal section these have the appearance of narrow fjords (Figs 10.7–10.9) but in transverse section are seen almost completely to encircle the entrapped fibres (Figs 10.10 and 10.11).

In phase 2 (Fig. 10.12) there appears to be a release of intact membrane-bound vesicles into these extracellular clefts around the collagen fibres. Release of the vesicle contents into the confined microenvironment of the extracellular cleft produces preliminary breakdown of the entrapped collagen fibres into smaller segments in preparation for internalization.

In phase 3 (Fig. 10.13) segments of collagen from the phase 2 predigestion are totally enclosed by constriction of the cell membrane around the extracellular cleft. The collagen fibres thus become truly internalized. Once internalized, the collagen segments fuse with the dense primary lysosomes from the Golgi to form a secondary lysosome which completes the disaggregation and denaturation of the collagen in preparation for synthetic recycling.

Similar zones of connective tissue remodelling have been observed within samples of apparently normal longitudinal palmar fascial bundles taken from adult post-mortem palmar samples, even from subjects in their mid 20s (see Fig. 10.6). We

CONTRACTION AND CONTRACTURE 113

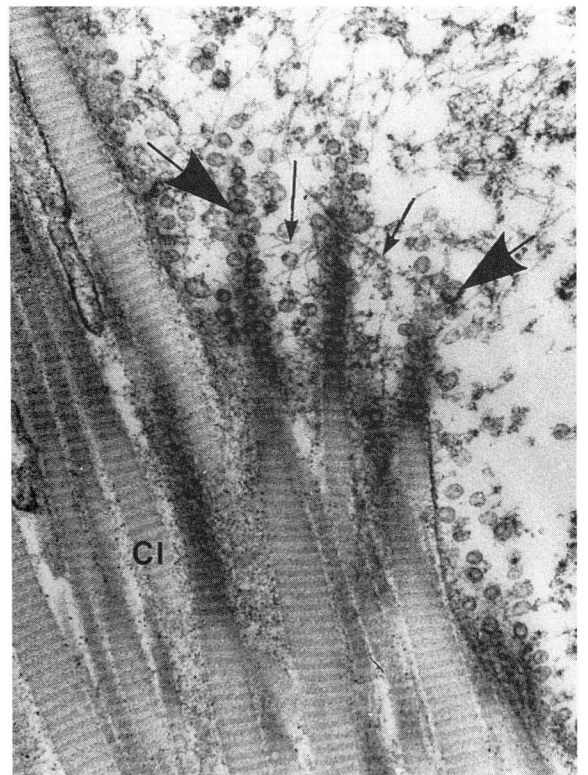

feel that the observation of intense connective tissue remodelling within apparently clinically normal and shiny, unaffected palmar fascial bundles provides a satisfactory explanation for the previous reports of increased type III collagen and increased glycosaminoglycan levels in apparently uninvolved palmar fascial fibres (Bailey et al 1977; Bazin et al 1980; Brickley-Parsons et al 1981). It is interesting in this regard that these changes have only been found in longitudinally running fascial fibre bundles and not in the transverse fibres (see Chapters 12 and 26) which are reportedly not primarily involved in the disease process (Skoog 1963). We would suggest that the apparently normal uninvolved fibre bundles examined biochemically in previous studies also contained microscopic zones of connective tissue remodelling

Fig. 10.8 Detail from remodelling rabbit FDP tendon illustrating the primary phase of collagen phagocytosis characterized by the aligment of many small vesicles along collagen (Cl) fibres closely opposed to the cell surface (large arrows) and the attachment of random actin filaments to the cell membrane in the vicinity of the collagen fibre and the small vesicles (small arrows). Magnification × 29 000.

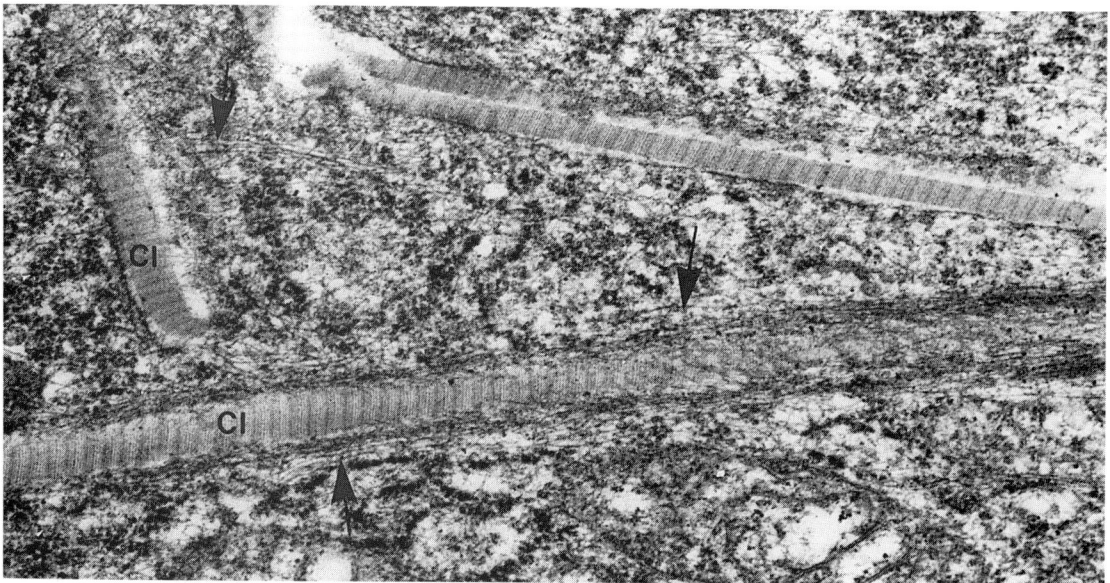

Fig. 10.9 Transected rat tail tendon 7 days postoperatively. Collagen fibres are enclosed within deep clefts in the cytoplasm. During the initial phase of phagocytosis, internalized collagen fibres (Cl) are often associated with and surrounded by numerous actin filaments (arrows). These appear to pull the collagen fibres into an extracellular cleft in preparation for the secondary phase of phagocytosis. Magnification × 38 000.

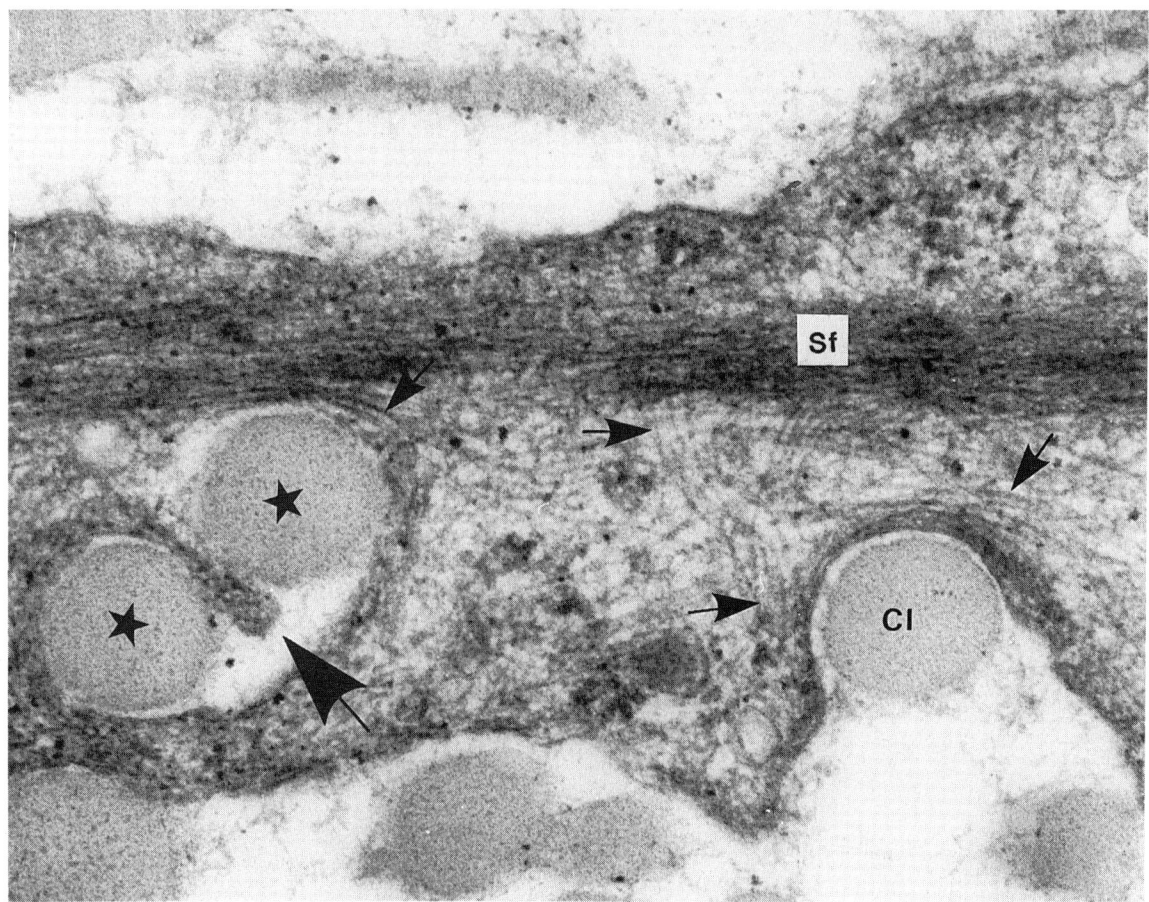

Fig. 10.10 Rat tail tendon experiments: a partially enveloped collagen fibre (Cl) forms an intimate contact with the cell membrane of a developing cleft, while two other collagen fibres (stars) appear totally enclosed within an extracellular cleft (large arrow) projecting into the cytoplasm. An important feature to note is the branching off from the stress fibre (Sf) of numerous actin filaments (small arrows) which make contact with the dense cell membrane adjacent to the collagen fibre, about to be internalized. This may suggest an active role for actin filaments during the initial phase of collagen internalization phagocytosis and remodelling. Magnification × 90 000.

and repair and thus could be expected to demonstrate changes in collagen type and glycosaminoglycan.

In the case of established DD the tendency for the hand to assume a finger-flexed posture provides no resistance or corrective signalling to prevent the effect of this constant reorganization and remodelling (Hueston 1975). As a result, the tissues on the volar surface of the hand and fingers, may actually remodel into a progressively shorter fabric length at an alarming rate to produce an actual skin or soft tissue deficit once a critical degree of flexion deformity has occurred.

Once the fingers and the Dupuytren's tissue have shortened and remodelled into a rigid fibrous mass, it is generally counterproductive to try to overcome the condition by forcible stretching over either a short or long time span. Increasing the distractive tensional loading by forcible stretching will generally induce a further accretion of collagen. This occurs as a result of the normal, biological feedback response by which increased loading induces collagen accretion and aggregation. If the stretching is even more forcible, leading to disruption and tearing, it will of course produce a new fascial wound repair situation, leading to further contracture and shortening.

However, if the tensional load is removed from

Fig. 10.11 Rat tail tendon cultured in vitro for 7 days begins remodelling of the matrix by extending long thin cell processes (Cp) along and around selected collagen fibres (Cl) and extracellular microfilament bundles (Mf). Magnification × 61 000.

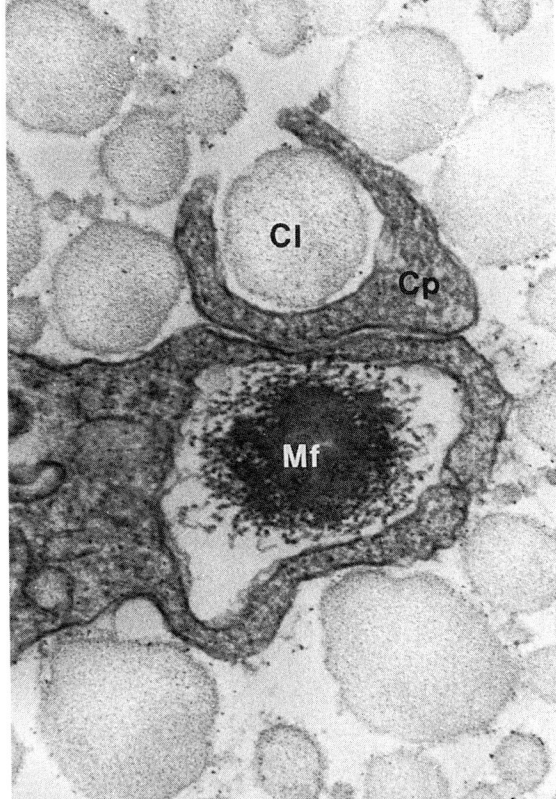

Fig. 10.12 Photomicrograph from remodelling rat tail tendon in vitro, illustrating the second phase of collagen phagocytosis. An active segment of the Golgi apparatus (G) is seen forming vesicles at its trans face (large arrow), while many small vesicles (small arrows) have now entered the space of the extracellular cleft formed during the primary phase of internalization. These vesicles are thought to act to partially digest the collagen fibre (Cl) within the confined environment of the extracellular cleft prior to complete internalization and digestion by primary lysosomes (during the third and final stage of collagen phagocytosis). Mt = Mitochondria. Magnification × 48 000.

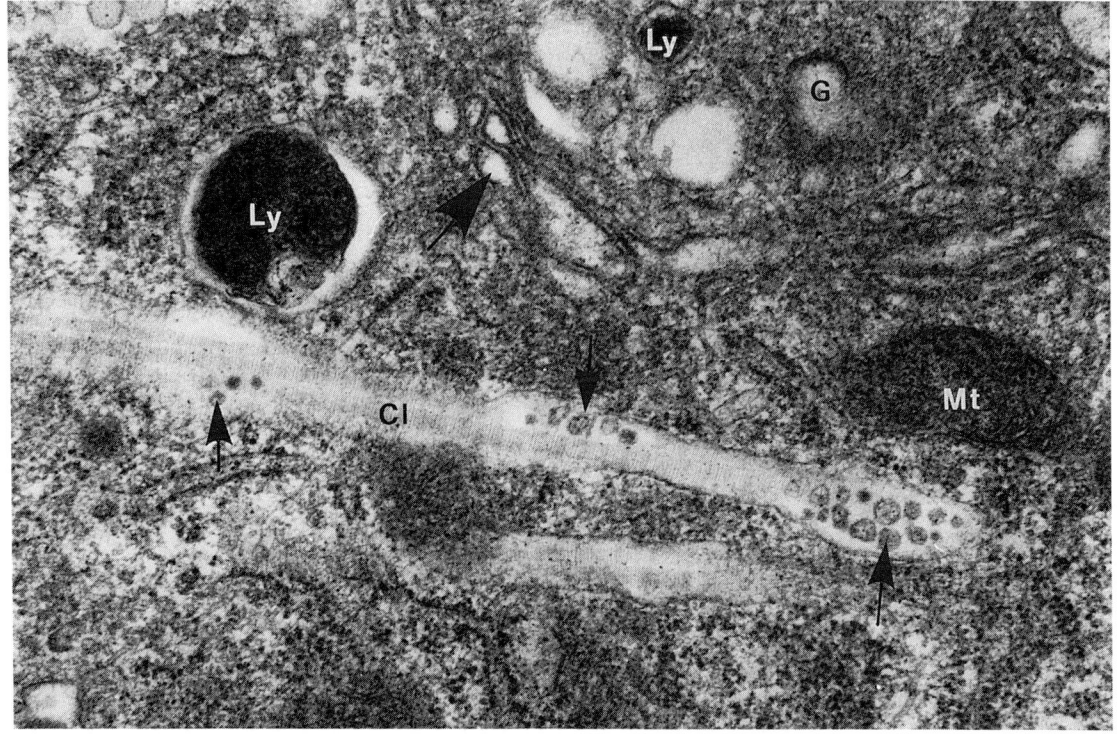

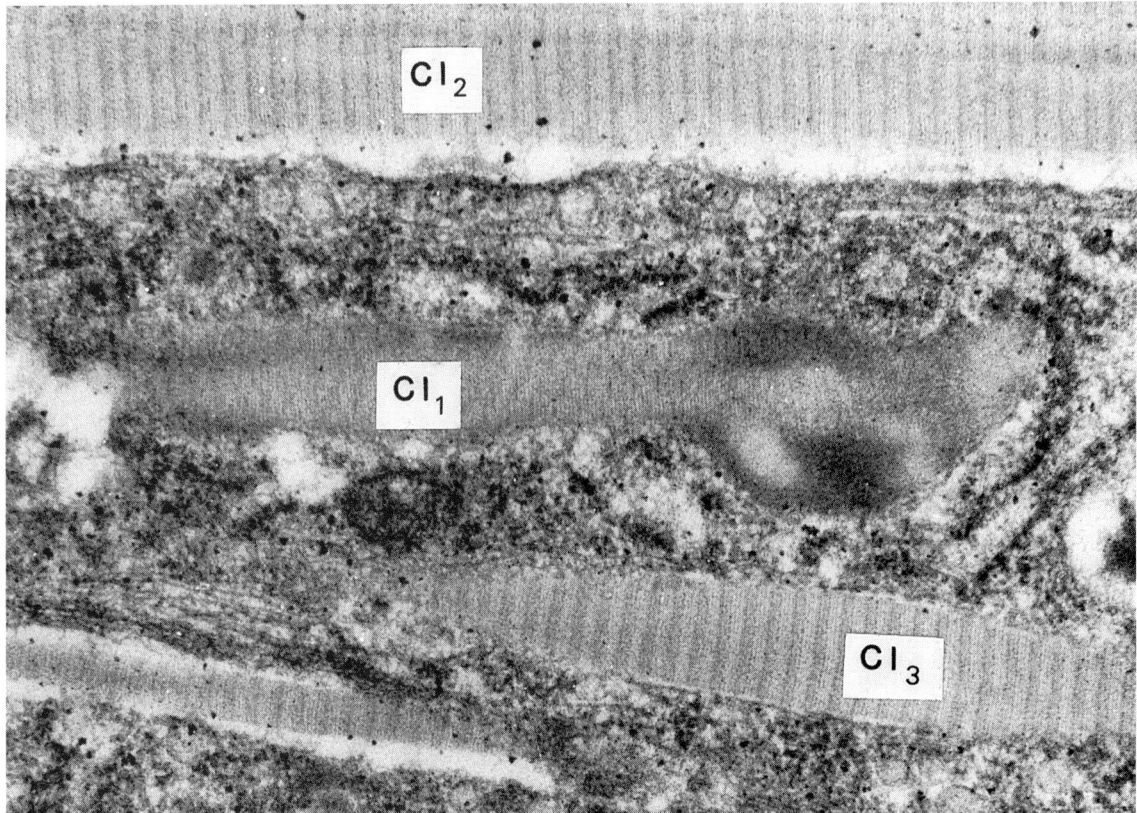

Fig. 10.13 Photomicrograph of a segment of collagen (Cl_1) during the third and final phase of phagocytosis. Note the loss of periodic striations of the collagen fibre in the secondary lysosome compared with those of extracellular collagen fibrils (Cl_2) and those internalized (Cl_3) awaiting the completion of phagocytosis. Magnification $\times$ 61 000.

the thickened fibrous cords or skin by tenotomy or Z-plasty, the cords are likely to soften spontaneously. This occurs by connective tissue remodelling following the release of tension (McGregor 1967; Flint 1972; Watson 1984; Thurston 1987). This effect is akin to, and governed by, the same laws of remodelling by which John Hunter, a surgical biologist in the late 18th century, had explained the growth and reshaping of long bones, and which was further developed in the framework of Wolff's law (Wolff 1892), and more recently in several writings by Frost (Frost 1964, 1988). In recent years it has been demonstrated that simple division or segmental removal of the fibrotic contracture (Kelly & Clifford 1959; Moermans & Duchateau 1984; Rowley et al 1984; see Moermans, Chapter 32) or the insertion of additional grafted skin after segmental division of contractures may satisfactorily promote a dissolution of the intrafascial nodules and the contractural process by allowing connective tissue remodelling to occur (Gonzales 1971; Ketchum & Hixson 1987). We believe that these effects are due to the release of longitudinal tension from the peripheral collagen fibres surrounding the intrafascial nodules and thereby the concomitant removal of centripetal pressure forces from the 'chondroid' cells of the nodule (see Chapters 2 and 12). The resultant cellular reorganization and synthetic maturation leads to softening and eventually to dissolution of the residual nodules. Hueston (1984) made use of similar biological effects in utilizing 'fire-break' grafts to prevent recurrence after excision of the contractural mass.

We believe that a proper understanding of the biological basis of contraction, contracture and connective tissue remodelling is essential to the correct clinical management of DD.

SECTION 2

Normal and pathological anatomy

K. A. Caughell and R. M. McFarlane

11 The development of the palmar fascia

INTRODUCTION

In spite of exhaustive anatomical studies of the palmar fascia there remain some points of controversy which are not only of academic interest but pertain to the onset and progress of Dupuytren's disease (DD). Is the palmar aponeurosis a disappearing structure or is it an important part of the supportive tissue of the palm? According to Stack (1973), Albinus described the palmar aponeurosis as an extension of the palmaris longus tendon in 1734. Wood Jones (1941) wrote:

The palmaris longus exists in ninety out of every hundred persons, but its function of flexing the metacarpophalangeal joint has been taken over by other muscles. Its degenerated tendons are now represented by a tendinous fascia which spreads fan-like in the palm but still divides into five slips, one slip running to the base of each digit.

Kaplan (1966) presents the opposite view:

If the midpalmar fascia, together with the palmaris longus tendon, would represent a remnant of a flexor superficialis there would have been, perhaps occasionally, instances where the midpalmar fascia would be absent in a way similar to the absence of the palmaris longus. . . . The connection of the midpalmar fascia with the palmaris longus tendon is incidental, inconstant and without particular significance.

Shrewsbury (personal communication) agrees that the palmaris longus tendon and palmar aponeurosis are only morphologically related but believes that the latter is a disappearing structure. His concern is that the pretendinous bands of the palmar aponeurosis bifurcate to pass on either side of the metacarpophalangeal joint and he believes that these terminal parts represent the remnants of paired superficial flexors. Weitbrecht (1742) described this distal bifurcation and Dupuytren (1832) stated that these slips contributed to the contraction.

If the palmar aponeurosis is disappearing then presumably it has no significant function. It is stated repeatedly that the palmar aponeurosis can be removed in patients with DD with no loss of function. The patients however do not necessarily agree and many of them will assert that 'something is missing' in the palm. Kaplan (1966) stated that the palmar aponeurosis functions to fix the metacarpus. Manske & Lesker (1983) showed that the transverse fibres of the palmar aponeurosis have a small but nevertheless significant retinacular function on the flexor tendons just proximal to the A_1 pulley. Two papers (Nieminen 1986; Powell et al 1986) suggest that DD does not appear in the absence of the palmaris longus tendon, that tension applied to the palmar aponeurosis by the palmaris longus may be a causative factor in DD and that resection of the tendon will reduce the incidence of recurrent disease.

If proximal tension upon the palmar aponeurosis contributes to DD then the observation of Fahrer (1980) must also be considered. He noted terminal fibres from the flexor carpi ulnaris tendon joining the palmar aponeurosis and concluded that in the absence of the palmaris longus tendon the flexor carpi ulnaris completely takes over as the longitudinal tensor of the palmar aponeurosis.

TERMINOLOGY

The varying descriptions and terminologies of the individual ligamentous components of the palmar fascia are described in Chapter 12.

Of particular interest is the fundamental difference of opinion about the septal partitions in the palm. Legueu & Juvara (1892) described septa passing deeply from the pretendinous bands of the palmar aponeurosis to form eight narrow compartments, four contained the digital flexor tendons and four the lumbrical muscles and neurovascular bundles. Kaplan (1966) denies the existence of these septa other than to say that they may be present as abnormal fascia in patients with DD. They are not mentioned by Wood Jones (1941) or Gray (1973). Bojsen-Moller & Schmidt (1974) demonstrated them in a precise anatomical study. They emphasized that the septa are of variable length and are most well developed distally. Further, they showed that distally these septa blend with the transverse metacarpal ligament. Two of their figures are reproduced here to show that these septa do exist (Figs 11.1 and 11.2). At operation, when the palmar aponeurosis is removed these septa are always seen and in fact are a guide to the preservation of the neurovascular bundles as the fascia is removed from one side of the palm to the other. It is interesting to note that these fascial septa are never diseased.

EMBRYOLOGICAL AND FETAL DEVELOPMENT OF THE PALMAR FASCIA

The early development of the limb bud is described according to Kuczynski (1972). The upper limb appears at the 26th day post fertilization opposite the lower cervical somites and is initially represented as a condensation of mesoderm which extends as a longitudinal crest on the lateral surface of the embryo. The cranial end of this crest proliferates to form the upper limb bud while the caudal end gives rise to the lower limb bud somewhat later. The limb bud grows rapidly. Initially it appears as a paddle but later becomes scalloped as the digital rays appear. By 5 weeks nerves have grown into the hand; by 6 weeks the digits have separated. They are fully

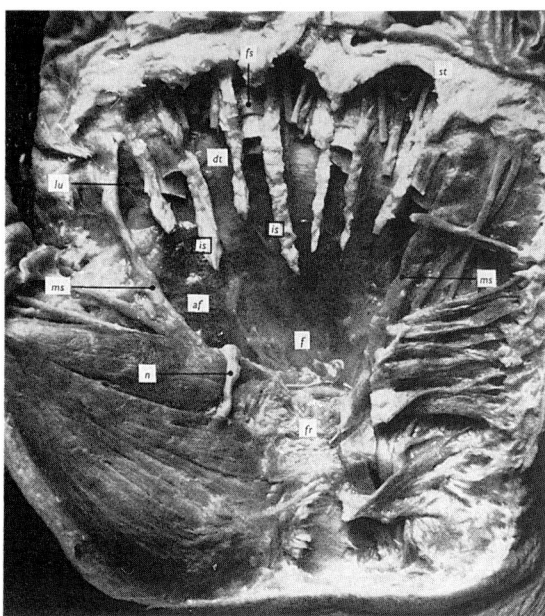

Fig. 11.1 The two marginal (ms) and seven intermediate (is) septa of Legueu & Juvara (1892), creating eight compartments. From the radial side the second, fourth, sixth and eighth compartments contain flexor tendons; the others contain lumbricals and neurovascular bundles. af, adductor fascia; lu, lumrical canal; dt, deep transverse metacarpal ligament; f, fat body; fr flexor retinaculum; fs, fibrous flexor sheaths; n, nerve to thenar muscles; st, superficial transverse metacarpal ligament. From Bojsen-Moller & Schmidt (1974).

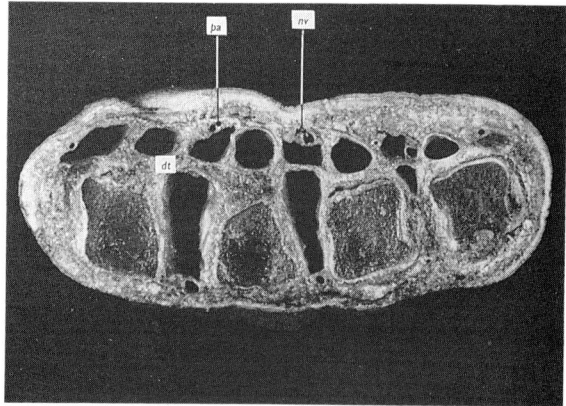

Fig. 11.2 Cross-section of the septa and compartments. From Bojsen-Moller & Schmidt (1974). nv, interdigital nerves and vessels; dt, deep transverse metacrapal ligament; pa, palmar aponeurosis.

THE DEVELOPMENT OF THE PALMAR FASCIA 121

formed and ossification has begun by the 8th week. This marks the end of the embryonic period and the beginning of the fetal period, at which time all structures and organs are present. During the fetal period further changes consist primarily of an increase in size and proportion of parts.

Our own studies (Caughell et al 1987) have examined hands from 5 weeks' gestation to term to identify the various components of the palmar fascia and, in particular, to determine the relationship between the palmar aponeurosis and the palmaris longus tendon. Thirty-three hands were examined. Gestational ages of the specimens were calculated by using the crown–rump length and dates from the last menstrual period. Once specimens were obtained, they were placed in either 10% formalin or 3% buffered gluteraldehyde solution, depending upon whether they were to be processed for light or scanning electron microscopy respectively. Twelve specimens were examined with the scanning electron microscope and 21 with the light microscope. In those specimens selected for light microscopy the hands, after fixation, were embedded in paraffin and sectioned either longitudinally or in cross-section. Sections of 15 μ thickness were obtained and stained with trichrome stain which differentiates between nerve, muscle, tendon and fascia. In those specimens selected for scanning by electron microscopy, a critical point freeze-drying technique was used and specimens were coated with gold using a Polaron Sputter Coater.

The palmar aponeurosis

The earliest hand examined was of 5 weeks' gestational age (Fig. 11.3). The palmar aponeurosis was present. Light microscopy revealed that the palmar aponeurosis consisted of longitudinal and transverse layers which were very thin and predominantly cellular (Fig. 11.4). The vertical

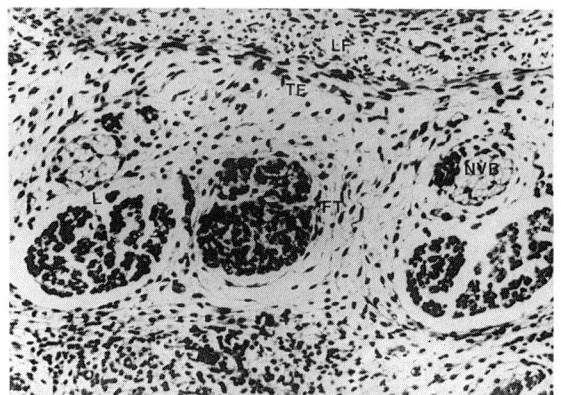

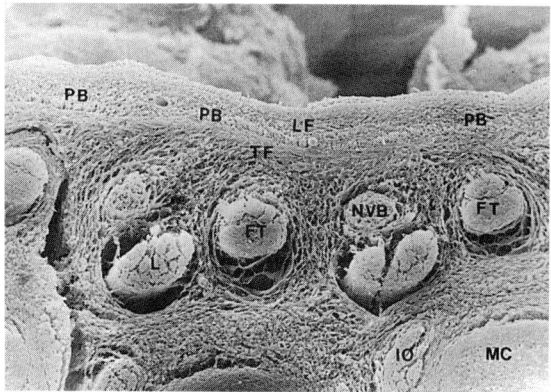

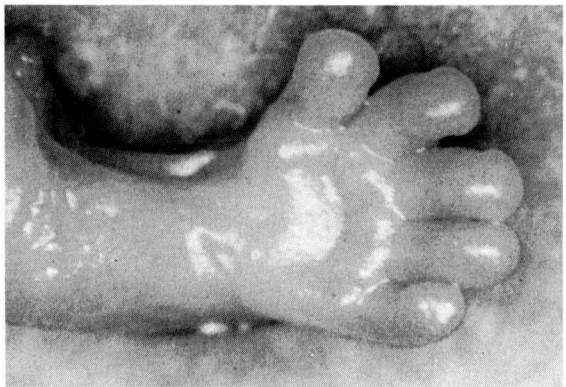

Fig. 11.3 A 5 weeks' gestation hand. It measures 2 mm in length. Note the absence of palmar and digital creases.

Fig. 11.4 A Light micrograph of a 5 weeks' gestation hand in cross-section at the level of the mid-palm. Both longitudinal (LF) and transverse fibres (TF) of the palmar aponeurosis are present, but both layers are predominantly cellular. The flexor tendons (FT), lumbricals (L) and neurovascular bundles (NVB) are indicated. Original magnification × 250. B The corresponding scanning electron micrograph. Longitudinal fibres (LF) and transverse fibres (TF) are more clearly demonstrated. Even at this early stage of development the longitudinal fibres are concentrated into pretendinous bands (PB). Note the loose areolar tissue between the flexor tendons (FT) and lumbricals (L). This areolar tissue represents the septa of Legueu & Juvara (1892). The deeper structures of metacarpal bone (MC) and interosseous muscle (IO) are marked. Original magnification × 45.

septa of Legueu & Juvara (1892) were seen in this specimen as loose areolar tissue coursing between the flexor tendons, the lumbrical muscles and neurovascular bundles. These septa appeared to arise from the transverse fibres of the palmar aponeurosis. At 12 weeks' gestation the septa were well developed and were distinct anatomical structures, as shown by scanning electron microscopy (Fig. 11.5).

The presence of the palmaris longus tendon

When the tendon of the palmaris longus muscle was present, longitudinal sections revealed that the tendon was in direct continuity with the longitudinal fibres of the palmar aponeurosis. With trichrome stain (Fig. 11.6) the tendon of the palmaris longus muscle stained black similar to the flexor tendons, whereas the palmar aponeurosis stained a blue-green like that of the transverse carpal ligament and antebrachial fascia. The transformation from tendon to fascia occurred gradually over the area of the transverse carpal ligament, as shown in the series of scanning electron micrographs in Figure 11.7.

The absence of the palmaris longus tendon

It was not difficult, even in early specimens, to determine the presence or absence of the palmaris longus tendon (Fig. 11.8). In five specimens the tendon was absent. Both longitudinal and transverse layers of the palmar aponeurosis were present. Proximally the longitudinal fibres blended with the transverse carpal ligament or antebrachial fascia. Distally they terminated at the level of the metacarpophalangeal joint by passing both deep and superficial to the natatory ligament (Figs 11.9–11.11).

The natatory ligament and Cleland's and Grayson's ligaments

In early specimens these structures are not present as definite fascial entities but abundant tissue is present to account for their later development. In Figure 11.12 the natatory ligament is identified as a layer of fascia that passes transversely from one tendon sheath to another as it does in the adult. The fibres of Cleland's and Grayson's ligaments are not clearly defined, although Figure 11.13 clearly shows fibres and cells from the core of the digit, surrounding the neurovascular bundle and related to the skin. In the same way, the vertical fibres of the palmar aponeurosis, described by Mc-

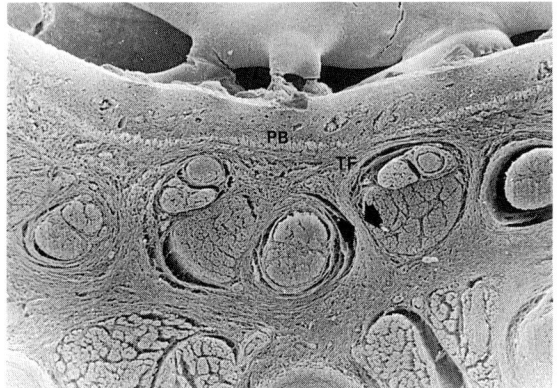

Fig. 11.5 Scanning electron micrograph of a 12 weeks' gestation hand in cross-section at the level of the distal palm. The pretendinous bands (PB) are now clearly seen. Transverse fibres (TF) are located immediately deep to the longitudinal fibres and appear to sweep downwards (arrows) to form the vertical septa of Legueu & Juvara (1892). Original magnification × 45.

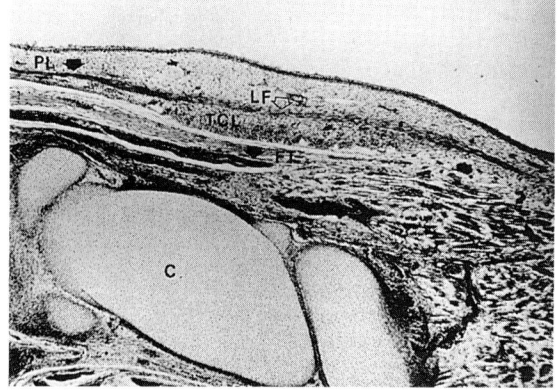

Fig. 11.6 Light micrograph of an 8 weeks' gestation hand at the level of the carpus (c) in longitudinal section. The longitudinal fibres (LF) of the palmar aponeurosis stain like fascia, similar to the transverse carpal ligament (TCL). The fibres of the palmaris longus, (PL) tendon stain dark, similar to the flexor tendons (FT and arrow). This trichrome stain actually stains tendon black and connective tissue green. Note that the palmaris longus tendon is in direct continuity with the longitudinal fibres of the palmar aponeurosis. Original magnification × 18.

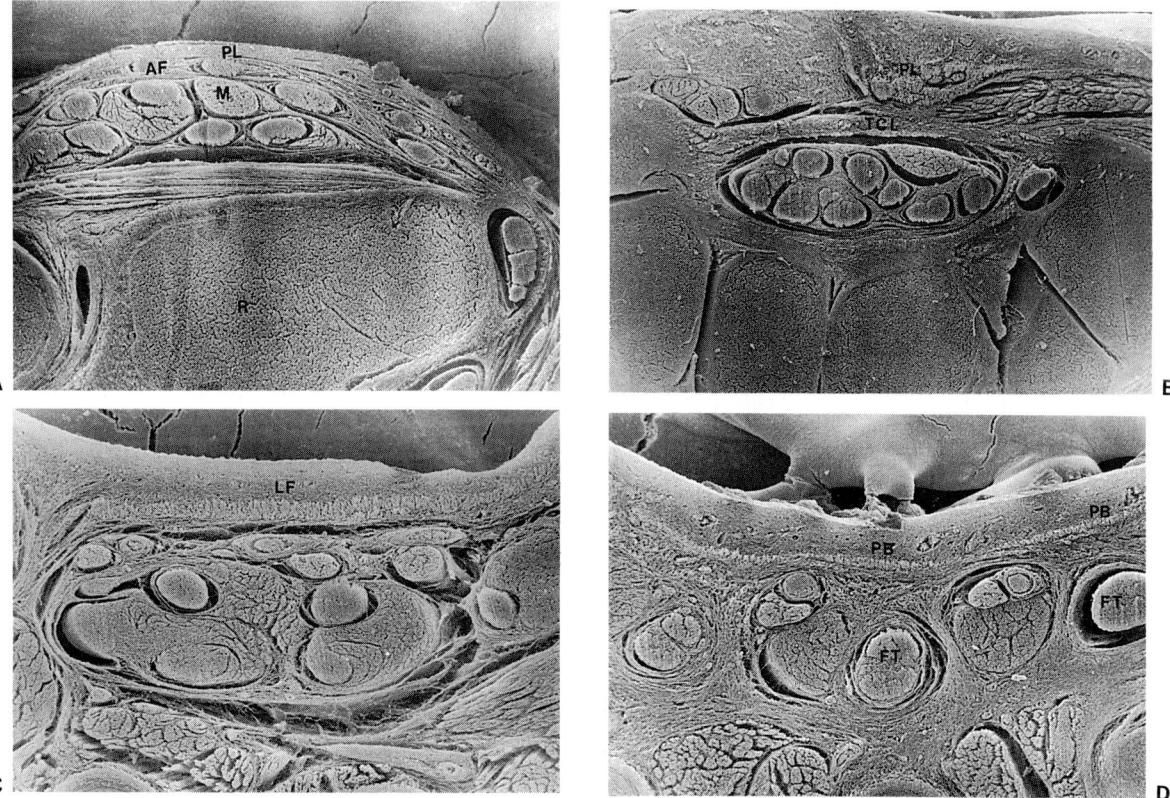

Fig. 11.7 Scanning electron micrograph of a 12 weeks' gestation hand at four levels. **A** Distal radius (R). The palmaris longus, (PL) tendon is superficial to the antebrachial fascia (AF) and median nerve (M). **B** Carpal tunnel. The palmaris longus (PL) tendon is beginning to flatten out. The transverse carpal ligament (TCL) is shown superficial to the contents of the carpal tunnel. **C** Proximal palm. The tendon of the palmaris longus is now represented by the longitudinal fibres (LF) of the palmar aponeurosis. **D** Distal palm. Pretendinous bands (PB) are seen superficial to each flexor tendon (FT). Original magnification × 45.

Grouther (1982) were not seen early. However, by the 12th gestational week, concurrent with the appearance of dermal ridges and creases, the vertical fibres were apparent.

The fascial layers of the palm

In keeping with the 'continuous fascia' theory of Backhouse and the fascial layers described by Stack (1973), this study has identified in the longitudinal sections three layers of fascia: a superficial, a retinacular, and a deep layer. These layers are shown diagrammatically in Figure 11.14 but can also be identified in Figures 11.6, 11.9 and 11.11. This concept of layers is of more than academic interest. It seems that only the superficial layer — the pretendinous bands — the natatory ligament and Grayson's ligament are involved in Dupuytren's disease. This suggests that the anatomical location of the fascia is fundamental to the development of disease. Placing the transverse fibres of the palmar aponeurosis in the retinacular layer is consistent with Manske & Lesker's (1983) observation that these fibres have a pulley function, as well as with Kaplan's (1966) view that they retain the metacarpals.

DISCUSSION

The palmar aponeurosis is a constant structure. It is always present, whereas the palmaris longus tendon is absent in 11–23% of people (Kaplan 1966). Furthermore it is identifiable at the end of the

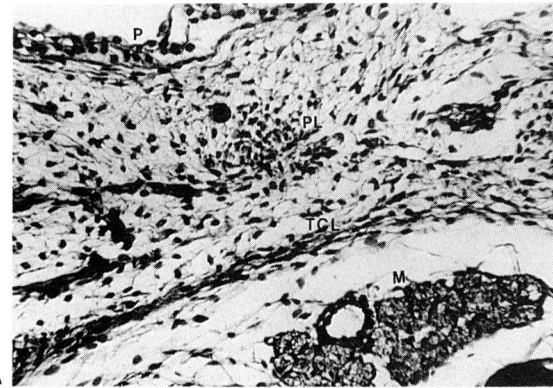

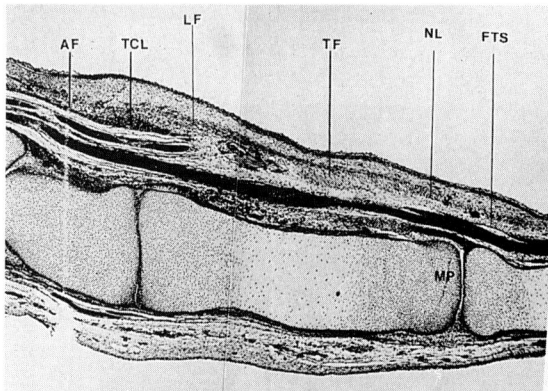

Fig. 11.9 Light micrograph of 8 weeks' gestation hand in longitudinal section. The palmaris longus tendon is absent. The longitudinal fibres (LF) of the palmar aponeurosis commence at the level of the transverse carpal ligament (TCL) and terminate at the metacarpophalangeal joint. The antebrachial fascia (AF) is seen proximally and is in continuity with the transverse carpal ligament and the transverse fibres (TF) of the palmar aponeurosis. The natatory ligament (NL) and flexor tendon sheath (FTS) are indicated. Original magnification × 18.

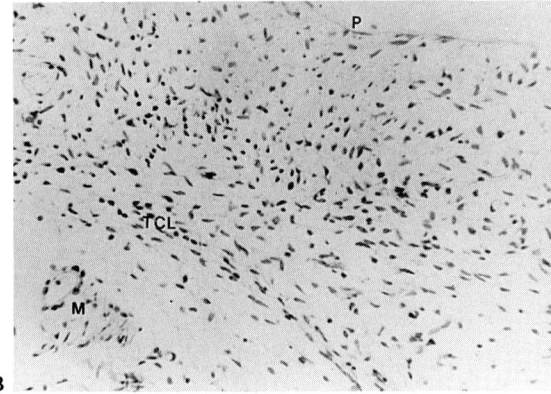

Fig. 11.8 A Light micrograph of a 6 weeks' gestation hand at the level of the carpal tunnel. The palmaris longus (PL) tendon is present, located superficial to the transverse carpal ligament (TCL). The median nerve (M) is located in the carpal tunnel. The palmar (P) surface of the hand is at the top of the figure. Original magnification × 18. B Light micrograph of a 6 weeks' gestation hand at the level of the carpal tunnel. The palmaris longus tendon is absent in this specimen. The transverse carpal ligament (TCL) and the median nerve (M) are seen. The palmar (P) surface of the hand is indicated. Original magnification × 18.

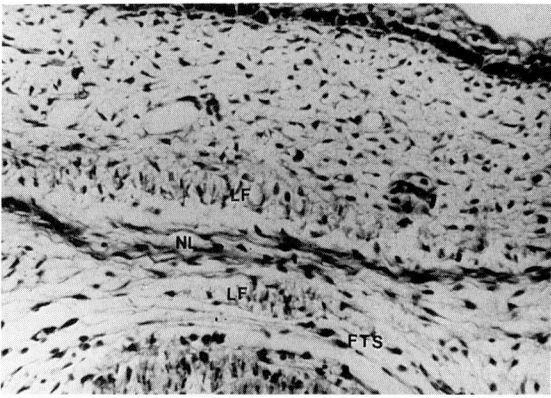

Fig. 11.10 Light micrograph of an 8 weeks' gestation hand at the level of the metacarpophalangeal joint. This cross-section illustrates the longitudinal fibres (LF) of the palmar aponeurosis coursing superficial and deep to the natatory ligament (NL). The flexor tendon sheath (FTS) is located at the bottom of the micrograph and the basal layer of the epidermis is at the top. Original magnification × 114.

embryonic period of development (6 weeks) as having both longitudinal and transverse layers. Zancolli & Zancolli (1984) felt that the palmar aponeurosis did not develop until later fetal life and that the transverse fibres appeared first. The aponeurosis at 6 weeks' gestation is just a few cells thick and can only be identified microscopically. The scanning electron microscope complements the light microscope in demonstrating these structures.

In a series of three papers Dylevsky (1968, 1969, 1973) described the phylogenetic development, the comparative anatomy and the association of DD with the palmar aponeurosis. He found that the longitudinal and transverse parts of the palmar aponeurosis developed simultaneously as an independent fibrous structure not related to any muscle layer of the palm. He studied the phylogenetic development of 55

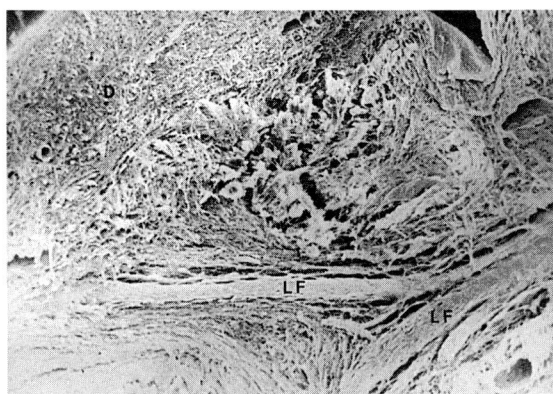

Fig. 11.11 Scanning electron micrograph of an 8 weeks' gestation hand in the longitudinal plane at the level of the metacarpophalangeal joint. The longitudinal fibres (LF) are diverging towards the dermis (D) and the deeper fibres towards the tendon sheath. Original magnification × 45.

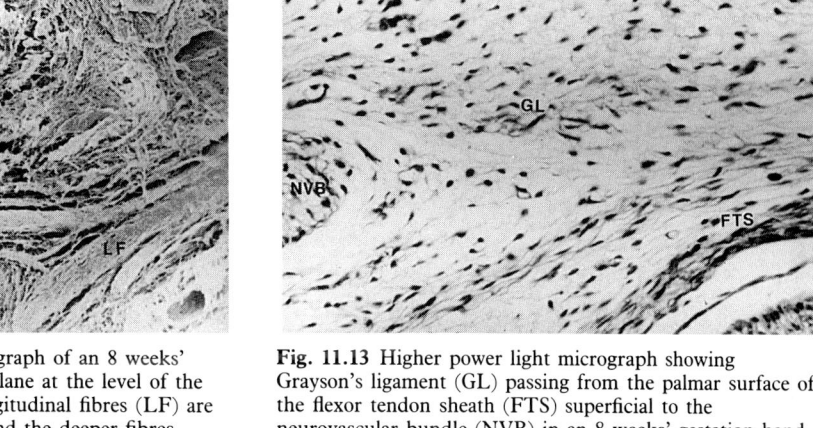

Fig. 11.13 Higher power light micrograph showing Grayson's ligament (GL) passing from the palmar surface of the flexor tendon sheath (FTS) superficial to the neurovascular bundle (NVB) in an 8 weeks' gestation hand. Original magnification × 114.

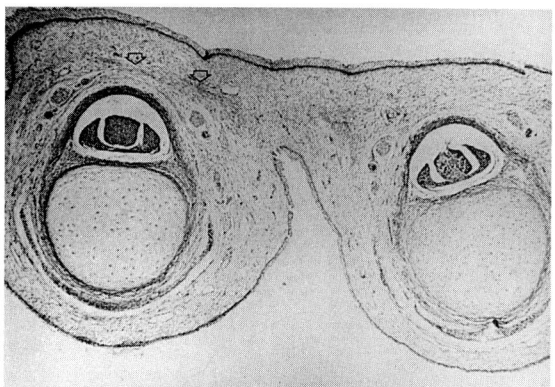

Fig. 11.12 Light micrograph of an 8 weeks' gestation hand at the level of the web space. The natatory ligament (arrows) courses from web space to web space. Original magnification × 18.

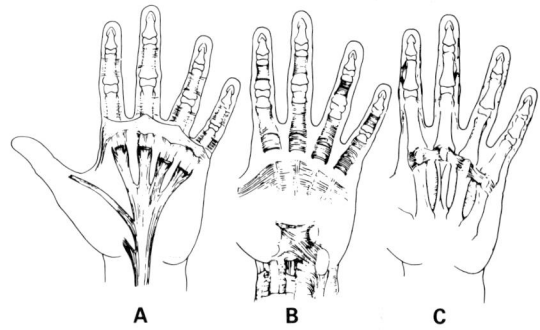

Fig. 11.14 The three layers of fascia in the palm and fingers. A The superficial layer consisting of Grayson's ligaments, natatory ligament and longitudinal fibres of the palmar aponeurosis. B The retinacular layer consisting of the flexor tendon sheath, the transverse fibres of the palmar aponeurosis and the transverse carpal ligament. C The deep layer consisting of Cleland's ligaments, the transverse metacarpal ligament and the interosseous fascia.

forelimbs in 22 species. The complete absence of the palmar aponeurosis was exceptional except in Monotremata. In Marsupialia, Insectvora and Tripaiidae there was a flexor brevis V as well as a differentiated palmar aponeurosis. He concluded that there was no relationship between the short flexors of the palm and the palmar aponeurosis and furthermore that DD does not arise from degenerated muscle layers of the palm, as had been proposed by Krogius (1921).

It is assumed by many authorities, and described best by Wood Jones (1941), that the original function of the palmaris longus muscle is to flex the metacarpophalangeal joint. In support of the adult appearance of the palmaris longus with a short muscle belly and a long tendon, as well as a well developed sheet of palmar aponeurosis, he writes:

Tendons may develop merely as a degenerative product of muscles which are waning in importance. We may say that muscle, tendon and fascia represent definite stages of degeneration, that is, muscle becomes more and more tendinous and tendon becomes more and more fascial.

Le Gros Clark (1958), discussing retrogressive variations of muscles, stated that the palmaris longus was a superficial flexor of the fingers in primitive mammals and the distal part has degenerated into the palmar fascia. However the earlier work of Lewis (1901) describes the embryological development of the forearm muscles as a superficial and deep group. The superficial group are the flexor carpi radialis, the pronator teres and the palmaris longus whereas the deep group consists of the flexor carpi ulnaris, the sublimis and profundus flexors. He noted the characteristic adult arrangement of the tendons in a 250 mm embryo. According to Lewis the palmaris longus develops with two other forearm muscles and is more likely to be a wrist than a finger flexor.

CONCLUSIONS

There are opposing views of the phylogenetic status of the palmar aponeurosis. We believe that it is not a disappearing structure because it has a definite function in maintaining the integrity of the palm. Also, we share Kaplan's view that the relationship between the palmar aponeurosis and palmaris longus tendon is only one of anatomical proximity. The evidence is as follows:

1. The palmaris longus develops from a muscle mass (with the flexor carpi radialis and pronator teres) which does not extend distal to the wrist.
2. There is no phylogenetic relationship between the short digital flexors and the palmar aponeurosis.
3. During embryonic development the palmaris longus tendon stains like tendon whereas the palmar aponeurosis stains like fascia.
4. The palmaris longus tendon may be absent but the palmar aponeurosis is never absent.
5. The morphology of the palmar aponeurosis is the same in the presence or absence of the palmaris longus tendon.
6. The palmar aponeurosis has a retinacular function to retain the metacarpals and the flexor tendons as well as to support the palmar skin against compressive and shearing forces.

D. A. McGrouther

12 The palm

'Le système fibreux de la paume de la main forme un tout continu dont on peut pour les besoins seulement d'une description dissocier les dieffrents éléments constituants' (Legueu & Juvara 1892).

These French authors, who produced a comprehensive description of the fascias of the hand, were well aware that the fibrous fascial systems form a continuum and that separation for the purposes of description is artificial.

The many published descriptions of the individual parts of the palmar fascial continuum have been confused by varying terminology and the use of eponyms, despite the recommendations of Nomina Anatomica. Confusion has arisen because individual fascial structures have been singled out by posterity, often without precise definition, and named in this way. By contrast the original anatomical reports have frequently presented comprehensive descriptions of the entire fascial network rather than of one fascial structure alone. The need for a standard terminology is apparent.

Even the terms palmar fascia and palmar aponeurosis are rather imprecise; the longitudinal fibres in the midpalm have been variously termed the central portion of the palmar fascia (Wood Jones 1941) the mid palmar fascia or aponeurosis (Kaplan 1965) and the central part of the palmar aponeurosis (Gray 1973). All of these names give undue emphasis to this one part of the fascia of the hand. The term 'palmar' mistakenly implies confinement to the palmar area, whereas the digits and dorsal surfaces also have well defined fascias. It is better to consider the connective tissues of the hand as forming a fascial continuum or fibrous skeleton. It would therefore be more accurate to consider the site of DD as the fascial continuum of the hand; the portion in the central palmar area is best described according to the individual fibre bundles involved, for example, pretendinous longitudinal bands etc,

A working knowledge of the fascial ligaments of the palm is not just an academic pursuit but of practical value to the Dupuytren's surgeon who is thereby able to perform a more precise dissection, limiting tissue trauma, and securely preserving vital structures. The normal anatomy becomes distorted in a predictable fashion according to the particular fascial strands which are contracting; a precision approach to dissection of displaced neurovascular bundles is necessary.

The historical perspective is humbling. Detailed morphological description predated Dupuytren who had a much greater knowledge of the fascial anatomy than is often appreciated. An early account by Bartholinus (1668) is not only remarkable for its clarity and clear printing in the English language but is also far-seeing in its relationships of form and function: 'under the skin in the hollow of the hand is a broad tendon ... it seems to have been made that the hand might take the better hold, when the skin of the palm is wrinkled'.

In the 18th century, the loose subcutaneous planes (of the hand and elsewhere) were generally referred to as the 'cellular membrane', as mentioned in lectures by William Hunter. This term is no less vague but much more elegant than fascia. Fascial ligament or band are terms which seem to portray a well defined and orientated structure within the fibrous tissue continuum of the hand.

Goyrand (1834) considered that Dupuytren's contracture occurred in tissue *'de nouvelle formation*', but in a discussion of his paper, Sanson (1834) made the statement that the 'contracted bands were only the exaggeration by fibrous tissue of the aponeurosis which existed in health'. This was a clear statement (perhaps the first) that DD *follows anatomical pathways*. McFarlane (1974) has shown the precise way in which the contracture develops along anatomical structures.

In the 20th century standard reference texts have paid less and less attention to fine detail of gross anatomy where it does not seem to have immediate surgical application. Early this century anatomical interest was focused on the palmar spaces and potential spaces because of relevance to infection (Kanavel 1925; Anson & Ashley 1940). A decline in infections has rendered the anatomy of spaces of less immediate interest than the anatomy of the fascial structures themselves and this has been reflected in the literature. However, an excellent article by Bojsen-Moller & Schmidt (1974) reviews the spaces.

OVERALL PLAN OF ANATOMY

It is necessary to present a general plan which is comprehensible to the surgeon. Each fascial band will be considered in some detail with explanations of alternative descriptions and nomenclatures.

There is less controversy in relation to the structure of the transverse ligamentous systems, although there has been confusion in terminology (Table 12.1, Fig. 12.1). In particular, the term 'superficial' has been applied to a number of structures lying at different levels. The two main transverse fibre systems are the natatory ligament and the transverse fibres of the palmar aponeurosis.

The natatory ligament

These fascial ligaments span the distal palm at the palmar digital junction (Fig. 12.1). In all hands fibres run around the apex of the web skin from digit to digit but in some individuals there are also well defined transverse fibres running across the distal palm. These fascial structures have been described by Bourgery (1834) and Gerdy (cited by

Maslieurat-Lagemard 1839). Legueu & Juvara (1892) used the term 'interdigital ligament' and Grapow (1887) '*Schwimmband*'. Standard anatom-

Table 12.1 Transverse structures in the palm

Terminology			Corresponding diseased cords
Natatory ligament			
Wood Jones	—	ligamentum natorium or interdigital ligament	May form part of lateral cord
Kaplan	—	ligamentum natorium or interdigital ligament	
Gray	—	superficial transverse metacarpal ligament	
Transverse fibres of the palmar aponeurosis (TFPA)			Not involved
Wood Jones	—	superficial transverse palmar ligament	
Kaplan	—	superficial transverse palmar ligament	
Gray	—	transverse fibres of the palmar aponeurosis	
Skoog	—	transverse palmar ligament (superficial transverse ligament)	
Transverse metacarpal ligament			Not involved
Wood Jones	—	transverse metacarpal ligament	
Kaplan	—	deep transverse intermetacarpal ligament	
Gray	—	deep transverse metacarpal ligament	
Transverse structures in first web space			
Tubiana	—	**Proximal commissural ligament**	Proximal commissural cord
Tubiana	—	**Distal commissural ligament**	Distal commissural cord

Recommended terms are given in bold.
References: Wood Jones (1941); Kaplan (1965); Gray (1973); Skoog (1967); Tubiana et al (1982).

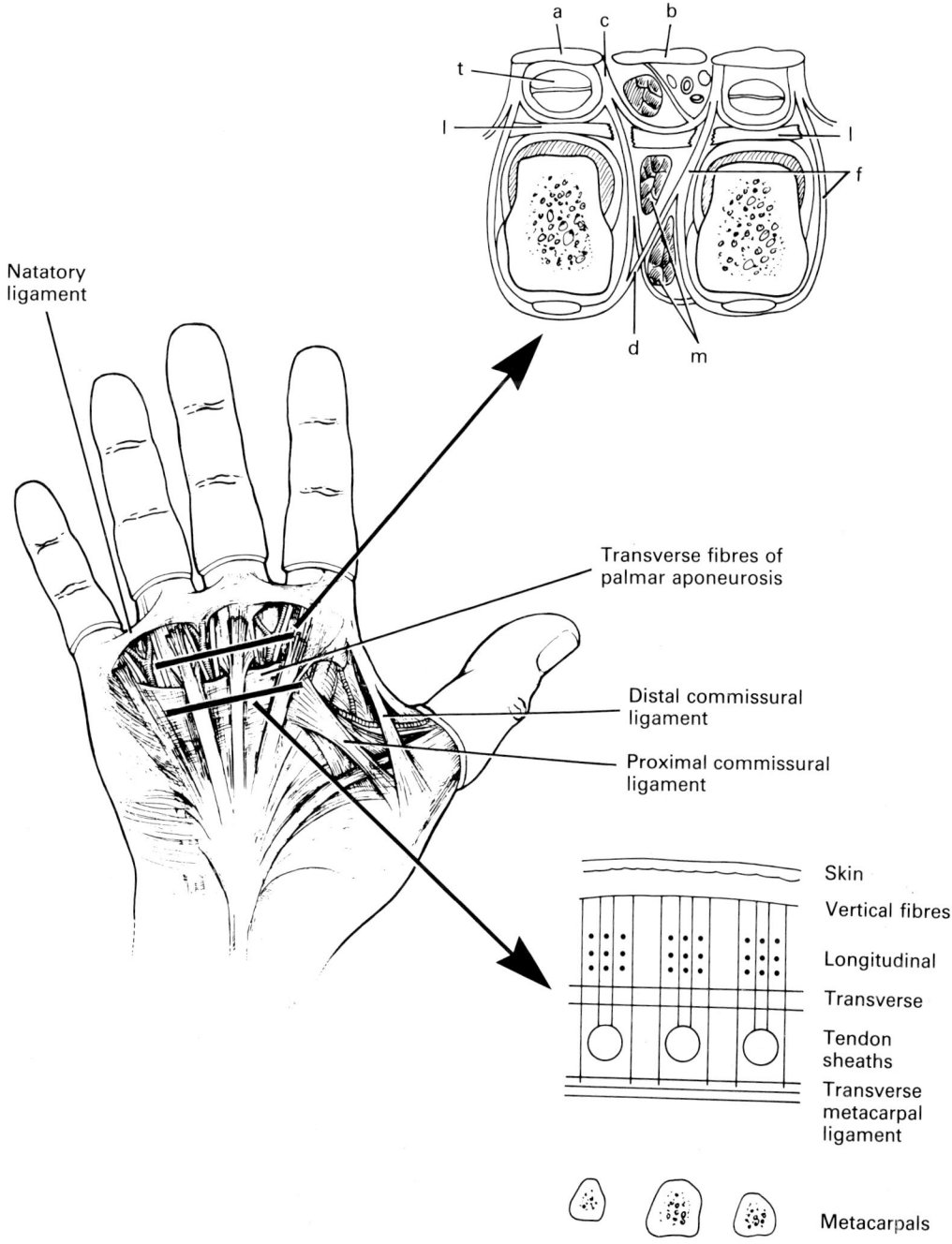

Fig. 12.1 Transverse fascial structures in the palm and first web space. **Top inset:** Cross-section of the hand at the level of the heads of the metacarpal bones. a = Pretendinous band; b = prelumbrical band (a and b together form the palmar aponeurosis); c = longitudinal septum penetrating the transverse metacarpal ligament (l), reaching the dorsal aspect of the hand (d). m = Interosseous muscles; t = flexor tendons. From Legueu & Juvara (1892). **Bottom inset:** The longitudinal fibres cut in cross-section, lying in channels between the skin superficially, transverse fibres deeply and vertical fibres laterally. From McGrouther (1982).

ical nomenclature recommends 'superficial transverse metacarpal ligament', which is confusing. The term most used by surgeons is the natatory ligament, or Schwimmband. The natatory ligament in the first web has also been called the distal commissural ligament (Tubiana et al 1982).

The natatory ligament is generally considered to limit the spreading of the skin of the palm and the separation of adjacent fingers. Grapow's (1887) concept of the function of the Schwimmband is interesting. He pictured four trapezoid web spaces lying between the transverse and longitudinal fibre systems. He described this area as forming a bellows mechanism for the pumping of blood and lymph out of the fingers, with suction being applied when the fingers are spread. This concept has received little attention since then.

The transverse fibres of the palmar aponeurosis (TFPA)

These fibres, which are well developed discrete unbranching silvery glistening tendinous structures, lie more proximally than the natatory ligament and on a deeper plane. The longitudinal pretendinous fibres lie anterior to the TFPA and their distal extensions (layers 2 and 3, see below) are posterior to the natatory fibres. Thus the different transverse fibre systems can be readily distinguished.

Legueu & Juvara (1892) and Skoog (1967 ab) used the term superficial transverse ligament. However, 'superficial' has been confusing and these fibres have been termed in Nomina Anatomica the transverse fibres of the palmar aponeurosis. Skoog considered that these fibres were never contracted in DD and advised their careful preservation during selective fasciectomy. The distal edge of the fibres underlies the distal palmar crease and they have been attributed a retinacular role (Manske & Lesker 1983). Legueu & Juvara (1892) considered that the TFPA together with the bifurcating pretendinous languettes (see below) contributed to the formation of a *palmar tendinous sheath*. Medially and laterally the TFPA extend to fascias over the thenar and hypothenar muscles. A radial extension to the first ray has been called the proximal commissural ligament by Tubiana et al (1982, 1985). This is fully described in Chapter 16.

Transverse metacarpal ligament

This deep layer has been beautifully illustrated by Weitbrecht (1742; see Fig. 12.2); and Zancolli (1979). It consists of strong transverse fibres deep to the flexor sheaths in continuity with the volar plates.

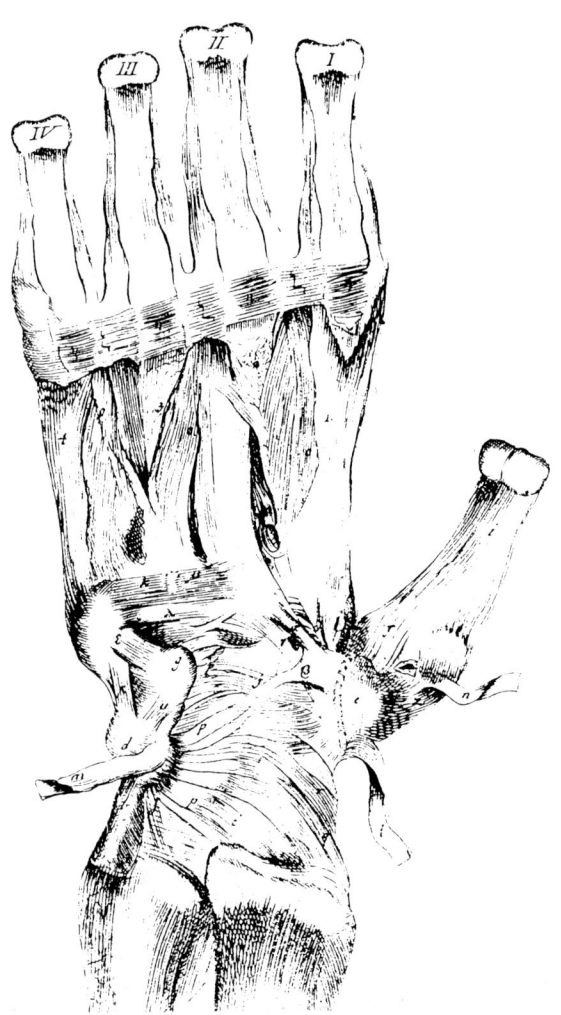

Fig. 12.2 Weitbrecht (1742) described in detail the ligamentous structures within the hand. Here the transverse metacarpal ligament is shown.

LONGITUDINAL FIBRE SYSTEMS

Proximal palm — Longitudinal pretendinous fibres

Albinus (1734), Weitbrecht (1742) and Dupuytren (1831) recognized four longitudinal pretendinous bands of palmar fascial fibres, one for each digital ray, passing distally from the wrist in a plane anterior to the flexor tendons and seeming to bifurcate in the distal palm to pass on either side of the flexor tendons. (The original accounts have been translated with great care by Stack 1973.)

This general plan (Fig. 12.3; Table 12.2) has been agreed by most subsequent anatomists with the added appreciation of a band to the thumb. Kalberg (1935) classified the palmar fascia according to the different patterns of pretendinous fibres to each digit in an examination of 400 hands. He found that not all digital rays had a unique pretendinous band; some rays had more than one, whereas a Y-shaped arrangement sometimes served more than one digital ray. Millesi (1959) confirmed this, referring in particular to the possibility of the pretendinous bands of the ring and little finger arising together. Kalberg's paper has served to underline the individual variation in fibre arrangement rather than highlighting any anatomical differences relevant to the onset of DD.

Legueu & Juvara (1892) used the term 'vertical' (anatomically correct but confusing) superficial palmar ligament for the longitudinal pretendinous fibres and emphasized that between the well defined fibre bundles to each ray were prelumbrical areas. This whole part of the middle hand has often been simplified by being described as a triangle.

All the longitudinal fibres have insertions distal to the TFPA; none insert into these transverse fibres or into the skin creases. Wood Jones (1941) suggested that they may represent a phylogenetically degenerate metacarpophalangeal flexor. Their proximal origin is from the palmaris longus or in its absence, from a fascial layer which overlies the flexor retinaculum (Chapter 11).

Distal palm

It is the arrangement of the longitudinal fibres in the distal palm and palmar digital junction that has given rise to the greatest number of varied descriptions and interpretations. There are however common features, such that a uniform plan can be described. Just distal to the distal free edge of the TFPA the pretendinous fibres separate into groups or layers, with different distal insertions. For descriptive purposes these will be numbered from superficial to deep.

Layer 1: superficial pretendinous insertion

The most superficial pretendinous fibres have a strong and definite insertion into the dermis of the

Table 12.2 Longitudinal structures in the palm

Terminology		Corresponding diseased structures
Palmar aponeurosis		
Wood Jones	— central portion of the palmar fascia	
Kaplan	— mid palmar fascia or aponeurosis	
Gray	— central part of the palmar aponeurosis	
Proximally		
Pretendinous bands of the palmar aponeurosis		Pretendinous cord
Wood Jones	— radiate longitudinal bands	
Kaplan	— pretendinous bands of the mid palmar fascia	
Gray	— slips	
Distally		
Layer 1		
Insertion in the dermis (Thomine, McGrouther)		Nodule
Central fibrofatty tissue or continuation of pretendinous band		Central cord
Layer 2		
McFarlane	— spiral band	Spiral cord
Gosset	— bifurcation of pretendinous strips	
Layer 3		
Legueu & Juvara	— perforating fibres	Un-named deep cord

The recommended term is given in bold.
References: Wood Jones (1941); Kaplan (1965); Gray (1973); Thomine (1965); McGrouther (1982); McFarlane (1974); Gosset (1985), Legueu & Juvara (1892).

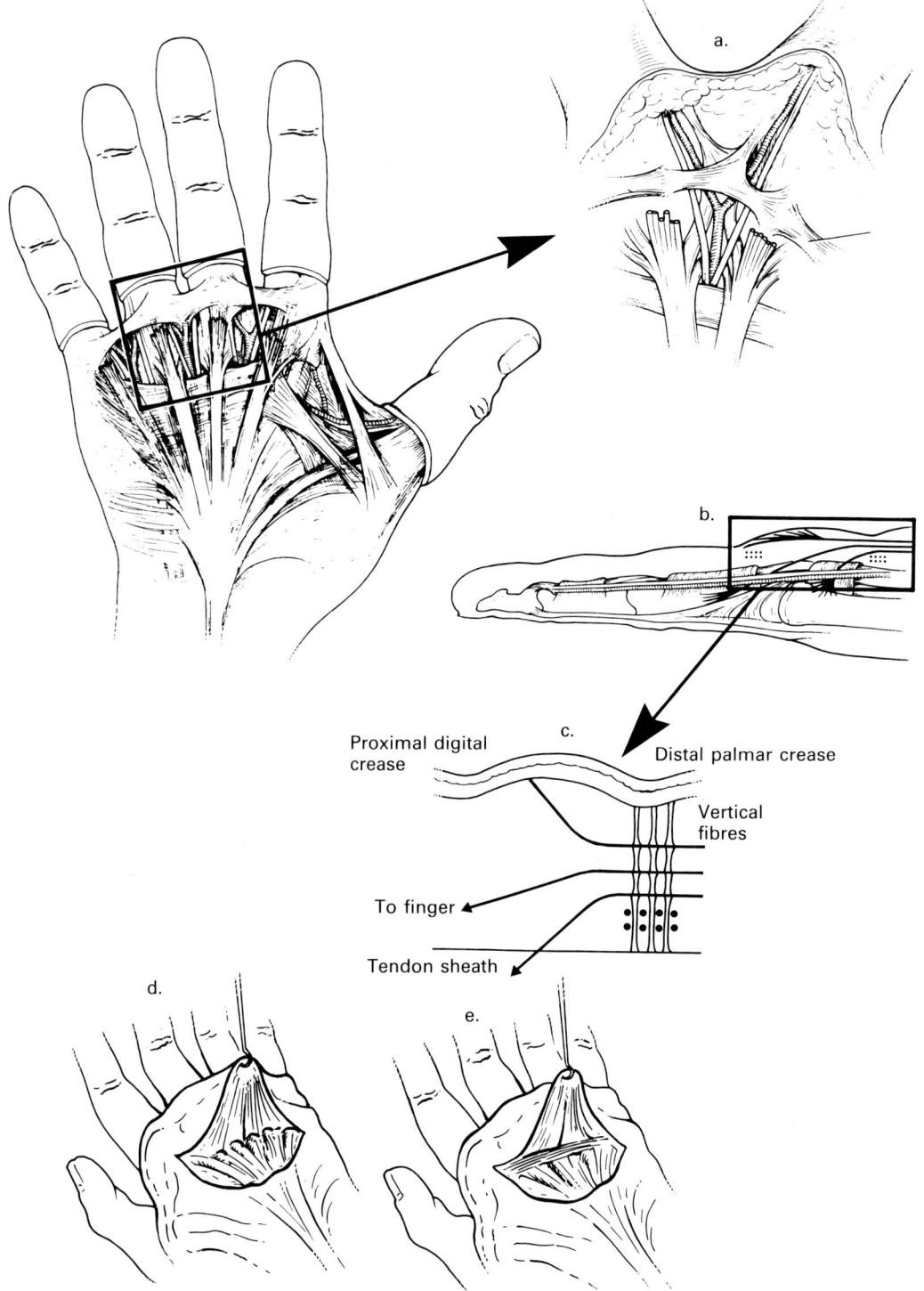

Fig. 12.3 Longitudinal fascial structures. **inset a, b, c** Distal insertions of the pretendinous longitudinal fibres. The most superficial fibres (cut end illustrated) insert into the dermis. Deep to the above, fibres pass deep to the neurovascular bundles and pass to the lateral digital sheet. The deepest fibres pass on either side of the metacarpophalangeal joint. **Inset d**: The arrangement suggested by Legueu & Juvara (1892). **Inset e**: The author has found however that the pretendinous fibres can be elevated from the transverse fibres and that the pretendinous fibres do not pass deeply until a point distal to the transverse fibres.

skin at a point midway between the distal palmar crease and proximal digital crease. This insertion is best developed in the middle and ring fingers but is also apparent in the little finger ray. In the index finger the skin insertion is more proximal, tending to be in the region of the proximal palmar crease. This layer of skin insertion was dissected by the author (McGrouther 1982) and at the same time Michael Flint, working quite independently in Auckland, New Zealand, demonstrated this in a histological study. Readers can observe from their own hands an indentation on flexing the hand slightly. Maslieurat-Lagemard (1839) suggested a longitudinal depression at this point on full digital extension due to attachment of fibres to the flexor sheath with exaggeration of the monticuli or fatty swellings on either side.

This insertion has been controversial. Thomine (1965) suggested an abrupt stopping of longitudinal fibres by insertion of all of these into the skin. Gosset (1967, 1985) by contrast found that all the pretendinous fibres passed deeply and did not recognize any skin insertion; this seems a minority view. Other anatomists have shown pretendinous fibres running distally underneath the proximal digital crease to the palmar surface of the digits. This plan has been illustrated by Wood Jones (1941) and Zancolli (1979) but in the author's view this plan is not usual and may even represent one of the very earliest changes of DD.

Involvement of layer 1 in DD. The effects of contracture along the line of these fibres can best be appreciated by reference to Figure 12.4. The earliest sign is an approximation of the dermal attachment point to the distal palmar crease with bunching of the skin between to form a nodule. This site of an early Dupuytren's nodule is characteristic. Distally there is skin blanching on digital extension. A pit may develop at the skin attachment point, inclined proximally by traction. Contracture of the fascia proximal to the distal palmar crease will be obvious as a cord and a pit may develop at the distal palmar crease itself (some vertical fibre shortening must be associated). Further nodules may develop in the line of the pretendinous cord and there will be vertical and horizontal distortion of the palmar creases (Chapter 18).

Contracture of this layer need not necessarily be associated with joint contracture. The contracture line may propagate distally from the dermal attachment point through dermis (skin involvement) or fibres just deep to the dermis. This pretendinous cord may run superficial to the natatory fibres, or involve and tether these. With an isolated central cord, there is no neurovascular bundle displacement (Chapter 14).

Layer 2

The next deep layer of pretendinous fibres passes deep to the natatory ligaments and deep to the neurovascular bundles towards the digits. In the normal hand there is an extensive loose meshwork of fascia in the web which becomes well oriented as a fascial cord in DD. It has been well illustrated by Gosset (1967) and McFarlane (1974) has used the term 'the spiral band of Gosset'.

On reaching the digits these fibres merge with longitudinally running fascia on the side of the digit; Gosset (1967) has interpreted this as a lateral digital sheet and Thomine (1965) as a retrovascular band.

Involvement of Layer 2 in DD. Contracture extending along the line of the spiral band of Gosset gives rise to a risk of displacement of the neurovascular bundle in the region of the palmodigital junction. Contracture along this layer of fascia is likely to flex the metacarpophalangeal and proximal interphalangeal joints due to traction via the lateral digital sheet to the distal insertion on the middle phalanx.

Layer 3

The deepest layer of longitudinal fibres passes around the sides of the flexor sheath and metacarpophalangeal joint. Legueu & Juvara (1892) followed these fibres which perforated the deep transverse metacarpal ligament and passed around the sides of the metacarpophalangeal (they used the term 'perforating fibres'). These fibres have been shown histologically by Stack (1973) and have been well illustrated by Kaplan (1938) and Zancolli (1979). By contrast, Horwitz (1942) and Landsmeer (1949) have been unable to

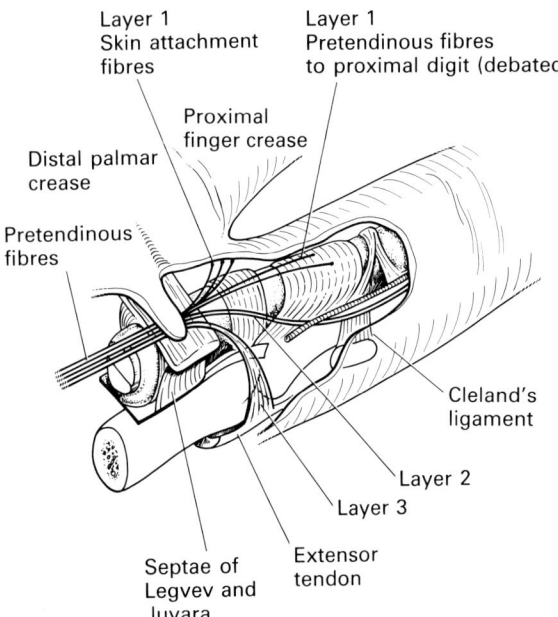

Fig. 12.4 Distal insertions of the palmar fascia.

demonstrate these fibres and Kempf & Gonzalo-Vivar (1962) considered them rare structures. They pass around the metcarpophalangeal joints inserting into the extensor tendon and are best known to the surgeon undertaking metacarpophalangeal joint replacement arthroplasty as the transverse retinacular fibres.

It is valuable for the reader to formulate a mental picture of the distal insertions of the palmar fascia (Fig. 12.4). Kempf & Gonzalo-Vivar (1962) described the fibrous tissue systems surrounding the head of the metacarpals with the extensor expansion linked to the palmar plates and the deep transverse ligaments of the palm. They described this junction of the fascia as a goose's foot, the fibrous cross-roads on either side of the flexor tendon sheaths, with articular capsule lamina transverse, the intermetacarpal ligament and the intertendinous partition. They remark on the importance of this junction; the whole system stabilizes the flexor, extensor and interosseous muscle systems together and unites the systems with the bone. They emphasize, however, that this system surrounds the metacarpal heads, without an actual attachment to them.

There has often been confusion between the perforating fibres described by Legueu & Juvara and the structure which has been termed the vertical septae of Legueu & Juvara. As described above, the perforating fibres are a distal continuation of the pretendinous fibres which turn down distal to the TFPA to perforate the deep transverse fibres. By contrast the vertical septae lie deep to the TFPA (Fig. 12.4). The orientation of fibres within these septae is uncertain. Chapter 11 suggests that the fibres are largely vertical — lying at right angles to the plane of the palm and tending to encircle the flexor sheaths merging with TFPA superiorly and deep transverse fibres in the depths of the hand.

Legueu & Juvara (1892) and Gosset (1985) by contrast have shown by dividing the palmaris longus proximally and reflecting it distally that there are deep extensions from the pretendinous fibres running longitudinally down into the vertical septae between the flexor tendons. This has not been the author's impression, but further dissection is being undertaken in this area. The confusion between perforating fibres and vertical septae has been heightened by the suggestion of Gosset that at the distal edge of the TFPA these two layers are in continuity, as shown in Figure 12.4.

Involvement of layer 3 in DD. When layer 3 contracts, the more distal perforating fibres distal to the metacarpophalangeal joint cause its contracture. This type of cord cannot readily be divided by a subcutaneous fasciotomy.

DISCUSSION

The description of distal insertions of the longitudinal fibres in layers is a simplification of a three-dimensional arrangement for the purposes of description. Maslieurat-Lagemard (1839) rather viewed the separation of the fibres in the distal palm as forming gutters concave posteriorly which inserted into the flexor sheaths at the palmodigital junction. This gutter concept allows the reader a mental picture of how layers 1, 2 and 3 surround the flexor sheaths. His particularly thorough and clear account was published from the Hôtel-Dieu but regrettably, no illustrations have been found. This precise work, together with that of Bourgery

(1834), Cruveilhier, Gerdy and Blandin, which he cites, shows the considerable interest in palmar anatomy in Paris at the time of Dupuytren. Maslieurat-Lagemard also considered that the lumbrical canals allowed the cellular tissue at the base of the fingers to continue with that occupying the central and subaponeurotic parts of the hand. He therefore presented a very clear picture of the palmar fascial continuum which has been modified little since that time.

Vertical fibres

The term 'vertical' is taken to be at right angles to the skin surface and, although anatomically imprecise, it is a term readily appreciated by surgeons. Over the thenar and hypothenar eminence there are numerous vertical skin attachments which, with fat loculation, contribute to the shock-absorbing role of the palm. In the central palm there are scattered vertical fibrous connections but these are particularly concentrated for a few millimetres on either side of the palmar creases rather than in the apex of the creases themselves. These attachments anchor the skin adjacent to the creases and form part of the skin joint mechanism. These vertical fibres are much more flimsy than the longitudinal or transverse ones. The vertical fibres run down through the TFPA to unite with deep structures. Deep to the TFPA, as described above, the vertical partitions which separate the spaces for the tendons from the spaces for the neurovascular bundles have a vertical orientation.

Significance of palmar fascial anatomy in relation to DD

The palmar fascial continuum is seen to be a complex three-dimensional arrangement of fibres which can be described as longitudinal, transverse and vertical fibres. This is a complex system of retinacular function and mobile skin anchorage which is effective in any posture of the hand. The inelastic palmar skin is draped in a precise and complex fashion. The hand must comply with the rule of natural physics that to every force there is an equal and opposite reaction and the internal anatomical arrangement is ideally suited to balance external forces. Callosities or blisters map out areas of skin which are immobilized by fascial anchorage. *This complex system requires relative motion between the individual fascial structures, which is lost in DD*. The complex channel system underlying the skin creases is especially vulnerable.

13 The genesis of the palmar lesion

M. H. Flint

It is frequently stated that the primary lesion in Dupuytren's disease (DD) is the palmar nodule (Luck 1959; Gabbiani & Majno 1972; Hueston 1975). However, the term 'nodule', which is commonly used, is really a clinically descriptive term for a localized palmar thickening which although clearly palpable is not always clearly defined. The use of the term 'nodule' in this clinical context must be carefully differentiated from the biological or pathological use of the word 'nodule' in DD. The differences in the usage of the term 'nodule' in the clinical and pathological or biological sense have probably contributed to some of the differences of opinion about the aetiology or pathogenesis of DD. Few would argue that a palpable nodule — often localized to the proximal side of the distal palmar crease — is one of the most frequent and well recognized early clinical manifestations of the disease. Histological examination of one of these clinically manifest early 'nodules' from the palm shows that it is really a composite structure of thickened, coalesced, longitudinally running fascial fibres exhibiting patches or localised zones of intrafasicular cellularity collagenolysis and connective tissue remodelling. In reality, it represents a series of progressive changes which have been developing long before the thickened nodule became clinically apparent and which have gradually transformed the soft, plump, compliant palm of the child into the more fibrotic, inelastic and non-compliant material of the adult (Table 13.1).

In some circumstances, a clinically apparent nodule may appear to have developed locally without any obvious connection with a previously thickened band of fascia. However, the slowly developing fibrous plaques which are found in the region of the distal palmar crease are usually associated with more widespread thickening of the palmar fascial fibres and present either as a diffuse resistance to pressure on the palm or as a localized subcutaneous thickening in the distal palm. This type of localized subcutaneous thickening may also be associated with pits in the skin where the dermis is apparently tethered to the deeper fibres (Fig. 13.1). These dermal pits arising on the distal side of the distal palmar crease may be the first and only manifestation of underlying fibrosis.

Previous writers have described changes found in the dermis and palmar fascial fibres in samples of palm skin taken at operation from patients undergoing surgery for DD (Meyerding et al 1941; MacCallum & Hueston 1962; Chiu & McFarlane 1978; Bazin et al 1980; Ushijima et al 1984; Nezelof 1985). Whilst these samples have provided a fund of information about the nature and progression of the disease process they have not — because of their very nature — provided much information about the origin of the biological or

Table 13.1 Biological events in Dupuytren's disease

Primary thickening of superficial palmar fascia, especially superficial longitudinal bands
Matting of longitudinal vertical and oblique fibres and loss of compliance
Loss of hyaluronate from fascial fibres?
Development of intrafascial cellular lesions
Secondary fascial thickening
Contraction — cellular and extracellular
Contracture — connective tissue remodelling

THE GENESIS OF THE PALMAR LESION 137

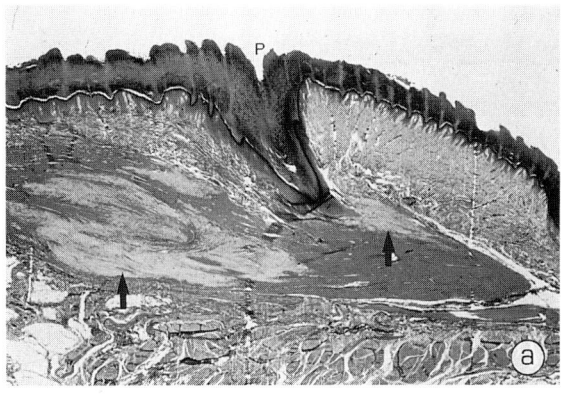

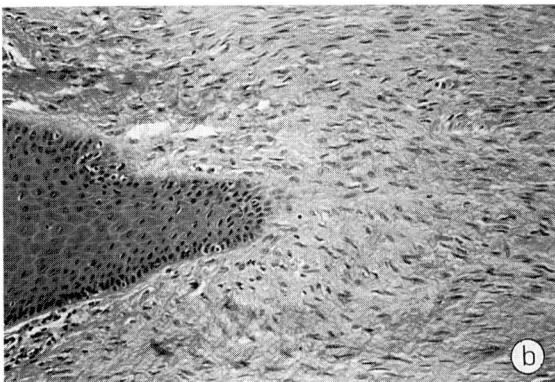

Fig. 13.1 Dermal pit. **a** Longitudinal histological section of thickened superficial pretendinous fascial band in distal palm showing pale staining intrafascicular cellular nodules (arrows). The proximal nodule is causing an invagination of the epidermis and overlying keratin, forming a dermal pit (P). **b** Higher power view of the indrawn tip of the invaginated epidermis in Figure 13.1a, showing cellularity of the contractile tissue of the nodule.

layers of the hand under the dissecting microscope (McGrouther 1982) or by the histological examination of serial longitudinal sections of palm skin and the underlying fascia from a wide variety of post-mortem subjects (Millesi 1959, 1985; Flint, unpublished observations — see also Chapters 10 and 28), have provided a better understanding of the microstructure of the apparently uninvolved palm and an opportunity to observe the development of changes within these normal structures which presage the later development of DD.

THE NORMAL PALM

In Chapter 2 the close interrelationship between connective tissue form and function has been stressed. Many features of this interdependent relationship are apparent in the specific adaptations to prehensile gripping of the superficial palm and its connective tissues.

The surface skin of the hand and fingers is covered by fine antiskid channels — the dermal ridges — the functional capability of which is enormously increased by the secretion of sweat from the apices of these ridges. Whilst the skin of the hand and fingers may undergo spontaneous hyperkeratosis as a self-protective mechanism when subjected to chronic localized frictional, torsional or pressure forces, the ability of the specialized integument to absorb these forces is enormously increased by its firm attachment to the underlying palmar aponeurosis by a honeycomb of interlocking fascial fibres. Grapow (1887) emphasized this relationship and noted that the palmar fascia 'secures grip through its intense surface connections with the overlying skin which might otherwise slide off the hand like a glove'. Millesi (1959, 1985) and Thomine (1965) also stressed the importance of this firm fibrous attachment in preventing avulsion of the skin during torsional and compressive movements. They pointed out that from a comparative anatomical viewpoint the palmar aponeurosis is a late phylogenetic development and is best developed in climbing animals. Millesi (1959) also noted the cushioning effect of the fat lobules laid down in the fibrous tissue network immediately beneath

pathological changes preceding the clinical appearance of the disease. Some workers have occasionally been able to obtain biopsy samples of clinically asymptomatic palmar nodules at the time of operative treatment of some other lesion on the hand, such as a trigger finger (Chiu & McFarlane 1978). Although histological studies of these nodular biopsy samples describe changes which could justly be regarded as being earlier than those in clinically troublesome lesions, they do not necessarily describe the primal changes in the disease process.

However, the anatomical and histological studies of apparently normal, uninvolved hands, either by meticulous dissection of the surface the dermis in the superficial palmar connective tissue continuum.

LOAD BEARING AND MOBILITY

The load-bearing fibrofatty subcutaneous tissues of the palm, the heel and the plantar surface of the foot under the metatarsal heads are quite different from other subcutaneous fatty tissues (Gillard et al 1977). In load-bearing situations the subcutaneous fat cells are arranged in groups within fibrous compartments made up from collagen and elastic fibres embedded in a proteoglycan matrix, particularly rich in chondroitin sulphate (Fig. 13.2). The containment of the fat within relatively non-extensible fibrous boundaries makes it more efficient as a pressure absorptive structure. In the palm, anchoring of the skin is achieved by means of the interlacing three-dimensional fibrous network of 'the palmar connective tissue continuum' (see Chapter 2) which stabilizes the palmar skin during gripping and ensures that the skin does not fold or roll when subject to shearing or compressive forces. The hypodermal fat pads occupying the spaces within and around the three-dimensional fibrous network serve to absorb the energy of such forces.

I believe that these fibrous attachments, particularly of the fine, superficial longitudinal and oblique fibres, and the surrounding fibrofatty compartmentalized shock-absorbers, hold the key to the early pathogenesis of Dupuytren's contracture and also allow the apparently divergent views of Millesi (1985) and Hueston (1985) or Dupuytren (1834) and Goyrand (1833) to be more easily reconciled.

The situation is compounded by the increased mobility of the fourth and fifth metacarpal rays, particularly around the metacarpophalangeal joints, which leads to increased excursion of and stress upon the skin, the subcutaneous tissue and the longitudinal fascial bundles on the ulnar side of the palm. In this region the superficial pretendinous longitudinal fibres inserting into the skin beyond the distal palmar crease form part of a complex fasciocutaneous anchoring system which controls the folding of the skin at the distal palmar crease during hand flexion. It is interesting that DD typically occurs in areas of the palm skin which are 'loose' in the resting flexed posture and where anchoring systems are more highly developed (McGrouther, personal observation).

Hueston (1977) has stressed that the transverse distal palmar crease is retracted and hidden when the fingers are flexed into a gripping position. However, if one marks the palmar skin whilst the fingers are flexed at the metacarpophalangeal and interphalangeal joints it will be observed that the contact areas lie proximal and distal to the distal palmar crease, exactly coincident with the site of development of palmar nodules (Fig. 13.3). Whilst I would agree with Hueston that the distal palmar crease retracts out of the zone of contact loading, it should be remembered that the distal palmar crease itself is rarely the site of development of the initial palmar nodule.

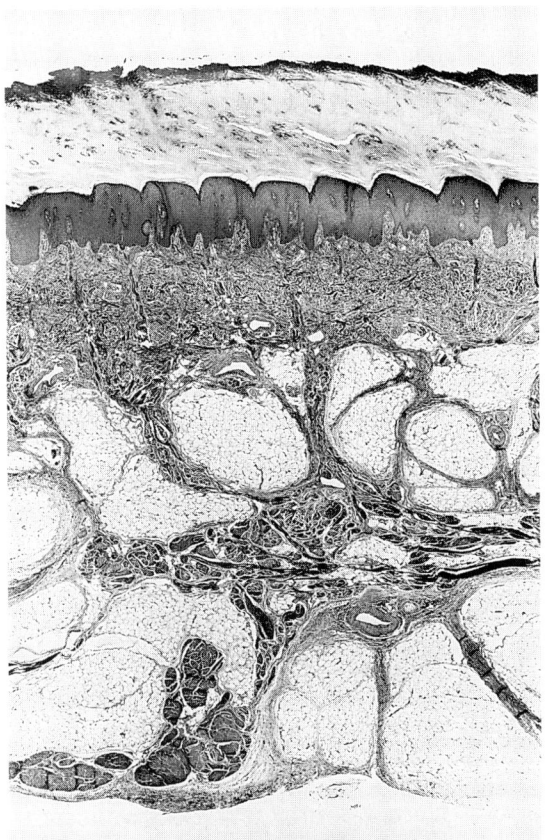

Fig. 13.2 Load-bearing skin of the heel showing the thickened keratin and epidermis and the loculated fibrofatty shock absorbers beneath the dermis.

Millesi (1959) emphasized that by ordinary methods of dissection, the skin and subcutaneous fascia of the palm are removed together, revealing the so-called 'palmar aponeurosis'. As a result, the superficial longitudinal fibres are usually removed or lost and thus are ignored or only briefly described in most textbooks. By removing only a fine layer of corium from the palm and dissecting individual fat lobules, Millesi was able to reveal the whole of the 'binding tissue system' of the superficial palmar aponeurosis. By carefully dissecting hand specimens under water whilst viewing them through the dissecting microscope, McGrouther (1982) was able to show the course and attachment of the superficial longitudinal fibres and their relationship to the deep longitudinal fibres of the aponeurosis. He also demonstrated their close blending with the deeper aspects of the dermis beyond the distal palmar crease. McGrouther's dissections enabled him to develop a much clearer understanding of the three-dimensional interrelationships of the longitudinal, vertical, oblique and transverse fibre components of the palmar fascia and relate them to the distribution of the known thickened cords of Dupuytren's disease.

SUPERFICIAL LONGITUDINAL PALMAR FASCIAL BUNDLES

A histological study of specimens of palm skin taken from the fourth ray of a large number of post-mortem subjects ranging from mid-term fetus to old age, which I carried out in Auckland, demonstrated that from a very early stage of fetal development it is possible to trace a constant band of fascial fibres branching from the superficial surface of the deep longitudinal pretendinous fascial bands. These branching fibres run obliquely distally and progressively superficially to blend with the deep dermis beyond the distal palmar crease (Fig. 13.4).

At birth, this superficial longitudinal fibre bundle is well defined approximately 30–50 μ wide, running in its own fine paratenon sheath between two layers of loculated fibrofatty pads (Fig. 13.5). The form of this arrangement was found to be so constant that for the purpose of description, the hypodermal fat pads lying proximal to the distal palmar crease may be regarded as a superficial and a deep group

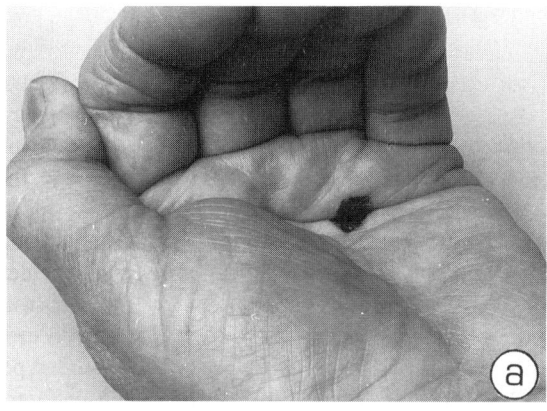

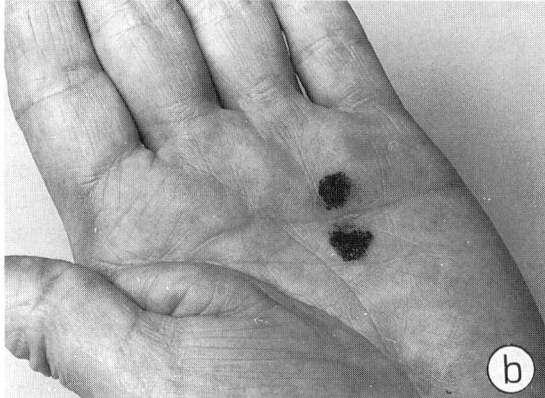

Fig. 13.3 a Ink spot marking impact area in fourth ray of palm of flexed hand. **b** Separation of spots on opening the hand demonstrate that the impact area in the flexed palm is coincident with the common sites of nodular thickening on either side of the distal palmar crease.

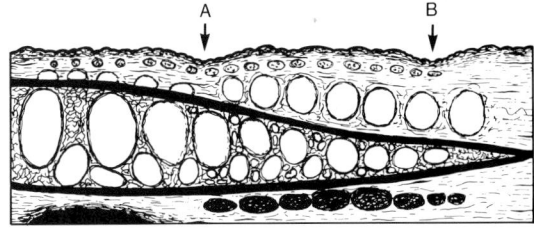

Fig. 13.4 Superficial and deep longitudinal pretendinous fascial bands. The fibres may separate more proximally at the level of the distal carpus. The subcutaneous fat pads lie superficial and deep to the superficial longitudinal bundle. (A) Distal palmar crease (B); proximal palmar crease.

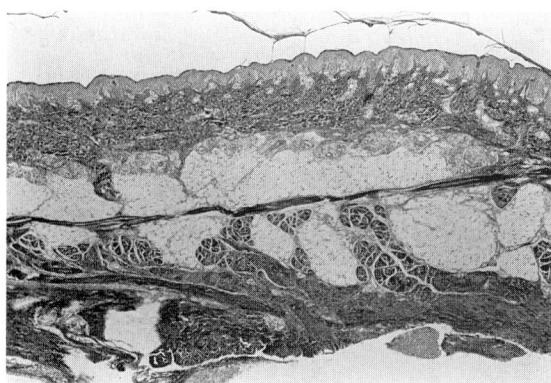

Fig. 13.5 Longitudinal section of palm skin of fourth ray of 1-day-old child showing superficial longitudinal fascial bundle running obliquely upwards towards the palmar crease, sandwiched between superficial and deep fibrofatty loculi.

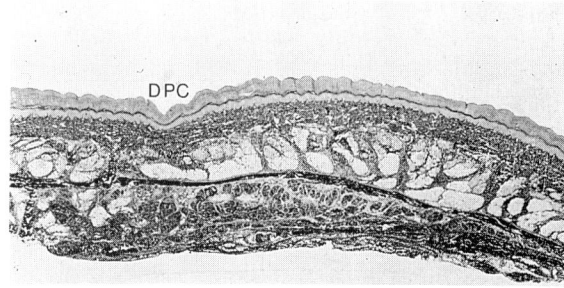

Fig. 13.6 Longitudinal section of adolescent fourth ray palm skin. Superficial longitudinal pretendinous fascial band separating from deep pretendinous fibres and passing forwards and upwards towards the distal palmar dermis. Note thickening of superficial longitudinal bundle and that the deep layer of fat pads proximal to the distal palmar crease (DPC) is not so apparent as the superficial group or as in Figure 13.5.

separated from each other by the obliquely running fibres of the superficial longitudinal fascial bundles (Fig. 13.6).

During late adolescence or early adult life, the fibre bundles were frequently more than a millimetre wide, and by the fourth or fifth decade were in some instances thickened and coalesced to 2–3 mm (Fig. 13.7). In such cases patches of intrafasicular cellularity or areas of apparent tissue repair or remodelling were sometimes evident within the fibre bundles. In some instances there was clear evidence of fibre rupture and connective tissue remodelling occurring within the substance of the 'microtendon' (Fig. 13.8). These regions of internal damage ranged from small discrete areas of change only discernible at higher magnification to large areas which were clearly discernible under the low power dissecting microscope (Fig. 13.9b). These larger zones were indistinguishable from classical Dupuytren's nodules.

As more specimens were examined, it became increasingly apparent that there was a progressive spectrum of change occurring within the fibres of the superficial longitudinal bands and that the thickened cords of fascial fibres containing the Dupuytren's nodules were generally anatomically coincident with the superficial longitudinal fibre bundles. This supports the concept that Dupuytren's cords and nodules developed in pre-existing fascial bands.

SUBDERMAL FIBROFATTY LOCULI

The importance of the attachment of the pretendinous fascial bands to the skin in maintaining the functional integrity of the palm has been stressed by a succession of writers (Grapow 1887; Legueu & Juvara 1892; Grodinsky & Holyoke 1941; Horwitz 1942; Skoog 1948; Iselin 1954a; Millesi 1959; McGrouther 1982), although few have recognized their role in the pathogenesis of the DD process. By contrast, there has over a corresponding period of time been much less mention of the subdermal fibrofatty loculi either in regard to their possible supportive functional role or in their relationship to the genesis of the palmar lesions.

In one of the earliest papers dealing with the anatomy of the palmar fascia, Maslieurat-Lagemard (1839) gave brief mention of these fibrofatty compartments, describing them as the 'soft pulpy tissue which contains a quantity of fat and numerous prolongations of fibres which come to adhere to the internal surface of the skin'. However, Madelung (1875), in what must now be considered to be a very enlightened work, graphically described the constancy and importance of the

'copious small fatty aggregations found in the palmar fascia of children and also of adults under the skin of the palm, ingrained as it were between the fibres of the connective tissue of the palmar fascia and the

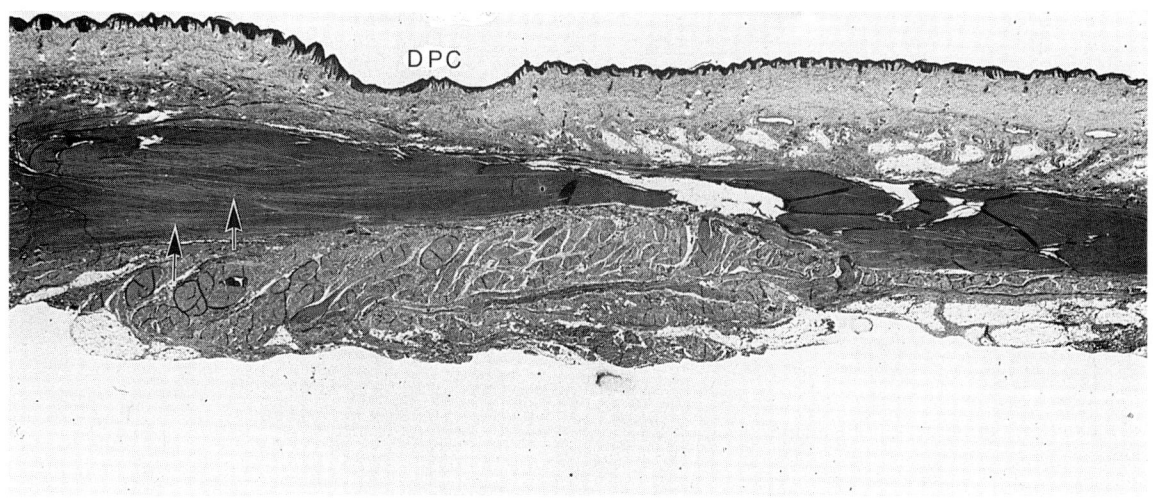

Fig. 13.7 Longitudinal histological section of palm skin of fourth ray of 47-year-old male showing marked thickening of superficial longitudinal band throughout its length. Distally note lighter streaks of intrafascial cellular reaction at site of small intrafascial ruptures (arrows). Note decreased size of fibrofatty loculi as compared with Figures 13.5 and 13.6. DPC = distal palmar crease.

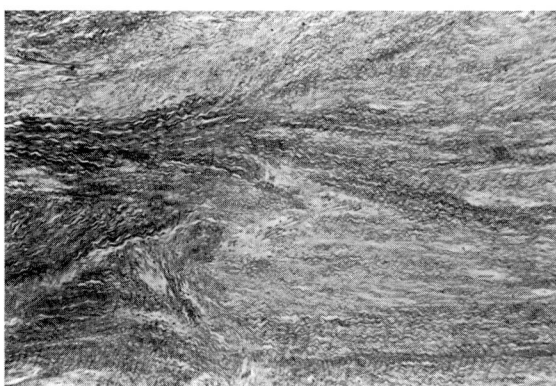

Fig. 13.8 Van Giesen stained longitudinal section of thickened superficial longitudinal pretendinous band showing zone of fibril discontinuity, collagen disaggregation and remodelling forming early cellular nodule.

numerous fibres ascending from it to the skin. Every interstice is filled with them, every bending of the hand causes shifting of these fatty particles within distinct limits'.

Madelung then clearly identified the probable function of the fatty pads, stating: 'it is clear that here as well as in other parts of the body, the function of the fat is to moderate pressure to which tissues of that part of the body are exposed and to distribute it over a larger area'. Since that time there have been few brief mentions of the existence of these subdermal fatty loculi, notably by Skoog (1948), Iselin (1955) and Thomine (1965). Millesi (1959), having meticulously picked out the small fatty globules from between the fine fibres of the superficial palmar fascia, was obviously well aware of their presence and indicated that they had a protective cushioning function.

Napier (1965) described the main fat pads of the palm under three headings — the thenar, the hypothenar and the metacarpophalangeal — and their function in accommodating the hand to grip. However, he specifically mentioned that the area of the palm overlying the palmar aponeurosis was relatively fat-free and formed the central anchorage for the skin and the rest of the palm. It may be that his observations were based on dissections of older hands in which the subdermal fat had disappeared. Certainly Madelung (1875) had also noticed the marked loss of subcutaneous fat in the mid-palm of older subjects; with great foresight he suggested that its absence could lead to increased stress on the more prominent fibres of the palmar fascia. In contrast to this, Iselin (1955) considered that the subcutaneous fatty pads were replaced as a *secondary* event by infiltration

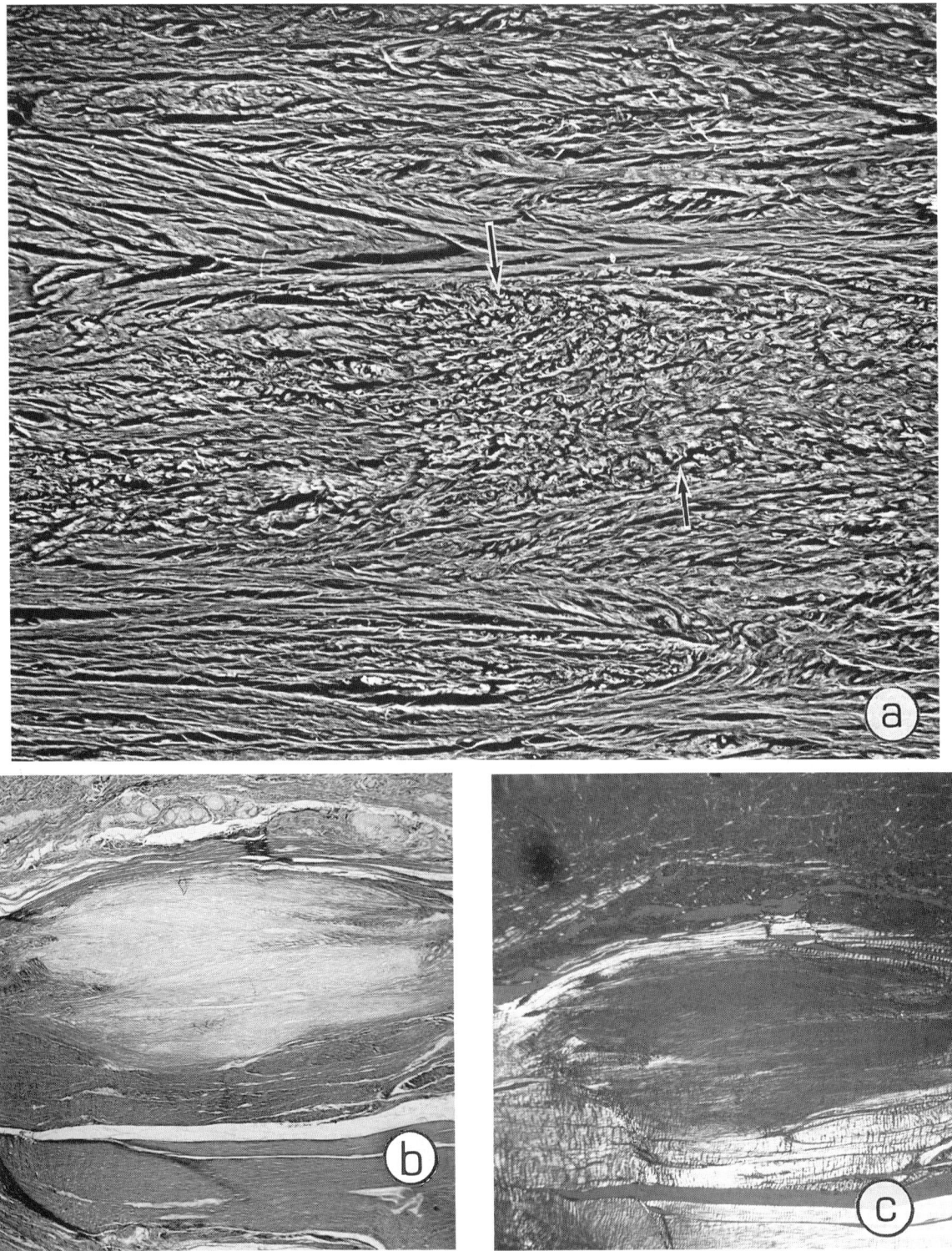

Fig. 13.9 a Small areas of cellular proliferation and fibril discontinuity observed in scanning electron microscope study of clinically unaffected longitudinal pretendinous fascial bands. **b** Longitudinal section of intrafascial cellular zone in longitudinal pretendinous band demonstrating fibril discontinuity across the lesion but fibril continuity peripherally. **c** Polarized view of same specimen showing fibril discontinuity within the central cellular zone but peripheral continuity.

of the Dupuytren's lesion extending superficially from the volar surface of the fascia. This idea is also expressed in many other writings dealing with the pathogenesis or histopathology of Dupuytren's disease (Meyerding et al 1941; Iselin 1954b; MacCallum & Hueston 1962; Nezelof 1985).

During the course of a comparative histological study of weight-bearing and non-weight-bearing skins (Gillard et al 1977), marked differences were observed in the size, shape, extent and distribution of the subdermal fibrofatty loculi in the palmar skin. At first it was thought that these differences were age-related, but further study demonstrated that this was not so. However, these studies indicated that there was an inverse relationship between the thickness and integrity of the subdermal fat and the thickness and compaction of the superficial longitudinal fibre bundles. In other words, loss or absence of the fat pads seemed to be associated with an increased thickness or compaction of the subdermal connective tissues and particularly of the superficial longitudinal pretendinous fascial bands.

The frequency of these histological observations prompted a more intense study of the structure of the superficial palm occupying the zone between the under-surface of the epidermis and the volar aspect of the thick, deep, pretendinous longitudinal fascial bands. In Chapter 2 this zone was referred to as the 'palmar connective tissue continuum' to emphasize the functional and structural integrity of the subepidermal and subcutaneous layers.

In surveying the vast literature that has accumulated on DD over the past few decades we have been struck by the paucity of information about the biology or even the morphology of the tissues within this important functional layer. There are numerous papers dealing in minute detail with the palmar fascia and the mode of its involvement in Dupuytren's disease (Luck 1959; Gosset 1967; Stack 1971; McFarlane 1974, 1985; Tubiana et al 1982; Gosset 1985; Strickland & Bassett 1985), but most of these, with the exception of papers by McGrouther (1982) and Millesi (1959, 1965, 1985), pay scant attention to this superficial layer of skin, fat and fibres, whilst providing exhaustive descriptions of the pretendinous fascial bundles, their extensions into the fingers and the effect of these on the development of deformity in DD. This is understandable because clinicians tend to be more interested in the treatment of the deformity and thus in the anatomical basis of the contractural bands. However, to understand the enigma of DD it must be appreciated that whilst the disease may sometimes start on or within the volar surface of the deep pretendinous bands of the palmar fascia, it probably more frequently has its beginnings in the connective tissues lying between these deep pretendinous bands and the epidermis, i.e. in the 'palmar connective tissue continuum' (see Chapters 2 and 28).

INTERRELATIONSHIP OF FASCIAL FIBRES AND FIBROFATTY LOCULI

The underside of the dermis is normally pegged into the underlying subcutaneous tissue by a honeycomb of fibrous compartments which on longitudinal section of the palm appear as fibrous bands running between the dermis and the pretendinous bands (Figs 13.6 and 13.10). Some of these vertical and oblique bands form septae between the fibrofatty compartments of the hypodermis and provide the hydroelastic shock-absorption system protecting the palmar connective tissues and the deeper neurovascular bundles and tendons from excessive compressive loading and shear stress. These fibrofatty compartments are particularly well developed in the palm proximal and distal to the distal palmar crease.

In longitudinal sections taken along the line of the fourth metacarpal ray, the fibrofatty pads proximal to the palmar crease are seen to be round or ovoid and packed closely together, being separated from each other by vertical or oblique fibrous septae (Figs 13.10 and 13.11). In fortunate planes of histological section of these palmar skin samples it is possible to observe that the fibrofatty compartments are separated into a superficial and deep group by the superficial pretendinous longitudinal fascial band (McGrouther 1982; Figs 13.6 and 13.11).

Distal to the distal palmar crease the superficial longitudinal band becomes progressively more superficial and blends with the dermis. Throughout its length this fascial bundle is surrounded by a

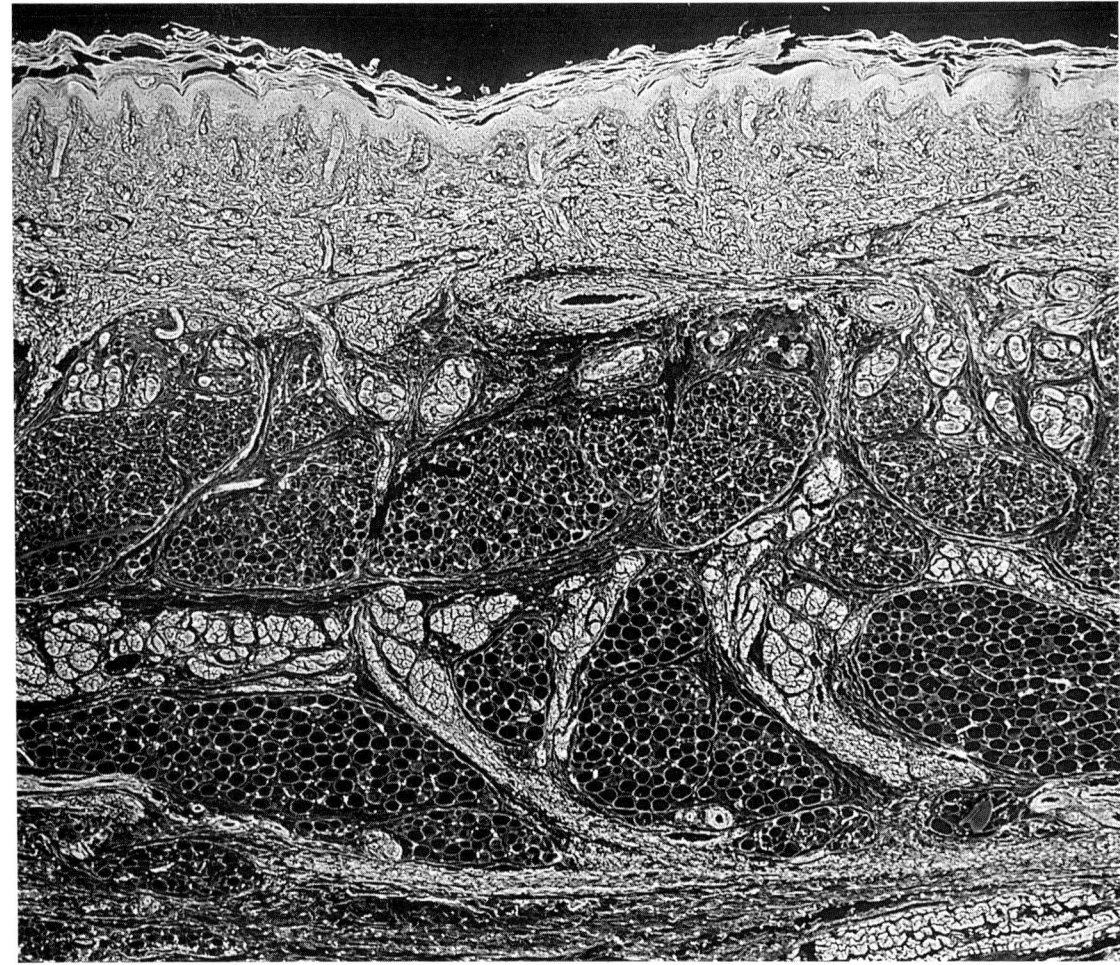

Fig. 13.10 Scanning electron microscope photomicrograph of longitudinal section of 1-day-old palm skin showing fibrofatty loculi, fibrous septae and attachment of the dermis to the longitudinal fascial strands by oblique and vertical fascial bundles.

thin paratenon-like sheath, indicating that there is normally a range of movement of this microtendon during flexion and extension of the hand and fingers (McGrouther 1982; Figs 13.5 and 13.11). Distal to the distal palmar crease, the fibrofatty compartments are often much larger, more ovoid and less compacted than those of the proximal group. The fibrous septae between them are also derived from vertical and obliquely running fibres extending between the dermis and the volar surface of the tendon sheath or the deep longitudinal fibres of the palmar fascia (McGrouther 1982; Millesi 1985).

There is considerable variation in the size and distribution of these fibrofatty compartments. In some instances the layer of fat pads may be twice or three times as thick as the dermis, whilst in others the dermis may equal or exceed their thickness. Initially, in our studies, it was thought that the difference in the size of the fibrofatty compartments was associated with ageing, but study of a large number of samples demonstrated that the differences were not age-related and that it was possible to have a very thick layer of fat pads in old people or alternatively pads that were almost completely obliterated in young people. We were

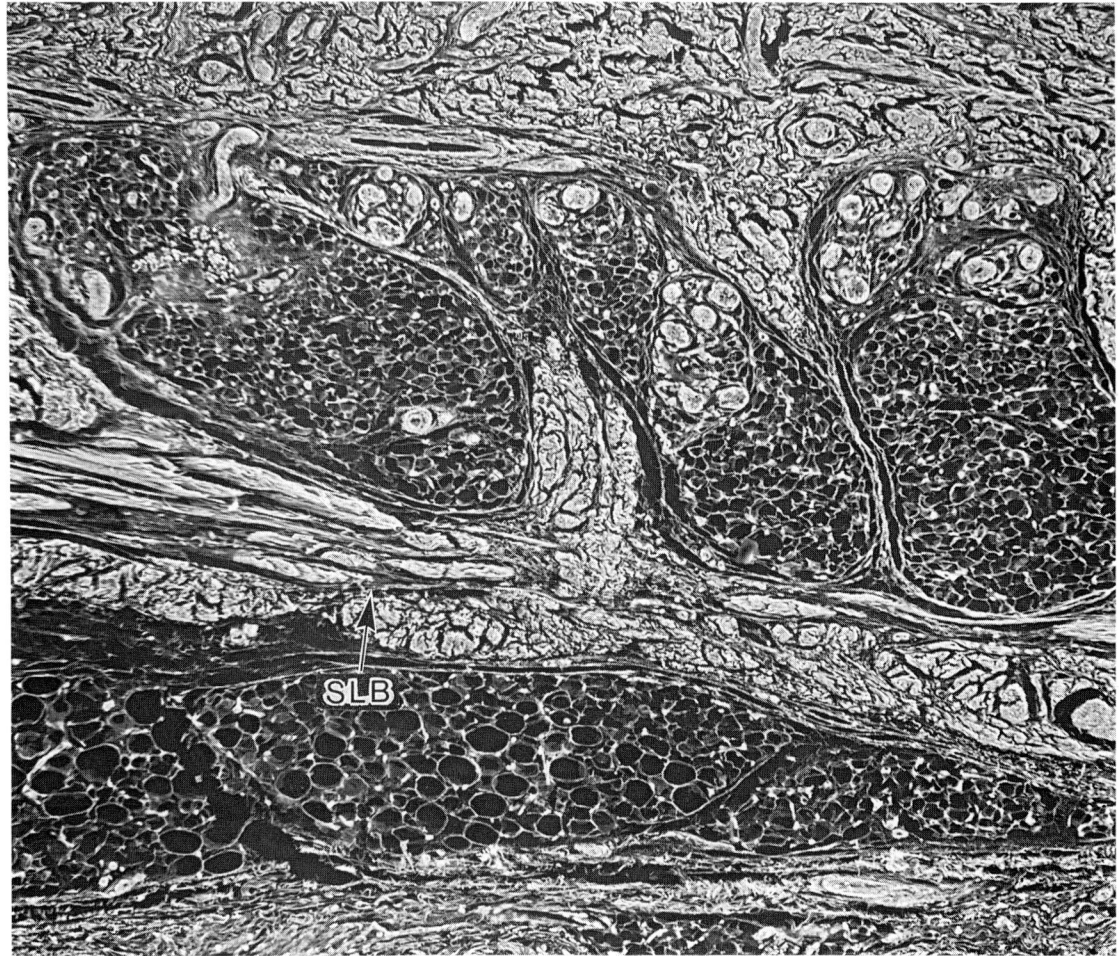

Fig. 13.11 Scanning electron microscope photomicrograph of longitudinal section of 1-day-old palm skin showing superficial longitudinal bundle (SLB) approximately 100 μ wide running between superficial and deep layers of fatty loculi within its paratenon sheath.

surprised to find the extent to which the fat pads were sometimes almost totally replaced by fibrosis in the palm and by the fact that this could happen over a wide age range.

At birth, or shortly thereafter, the fat pads are arranged like a closely packed honeycomb (Fig. 13.10). However, in some instances by early adult life or even in adolescence, the fibrofatty compartments in the specimens we examined had apparently been replaced by progressive fibrosis which appeared to have its origins in the loose connective tissue around the fatty loculi. This fibrosis was generally preceded by increased vascularity within the fatty loculi and by marked perivascular round cell response. Figure 13.12 shows the dramatic differences which were found between birth and early adolescence, with marked disruption of the fatty loculi and loss of the normal fibrous configuration. Figure 13.13 shows the increasing fibrosis and the gradual obliteration of the fatty loculi.

Fibrotic replacement

In many instances there was obvious fibrotic replacement of part or all of the deep or superficial

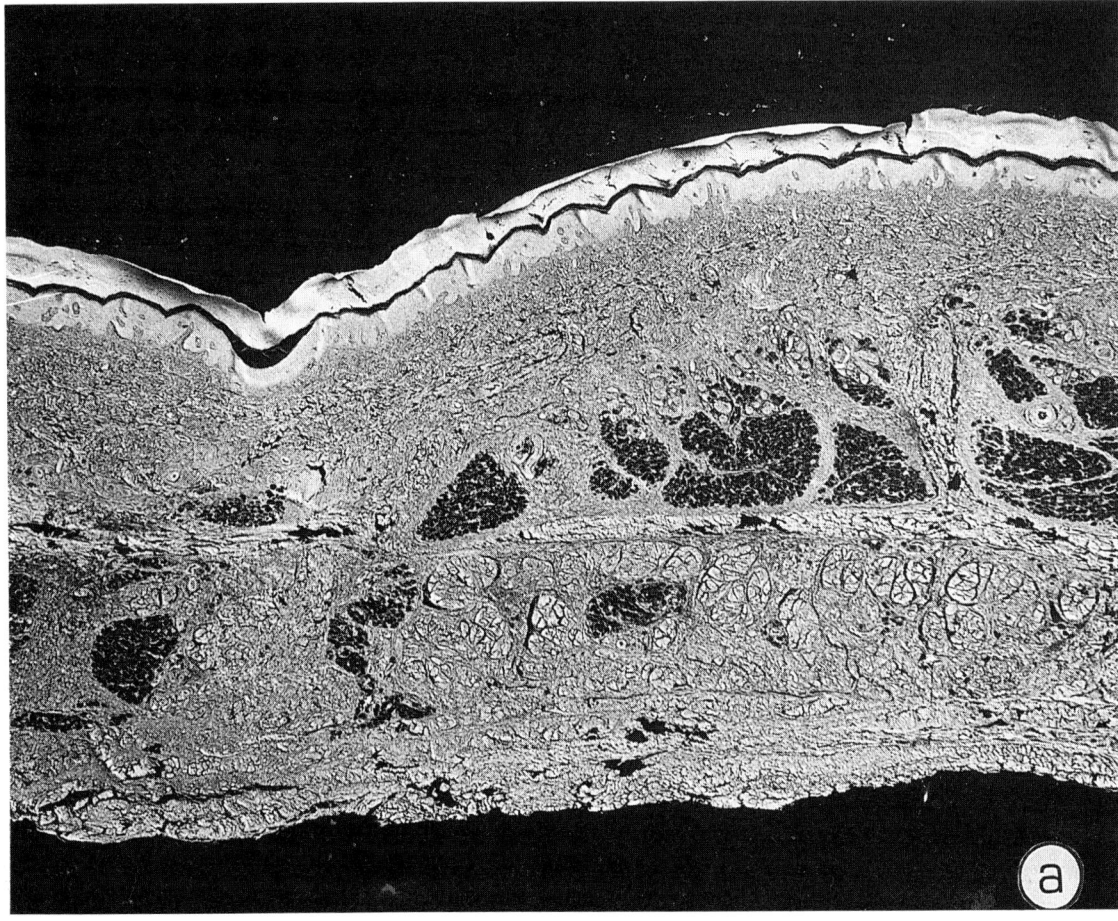

Fig. 13.12a Scanning electron microscope photomicrograph of longitudinal section of palm skin of a 15-year-old male. Note the marked relative decrease in size and integrity of fibrofatty loculi as compared to Figure 13.10. **b** Scanning electron microscope photomicrograph of longitudinal section of palm skin of an 18-year-old male. Note the marked fibrosis of palmar connective tissue and loss of fat as compared to Figure 13.10 at the same magnification.

layer of the fat pads proximal to the distal palmar crease. Examination of more than 250 samples of palm skin demonstrated a pattern of fibrous replacement which appeared to begin in the deeper layer just proximal to the distal palmar crease and which progressively extended backwards, i.e. proximally, throughout the whole of the deep layer. Fibrotic replacement of the deep layer of the proximal group of fat pads often appeared to be followed by fibrotic replacement of the superficial layer, progressing in a similar manner proximally from the distal palmar crease (Fig. 13.13).

Although it is not possible to be certain that these progressive changes always took place in this order, it was unusual to find isolated fibrotic replacement of the proximal or superficial fat pads without involvement of those adjacent to the distal palmar crease. It was also unusual to find replacement of the superficial layer if the deep layer fat pads were still intact.

Increased vascularity

The fibrotic replacement of the fibrofatty compartments appeared to be preceded by, and associated with, increased microvascularity of the

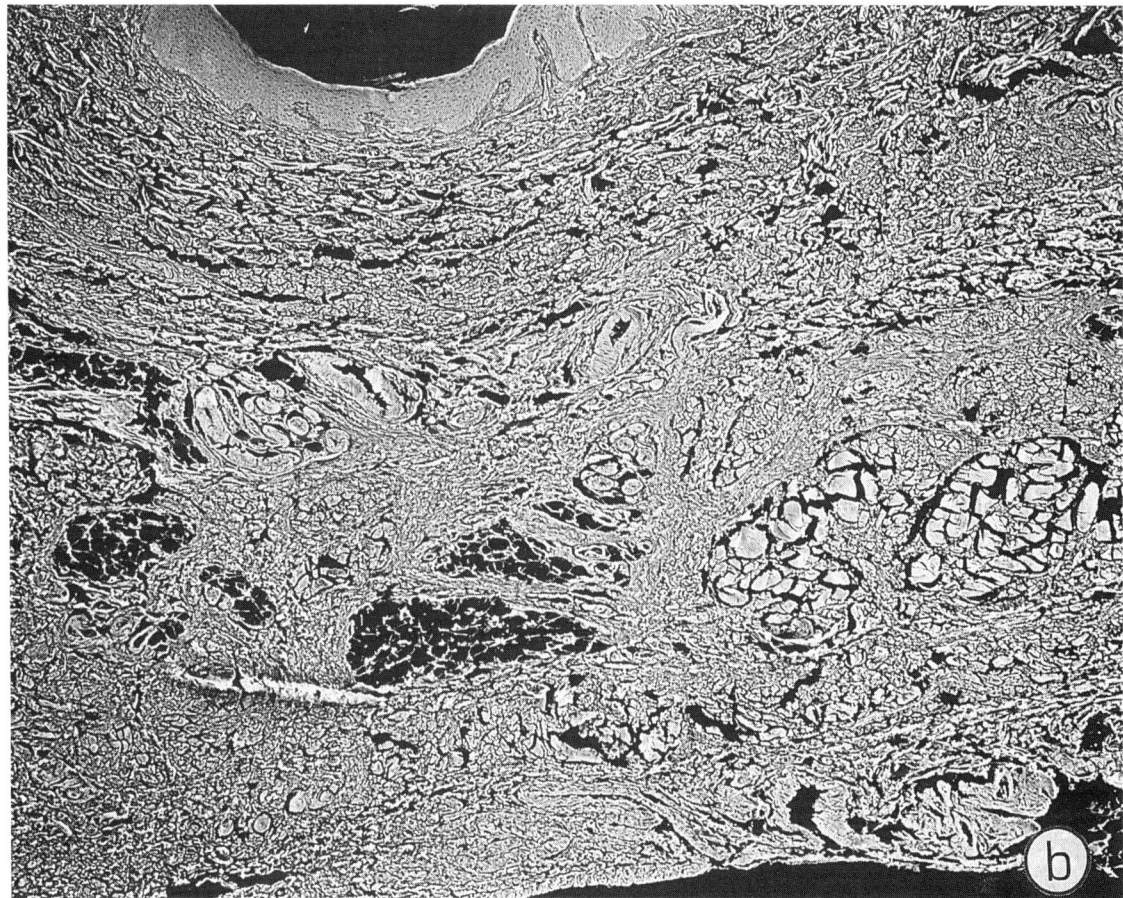

Fig. 13.12b

connective tissues within and between the fatty compartments and by perivascular fibroblastic activation (Fig. 13.14). Sometimes the replacement was associated with perilobular fibrosis and there often appeared to be periacinar and periductal fibrosis spreading centrifugally from the sweat ducts. The increased vascularity and perivascular reaction observed at the onset of the fibrotic replacement agreed with the observations of Meyerding et al (1941) but was at variance with the suggestion of Kischer & Speer (1984) that the excessive fibrosis of Dupuytren's contracture and hypertrophic scarring is due to, or associated with, tissue anoxia, occurring as a result of microvascular occlusion (Kischer et al 1982).

In ideal circumstances the young fibrofatty loculi exhibited well formed fat cells with intact microseptae surrounded by a thicker peripheral fibrous boundary composed of collagen and elastic fibres (Figs 13.10 and 13.11). The progressive fibrosis of the shock-absorbing system in the palm skin was associated with disaggregation, fragmentation and clumping of the elastic fibres in the fibrous septae between the fatty loculi and also with changes in the microarchitecture of the collagen fibres. Scanning electron microscopic photographs of specially prepared paraffin-embedded sections of palm skin graphically demonstrated marked disaggregation of the fibrous walls and septae of the fatty loculi and dense compaction and thickening of the collagen fibre bundles (Fig. 13.15). These findings support the observations of Millesi (1985) of compaction and changes in the viscoelastic properties of some of the collagen fibres in the superficial palm before the onset of any of the classical features of Dupuytren's disease.

Consequence of fibrosis

Although no biomechanical studies have been done to assess the resilience or compliance of fibrotic palms as opposed to those containing normally intact fat pads, it is likely that the progressive loss of the fibrofatty shock absorbent layer would be followed by progressive alterations in the distribution and dissipation of pressure and shearing forces in the palm. These changes would be compounded by the loss of free movement of the fascial microtendons within their paratenon sheaths which would follow their involvement in the progressive fibrotic process (McGrouther 1982). Compressive, or more particularly, compressive shearing forces applied to regions of the palm unprotected by an efficient elastic recoil system, especially in regions of greatest anteroposterior mobility, as in the fourth and fifth rays, could produce marked alterations in the longitudinal fibrous elements of the palmar connective tissue continuum.

As long as the protective insulation of the fat pads remained relatively intact and the longitudinal fascial fibres were still relatively mobile, increased compressive or shearing load on the palm would induce increased tensional loading on the longitudinally running fascial fibres leading to their compensatory thickening and hypertrophy. On the other hand, once the compressive absorptive capacity of the fat pads had been more profoundly affected by the increasing fibrosis, the longitudinally running collagen fibres would become less compliant and less able to slide or deform to accommodate the applied stress. This would be compounded by the glueing together and compaction of the fibre bundles which follow inflammatory oedema. These various factors would subject the fibre bundles to localized areas of high stress loading. The biological effect of this is discussed more fully in Chapter 26.

Although collagen fibres are extremely strong in transmitting or withstanding tensional forces they are notoriously weak when subjected to compressive or shearing stress (Parry 1988). It is for this reason that the collagen fibres in cartilage are embedded in a proteoglycan-rich matrix which absorbs and dissipates the compressive loads. If the longitudinally running collagen fibres in the superficial pretendinous bands are deprived of their protective fat pads, or the concentration of the glycosaminoglycan hyaluronate within the fibre bundles decreases (Flint et al 1982), making them

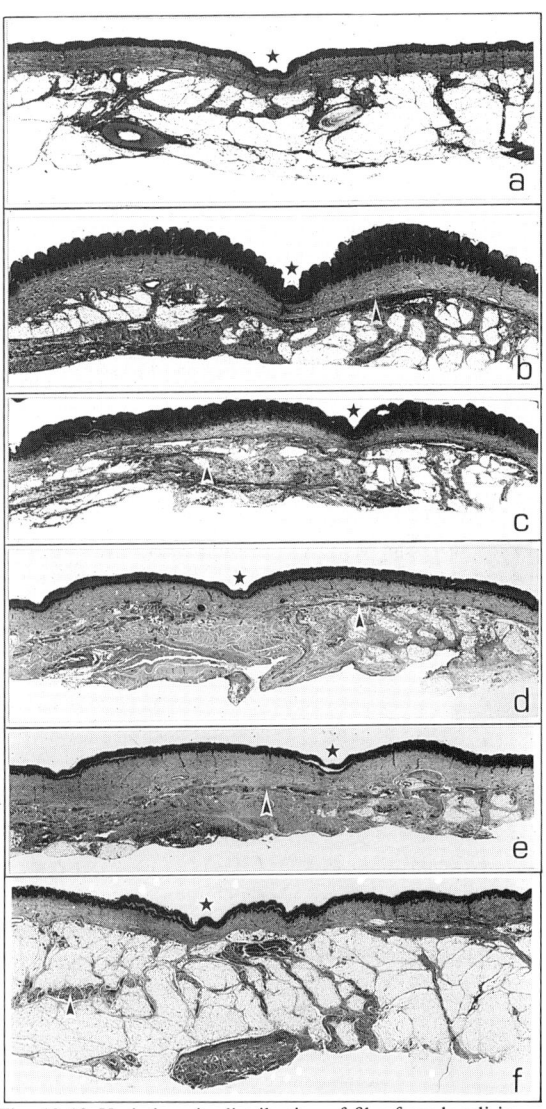

Fig. 13.13 Variations in distribution of fibrofatty loculi in longitudinal sections of palm skin taken along the fourth ray of individuals of various ages: **a** 17-year-old female; **b** 18-year-old male; **c** 16-year-old male; **d** 83-year-old male; **e** 80-year-old female. Star = Distal palmar crease; arrow = superficial longitudinal bundle, where discernible. **f** Intact fibrofatty loculi in an 83-year-old female, showing that the loss of fibrofatty loculi does not inevitably occur during ageing.

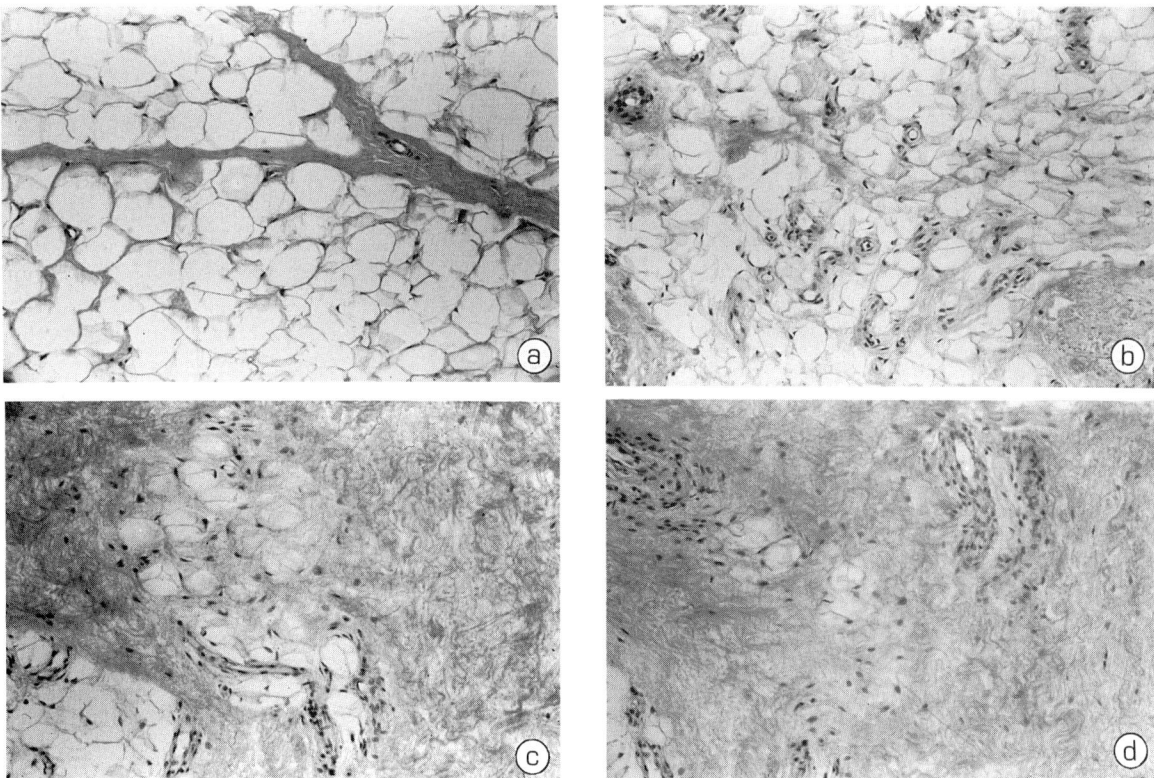

Fig. 13.14 Vascularity and fibrosis of fatty loculi. **a** Normal fatty loculi; **b** increasing vascularity amongst subdermal fibrofatty loculi in the palm of a 15-year-old male; **c** perivascular cellularity and fibrosis in fatty loculi in another area of the same palm; **d** area of fibrous replacement with faint ghosts of fatty loculi.

less compliant and stiffer, they become more vulnerable to these vertically applied compressive and shearing loads. As a consequence they are more likely to sustain stress or fatigue fractures and cracks, especially when the longitudinal bands are repeatedly flexed by the impact loading.

I believe that the palmar lesions of DD arise as a direct consequence of one or other of these biological responses. It has been well documented in other biological situations that the application of increased tensional loading to longitudinally running collagenous structures such as tendons inevitably leads to concomitant progressive increases in the thickness of the tension-transmitting collagen fibres (Buck 1953; Viidik 1967, 1968; Tipton et al 1967, 1970, 1975; Arem & Madden 1976). Such progressive thickening of the longitudinal fibre bundles was very evident in our studies. Figure 13.16 shows the increase in thickness from the normally very thin superficial pretendinous band of the child to the thickened palmar cords of the adult. It is apparent from our studies that the thickened cords run in the same direction and between the same anatomical layers as the thin superficial pretendinous bands and that they are in reality variations of one and the same structure. The observation of cellular nodule formation within these thickened bands (Figs 13.1 and 13.9) demonstrates that the DD process, on occasions at least, has its origins within abnormally thickened, but normally occurring, anatomical structures (Stack 1971; McFarlane 1974, 1985; Tubiana et al 1982).

Histopathological nodule development

In previous chapters it has been noted that the nodular areas which develop in the thickened fascial cords appear to be similar in biochemical content and cellular morphology to hypertrophic

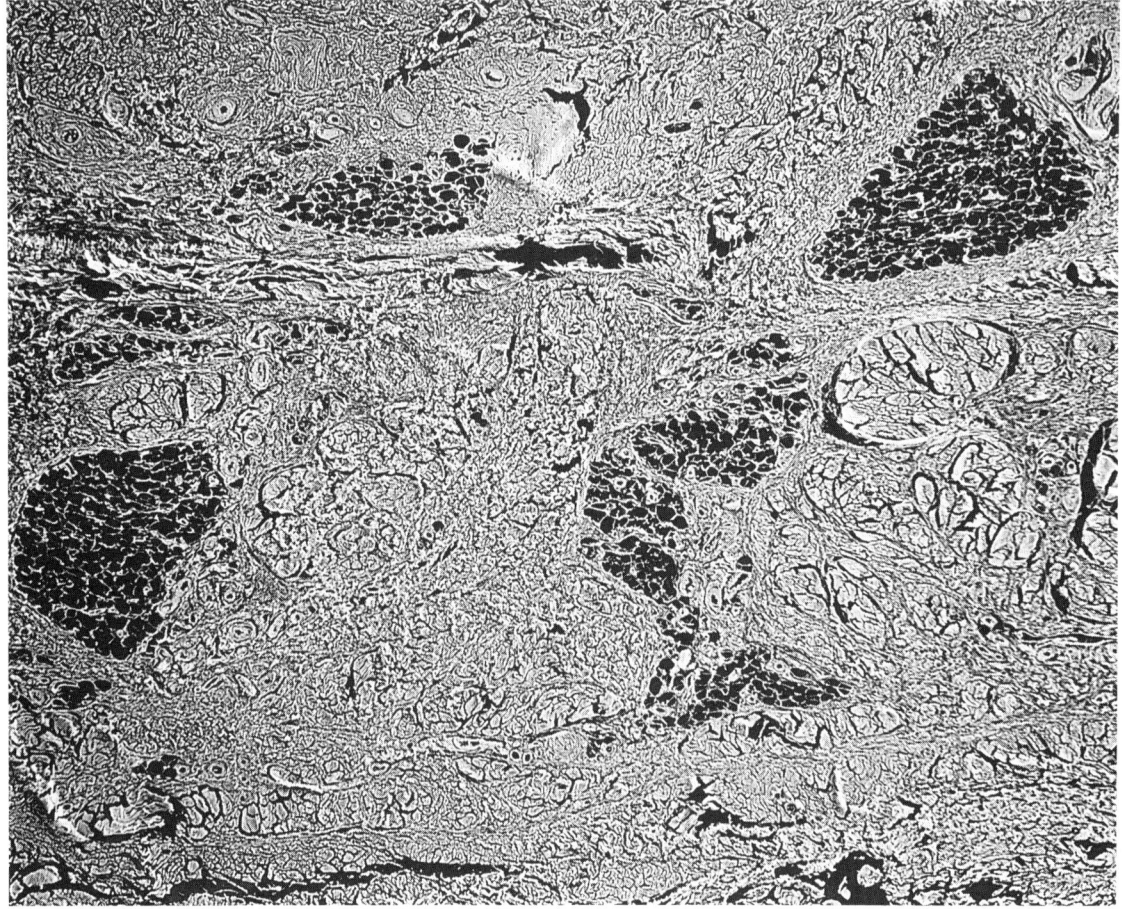

Fig. 13.15 Scanning electron microscope photomicrograph of the palm of an 18-year-old male showing loss and disaggregation of most fatty loculi and marked fibrosis of deep layers of the palm.

scars. Careful consideration of all the available data indicates that they are likely to be areas of reparative response or at least active tissue remodelling which develop as the result of a wound healing repair *within* the microtendon-like structure of the fascial bundle. How do these changes come about?

I believe that the changes in the physical characteristics and biomechanical properties of the palm — either by loss of the protective fat pads or by changes in the physicochemical and biomechanical properties of the fat contained within the fibrofatty lobules — will lead to an increased loading of the longitudinally running strands. In some instances, the increased intermittent tensional loading may simply stimulate collagen synthesis and collagen accretion by giving rise to increased fibril and bundle diameters (Parry et al 1982). However if the physical properties of the collagen fibres are less than ideal, perhaps due to changes in nutrition, changes in intrafascial hyaluronate levels, the effects of frictional heating (Harkness 1961, 1979, Rigby 1977) or the local accumulation of free radicals (Murrell et al 1987a, b; Outhwaite et al 1988), or if the increased tensional loading is more sudden and acute, there may be localized tearing or shredding of some of the collagen fibres within the substances of some of the longitudinally running bundles. If the tearing or shredding produces complete separation of the fibres, leaving a gap between the fibre ends such as is found following division of a tendon, one

THE GENESIS OF THE PALMAR LESION 151

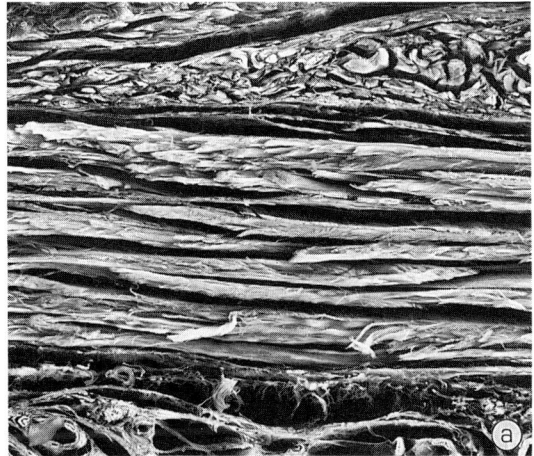

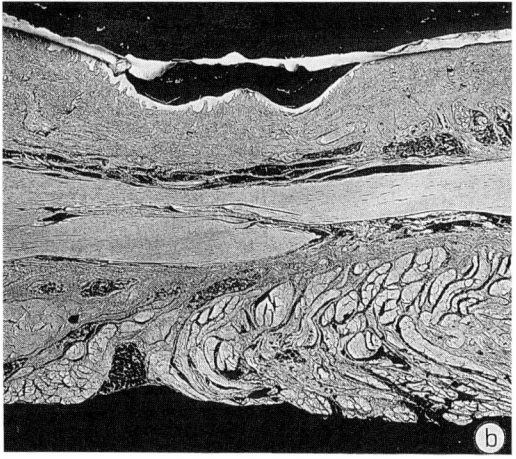

Fig. 13.16 a Scanning electron microscope photomicrograph of 3-month-old child: superficial longitudinal fascial strands approximately 100 μ thick lying within paratenon sheath. **b** Thickened superior longitudinal fascial band approximately 2 mm thick in 67-year-old male.

would anticipate that the normal processes of tendon repair would be set in motion with division and migration of cells from the paratenon-like structure covering the fascial strand. In this way the fibril continuity would be re-established without nodule formation, under the stimulation and guidance of the tensional forces (Fig. 13.17).

However, if the tearing of the fibres within the bundle was only partial, leaving an intact outer rim of fibres around an internal tear (Figs 13.9 and 13.18), then the repair process would be subject to entirely different forces. Cells coming into the reparative area would not then be subjected to longitudinal tensional forces and as a result would tend to form a diffuse cellular mass which would gradually increase in size to produce an obvious thickening within the fibre bundle. As the tensional forces would be still transmitted along the intact fibres in the periphery of the damaged bundle, the cells in the centre of the divided repair area would be deprived of the necessary controlling sensory input. In fact, they would probably be subjected to increased *compressional* forces induced by the pressure and constraint of the intact outer fibres as they were placed under tensional load (see Fig. 13.19). As a result, a cellular hypertrophic area would develop within the cord reminiscent of the hypertrophic callus which develops around a poorly immobilized limb fracture. As the developing wound repair lying within the substance of the palmar fascial bundle would be deprived of uniaxially directed tensional forces, the cells within their reparative area would continue to divide (hence their dense aggregation), and would continue to synthesize increased amounts of glycosaminoglycans, particularly chondroitin sulphate, and type III collagen. This situation would be continually self-perpetuating unless it was interrupted by changes in the physical loading of the tissue, or by treatment such as triamcinolone injections aimed at halting or reversing the cellular reaction (Ketchum 1971).

Research in other areas has indicated that tendons or skin wounds which are subjected to uniaxial longitudinal tension along their length, with little or no distractive tension from either side, are likely to contain lesser amounts of total glycosaminoglycan and lower levels of chondroitin sulphate (Flint et al 1980). The fact that the nodular areas of Dupuytren's contracture have quite high levels of total glycosaminoglycans with a greatly increased proportion of chondroitin sulphate adds weight to the suggestion that the repair tissue within the nodule is not subject to longitudinal tensional forces as one might expect, but is subject to laterally applied compressional forces.

Our previous research work on tendons and sesamoids (Gillard et al 1979) demonstrated that applied compressional forces encourage the development or persistence of round chondrocytic-like cells which synthesize increased amounts of glycosaminoglycans, particularly chondroitin sul-

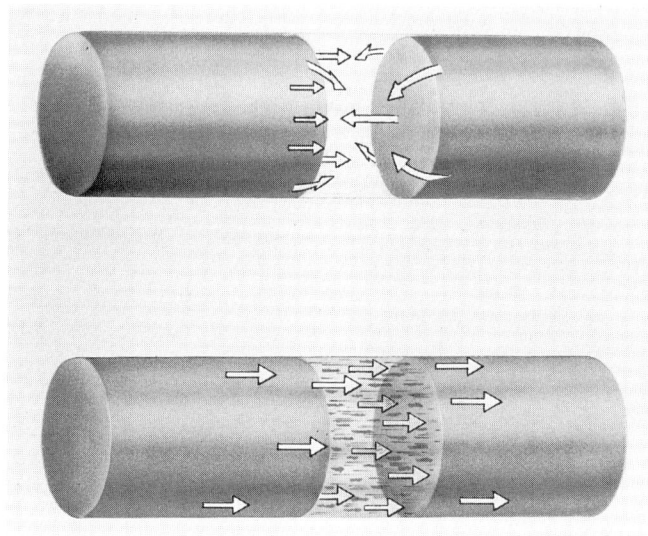

Fig. 13.17 Complete division of tension-transmitting fibres stimulates cellular organization and repair of the gap (top) which becomes organized and aligned by uniaxial tension forces (bottom).

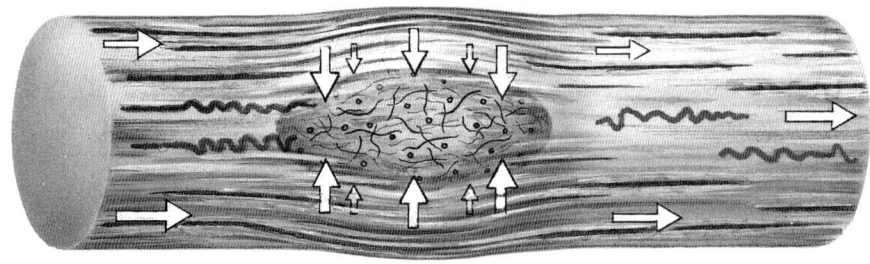

Fig. 13.18 The result of an incomplete intrafascial (or intratendinous) central tear or fibre division: fibres are intact peripherally. The central repair would lack the uniaxial tensional forces necessary for cellular and scaffold alignment and would be subject to additional lateral compressional forces from the intact peripheral longitudinal fibres.

phate, with the result that there is less compaction and organization of the collagen fibres (Merrilees & Flint 1980). In the Dupuytren's nodule the greatest increase in glycosaminoglycan is in the chondroitin sulphate fraction. This and the chondroid morphological features of the cellular response support the suggestion that the tissues within the nodule are subjected to lateral compressional forces as a result of the longitudinal tensional forces still exerted on the peripheral fibres (Fig. 13.20).

Previous research has demonstrated that the red staining of collagen fibres of mature intact cords by the Masson trichrome procedure indicates that they are subject to longitudinal tension (Flint & Lyons 1975; Flint et al 1975) whereas the retention

THE GENESIS OF THE PALMAR LESION 153

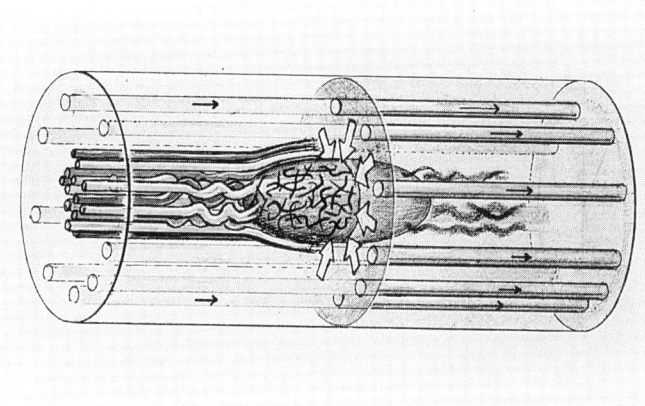

Fig. 13.19 Centripetal pressure forces acting on the intrafascial repair will perpetuate the lack of longitudinal orientation of cells and collagen fibres and stimulate continued synthesis of chondroitin sulphate and type III collagen.

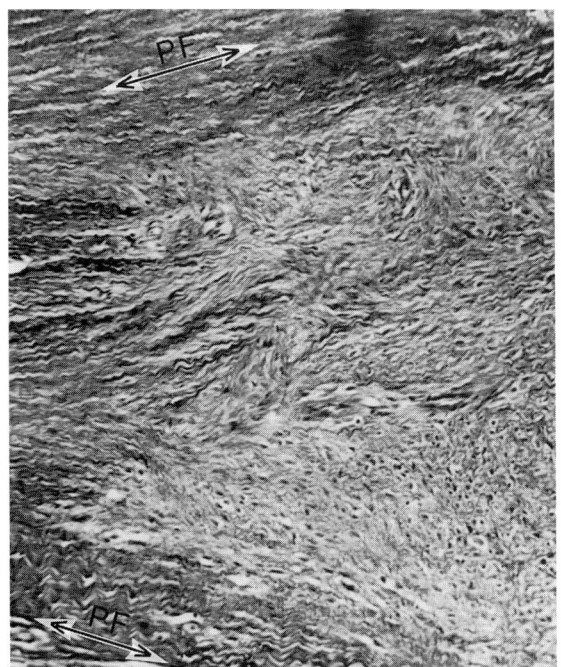

Fig. 13.20 Photomicrograph of longitudinal section of edge of intrafascial lesion in superficial longitudinal band showing peripheral fibre (PF) continuity, central fibre discontinuity and chondroid-like cells within the reparative zone.

mature fibrous cords confirms their tensional state whilst the green staining of collagen fibres within the nodules or in the bands adjacent to the nodule supports the concept that these fibres have been severed at the level of the nodule and demonstrates that there is little or no uniaxial tensional force acting upon them. Polarized light studies also demonstrate the disaggregation and separation of collagen fibres in the centre of the nodules with the maintenance of a rim of old intact fibres around the periphery (Fig. 13.21).

It is now over 40 years since Tord Skoog postulated that the cellular nodular areas developed in regions where the collagen fibres had been disrupted (Skoog 1948, 1963, 1967). Unfortunately, his ideas and those of supporting workers such as Larsen (Larsen et al 1960) have been severely criticized (Hueston 1975, 1985) and almost rejected. It is now over 100 years since Madelung (1876) suggested that as a result of the loss of the subdermal fat,

of the green dye of the Masson trichrome procedure by collagen fibres indicates that they are not subject to these forces. In many Dupuytren's nodules and bands the red Masson staining of the

single regions of the palm would become more exposed to a constant pressure, become more easily injured, especially those which are situated opposite the firm part of the bony structure of the hand, e.g., the heads of the metacarpal bones and the flexor tendons. The frequent injurious exposure evidently excites the now unprotected tense connective tissue of the palm to a state of chronic inflammation, leads to hyperplasia of the normal fibres and finally to their shrinking with consequent permanent bending of the

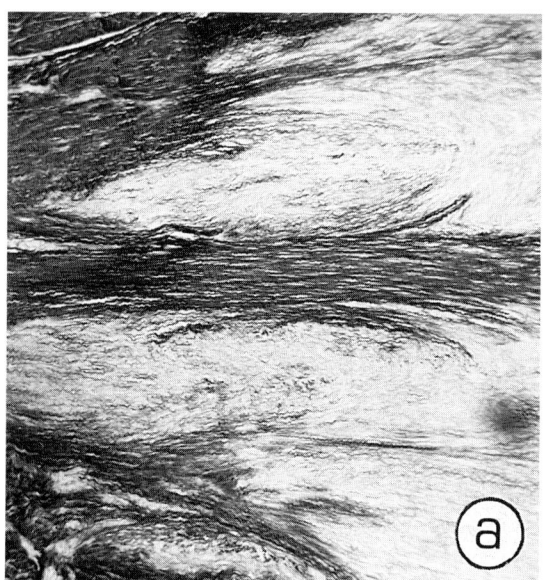 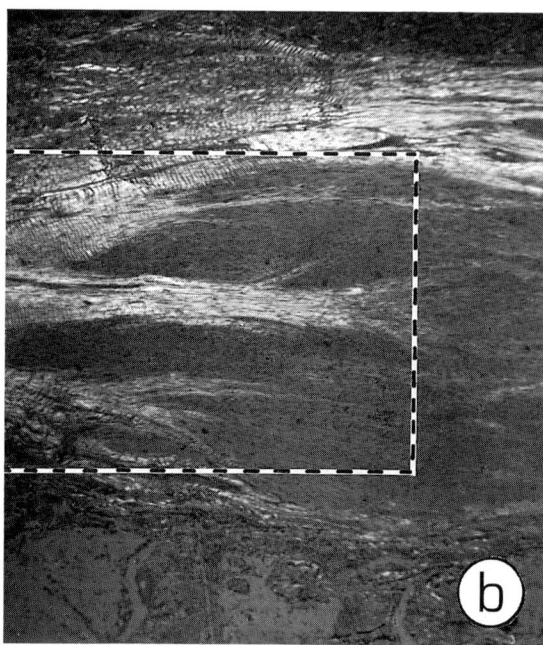

Fig. 13.21a Photomicrograph of Van Giesen stained histological section of the superficial longitudinal band showing a composite intrafascial lesion partly divided by a band of fibres. These fibres probably previously served as the peripheral fibres of two adjacent lesions which have become confluent as the result of secondary fibril rupture. b Adjacent section, viewed through crossed polarizing prisms, shows the composite nature of the lesion with residual birefringent collagen fibres surrounding the island of frustrated repair. The field demonstrated in Figure 13.21a is indicated by dashed lines on Figure 13.21b.

fingers . . . *and that the numerous consequent exposures to injury* will act more and more on the individual diseased part and incite it to further change.' (Madelung, 1876).

Whilst we acknowledge that DD may have a multifactorial basis, we feel that it is now essential to reconsider the role of mechanical factors in the induction of the palmar lesion. We believe that with the application of biological principles to an understanding of DD we are now able satisfactorily to integrate the observations of Dupuytren, Goyrand, Madelung, Meyerding, Skoog, Hueston, Millesi, McFarlane, McGrouther and Flint into a more meaningful and understandable integrated montage.

R. M. McFarlane

14 The finger

The key to treatment of Dupuytren's disease (DD) is a clear understanding of the normal and pathological anatomy of the fascia that is involved. This is especially true in the finger where the anatomy of the fascia is complex and other structures such as neurovascular bundles, tendons and tendon sheaths, joint capsules and ligaments as well as the overlying skin are intimately related to one other. The following account is provided according to the thesis that all of the finger contractures that occur in DD can be explained on the basis of pathological shortening of the normal fascial structures.

THE DIGITAL FASCIA

Our understanding of digital anatomy is provided by classical anatomists and embellished by the detailed studies of Gosset (1972) and Landsmeer (1976). Stack (1971) and Thomine (1972) paid special attention to the fascia in Landsmeer's preparations of fetal hands. It is difficult to interpret fascial anatomy because the usual methods of dissection destroy the very tissue that is to be studied. In the finger, a somewhat different interpretation will be made if the dissection proceeds from the dorsum, the side, or the palmar surface. It is for this reason that Landsmeer prepared longitudinal and transverse sections of small hands which could be studied serially.

Ideally, the diseased fascia should be studied in fresh cadaver hands, as reported by Dupuytren (1832), Goyrand (1833), Adams (1879), and Kaplan (1965) but sufficient material is not often available. My own observations have been made in

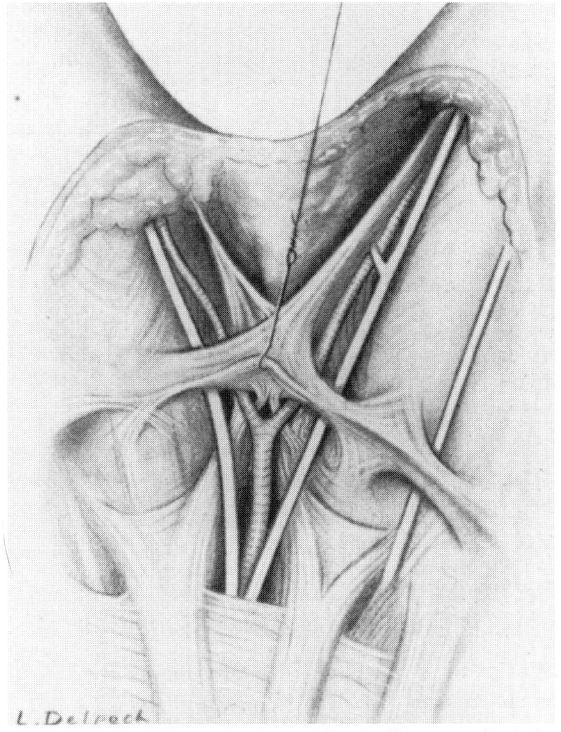

Fig. 14.1 Even though this illustration is diagrammatic, it is anatomically accurate and extremely helpful in understanding the pathological anatomy of the palmar digital area. The various components of fascia are clearly shown because all of the fat that normally occupies this area has been removed. Proximally the transverse fibres of the palmar aponeurosis are shown and just distal to them the pretendinous bands of the palmar aponeurosis bifurcate and pass on either side of the capsule of the metacarpophalageal joint. The fibres then enter a three-dimensional chiasm to which fibres of the natatory ligament contribute and more distally these fibres form the lateral digital sheet of finger fascia. Note the very proximal bifurcation of the digital nerve whereas the digital artery only bifurcates because the fibres of the natatory ligament demand it. It is at this site that the artery and sometimes the nerve are frequently cut. From Gosset (1972).

the operating room and recorded not only by photography but also by a medical illustrator who was present at the operation and capable of highlighting the essential anatomical features.

THE PALMAR DIGITAL AREA

A knowledge of the anatomy at the junction of the palm and finger, that is, the palmar digital area, is essential in the treatment of DD because this is the commonest site of injury to the neurovascular bundle. The normal anatomy of this area was described by Gosset (1972). His description is the basis of my interpretation of the pathological changes that occur. The normal fascial structures are clearly demonstrated in Figure 14.1, taken from Gosset's original paper. The more superficial fibres of the pretendinous band of the palmar aponeurosis terminate in the skin near the distal crease of the palm. They are not shown in Figure 14.1. The deeper fibres pass on either side of the metacarpophalangeal joint, deep to the neurovascular bundles, to reach the side of the finger. They are band-like and are very obvious in the normal state. Because these fibres spiral around the neurovascular bundle they are called the spiral bands of Gosset; in disease they are called the spiral cords.

At this same level the natatory ligament consists not only of fibres passing across the distal palm but also of fibres passing down each side of each finger. These fibres blend with the spiral band to form what Gosset called the lateral digital sheet. In the normal state this structure is also band-like, easily identified, and readily dissected from the overlying skin. In disease it becomes the lateral cord. Thus a three-dimensional chiasm is formed by the fascia in the palmar digital area and through this chiasm pass the digital nerves and vessels. In the normal state these components of fascia never interfere with the dissection of important structures such as nerve and vessel. In disease not only is the fascia thickened but there is joint contracture, altering normal relationships. Unless the normal state is understood it is very difficult to dissect with safety through this area.

THE FINGER FASCIA

Within the finger the fascia consists of an outer tubular sheath of superficial fascia which is fibrofatty on the dorsal and palmar surfaces, but more sheet-like laterally where it is called the lateral digital sheet (Gosset 1972). Within the core of the finger are condensations of fascia such as the flexor tendon sheath, Cleland's, Grayson's, and Landsmeer's ligaments (Fig. 14.2). As in the palm, only certain components of this fascia become diseased and one would expect this fact to be a clue to the pathological process. It does suggest that biomechanical forces play a role.

The palmar and dorsal superficial fascia is fibrofatty, containing more or less fat in different individuals. The palmar fascia is often diseased and forms the central cord which is a common cause of proximal interphalangeal joint contrac-

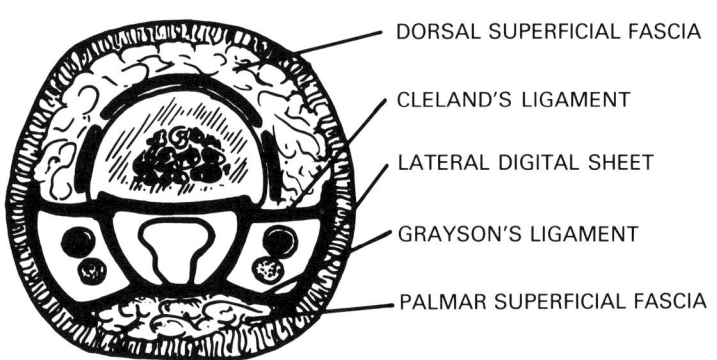

Fig. 14.2 Cross section of the finger.

ture. The dorsal fascia is the site of knuckle pads which usually appear over the proximal interphalangeal joint. They do not cause contracture per se, probably because of the different forces applied to the diseased tissue by flexion and extension.

Figure 14.2 shows Cleland's and Grayson's ligaments. Cleland (1878) reported that:

> strong ligaments, hitherto undescribed, extend from the sides of the phalanges, near the phalangeal articulations, and are inserted into the skin, helping to retain the different parts of the integument in the positions which they are adapted to occupy.

These observations were corroborated by Grayson (1940) who wrote:

> The ligaments arise from the sides of the phalanges and are inserted into the skin over the interphalangeal joints. But in addition to these structures it was apparent that there is also a fibrous septum volar to the digital vessels and nerves. This septum forms a series of retinacula which, if we refer to Cleland's ligaments as the deep digital skin retinacula, might well be termed the superficial or volar retinacula. Their distribution is such that they could obviously subserve precisely the same function as their deeper fellows.

Grayson's figure is reproduced here as Figure 14.3 and shows — of particular importance in DD — that the neurovascular bundle is deep to Grayson's but superficial to Cleland's ligament. The figure does not show that in the normal state Grayson's ligaments are delicate and sheet-like whereas Cleland's ligaments are thick, firm, and ligamentous in appearance (Fig. 14.4). It is my observation that Grayson's ligaments are frequently, if not always, diseased in DD whereas Cleland's ligaments are not.

Thomine (1972) did not observe Cleland's ligaments but interpreted the fascia deep to the neurovascular bundle as a retrovascular band of tissue attached to the side of the proximal phalanx as well as the distal phalanx but running in a proximal–distal direction. He cites the observations of Legueu & Juvara (1892) to corroborate his views. It is probable that what was observed by Thomine in the fetal hand and Cleland in the adult hand was similar tissue, altered by function in the adult. However, in disease, I have observed the retrovascular cord of Thomine lying superficial

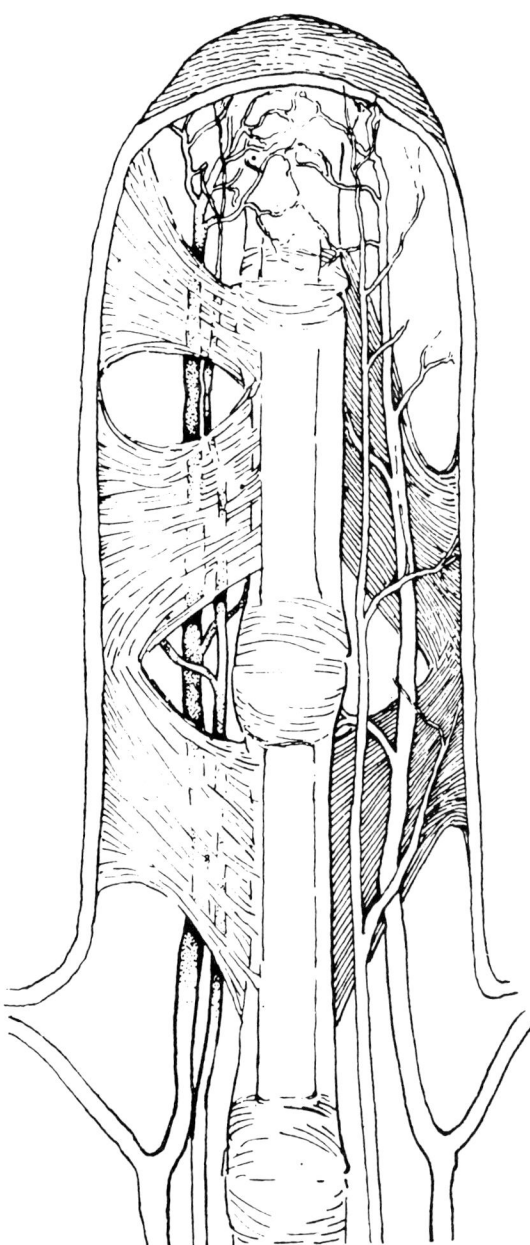

Fig. 14.3 From Grayson (1940), showing the attachment of Cleland's and Grayson's ligaments and their relationship to the neurovascular bundles. In the fetus these structures are continuous sheets of fascia and are not distinguishable from other fascia. Their adult appearance is due to stresses applied by joint movement; Cleland's ligaments are much stronger than Grayson's ligaments, which retain the appearance of a discontinuous fascial sheet.

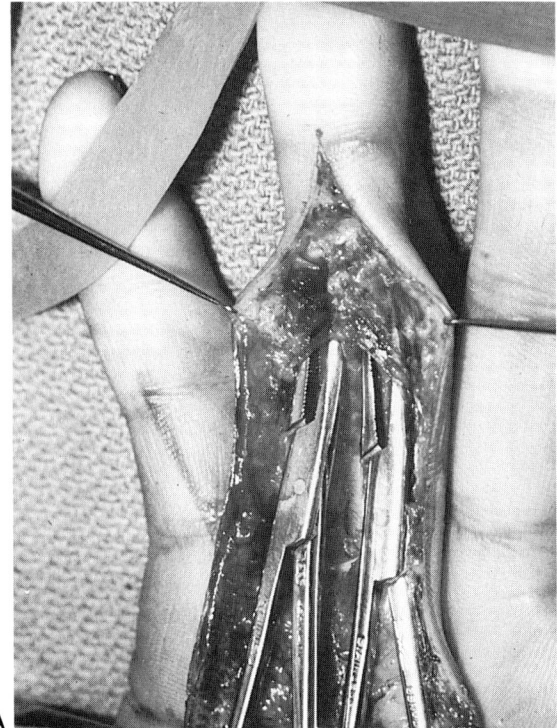

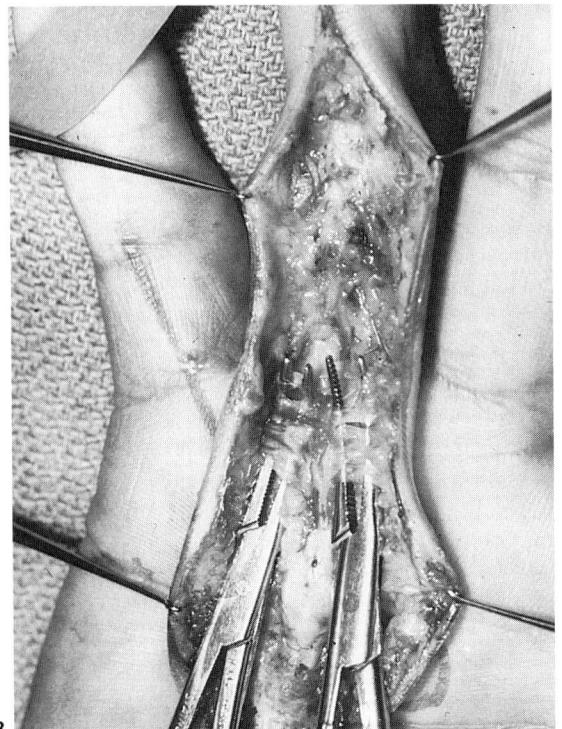

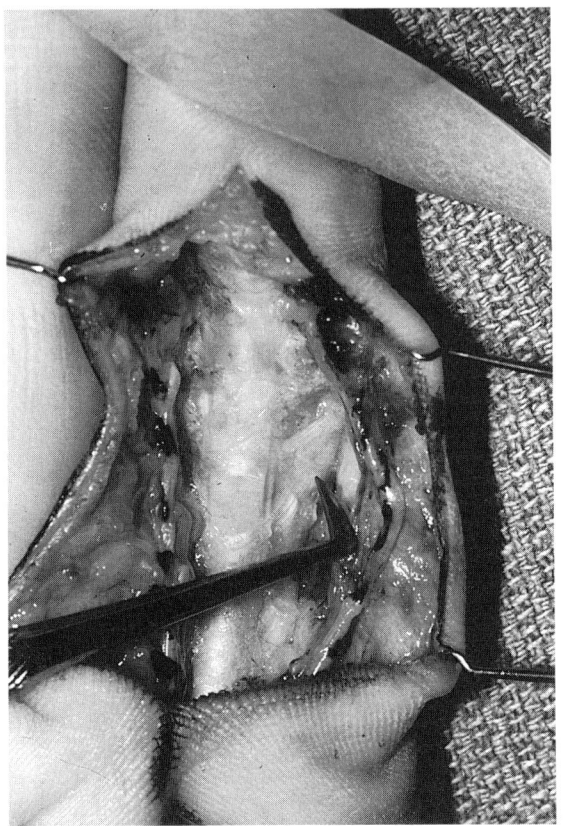

Fig. 14.4 A comparison of Grayson's, Cleland's and the natatory ligament. **A** Grayson's ligaments are shown over the middle phalanx bilaterally. Centrally they are attached to the flexor tendon sheath and laterally to the skin. The haemostats are deep to each ligament which is thin and translucent in the normal state. **B** The natatory ligament in the same patient. The texture of the fascia is the same because Grayson's ligaments and the natatory ligament are derived from the same embryological layer. **C** In another patient Cleland's ligament is shown on the ulnar side of the little finger at the tip of the probe. It is discrete, thick and ligamentous.

to normal-seeming Cleland's ligaments. Thus there is abundant fascia in this retrovascular area of the digit to account for the retrovascular band of Thomine and Cleland's ligaments. Whether both structures exist or are simply different interpretations of the same tissue and whether or not Cleland's ligaments are involved in the process of DD are academic arguments. What is important is that diseased tissue resides dorsal to the neurovascular bundles. It must be found and removed at operation.

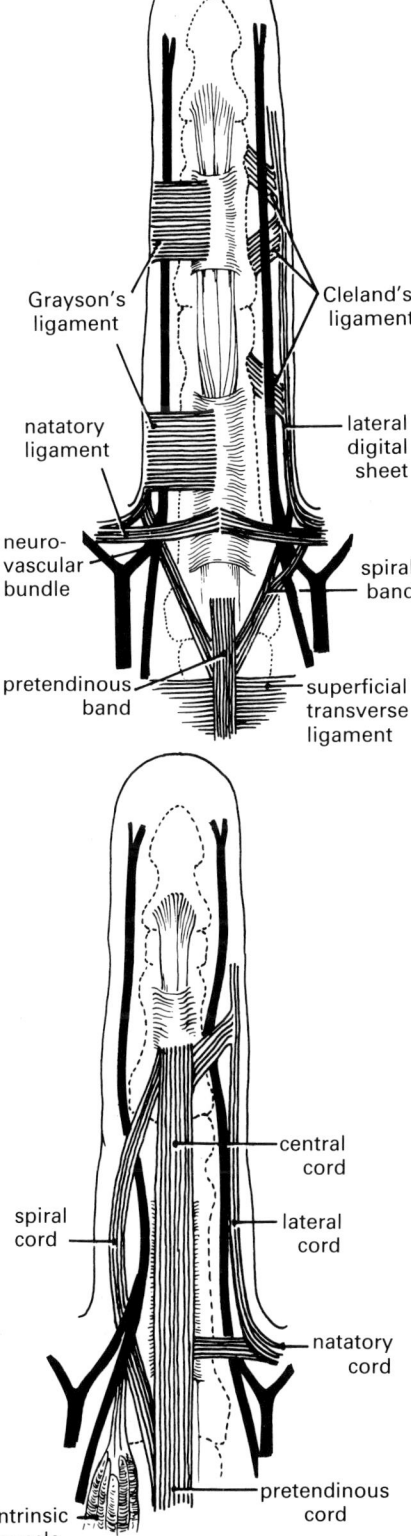

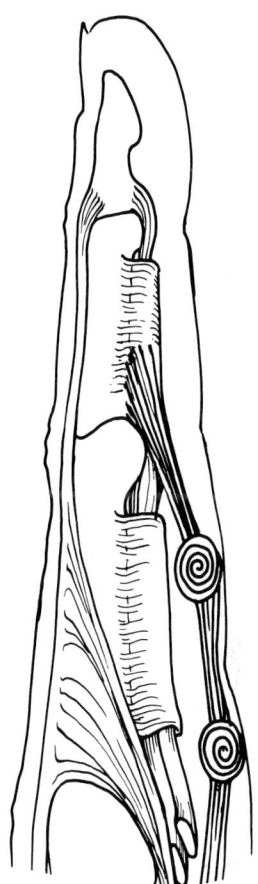

Fig. 14.6 The relation of diseased fascia to skin in the finger, in particular, as it pertains to the central cord. Over the proximal phalanx the fascia is intimately related to skin and a nodule is often present just distal to the proximal crease or just proximal to the middle crease of the finger. The fascia is free of the tendon sheath. Distal to the proximal interphalangeal joint the converse is true. The fascia attaches to the tendon sheath but is free of the skin.

THE DISEASED FASCIA

There are four cords which alone or in combination contract the interphalangeal joints (McFarlane 1974). Each one originates in fascia that is normally present and, except for the central cord which arises from the palmar superficial fascia, the fascia is band-like in its original state (Fig. 14.5). The fascia from which these cords arise is present bilaterally but invariably the diseased cord appears

Fig. 14.5 A The normal components of the finger fascia; **B** the change in this fascia to form the central, lateral, and spiral cords that contract the proximal interphalangeal joint. (The retrovascular cord is shown in Figure 14.12.)

160 DUPUYTREN'S DISEASE

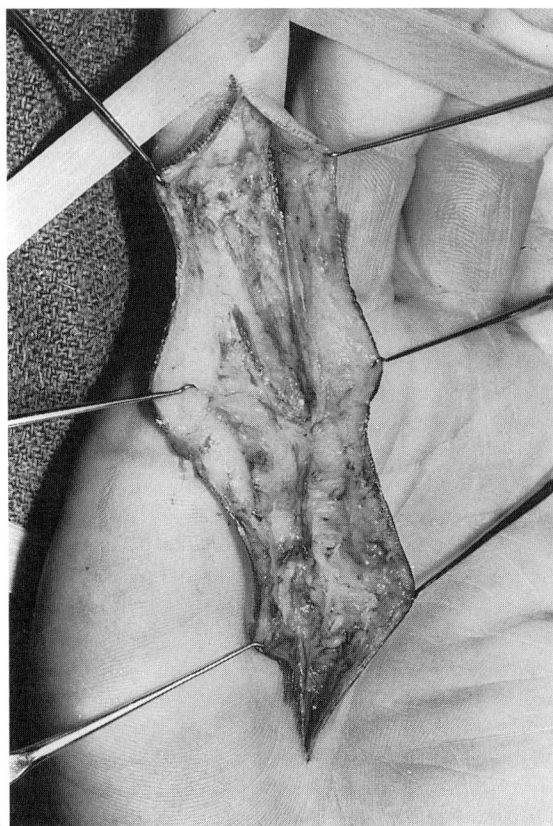

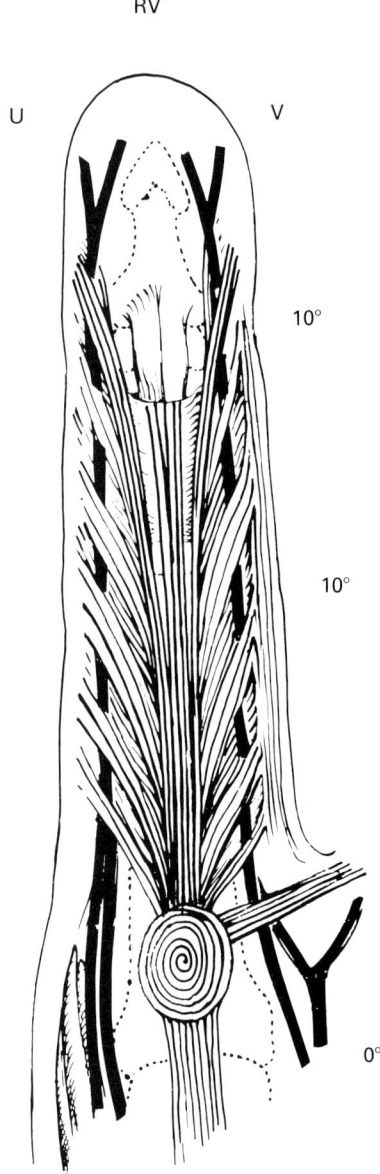

Fig. 14.7 A and **B** The right little finger in early disease. Note the diffuse nature of the fascia but orientation is still longitudinal. **C–E** The left little finger in advanced disease. The central cord is well developed and attaches to the tendon sheath and bone on the radial side of the middle phalanx. The radial neurovascular bundle is tethered to the side of the phalanx by diseased fascia. In the little finger there is usually diseased fascia on the ulnar side; however, it was absent in this patient.

only on one side. This is another observation that supports the view that biomechanical forces contribute to the progress of disease. The diseased cords lie palmar to the mid lateral line of the finger. There is fascial continuity from the palmar to the dorsal surface of the finger, notably through Landsmeer's ligaments and the lateral peritendinous cutaneous fibres described by Stanisavljevic & Pool (1962), Milford (1968) and Law & McGrouther (1984). These structures are not diseased but with abnormal tensions applied, Landsmeer's ligaments are involved in the development of the boutonnière deformity of DD and the peritendinous fibres may contribute to the development of knuckle pads.

It is important to appreciate that the diseased fascia in the finger is not distributed haphazardly but rather appears as four cords which are present singly or in combination. Since my description of these cords in 1974 I have expected others to report new patterns of disease or variations of this pathological anatomy. White (1984) has detailed the normal anatomy of the ulnar side of the hand as it pertains to DD and Barton (1984) has studied

THE FINGER 161

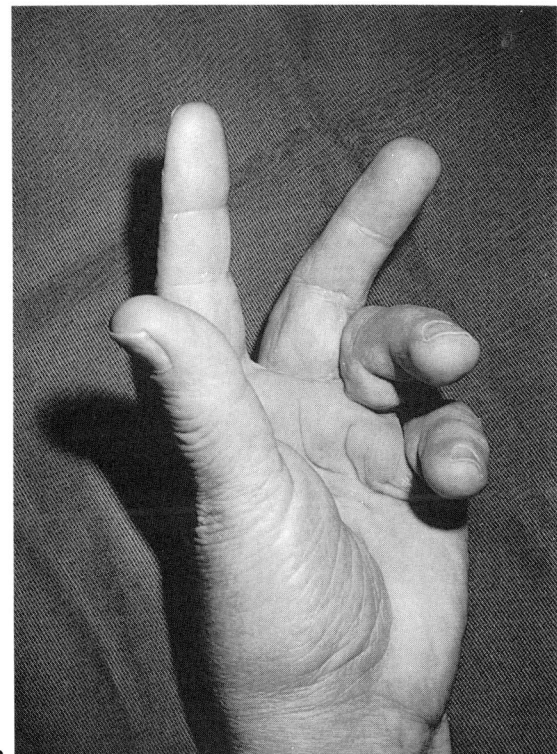

C

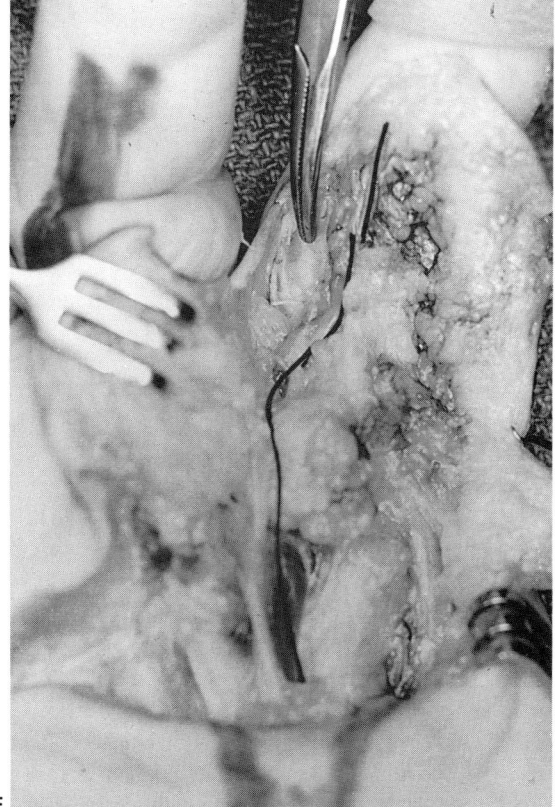

E

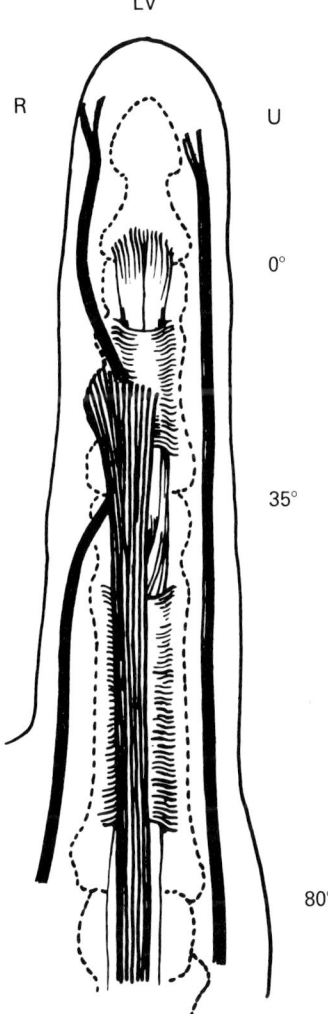

D

the diseased tissue in the same area. Strickland & Bassett (1985) described cords within the digit arising from periosteum, ligament and intrinsic tendon; this is a somewhat different interpretation of the origin of the spiral cord and also implies that Cleland's ligaments are involved in DD. Recently Cleland (an appropriate name!) & Morrison (1986) reported the presence of a central cord in the thumb. Further observations are inevitable but the point has been made that the diseased tissue appears in a predictable rather than a haphazard fashion from pre-existing normal fascia.

A clear understanding of each cord of diseased fascia will help the surgeon to correct joint con-

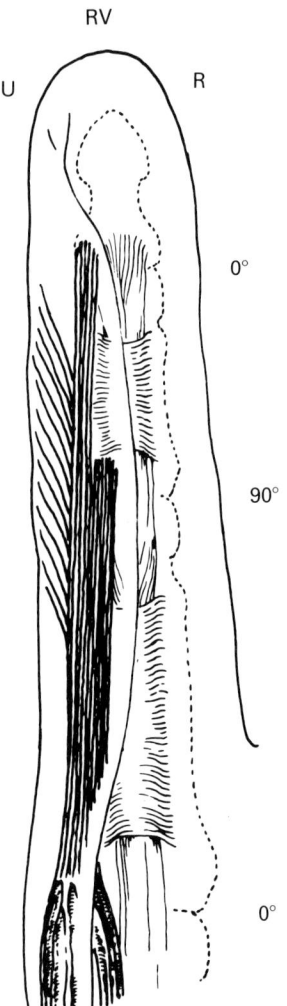

Fig. 14.8 An example of a lateral cord pushing the ulnar neurovascular bundle of the little finger toward the midline. The cord arose in the abductor digiti minimi tendon and was attached not only to skin but also to the bone of the middle and distal phalanges. This patient had 90° proximal interphalangeal joint contracture but no contracture at the distal interphalangeal joint, although the diseased fascia was present.

tracture and avoid damage to the neurovascular bundles.

The central cord

The central cord is a direct extension of the pretendinous cord in the palm and is the commonest cause of proximal interphalangeal joint contracture. It arises from the palmar superficial fascia and lies between the neurovascular bundles. Over the proximal phalanx the cord is intimately attached to skin but not to tendon sheath (Fig. 14.6). It attaches to tendon sheath and periosteum of the middle phalanx, usually on one or other side but a symmetrical attachment is seen occasionally. The development of this cord from the fibrofatty superficial fascia is apparent from its appearance in early and advanced disease, as illustrated in Figure 14.7. The central cord does not displace the neurovascular bundle but some fibres of Grayson's ligament invariably became involved and tether the bundle closer to the phalanx.

The lateral cord

The lateral cord arises from the lateral digital sheet and therefore receives fibres from the natatory ligament and the spiral band. On the ulnar side of the little finger the natatory ligament does not contribute but a well developed band is present in the normal state and a diseased cord frequently arises from the tendon of insertion of the abductor digiti minimi muscle (Fig. 14.8). On the radial side of the index finger a lateral cord, coursing from the base of the thumb, through the first web space and into the index finger is not uncommon. The lateral cord attaches primarily to skin and generally does not cause severe proximal interphalangeal joint contracture. Through Grayson's ligament it attaches to the tendon sheath distal to the proximal interphalangeal joint and in the little finger can cause severe proximal interphalangeal joint contracture. The distal extension of the lateral cord causes distal interphalangeal joint contracture. The cord does not disturb the neurovascular bundle, except in the little finger where its bulk can push the neurovascular bundle toward the midline.

The spiral cord

The spiral cord is a composite structure which arises from the pretendinous cord and terminates on the middle phalanx through Grayson's ligament, as illustrated in Figure 14.9. Occasionally it seems to arise from an interosseous tendon of the ring or middle finger, especially the tendon of the fourth dorsal interosseus muscle, but the spiral

THE FINGER 163

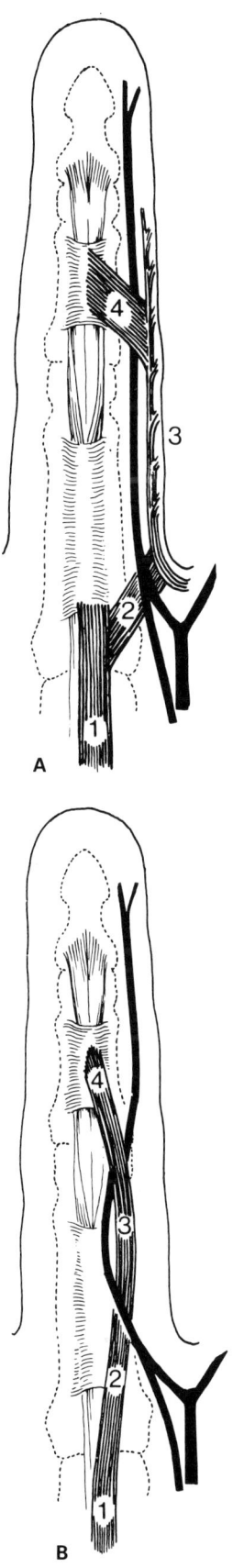

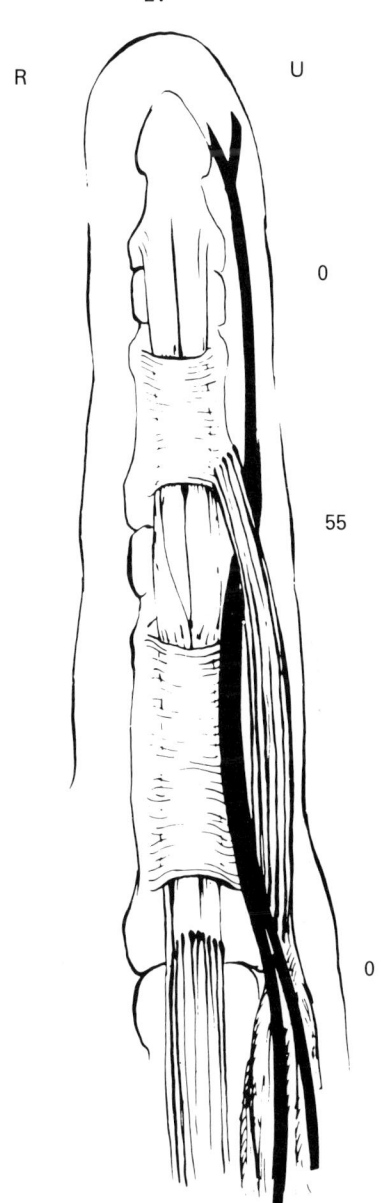

Fig. 14.9 A The four normal fascial components forming the spiral cord. 1 = pretendinous band; 2 = spiral band; 3 = lateral digital sheet; 4 = Grayson's ligament. **B** As these structures shorten with disease and form a cord-like structure the neurovascular bundle is displaced toward the midline of the finger.

Fig. 14.10 A spiral cord arising from the abductor digiti minimi tendon. This pattern is similar to Figure 14.8.

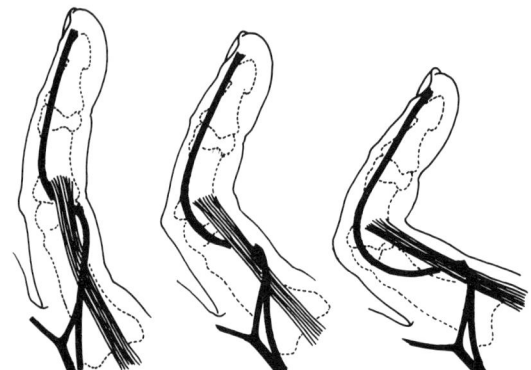

Fig. 14.11 From left: proximal, superficial and central displacement of the neurovascular bundle with increasing flexion contracture at the proximal interphalangeal joint.

band is also involved. Strickland & Bassett (1985) observed similar cords, frequently arising from the periosteum of the proximal phalanx as well as intrinsic tendons. Because the spiral band is always present in the normal state and because its anatomical course is close to the capsule of the metacarpophalangeal joint, the base of the proximal phalanx, and interosseous tendons, I believe that it is the spiral band that is involved in every instance and the band has become more or less adherent to one or other structure in the area.

On the ulnar side of the little finger there is a spiral band and therefore a spiral cord can appear in the usual way. In addition, a type of spiral cord can arise from the tendon of the abductor digiti minimi muscle in the sense that the neurovascular bundle is superficial to the muscle belly in the palm but passes deep to the diseased cord over the proximal phalanx (Fig. 14.10).

The spiral cord usually causes severe proximal interphalangeal joint contracture. Therefore, with severe contracture, one should suspect a spiral cord. I know of no other way of predicting a spiral cord contracture. With severe metacarpophalangeal joint and proximal interphalangeal joint contracture the spiral cord is invariably present and the neurovascular bundle is displaced. The more severe the contracture, the more proximal and superficial is the point of displacement of the neurovascular bundle so that the bundle could be divided during the skin incision (Fig. 14.11).

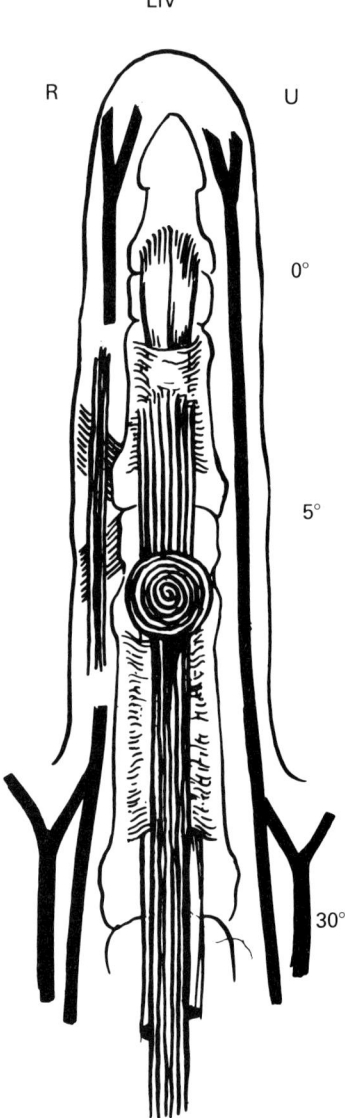

Fig. 14.12 The retrovascular cord. It attaches to the proximal, middle and distal phalanges and it is well developed at the level of the proximal interphalangeal joint. It lies superficial or palmar to Cleland's ligaments.

The retrovascular cord

The retrovascular cord is located dorsal to the neurovascular bundle. The fibres are oriented longitudinally and therefore are distinct from Cleland's ligament. In the diseased state the cord is most prominent at the level of the proximal in-

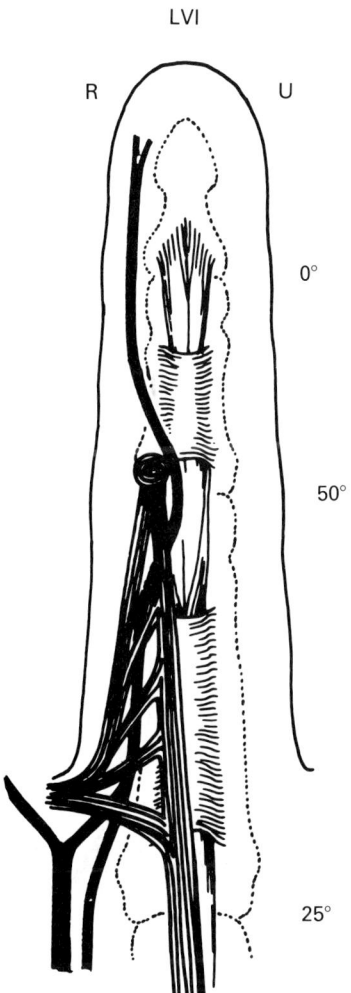

Fig. 14.13 An example of combination of a central and lateral cord causing 50° flexion contracture at the proximal interphalangeal joint of the left ring finger. Note how the lateral cord arises from the natatory cord. The neurovascular bundle is deep to the diseased cords but becomes centrally displaced at the level of the proximal interphalangeal joint because most of the fascia attaches to the base of the middle phalanx lateral to the bundle. A nodule was present at the attachment of the fascia.

terphalangeal joint (Fig. 14.12). The retrovascular cord has not been found to be the sole cause of proximal interphalangeal joint contracture but it is often present in combination with other cords and is often seen with recurrent proximal interphalangeal joint contracture. This cord proceeds distally

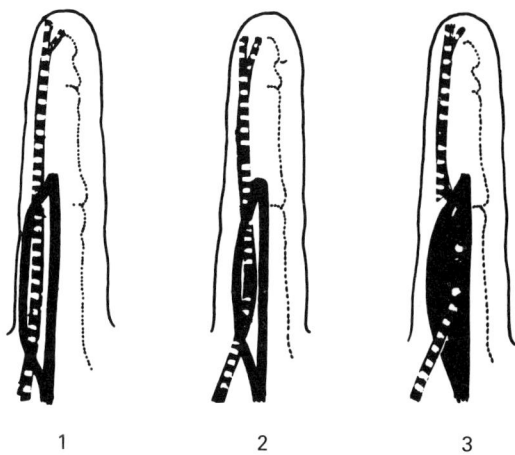

Fig. 14.14 The process of encasement of the neurovascular bundle by a central and spiral cord. **1** Early in disease the two cords are separate. **2** With contracture the spiral cord approaches the central cord and displaces the neurovascular bundle. **3** The two cords form a mass of tissue through which the neurovascular bundle passes. There is always a plane in which to separate the neurovascular bundle by blunt dissection. The surgeon can proceed with confidence if the mechanism of this displacement is understood.

beyond the distal interphalangeal joint where it blends with the lateral cord and terminates on the side of the distal phalanx. Therefore, it can contract the distal interphalangeal joint with the lateral cord.

COMBINATIONS OF CORDS

Usually one cord is the prime cause of proximal interphalangeal joint contracture but others are present. This is especially so of the central cord which is the most common cause of proximal interphalangeal joint contracture. With excision of the cord which seems to be the prime offender, it is not uncommon for the proximal interphalangeal joint to remain flexed until the less well developed cords have also been removed. It is for this reason that I recommend block excision of the diseased fascia rather than removal of one cord at a time (see Section 5). The two common combinations are a central and lateral cord (Fig. 14.13) and a central and spiral cord (Fig. 14.14).

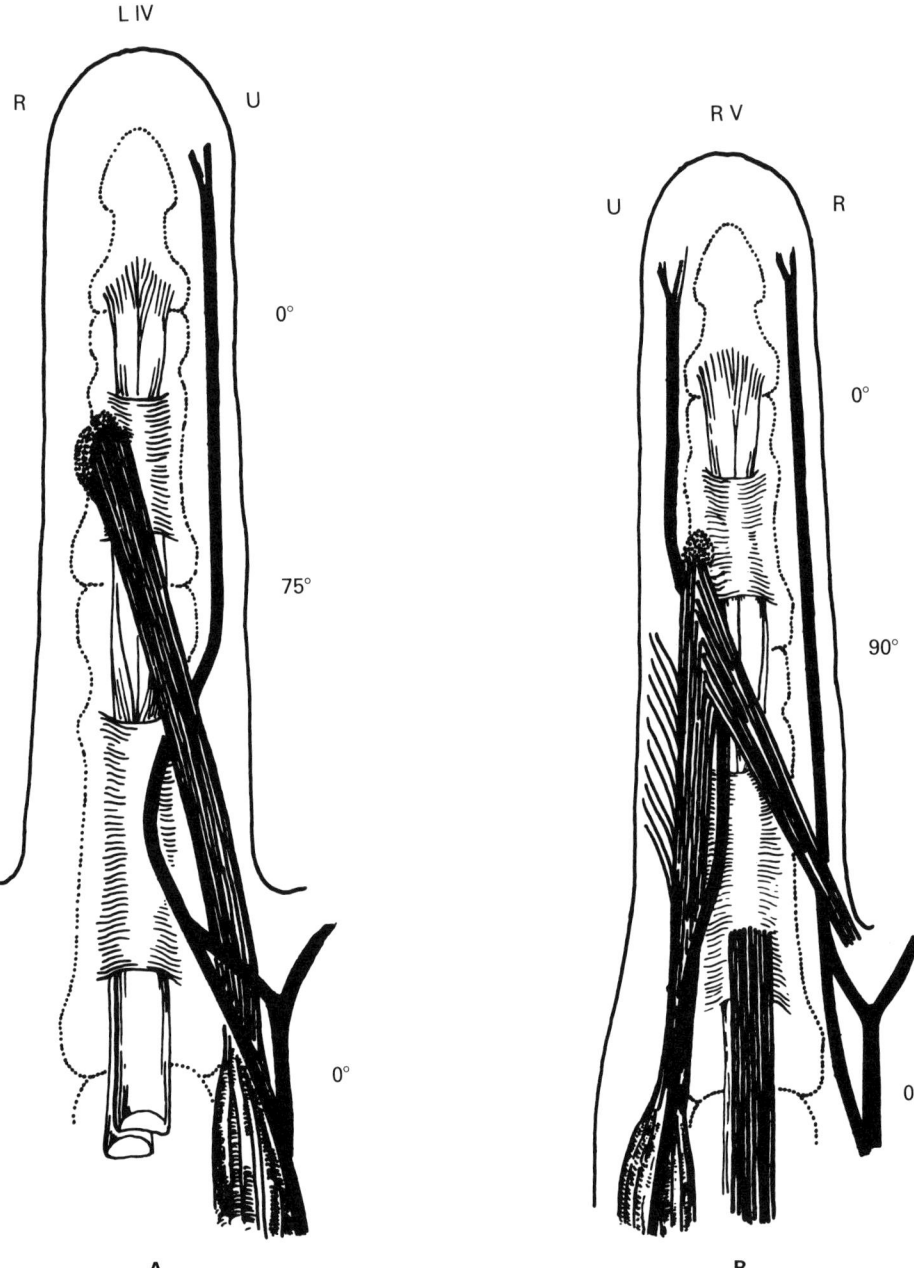

Fig. 14.15 Three examples of unusual fascial patterns. **A** A spiral cord in the left ring finger arising from the fourth dorsal interosseous tendon, displacing the neurovascular bundle in the usual way, but attaching to the middle phalanx on the opposite side of the finger. **B** An oblique cord in the right little finger arising in the natatory cord and passing to the other side of the finger to blend with a lateral cord and attach to the side of the middle phalanx. **C** A 'reverse' spiral cord originating in the lumbrical tendon of the right index finger, spiralling around the neurovascular bundle and attaching to the base of the middle phalanx. The neurovascular bundle was not displaced. R, right hand; L, left hand; V, little finger; IV, ring finger.

THE FINGER 167

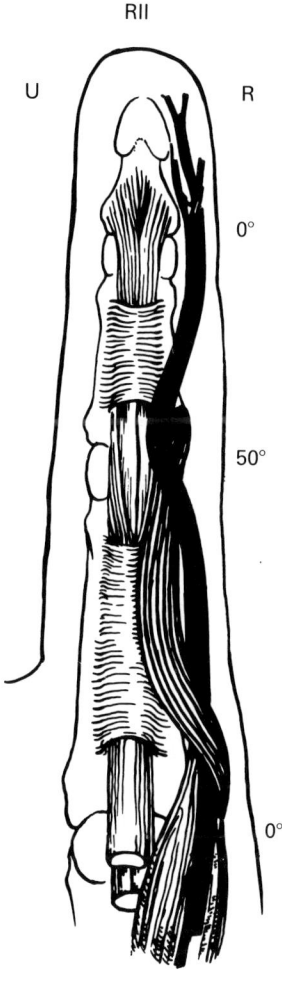

UNUSUAL PATTERNS

Fascial patterns which are inconsistent with the four basic patterns causing proximal interphalangeal joint contracture are bound to occur. Three examples are shown in Figure 14.15. Exceptions are uncommon and are of no concern surgically because they will be observed in the course of complete excision of the diseased fascia.

D. A. McGrouther

15 The extensor mechanism and knuckle changes

Swellings over the finger joints in association with Dupuytren's disease (DD) were noted in 1893 by Archibald E. Garrod, Assistant Physician at St Bartholomew's Hospital, and later described by Garrod in the British Medical Journal (1904) as 'pads' (Fig. 15.1).

Sir James Paget (1875) had previously written in the same journal an article entitled 'On the minor signs of gout in the hands and feet' and wrote of the 'formation of abnormal bursae'. He described the evolution of such a swelling as follows:

this soon became thickened and hardened, and almost rigid, and all the integuments over it grew thick and dense, so that a considerable nodular mass was the result; not, however, let it be observed, connected at all with a diseased articulation, but situated only in the subcutaneous tissue just beneath the integument.

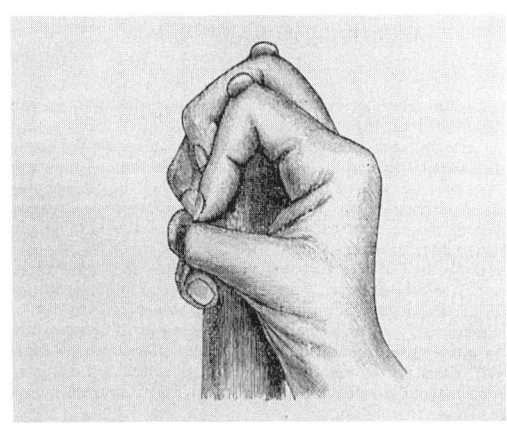

Fig. 15.1 Illustration from Garrod (1893); On an unusual form of nodule upon the joints of the fingers.

This curious description may today be confusing unless one appreciates the rather wider scope of the diagnosis 'gout' in the 19th century; contracture of the palmar fascia 'was often characteristic of gout'.

Skoog (1948) has reviewed the literature of this condition and the origins of the terms '*Fingerknockelpolster*', '*coussinets des phalanges*', '*symmetrischer Fibromatose*', '*helodermia*', '*callosités dorsodigitales*', '*keratomes en nappe de mains*', '*keratosis supracapitularis*'.

It has been suggested that knuckle pads occur in sheep shearers (Wilson 1972) and other occupations (Hueston & Wilson 1973), but epidemiological evidence is lacking.

The incidence of knuckle pads in association with DD has been variously reported to be 44% (Skoog 1948), 20% in primary cases and 75% in those with recurrence (Hueston 1963), and in 45% of men and 62% of women operated on for DD (Mikkelsen 1977).

In his general population group Mikkelsen noted 9% of men (women 8.6%) to have knuckle pads and Lund (1941) found 29% of epileptic men to have these changes; most also had palmar contractures.

Hueston (1963) considers this physical sign to indicate a strong diathesis or tendency towards DD, but Mikkelsen (1977) disagrees.

These accounts, however, do not seem adequate to describe the clinical signs present in the wrinkle skin. A study was undertaken (McGrouther & Walton, unpublished observations) to describe knuckle pads and other knuckle changes and record their frequency. Readers will note from their own hands that the wrinkle skin over the dorsum of the proximal interphalangeal joint,

THE EXTENSOR MECHANISM AND KNUCKLE CHANGES 169

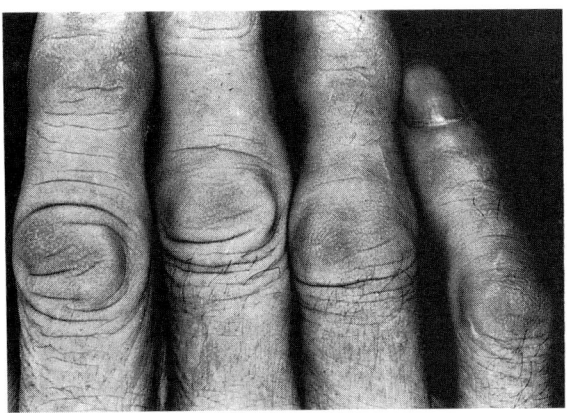

Fig. 15.2 The middle finger shows a common pattern of loss of the distal skin wrinkles and slight tethering of the proximal wrinkles. Hyperkeratosis is most marked in the index finger.

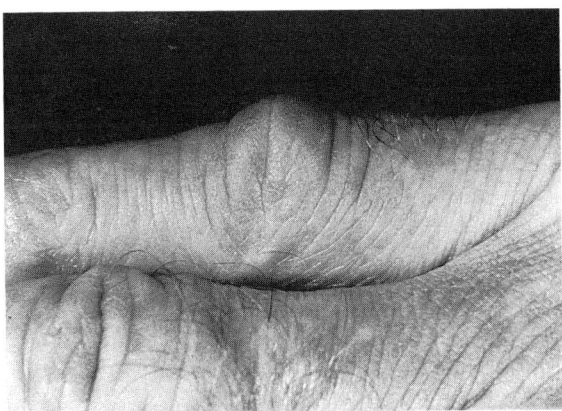

Fig. 15.4 A knuckle pad.

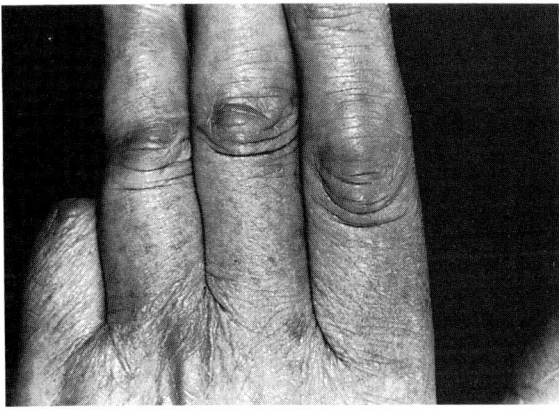

Fig. 15.3 A skin thickening is apparent in the index finger. In the middle and ring fingers a discrete lump is palpable.

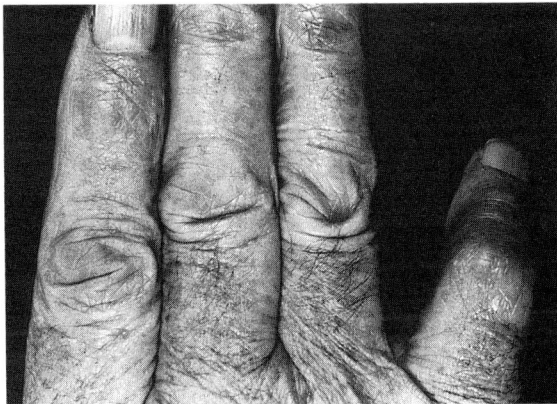

Fig. 15.5 Marked skin tethering in the ring finger.

which is apparent on full extension of the digit, is much less obvious when the hand is in the neutral resting position (semi-flexed). There is considerable individual variation in the development of these wrinkles. The appearance of the wrinkle skin reflects the range of motion in the underlying joint; it disappears in the stiff or arthrodesed joint. In the normal hand the skin is thrown into a series of wrinkles forming a transverse oval ellipse. The skin wrinkles proximal and distal to the joint are concave towards the joint line and the centre of the wrinkle skin area.

In DD there was a tendency towards loss of the distal wrinkles (83% of digits in a series of 50 patients; Fig. 15.2). This loss was associated with either skin thickening or a discrete nodule in 45% of digits (Figs 15.3 and 15.4). The site of the thickening or nodule varied, being either in the digital midline or off-centre in the radial or ulnar aspects. Proximal tethering of the proximal wrinkles was noted in 56% (Fig. 15.5) with deeper valleys between the skin wrinkles and a suggestion of tethering of the skin by a deep contracture process.

There was frequently a degree of hyperkeratosis of the skin apparent on clinical examination (see Fig. 15.2). Sequential examination in a few patients over 5 years showed that the knuckle pads may develop, regress, or show little change.

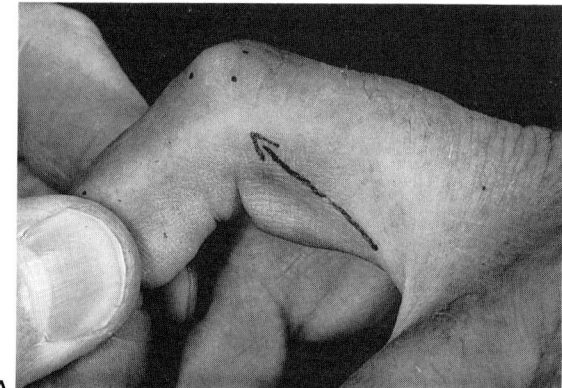

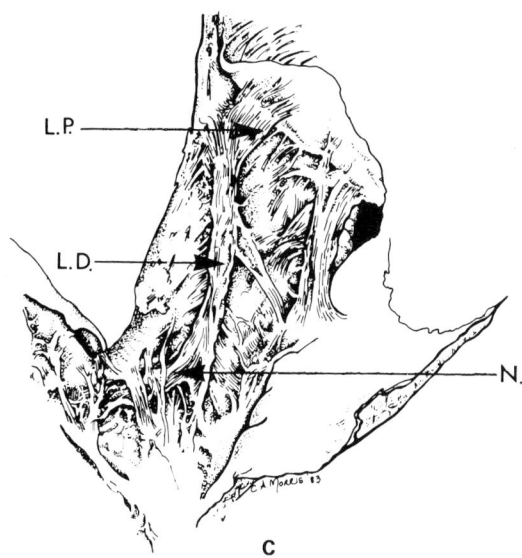

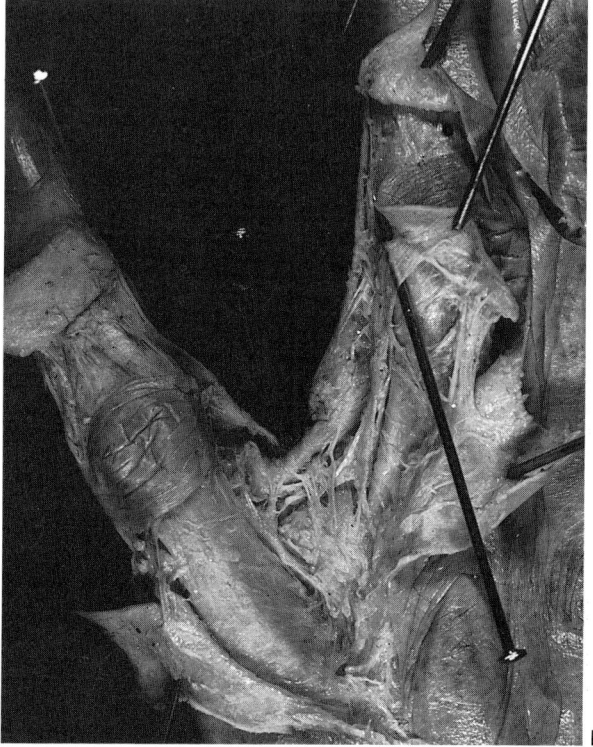

Fig. 15.6 A The arrow indicates the line of the natatory ligaments extending via the lateral peritendinous cutaneous fibres to the dorsal skin over the proximal interphalangeal joint. Contracture of these structures may be the cause of proximal tethering. **B** and **C** Dissection of ring finger with pin marking lateral peritendinous (LP) cutaneous fibres. Continuity of these with the lateral digital (LD) sheet and dorsal extent of the natatory (N) ligament is shown.

This study suggested that knuckle pads are part of a spectrum of *knuckle changes* which occur frequently — in 87% of digits — in Dupuytren's patients and that they are not indicative of the stage of palmar disease or its severity. There is a spectrum of change from the normal appearance through skin thickening to a palpable nodule and there is therefore some debate about what exactly constitutes a 'pad', which may explain the wide difference in reported incidence. Changes in the skin wrinkle pattern have received little attention, except in a case report by Hueston (1985) in which he suggests that tethering may be a precursor of knuckle pads. It is possible that the proximal tethering is due to contracture in the ligamentous system, described by Law & McGrouther (1984) as the lateral peritendinous cutaneous fibres (Fig. 15.6). These fibres, inserted into the outer part of the wrinkle skin, are continuous proximally with the lateral digital sheet which in turn is continuous with the natatory ligament and spiral cord of Gosset. Thus there is a fascial continuity between palmar structures and the dorsal wrinkle skin over the proximal interphalangeal joint.

The frequent finding of knuckle changes in patients with DD suggests that palmar contracture, although being of considerable functional significance to the patient, is not an indication of the extent of pathological change. Knuckle changes are present even in non-contracted fingers. DD therefore seems to be a more widespread affliction of the connective tissues than is immediately apparent from study of the palm of the hand.

The importance of knuckle changes requires further clarification by epidemiological survey in different parts of the world. The recognition of a diffuse set of knuckle changes may prove useful in recognizing the Dupuytren's-prone patients long before Garrod's nodules become apparent and before the palmar changes develop.

E. J. Hall-Findlay

16

The radial side of the hand

We are all familiar with drawings of the palmar aponeurosis of the hand. But if you look at the drawings again, you will notice that the fibres seem to fade into obscurity as they approach the first web space.

Only a few authors have discussed this region, whereas there is an abundance of articles on the palmar aponeurosis of the rest of the hand. Descriptions of the fascial anatomy of the first web space seem confused.

ANATOMY

The normal anatomy of the radial side of the hand was examined in both fresh and fixed specimens.

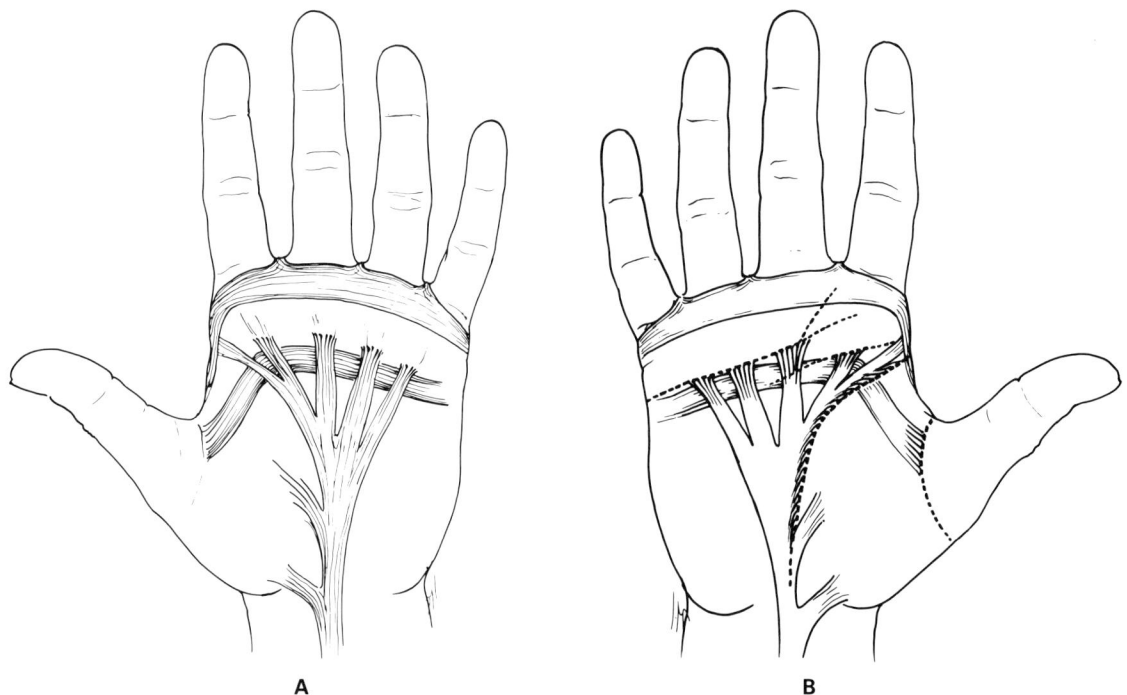

Fig. 16.1 A The normal pattern of fascia in the hand, including the thumb and first web space. There are three fascial systems: the pretendinous bands, the transverse fibres of the palmar aponeurosis and the natatory ligament. **B** Note how the fascia of the palmar aponeurosis, both pretendinous bands and the transverse fibres are related to and contribute to the palmar crease, the thenar crease and the basal thumb crease. Note also how the pretendinous band to the index finger attaches to the radial border of the hand rather than extending into the index finger.

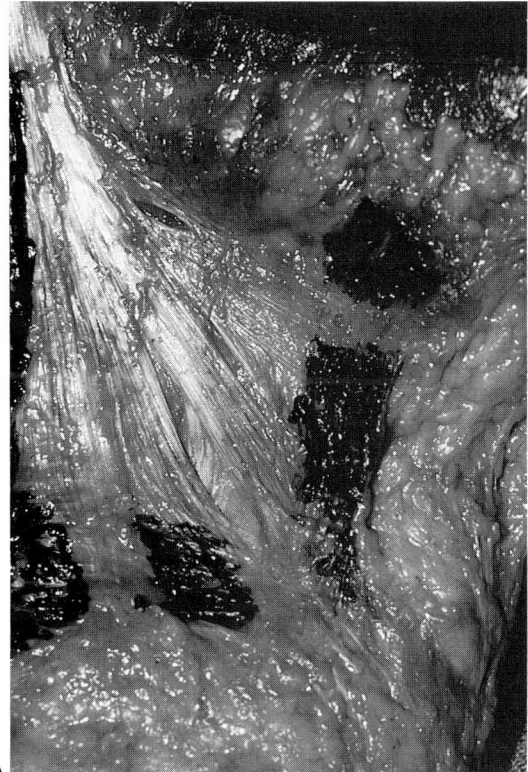 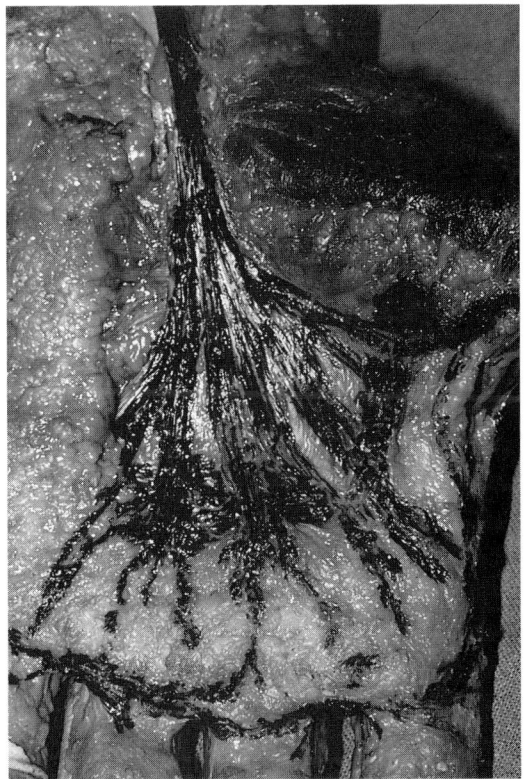

Fig. 16.2 A Cadaver dissections with the transverse fibres marked. Note how the fibres sweep across the palm and into the first web space and base of the thumb. **B** Cadaver dissection outlining the three fascial systems involved in the normal anatomy of the thumb and first web space. The transverse fibres are part of the palmar aponeurosis. The natatory ligament sweeps across the web spaces and interdigitates with the fascia going into the fingers.

We wanted to discover the relationship between the normal fascia in cadavers and the diseased fascia in clinical cases of Dupuytren's disease (DD). As pointed out so aptly by Stack (1971), dissection of fascia is difficult because it involves, by definition, cutting those very fibres one is attempting to identify.

The palmar fascia fans out as an inverse triangle from the base of the hand. It forms a sheet over the palm of the hand, with fibres concentrated in what have been called pretendinous bands. The number, density and direction of these bands are highly variable. There are pretendinous bands to the thumb in some hands, but often these are quite thin and attenuated.

There appear to be three definable systems of fascia in the first web space and base of the thumb (Figs 16.1 and 16.2):

1. The pretendinous band.
2. The transverse fibres of the palmar aponeurosis.
3. The natatory ligament.

The pretendinous band

The pretendinous bands send fibres to the skin throughout their length, but these skin fibres are densely concentrated at the distal skin creases, just at the level of the transverse fibres of the palmar aponeurosis. The pretendinous bands then dip down on either side of the metacarpal and extend into the fingers deep to the neurovascular bundles as the spiral bands (Gosset 1966). As mentioned by Thomine (1972), our dissection also showed few but definite fibres extending across the fat pad to the base of the fingers.

A few fibres would occasionally be sent to the base of the thumb as a pretendinous band. These were at times indistinct and did not travel far into the thumb, with the exception of a few isolated fibres which extended toward the basal crease. The pretendinous band which was directed toward the index finger sent a high density of fibres along its entire length to insert into and form the thenar crease.

The transverse fibres of the palmar aponeurosis

These fibres run deep to the pretendinous bands and form a continuous sheet beneath them, with some fibres woven among the longitudinal fibres. It was interesting to note that these transverse fibres also sent extensions to the skin throughout their length.

The transverse fibres continued radially from the pretendinous band to the index finger to insert into the skin crease at the base of the thumb. It was easier to see in a fresh hand that these transverse fibres did not take an abrupt change in direction from the palm of the hand, but formed a continuous arc from the palm to the thumb.

The natatory ligament

These are superficial fibres that spread across the base of the fingers and cross the web spaces in an interdigitating chiasmic fashion. These merge with the digital fascia and form the natatory ligaments of the web spaces (Grapow 1887).

The natatory ligaments also send interdigitating fibres between the index finger and the thumb. Some fibres extend toward the skin at the base of the index finger while some are sent across the web space. These pass toward the thumb along the web fold and merge with the fascia of the thumb. It is the natatory ligament to the thumb that Tubiana and DeFrenne (1976) call the distal commissural ligament.

PATHOLOGY

DD of the thumb and first web space is not rare. It is often overlooked. As pointed out by Tubiana & DeFrenne (1976), disease in the radial aspect of the hand rarely expresses itself to the point of disability. In an analysis of 152 cases at the Institut

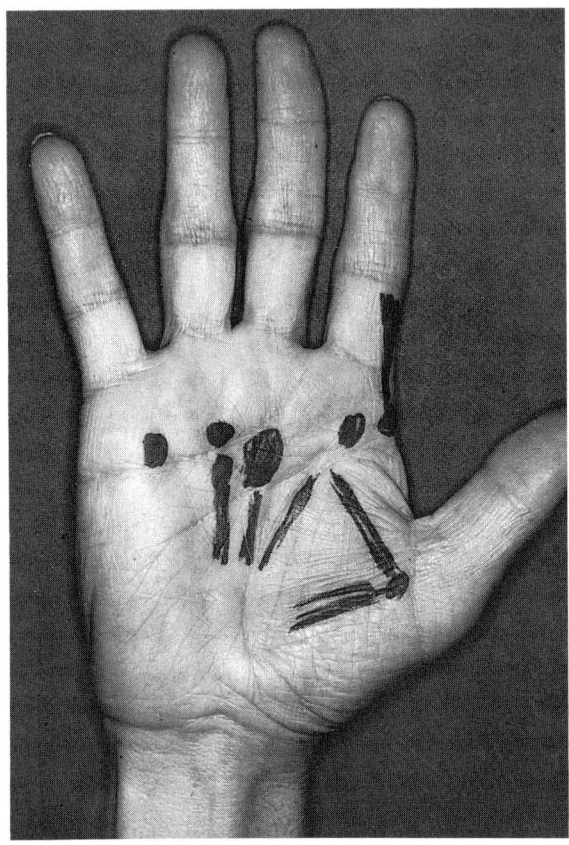

Fig. 16.3 Patterns of diseased fascia show involvements of the radial side of the hand. Here the pretendinous cord is evident, together with disease in the transverse fibres of the palmar aponeurosis. (Proximal commissural ligament, Tubiana and DeFrenne, 1976)

de la Main, they found radial involvement in 39% of hands.

Usually the first sign of disease is a nodule at the proximal crease of the thumb; this nodule may be connected with one or any combination of the three fascial bands described above (McFarlane 1974; (Fig. 16.3).

Disease of the pretendinous cord rarely causes metacarpophalangeal joint flexion, but it can limit both extension and abduction of the thumb. DD in the radial side of the hand often forms an L-shaped cord, with one limb extending across the web space (corresponding to either the superficial transverse ligament or the natatory ligament) and with one limb extending toward the base of the thumb (corresponding to the pretendinous band). The diseased cords are superficial to the neurovas-

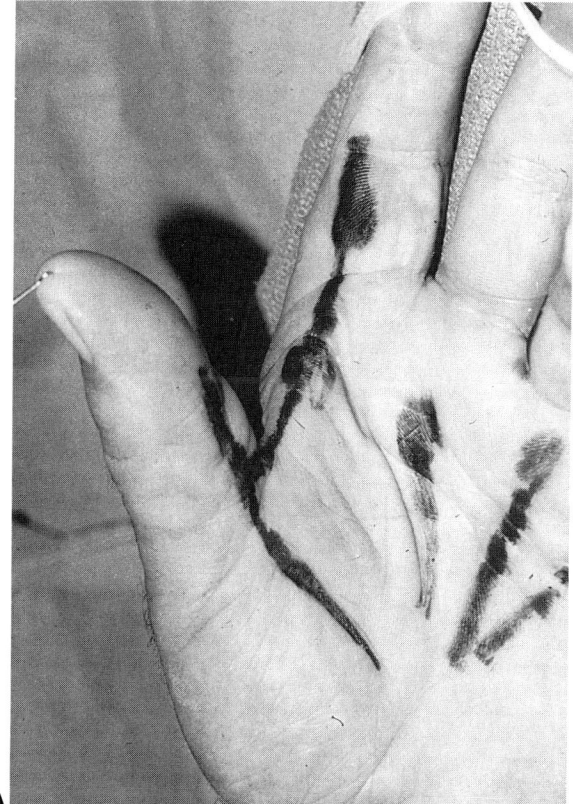 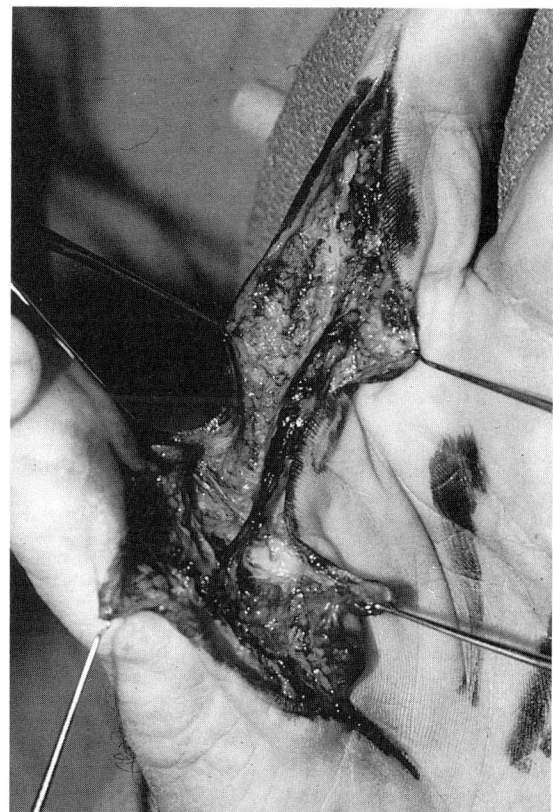

Fig. 16.4 A Disease of the radial side of the hand. The pretendinous cord is extending across the interphalangeal joint of the thumb. The natatory ligament in the first web space is involved. **B** The diseased cords are marked prior to excision. The neurovascular bundles are not displaced with this type of disease in the thumb and first web space.

cular bundles to the thumb and index finger and do not displace them (Fig. 16.4).

Cleland & Morrison (1986) have described two cases of a central cord in the thumb. Only one actually caused a contracture of the interphalangeal joint, but in both cases the central cord extended across the interphalangeal joint and was easily dissected off the flexor sheath without any evidence of displacement of the neurovascular bundles.

When a contracting cord develops through the thumb web and into the index finger, the web itself and the proximal interphalangeal joint of the index finger may become contracted, but the metacarpophalangeal joint of the index finger is not affected (McFarlane 1984). The lack of involvement of the index finger metacarpophalangeal joint can be explained anatomically. The pretendinous band to the index finger does in fact attach to the radial border of the hand rather than extend into the index finger itself.

CONCLUSIONS

The diseased patterns of fascia in DD involving the radial side of the hand can easily be related to the normal patterns of fascia. The diseased cords develop from three distinct systems of fascia: the pretendinous band to the thumb, the transverse fibres of the palmar aponeurosis and the natatory ligament.

The variability in expression of DD, apart from an individual's diathesis, may be due as much to variability in the concentration of the fascia normally present as to a peculiarity of the disease itself.

N. J. Barton

17 The ulnar side of the hand

Dupuytren's disease on the ulnar border of the hand is common, but has been strangely neglected in the literature. Hueston (1963) referred to and illustrated a distinctive type of Dupuytren's nodule 'found remote from the [palmar] aponeurosis and overlying the tendon of insertion of abductor digiti minimi'. Boyes (1969) pointed out that in contractures of the interphalangeal joints of the little finger there is often, in addition to the cord of diseased tissue running from the palm on to the undersurface of the finger, a second cord coming off the abductor digiti minimi (Fig. 17.1) and that 'many so-called recurrences of DD in the little finger are probably the result of an unrecognized lesion in the abductor digiti minimi band'. He recommended that in any operation for DD involving the little finger, the tendon of insertion of abductor digit minimi should be exposed so that any diseased tissue found in that area can be removed.

This paper by Boyes was not widely read and his message about DD arising from the abductor digiti minimi did not become widely known, despite the fact that he also mentioned and illustrated this in his fifth edition of 'Bunnell's Surgery of the Hand' (Boyes 1971).

Since then, little has been written about this common form of DD until the last few years. Although specialist hand surgeons are familiar with it, many general orthopaedic and plastic surgeons are not. This chapter attempts to summarize the known facts about the anatomy, pathology and prognosis of DD on the ulnar border of the hand.

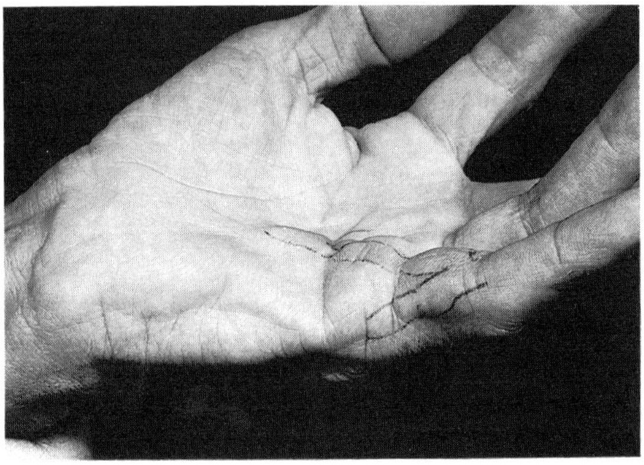

Fig. 17.1 This patient has two diseased cords of Dupuytren's tissue entering the little finger — one from the palm and the other from the area over the insertion of abductor digiti minimi. The outlines of the cords have been marked on the skin.

ANATOMY

As McFarlane (1974) has pointed out, the cords of diseased tissue 'do not arise de novo or haphazardly. Their anatomic configurations and relationship are predictable' and depend upon the normal anatomy of the fascia.

The most comprehensive work on the palmar fascia is by Stack (1973), based upon a detailed examination of fetal hands, prepared by Landsmeer, in the University of Leiden, Netherlands. Landsmeer (1976) found a set of fibres which he described as the 'ulnar root' of the palmar aponeurosis; these were 'derived from the flexor carpi-ulnaris-pisiform-hamate column'. He also stressed the presence of fibres anchoring the palmar fascia to the skin on the ulnar side of the hand, and described some of these as participating in a *Carrefour* (cross-roads) as seen on transverse section: from side to side the palmar aponeurosis continues as the superficial fascial investment of the hypothenar muscles, and from front to back the skin anchorages continue to form a septum between the flexor tendon compartment and the hypothenar muscles.

Distally, 'tendon formation in the abductor [digiti minimi] is extremely conspicuous and there is not another muscle in the midhand which shows such a variety of tendons and tendon fascicles. Most of these tendons become absorbed into the base of the proximal phalanx . . . the outer tendon of the abductor . . . merges into the outer root of the volar plate' of the fifth carpometacarpal joint (Landsmeer 1976).

The most detailed account of the fascial anatomy in this area is by White (1984) who studied 20 hands of cadavers by three methods. The first was simple *dissection:* this provides information which is readily applicable to surgical operations but some tissues must be destroyed to reveal others and it is possible to demonstrate sheets and bands which may not be entirely natural. Three frozen specimens were *cross-sectioned* at various levels and analysed under an operating microscope. This preserves normal relationships but as the structures are unstained it is difficult to assess the significance of some fine strands of connective tissue. Another three specimens were examined *histologically*. This involves decalcifying the bones first. (It was to avoid this difficulty that the Leiden specimens were of fetal hands where the bones had not yet ossified.)

White (1984) found that the area over the tendon of insertion of abductor digiti minimi is a meeting-place of fascial strands or bands which radiate from this central point in each of the six cardinal directions (Fig. 17.2) — in proximal, ulnar, radial, dorsal, volar and distal directions.

Proximally is the deep fascia which forms a sheath over the hypothenar muscles, just as that on the front of the forearm covers the flexor muscles. At the level of the fifth metacarpophalangeal joint, this merges with the short tendon of abductor digiti minimi although, as we shall see, another part of it continues distally into the finger. From this crucial point, fascial structures pass in ulnar, radial dorsal and volar directions (Fig. 17.3).

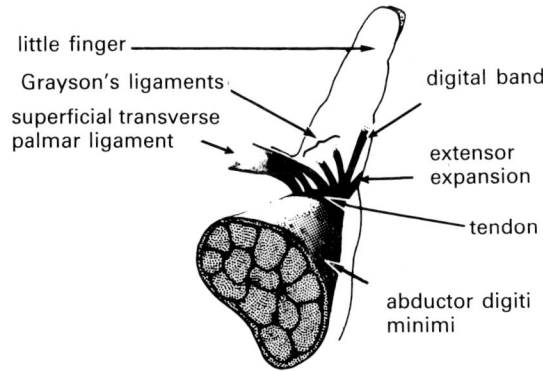

Fig. 17.2 The 'crucial area' on the ulnar side of the base of the little finger from where strands of palmar fascia radiate in all four directions. The superficial transverse palmar ligament is better called the natatory ligament. From White (1984) with permission.

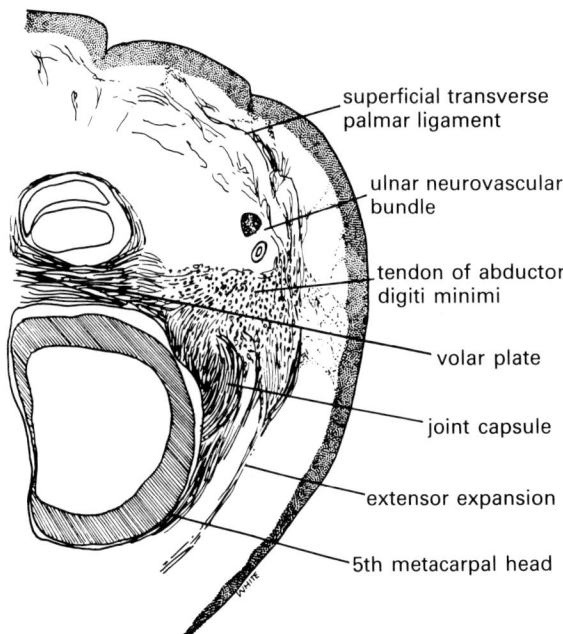

Fig. 17.3 Drawing of histological cross-section at the level of the distal palmar crease, showing again how elements of palmar fascia pass medially, laterally, anteriorly and posteriorly from the tendon of abductor digiti minimi. (The original histological section is reproduced in White's (1984) paper). From White (1984) with permission.

Radially, the tendon of abductor digiti minimi is attached to the volar plate of the fifth metacarpophalangeal joint and this in turn continues on the radial side as the deep transverse metacarpal ligament, which has also been described as the intervolar plate ligament.

Ulnarly, thin strands of fascia run superficially from the tendon of abductor digiti minimi to the deep surface of the skin. It is presumably here that the nodules arise to which Hueston (1963) referred.

Dorsally, the fascia merges into the extensor expansion or hood over the fifth metacarpophalangeal joint.

Volarly, a well developed band of fascia runs from the tendon of abductor digiti minimi in a radial direction and passes across the front of the palm proximal to the base of the fingers, superficial to the neurovascular bundles and the flexor tendons. White, following 'Gray's Anatomy' and Stack (1973), calls this the superficial transverse palmar ligament (and it is so labelled in Figs 17.2–17.4, reproduced from his paper), but this is a potentially confusing term as some authors apply it to the transverse fibres of the palmar aponeurosis. Amongst hand surgeons, the transverse fibroligamentous structure lying most distally and superficially in the palm, and in fact passing through the webs between the fingers, is usually called the natatory ligament.

Distally the situation becomes more complicated. White found that the digital sheet on the ulnar side of the little finger differed from that in the other fingers and from the radial side of the little finger in that it was 'larger, situated more anteriorly, and derived not from the anterior interosseous fascia but mainly from the tendon of abductor digiti minimi'. This continuity 'may be confirmed in the living hand by a simple manoeuvre. If one attempts to abduct the little finger against resistance, a palpable and visible ridge appears on the antero-ulnar aspect of the proximal segment. This corresponds to the tense digital band' (White 1984).

Since, as described earlier, the connective tissue of the tendon of abductor digiti minimi continues proximally as the deep fascia over that muscle, there is a continuous sheet of fascia running down the ulnar side of the hand into the little finger which, in its central part near the base of the finger, is anchored by the connections running forward, backwards and to either side, as described above.

The lateral digital sheet, running down the ulnar side of the finger, also has connections on either side. On the ulnar side it is loosely joined to skin, though in DD this become a close union, as surgeons know only too well. On the radial side it has connections at two levels. Superfically, volar to the digital nerve and artery, Grayson's ligaments run on to the front of the fibrous flexor sheath. This admittedly thin and discontinuous layer of tissue can be regarded as a distal continuation of the natatory ligament, as shown in Figure 17.4. Dorsally, deep to the ulnar nerve and artery, it is connected by Cleland's ligaments to the ulnar side of the fibrous flexor sheath. In Figure 17.5 the natatory and Grayson's ligaments have been removed to reveal the continuing course of the digital nerve and artery into the finger. Dorsal to them lie the oblique fibres of Cleland's ligaments. Proximally these fibres merge with the pretendinous fibres of the palmar aponeurosis.

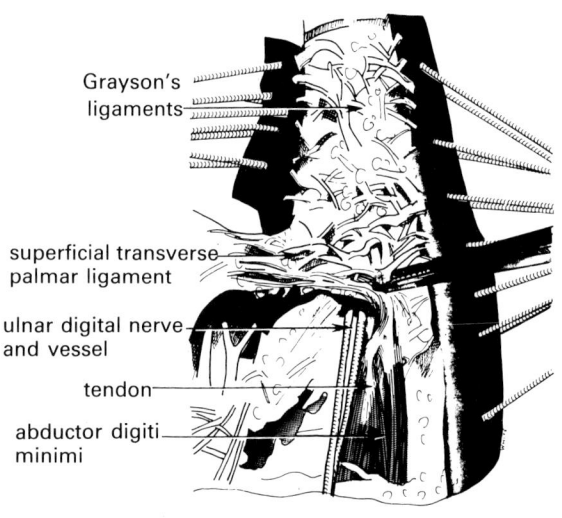

Fig. 17.4 Volar aspect of left little finger. The skin has been divided in the midline, freed from the subcorial fibrous tissue and retracted. The forceps are exerting traction on the tendinous extensions of abductor digiti minimi to the superficial transverse palmar (natatory) ligament and Grayson's ligaments. From White (1984) with permission.

PATHOLOGY

If patients with DD affecting the little finger are examined carefully, it will often be found that a diseased cord can be felt arising from the abductor digiti minimi. Moreover, even if it cannot be felt, exploration of this area at the time of operation may well reveal that there is a cord coming off the abductor digiti minimi.

The pattern of disease within the little finger varies. Figure 17.6 consists of drawings by White (1984); these are his interpretations of the brief written descriptions by the named authors. Figure 17.7 is a drawing by Dr William Littler showing in more detail a typical finger in which a cord coming off the abductor digiti minimi blends with another cord coming out of the palm.

In 1984, I studied 20 patients, to correspond to the 20 cadavers examined by White earlier in that year. At each operation, drawings and detailed notes were made (Barton 1984). The origin or proximal attachment of the cord on the ulnar side of the finger seemed to have three forms, as shown in Figure 17.8, the commonest being an origin from the tendon of abductor digiti minimi. However it was very difficult to distinguish that from an origin from the fascia overlying the abductor muscle, and this may be a distinction without a difference. The same may be said of the origin from the tendon and from its bony insertion on to the ulnar side of the base of the proximal phalanx.

The course of the diseased cord in relation to the ulnar digital nerve is shown in Figure 17.9. Usually the cord was superficial to the nerve, a safe arrangement for the surgeon. Subsequent experience has confirmed that this is nearly always the case, but not quite: I have now once encountered the nerve spiralling superficially over the cord, as it does in other fingers where the pathogenesis of this displacement has been so elegantly described by McFarlane (1974). Thus the surgeon cannot relax when working on the

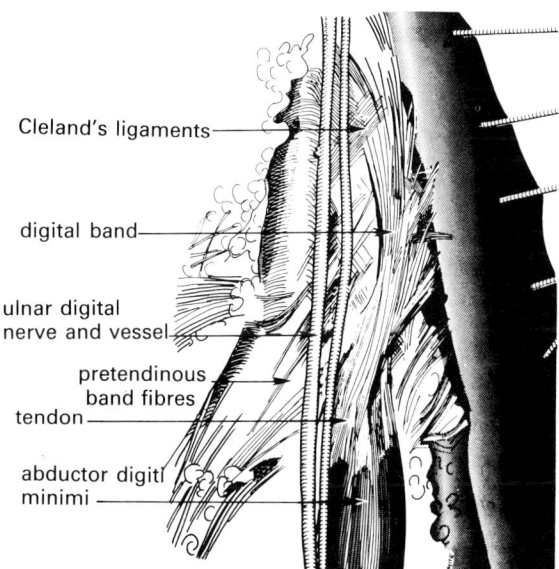

Fig. 17.5 Now the natatory ligament and Grayson's ligaments have also been removed, revealing the ulnar neurovascular bundle behind; this is a layer of fascia in which three elements can be identified. At the proximal interphalangeal joint level Cleland's ligaments predominate, whilst in the region of the metacarpophalangeal joint this layer of fascia is reinforced by fibres from the pretendinous band and fibres from the tendon of abductor digiti minimi which form a digital band running anteriorly down the ulnar side of the finger and attached to the skin. From White (1984) with permission.

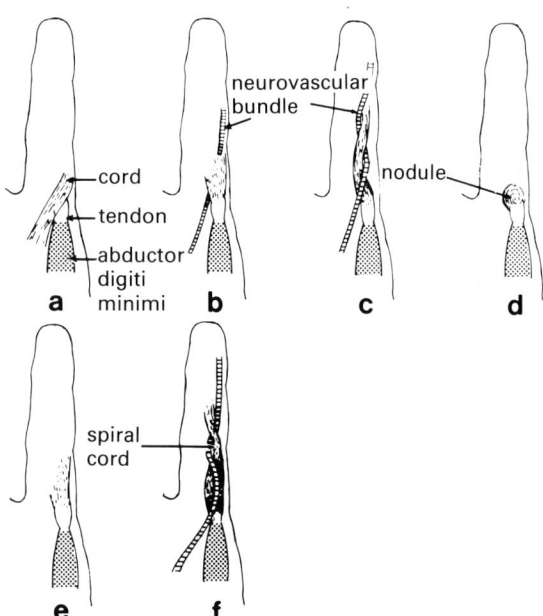

Fig. 17.6 White's (1984) interpretation of written descriptions by various authors of the pathological anatomy of on the ulnar border of the little finger. **a** Gosset (1974); **b** Tubiana & Thomine (1974); **c** Littler (1974); **d** Michon (1974); **e** Lamp (1981); **f** McFarlane 1974. From Barton (1984) with permission.

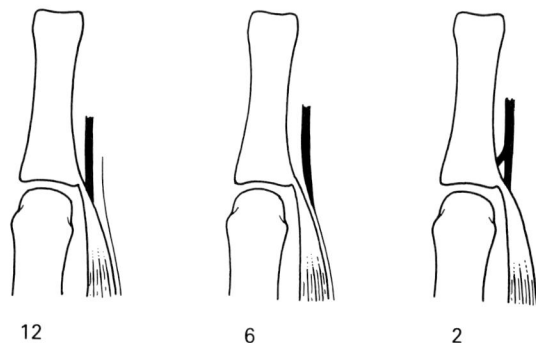

Fig. 17.8 Proximal origin of Dupuytren's tissue in 20 patients. Numbers indicate incidence. From Barton (1984) with permission.

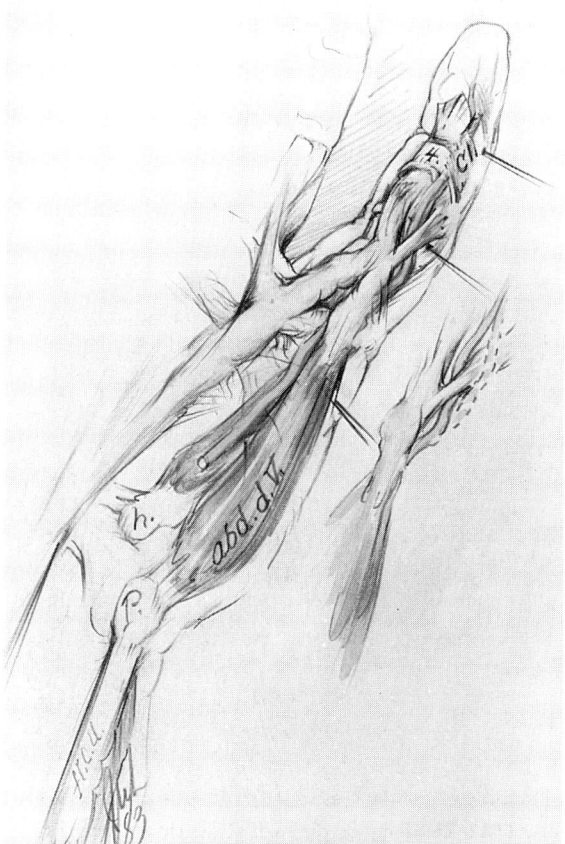

Fig. 17.7 Drawing by Dr J. W. Littler showing DD arising from the abductor digiti minimi and merging with another cord of diseased tissue coming from the palm. From Barton (1984) with permission.

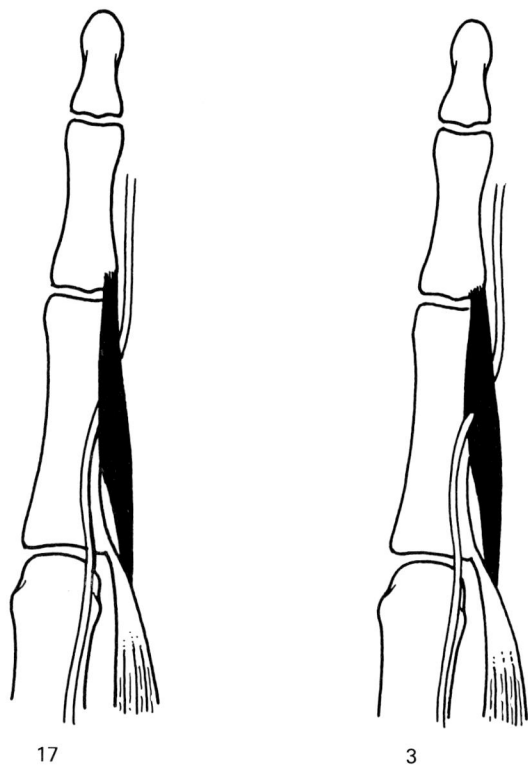

Fig. 17.9 Course of Dupuytren's cord and relationship to ulnar digital nerve in 20 patients. Numbers indicate incidence. From Barton (1984) with permission.

ulnar side of the finger but must follow the usual method of identifying the digital nerve in the distal part of the palm and tracing it distally. In some cases, as shown in Figure 17.9, the nerve will disappear into the midst of a mass of disease, presumably formed by the fusion of areas of disease arising in two originally separate parts of the digital fascia; the painstaking dissection required to trace the ulnar digital nerve and artery through this mass without damaging either can be very taxing.

The insertion or distal attachment of the cord showed the most variation, as shown in Figures 17.10 and 17.11. There is usually an insertion to the ulnar side of the base of the middle phalanx but this may be combined with other insertions, and occasionally the insertion is only to the fibrous sheath or to the base of the middle phalanx on the other side of the finger (Fig. 17.10). A particularly difficult type is that where the cord continues

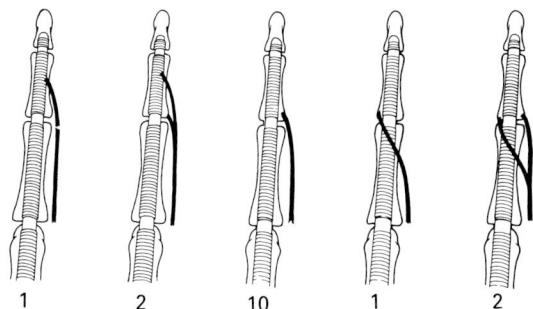

Fig. 17.10 Distal insertion of Dupuytren's cord in 16 patients in whom the disease terminated at the level of the middle phalanx. Numbers indicate incidence.

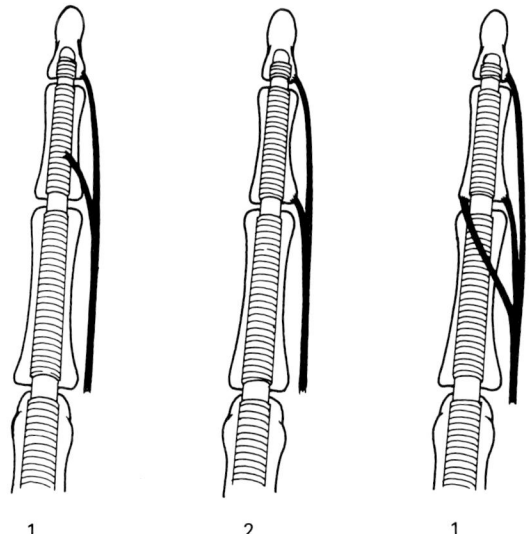

Fig. 17.11 Distal insertion of Dupuytren's cord in four patients in whom the disease continued into the distal phalanx. Numbers indicate incidence. From Barton (1984) with permission.

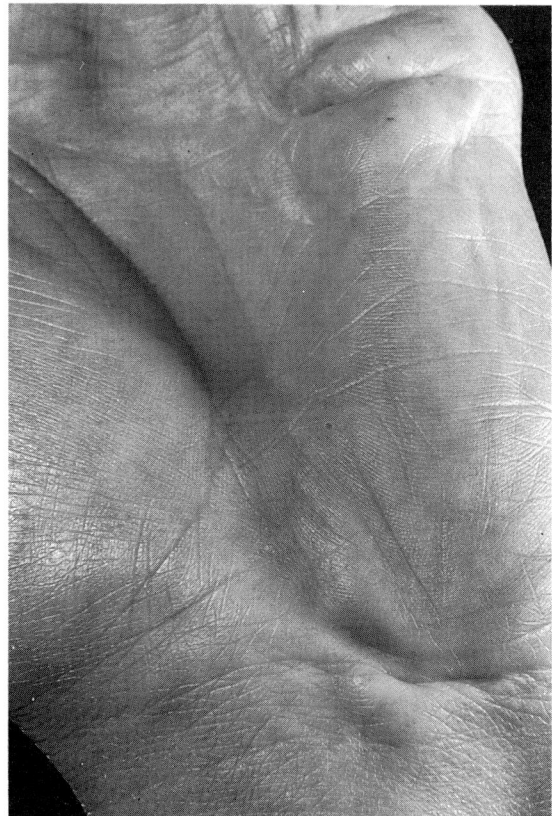

Fig. 17.12 This lump on the front of the wrist over the distal part of the tendon of flexor carpi ulnaris was exposed and histology showed the appearances of DD. There were similar changes in the other wrist; the patient also had more typical disease in both hands.

across the distal interphalangeal joint (Fig. 17.11); it is often said that in Dupuytren's disease the prognosis is worst for the fifth proximal interphalangeal joint but it is worse still for the fifth distal interphalangeal joint (Legge & Mcfarlane 1980) and unfortunately it is often in younger patients that this joint is affected.

Strickland & Bassett (1985) reported 32 patients with 37 cords of Dupuytren's tissue confined to the finger: 20 were in the little finger, and the remaining 17 in the other three fingers. There was no cord in the pretendinous fibres coming from the palm, and the disease arose proximally 'at the base of the proximal phalanges, with fibres emanating principally from the periosteum and from the intrinsic muscle-tendon insertion or from the lateral tendon to varying degrees'. The intrinsic tendon on the ulnar side of the little finger would include the insertion of the abductor digiti minimi. This origin from the periosteum at the base of the proximal phalanx and at the site of the tendinous insertion of the intrinsic muscle into bone was confirmed histologically. In addition, there were usually some fibres which appeared to emanate from the intrinsic tendon (lateral tendon) which did not insert into bone but joined the extensor apparatus (Strickland, personal communication).

A rare type of DD also affecting the ulnar side of the hand, is a plague of disease over the distal end of the flexor carpi ulnaris tendon (Fig. 17.12). This has also been described by Boyes & Jones, who reported two cases in 1968. It is particularly interesting since it is remote from the main palmar fascia; Boyes & Jones suggested that the tissue which was primarily involved was probably the deep fascia of the forearm, with secondary involvement of the tendon.

PROGNOSIS

The prognosis of DD on the ulnar border of the hand may be worse than that in the centre of the hand for two reasons.

First, this pattern of disease may have inherent properties which cause contractures to develop more quickly. Hueston (1963) writes:

> A central or radial band to the little finger can usually be expected to follow the same slow periodic progress of the rest of the palmar bands. The rapid progress of the deformity of both metacarpophalangeal and proximal interphalangeal joints once abductor digiti minimi is involved must be related to the muscular pull exerted on this shortening band which becomes virtually an insertion of the muscle.

This theory lacks statistical proof.

Second, the prognosis after operation may be worse because, as suggested by Boyes (1971), the operation is inadequate. The more obvious palmar cord is removed but the less obvious one arising from the abductor digiti minimi is left behind to work its evil will. This may explain why, in the little finger but not the other fingers, the prognosis for the proximal interphalangeal joint is related to the state, not only of the proximal interphalangeal joint itself, but also of the metacarpophalangeal joint.

If there is a cord coming from the palm, and causing contracture of the metacarpophalangeal joint too, a less obvious area of disease coming from the abductor digiti minimi can easily be overlooked, especially if the incision was not planned to give access to that area. However, those patients in whom the contracture is limited to the proximal interphalangeal joint often have disease limited to the ulnar side of the finger, with no cord coming from the palm. The

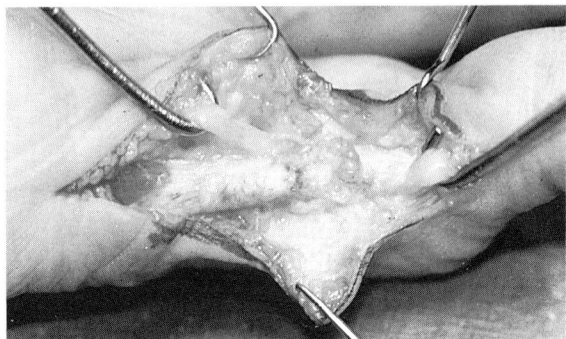
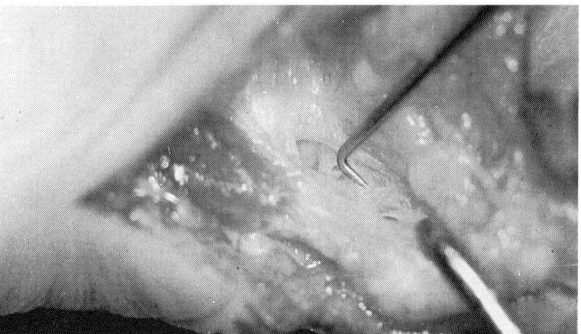
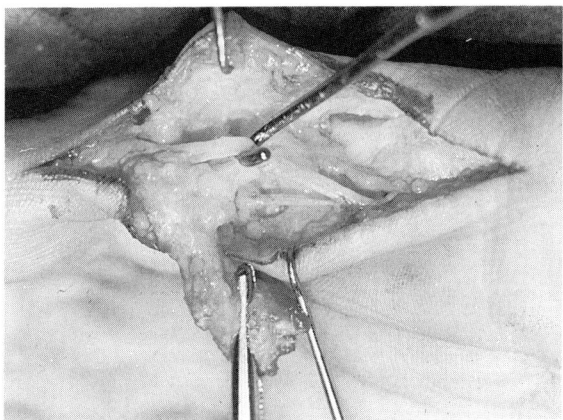

Fig. 17.13 Photographs taken at operation for removal of ulnar Dupuytren's cord in the left little finger: Volar above, proximal to the left. a The digital nerve has been identified volar to the tendon of abductor digiti minimi and is found to pass deep to the diseased cord on the ulnar side of the finger. b The diseased cord is pulled down by the blunt hook (bottom) to show that it arises from the tendon of abductor digiti minimi (indicated by the square hook). b c The proximal end of the diseased cord has now been detached (with a few fibres of abductor digiti minimi muscle) and pulled forwards with a clamp to reveal the digital nerve passing underneath (blunt hook from bottom left). A small anterior branch of the nerve can be seen passing into the diseased tissue.

cord arising from the abductor digiti minimi is therefore more evident and more likely to be removed (Barton 1984).

It is important to realize that ulnar disease may be impossible to detect by palpation before the operation, but it is usually there all the same. The lesson is clear. Every operation for DD of the little finger must include exploration of the area around the insertion of the abductor digiti minimi, even if it feels clinically normal, and the incision must be planned with this in mind (Fig. 17.13).

Acknowledgements

I would like to thank Graham Stack for his valuable comments.

SECTION 3

Epidemiology

D. A. McGrouther

18 The clinical diagnosis

The recognition of Dupuytren's disease (DD) has generally been considered straightforward, but it is much more difficult than it may seem. There is little confusion in the well developed case, at the stage when the patient frequently presents for treatment. By contrast in epidemiological surveys the minor signs challenge even the most experienced observer to distinguish between DD and the normal hand in which there is just thick skin or prominent fascia. There are no helpful ancillary diagnostic tests to resolve the problem. It can readily be appreciated that the precise point in the spectrum of clinical appearances at which a positive diagnosis of DD is made will alter considerably the reported incidence in the population under study. It is therefore important to consider how the early or minimal signs may be recognized and recorded.

The nodule has been central to most definitions: a 'simple nodular or banded thickening of fascia' (Lund 1941); a 'pathognomonic nodular thickening and retraction of the palmar aponeurosis' (Skoog 1948); the earliest stage being a nodule without finger contracture (Early 1962); 'a thickening in the palm fixed to the palmar fascia, either localised as a nodule or extending as a plaque or band to the fingers' (Hueston 1963).

Hueston recognized some diagnostic difficulties by specifically excluding paralysed hands where atrophy of fat and intrinsic muscles had rendered prominent the bands of the aponeurosis. He also considered that hands in which passive extension rendered the fascia palpable were a variant of normal. Ling (1963), in examining the families of Dupuytren's patients, reported: 'Although it might be felt that the diagnosis of DD presents no difficulty, in fact, in a number of relatives it was hard to be certain whether or not it was present'. Despite excluding patients with bands alone — nodules fixed to the palmar fascia with or without dimpling were regarded as essential for the diagnosis — he found that 68% of patients had affected relatives. This incidence may have been even higher with wider criteria. By contrast he accepted significant knuckle pads, even in the absence of palmar signs, as a sign of DD and many authors would disagree with this view (Mikkelsen 1972). In the largest and most authoritative study available of a general population group, Mikkelsen (1972; see Chapter 19, this edition) has based his diagnosis on the nodule, and considered it distinguishable from 'ordinary occupational indurations', but recognized the diagnostic problem of an extremely small nodule and excluded a few doubtful cases. Bands and contractures have served to provide further confirmation.

There has been a gradual evolution of perception of this curious malady with greater awareness of the signs preceding contraction. Noble et al (1984) have added tethering or a pretendinous band as definite indicators. They also report that in a pilot study of diabetic patients an 18% incidence of DD was noted on examination by a physician; this rate rose to 42% when the same hands were examined by an orthopaedic surgeon. It seems therefore that incidence depends very much on diagnostic criteria — how widely one chooses to cast the net — and observer interpretation.

The individual clinical signs found in DD and will be discussed in order. Associated fibromatous conditions outside the hand — plantar fasciitis or Peyronie's disease — lend strong support to the diagnosis.

THE NODULE

The pathogenesis of the clinical nodule must be understood (Chapter 12) to reflect either a bunching up of skin and subcutaneous tissue or the deposition of new cellular masses. Any palpable change in texture of the tissues is likely to be interpreted as a nodule (Fig. 18.1). This clinical sign must not be confused with the pathological description of a nodule — a histological feature of much smaller dimensions, representing a fibroblastic focus.

Is the clinically apparent nodule a certain sign of DD? Confusion may arise with other specific lumps in the hand, such as cysts, and ganglions, but distinction between these conditions and DD is generally not difficult as Dupuytren's nodules have a defined positioning, just proximal or distal to the distal crease of the palm, in the proximal segment of the finger, or at the base of the thumb. It is the nodule that appears in an unusual location, such as the base of the hypothenar eminence or at the distal crease of a finger, that poses a diagnostic problem.

Confusion may arise in the swollen hand where oedematous fat bulges between the inelastic fibrous fascial skeleton of the hand, with exaggeration of the normal fascial anchorage and of the normal monticuli in the distal palm. This lumpy thickening may be difficult to distinguish from DD (Fig. 18.2).

It is generally agreed that palpable nodules are diagnostic of DD, but they are not an invariable feature as they may disappear in the latter stages of the disease.

SKIN CHANGES

Various signs of DD are due to retraction or involvement of the skin (Chapter 12). Tethering has been used alone as a sign of DD by Noble et al (1984) without precise definition (Fig. 18.2). Loss of the normal mobility of the pretendinous bands upon the transverse fibres results in distortion of the palmar creases which may be vertical or horizontal. The former is a persistence of the flexed appearance of the palmar creases even on full digital extension; readers can observe from their own palms that the normal creases become flat linear marks on extension. Horizontal distortion is proximal or distal displacement of the creases depending on the direction of tethering (see Fig. 18.1). A particular result of tethering is the blanching sign (Fig. 18.3) apparent in the skin distal to the insertion of the longitudinal pretendinous fibres due to increased tension in the dermis on full extension. Pits or dimples are a

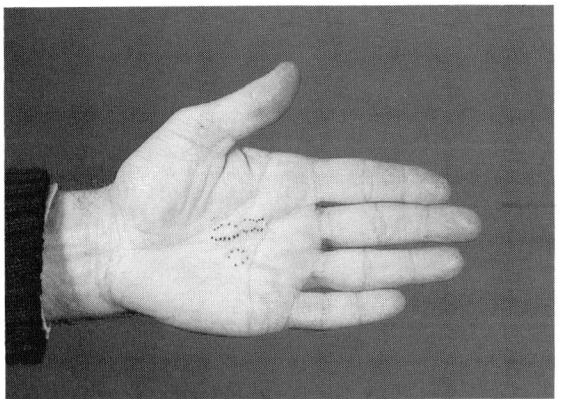

Fig. 18.1 Early palmar nodules. These are often the earliest sign of DD.

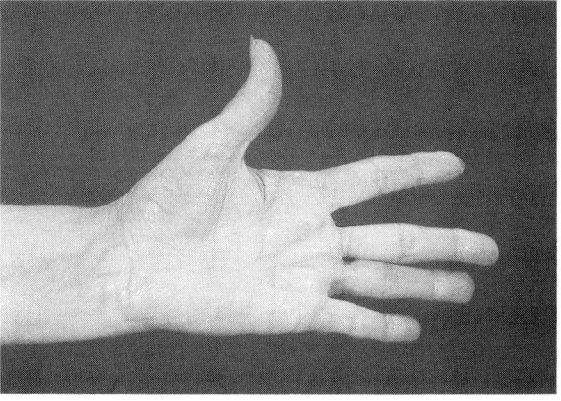

Fig. 18.2 Tethering. The logitudinal fascial bands are well defined in the distal palm and the fat of the web spaces bulges lateral to them.

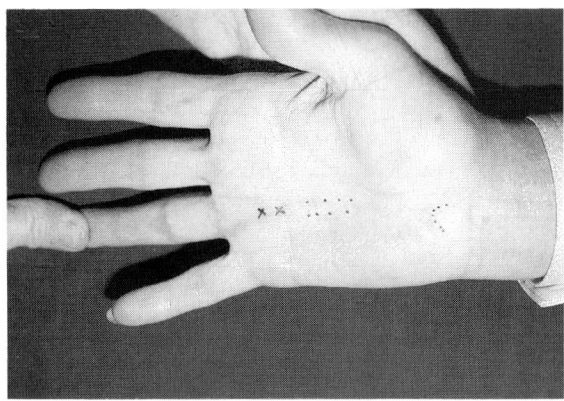

Fig. 18.3 The blanching sign. The skin of the distal palm blanches on full digital extension. A nodule is palpable just distal to the distal palmar crease.

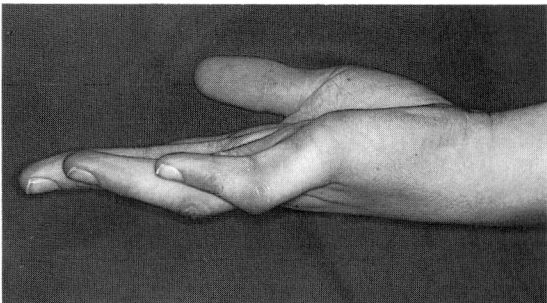

Fig. 18.4 Camptodactyly. The finger flexion can be mistaken for DD.

form of tethering where the contracting fascia inserts into the dermis: the pits are inclined towards the tethering fascial fibres. There may be thickening of the skin especially at the palmar digital junction, which indicates that the contracture is being propagated through the dermis. The various skin manifestations reflect pathological changes in the anchoring fascia.

CHANGES IN THE FASCIA (AND SUBCUTANEOUS FAT)

Cords are contracted bands. They may be palpable within the palm or digits or they may lie deeply within the tissues, and are found at operation to be more extensive than had been suspected. A clear distinction between a cord and a nodule is often not possible clinically because there is continuity of one to the other in series.

Bands are often found in the thumb web which may simply represent well defined anatomy; there appears to be a gradation between the anatomical band and the pathological cord. A source of confusion is adaptive shortening or remodelling of the bands which may occur from a long-standing position of flexion. Skoog (1948) has suggested this possibility in the senile hand. Ledderhose (1897) noted palmar bands in the hands of patients with rheumatoid arthritis, possibly from a prolonged flexion or ulnar deviation posture. The palmar contractures which accompany strokes or schizophrenia and also camptodactyly may be examples of adaptive shortening.

JOINT CONTRACTURE

Contracture of a joint may be defined as a loss of part of its range of motion. This may either occur from tethering outside the joint, as in the case of DD, or by contraction of the joint capsule or ligamentous components, which appears to occur in DD as a secondary phenomenon. There are certain specific causes of hand contracture which present as well defined clinical entities; these are unlikely to present difficulty to the experienced hand surgeon, but such cases have been referred to the author by the patient's family doctor as DD. These include congenital anomalies, such as congenital palmar contracture (the windblown hand), and camptodactyly. In adult life bilateral contracture of both little fingers may suggest DD but the contracture of camptodactyly will have been present from childhood or adolescence and no pathogenic nodules will be present. On occasion a palpable band will be present on the ulnar side of the proximal segment of the little finger but this band disappears with proximal interphalangeal joint flexion and it is not associated with a nodule. Zancolli (1979) has described multiple congenital finger contractures due to fascial shortening; this condition is seen in children.

Prolonged flexion is the common feature in patients who develop contracture secondary to the hand being habitually held closed. This posture may be adopted after organic disease of the central nervous system, strokes or spastic disorders, or in Psychoses, such as schizophrenia. The pattern of contracture is however different in that although the longitudinal pretendinous bands may be quite apparent on passively extending the digit, they are never as thickly hypertrophied as to develop typical cords. True nodules are not seen but distortion of palmar creases and shallow pits are found from adaptive shortening of the fascia. Fixed contracture of either the metacarpophalangeal or proximal interphalangeal joint may occur.

Following trauma to skin, bone or joint, the proximal interphalangeal joint in particular readily loses its extension range, and can progressively become stiff. Distinction between DD and trauma depends mainly on the history, but the question remains (see Chapter 25): Can trauma precipitate DD in some individuals?

Scleroderma involves many connective tissues and is often associated with severe proximal interphalangeal joint flexion. Tenosynovitis in rheumatoid arthritis may flex the digit and there are many causes of extension loss in this condition. A locked trigger finger can mimic DD. The fascinating condition of limited joint mobility has only recently been described by Rosenbloom & Frias (1974) and Ceruso et al (1987; see Chapter 22).

Interosseous paralysis, consequent upon ulnar nerve palsy, may result in a claw deformity, especially involving the ulnar digits. The similarity of distribution of these deformities has led many to speculate on a cause and effect relationship. Eulenberg (1864) felt that DD was due to an irritative lesion of the ulnar nerve. Bauer et al (1985) has presented an excellent review of this subject. Certainly a fixed claw deformity from interosseous paralysis may be mistaken for DD but in ulnar nerve lesions metacarpophalangeal joint hyperextension is always present.

Infections of deep spaces and cicatrization were important differentials for Dupuytren. Currently these are less frequent.

It is curious how little effect the masses of DD have on surrounding structures. It is difficult to demonstrate clinical dysfunction of nerve or vascular supply, but perhaps further experimental study may hold the key to future diagnostic testing. Meanwhile diagnosis depends on clinical judgement.

Epidemiology of a Norwegian population

POPULATION STUDIES REVIEWED

The nature and demography of Dupuytren's disease (DD) are still a challenge to medical researchers more than 150 years after the contribution of Baron Dupuytren (1834). Many of the statistics in use and commonly cited are based upon hospital patients, and in some respects they show conspicuous discrepancies. As will be seen from the present study, these patients are highly selected, and some bias can hardly be avoided. A comprehensive understanding of the epidemiological pattern may also lead to fruitful hypothesis on the aetiology of the disease (Lilienfeld 1960). The desire for further information initiated the present study, of which the main content has been published previously (Mikkelsen 1972, 1976, 1977a, 1977b, 1978). References used have been kept to a minimum; each is either comprehensive or submits a conspicuous statement.

MATERIALS

The field study was made in connection with a mass photofluorographic chest examination in Haugesund in 1969. Haugesund is a small coastal town in west Norway. Until that time few foreigners had moved to this area. The total population was 27 015 according to the last census. All inhabitants over 16 years of age were requested to attend the examination, and 15 950 complied. For practical reasons, ectopic sites of the disease, such as the penis and the soles of the feet, could not be covered by the study.

The diagnosis was usually straightforward in patients who had bands and finger contracture. In incipient stages diagnosis was based upon the finding of subcutaneous nodules located in the distal half of the palm or the fingers. The nodules were easily distinguishable from occupational skin indurations and from nodules in the underlying tendons. Diagnostic problems arose on a few occasions when the nodule was extremely small, and in some cases where there were scars left from earlier injuries or inflammation. In a few doubtful cases DD was not recorded. When there was no finger contracture but there was a band or nodule, the disease was linked to the corresponding finger of the affected ray of the palmar fascia. In those who had been operated upon and completely cured, digital distribution could usually be based upon the given information. If some doubt remained, this was solved by checking the hospital records.

The non-response problems have been analyzed in detail (Mikkelsen 1972), but these had only minimal effect on the results. The observed prevalence of DD may be slightly underestimated. Total attendance rate was 71% for men and 82.4% for women.

PREVALENCE OF DD

Of the 15 950 subjects examined, 647 men (10.5%) and 254 women (3.1%) had DD (Table 19.1). The youngest male was 24 and the oldest 91 years old. In women the corresponding ages were 42 and 90 years. In men the prevalence in-

Table 19.1 Ratio of men to women in those with DD, correlated with age

Age (years)	Men (%)	Women (%)	Ratio of men:women
20–24	0.19	0	∞
25–29	0.38	0	∞
30–34	0.23	0	∞
35–39	1.08	0	∞
40–44	2.50	0.29	8.4
45–49	4.95	0.95	5.2
50–54	9.95	1.73	5.8
55–59	14.42	2.28	6.1
60–64	21.87	3.74	5.8
65–69	27.01	8.00	3.4
70–74	36.67	13.45	2.7
75–79	33.66	16.48	2.0
80–84	22.99	17.78	1.3
85–89	30.77	25.00	1.2
Mean	10.5	3.1	3.4

Table 19.2 Number of men with Dupuytren's disease (DD) classified by age and hand affected

Age (years)	Number	DD	Right	Left	Both
20–29	1061	3	0	2	1
30–39	905	6	2	1	3
40–49	1288	50	19	6	25
50–59	1361	163	47	31	85
60–69	946	228	61	27	140
70–79	475	168	34	28	106
80–89	113	28	5	3	20
90–99	2	1	1	0	0
Total	6151	647	169	98	380

Table 19.3 Number of women with Dupuytren's disease (DD) classified by age and hand affected

Age (years)	Number	DD	Right	Left	Both
20–29	1510	0	0	0	0
30–39	1184	0	0	0	0
40–49	1650	11	5	6	0
50–59	1758	35	22	8	5
60–69	1320	76	30	14	32
70–79	667	98	26	18	54
80–89	171	33	11	4	18
90–99	10	1	0	0	1
Total	8270	254	94	50	110

creased steeply in the ages 40–70 years, peaking in the 70s (Fig. 19.1). For women, the steepest rise occurred in the ages 60–80, peaking in the 80s.

In all ages and both sexes the right hand was affected most frequently (Tables 19.2 and 19.3). The frequency of unilateral and bilateral DD in men aged under 60 was almost equal. In older age groups bilateral cases occurred nearly twice as often as unilateral cases. In women total unilateral cases exceeded the bilateral ones, but women also had a preponderance of bilateral incidence in the older age groups.

The ratio of men to women was infinite in the lower age classes as no women were recorded. After the age of 40, the ratio decreased gradually towards what seems to be a limiting value of unity (see Table 19.1).

INITIAL SYMPTOMS AND AGE OF ONSET

Some 90% of both sexes recognized nodules in the palm as the first symptom. Local tenderness was the first symptom in 5%, and finger contracture in 5%. Contracture as the first symptom was mentioned more often in older than younger people. A total of 98 men (15%) and 52 women (20.5%) were not aware of having the disease.

Two women and one man stated that the disease had started before the age of 10. In approximately half of the men, the disease started between 40 and 59 years of age, while in women it was between 40 and 69 years (Tables 19.4 and 19.5).

In bilateral disease approximately 10% of both sexes stated that it started bilaterally. Bilateral disease started most commonly in the right hand (Table 19.6).

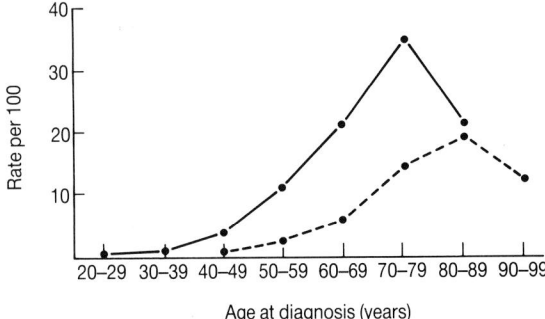

Fig. 19.1 The prevalence of DD in Norway. ——— Men; — — — women. From Mikkelsen (1972) with permission.

Table 19.4 Age of onset for 647 men with DD classified by presenting hand

Age of onset (years)	Right hand	Left hand	Both	Total
<10	1	0	1	2
10–19	3	3	4	10
20–29	10	1	10	21
30–39	14	10	49	73
40–49	39	16	88	143
50–59	36	27	96	159
60–69	22	12	60	94
70–79	5	4	18	27
80–89	1	1	1	3
?	2	2	13	17
Unaware	36	22	40	98
Total	169	98	380	647

? = Those who do not remember.

Table 19.5 Age of onset for 254 women with DD classified by presenting hand

Age of onset (years)	Right hand	Left hand	Both	Total
<10	0	1	0	1
10–19	0	2	0	2
20–29	0	0	1	1
30–39	1	0	2	3
40–49	15	13	5	33
50–59	19	8	15	42
60–69	18	11	30	59
70–79	11	5	18	34
80–89	2	7	1	10
?	4	3	10	17
Unaware	24	0	28	52
Total	94	50	110	254

? = Those who do not remember.

Table 19.6 Classification of 380 men and 110 women with bilateral Dupuytren's disease (DD) by age and hand where symptoms were first experienced

Age (years)	Right M	Right F	Left M	Left F	Both M	Both F	?	*Unaware of having DD
30–39	1	0	2	0	0	0	0	0
40–49	9	0	6	0	5	0	3	1
50–59	36	1	21	2	8	0	6	11
60–69	59	16	43	5	9	4	15	20
70–79	41	27	41	6	14	3	8	27
80–891	13	7	4	2	1	1	1	10
90–99	0	0	0	0	0	0	0	1
Total	159	51	117	15	37	8	33	70

? = Those who do not remember.

THE SPONTANEOUS COURSE

A slightly modified scheme proposed by Tubiana et al (1968) was applied to every affected ray or finger to assess the course of the disease:

Stage 1 — nodule and/or band without contracture.
Stage 2 — overall contracture 1–45° (total contracture of all joints of one finger).
Stage 3 — overall contracture 46–90°.
Stage 4 — overall contracture 91–135°.
Stage 5 — overall contracture more than 135°.

By adding together the score for each finger or ray, a score for the entire hand is obtained.

There was a trend towards more severe disease in men in the age group 40–79 years, compared with the onset of disease at younger or older ages. No particular pattern was seen in women.

The ring finger was affected most frequently in all groups — 85% of men and 92% of women had this finger affected (Figs. 19.2–19.5). The little finger was the second most affected one, and this was found in 45% of men and 40% of women. The frequency was higher in the left than in the right hand. Incidence in only one finger was also seen most frequently in the ring finger, and was definitely higher in unilateral disease. The thumb and index finger were rarely involved, and never alone. The most common combination of finger involvement was ring and little finger, followed by ring and middle finger, and middle, ring and little finger. Two men with bilateral disease had involvement of all fingers of the right hand. There was no significant difference as regards finger distribution in the different ages.

With the exception of the index finger, there was gradually increasing contracture from the thumb to the little finger (Tables 19.7–19.10). There was usually more contracture in the right hand than in the left, and the contracture was more developed in men than in women.

Correlating the mean stage of contracture with the duration of the disease, an idea of the spontaneous course is obtained (Fig. 19.6). In men, disease tended to increase during the first 20 years. This was followed by a more stationary phase of about 15 years, after which the disease regressed; however, there were large individual variations. In

194   DUPUYTREN'S DISEASE

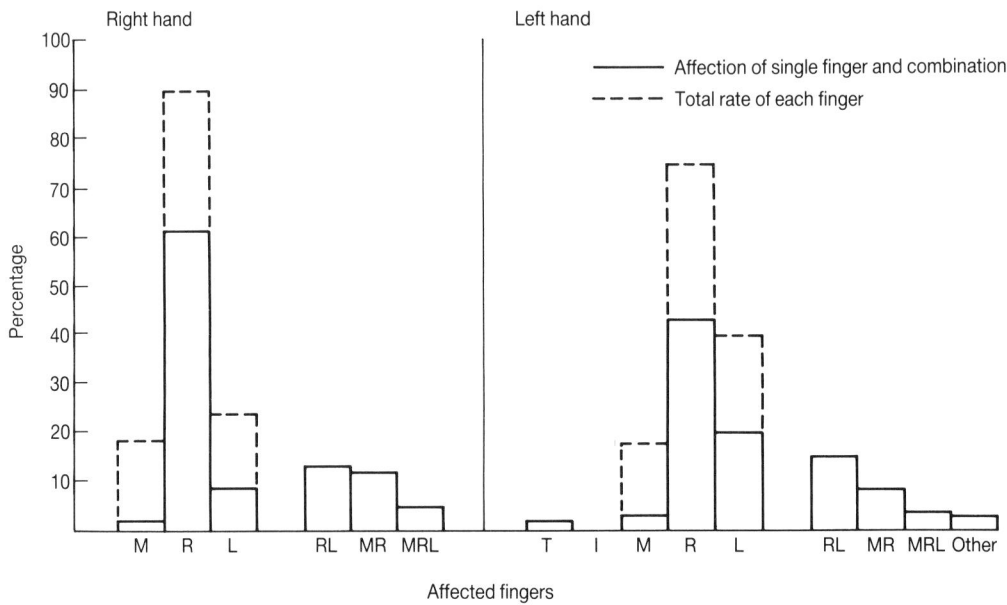

Fig. 19.2 The pattern of finger distribution in men with unilateral DD by percentage. Number of right hands = 169; number of left hands = 98. T = thumb; I = index, M = middle; R = ring; L = little finger. ———— Single finger or combination; — — — total for finger. From Mikkelsen (1976) with permission.

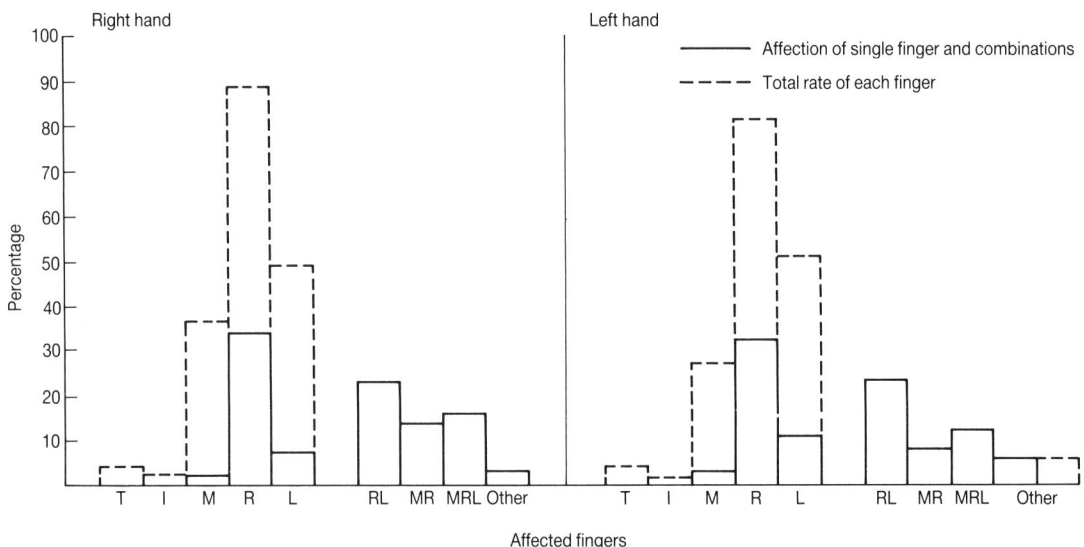

Fig. 19.3 The pattern of finger distribution in 380 men with bilateral DD by percentage of hands. T = Thumb; I = index; M = middle; R = ring; L = little finger. ———— Single finger or combination; — — — total for finger. From Mikkelsen (1976) with permission.

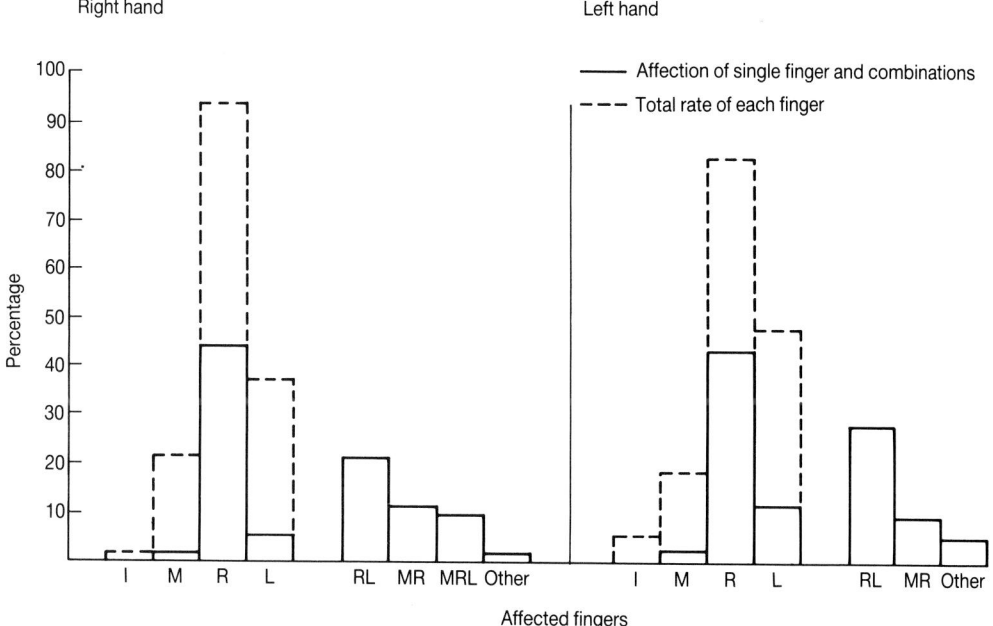

Fig. 19.4 The pattern of finger distribution in women with unilateral DD (93 right and 53 left hands), by percentage of hands. T = Thumb; I = index; M = middle; R = ring; L = little finger. ———— Single finger or combination; — — — total for finger. From Mikkelsen (1976) with permission.

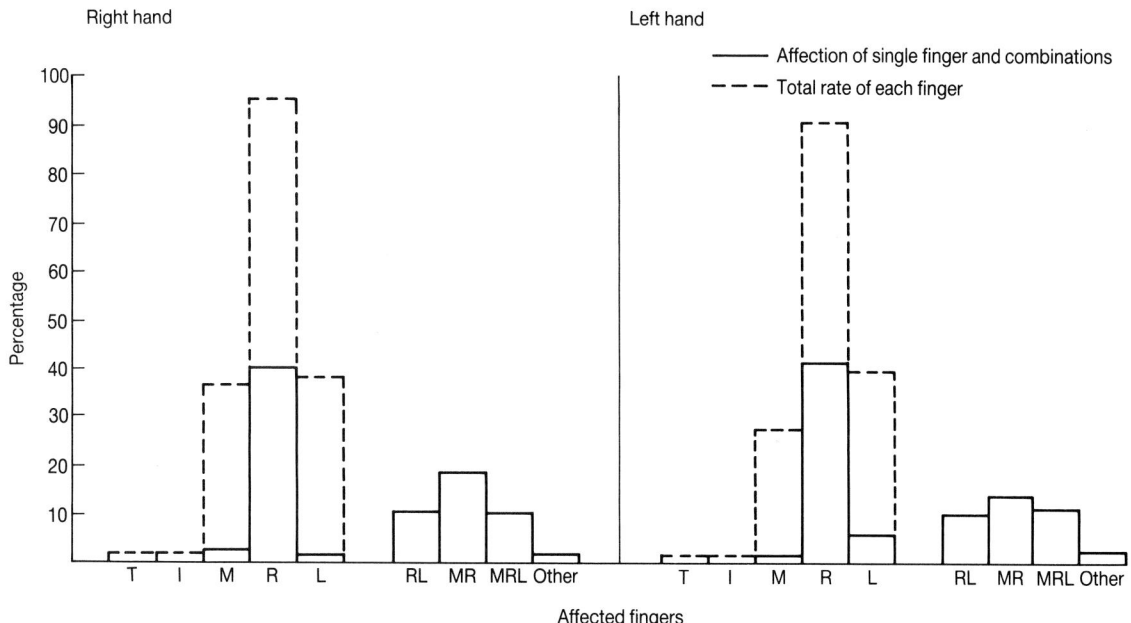

Fig. 19.5 The pattern of finger distribution in 110 women with bilateral DD by percentage of hands. T = thumb; I = index; M = middle; R = ring; L = little finger. ———— Single or combination; — — — total for finger. From Mikkelsen (1976) with permission.

196 DUPUYTREN'S DISEASE

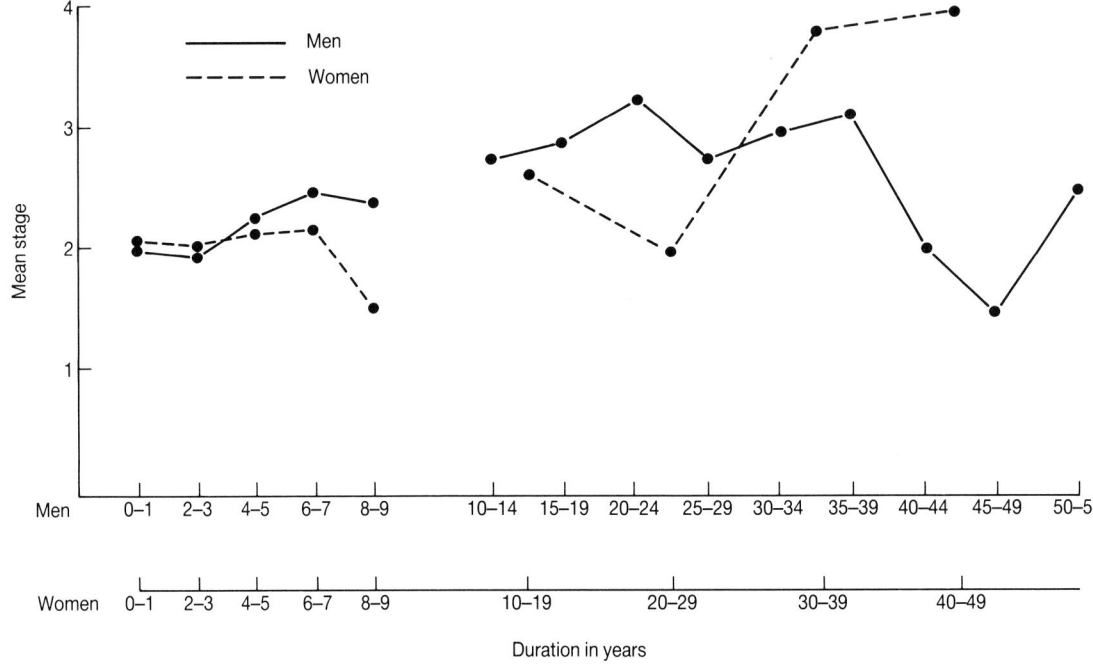

Fig. 19.6 Duration of DD by mean stage of contracture in 647 men (———) and 254 women (— — —). From Mikkelsen (1977a) with permission.

women there was even greater variation, but disease of higher stages was correlated with increasing duration of disease.

OCCUPATION AND PREVIOUS HAND INJURIES

Records were made of handedness and previous hand injuries for all those who had DD; occupation was noted for all participants in the study. (It was too complicated to record handedness and hand injuries for everyone.) The town was divided into districts, and the districts were requested to enter the examination separately. The characteristics mentioned were recorded for some of the districts selected at random. Pensioners and those who had changed their job during the last 5 years were registered under their previous occupation. Occupations were divided into four groups:

1. Heavy manual work (e.g. lumbarjacks, full-time farmers).
2. Medium-heavy work (e.g. bricklayers, most mechanics).
3. Light manual work (e.g. dentists, most industrial workers).
4. No manual work (e.g. clerks, vicars).

Table 19.7 Stage of DD in men with unilateral involvement, by number of digits

Digit	Right hand						Left hand				
	Stage						Stage				
	1	2	3	4	5	Mean	1	2	3	4	Mean
Thumb	0	0	0	0	0		1	0	0	0	1.00
Index finger	0	0	0	0	0		0	0	0	0	
Middle finger	21	9	0	0	0	1.30	14	3	0	0	1.18
Ring finger	80	74	0	0	0	1.48	45	28	0	0	1.40
Little finger	25	12	2	2	1	1.62	24	11	3	1	1.51

Table 19.8 Stage of DD in men with bilateral involvement, by number of digits

Digit	Right hand						Left hand					
	Stage						Stage					
	1	2	3	4	5	Mean	1	2	3	4	5	Mean
Thumb	13	0	0	0	0	1.00	13	4	0	0	0	1.24
Index finger	4	0	3	0	0	1.86	1	2	2	0	0	2.20
Middle finger	86	40	8	0	0	1.42	74	30	4	2	0	1.40
Ring finger	161	146	19	8	3	1.65	190	102	12	5	1	1.48
Little finger	96	56	19	11	4	1.77	133	31	20	12	3	1.60

Table 19.9 Stage of DD in women with unilateral involvement, by number of digits

Digit	Right hand						Left hand					
	Stage						Stage					
	1	2	3	4	5	Mean	1	2	3	4	5	Mean
Thumb	0	0	0	0	0		0	0	0	0	0	
Index finger	1	0	0	0	0	1.00	3	0	0	0	0	1.00
Middle finger	18	2	0	0	0	1.10	8	2	0	0	0	1.20
Ring finger	72	15	0	1	0	1.19	36	7	0	0	1	1.25
Little finger	31	2	1	0	0	1.12	18	3	0	2	2	1.68

Table 19.10 Stage of DD in women with bilateral involvement, by number of digits

Digit	Right hand						Left hand					
	Stage						Stage					
	1	2	3	4	5	Mean	1	2	3	4	Mean	
Thumb	1	0	0	0	0	1.00	1	0	0	0	1.00	
Index finger	1	0	0	0	0	1.00	1	0	0	0	1.00	
Middle finger	31	8	1	0	0	1.25	28	3	0	0	1.13	
Ring finger	66	33	2	2	0	1.42	83	14	2	0	1.18	
Little finger	30	6	3	1	1	1.46	35	4	2	2	1.33	

Groups 1 and 4 were clearly defined, but there was a more gradual transition between groups 2 and 3, and sometimes it was difficult to know which to choose.

Only definite, single injuries were recorded, such as fractures of the hand or wrist, tendon injuries, lacerations and deep infections or burns leaving visible scars.

DD was recorded in all kinds of occupation, but prevalence increased with increasing degree of heavy work (Table 19.11), although this statement must be qualified in the case of women doing heavy manual work because of the small number. Correlation of the prevalence of DD in men doing different kinds of work showed that the maximum prevalence occurred at a lower age in group 1 (heavy work) than in those groups doing less laborious work (Fig. 19.7). The hands of those involved in heavy labour also showed the highest degree of disease (Tables 19.12 and 19.13). In bilateral cases, the contracture was consistently worse in the right hand.

The rate of operations was almost equal within the four occupational groups — from 4.8 to 6.4%.

Table 19.11 The influence of different kinds of work on Dupuytren's disease (DD)

Type of work	Men			Women		
	Total	DD	%	Total	DD	%
Heavy	477	70	14.7	6	1	16.7
Medium	2304	262	11.4	4710	223	4.7
Light	2285	218	9.5	707	20	2.8
Non-manual	1805	96	5.3	1104	10	0.9
?	17	1	5.9	0		

? = Those who do not remember.

Table 19.12 The relationship between total stage of contracture and different kinds of work in 647 men with DD

Type of work	Stage of contracture											
	1	2	3	4	5	6	7	8	9	10	11	Mean
Heavy	46	33	15	14	6	6	4	0	0	1	1	2.67
Medium	129	137	60	38	18	12	7	4	5	3	3	2.61
Light	120	128	40	37	11	11	3	5	2	0	0	2.36
Non-manual	43	46	19	12	10	4	2	2	0	0	0	2.49

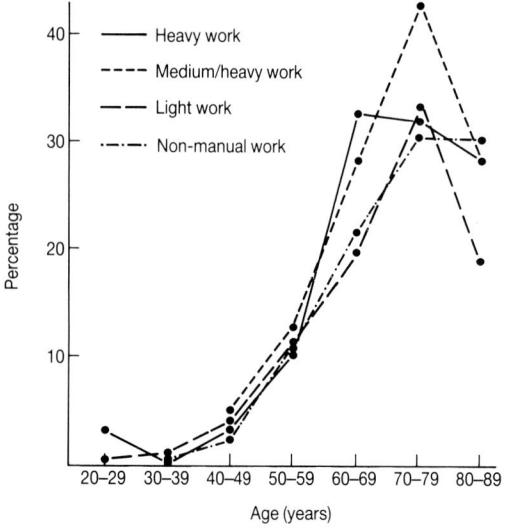

Fig. 19.7 Prevalence of DD in men by age and different kinds of work. ———— Heavy work; — — — medium-heavy work; — — light work; —.—. non-manual work. From Mikkelson (1978) with permission.

Table 19.13 The relationship between total stage of contracture and different kinds of work in 254 women with DD

Type of work	Stage of contracture										Mean
	1	2	3	4	5	6	7	8	9	10	
Heavy	0	1									
Medium	125	98	49	26	14	4	2	1	1	2	2.23
Light	13	13	2	0	0	0	0	0	0	0	1.60
Non-manual	7	4	1	1	1	0	0	0	0		1.93

An equal number of right and left hands were operated upon.

Previous hand injuries were recorded in 15.5% of the male population. In men with DD hand injuries were more common, and in bilateral cases the frequency was almost double that of the whole population (Table 19.14). Women with DD had approximately the same frequency of previous hand injuries as did the general male population. Each year a much lower number of hand injuries were seen in women in the local hospital. The conclusion, that women with DD had sustained previous hand injuries more often than the general population, therefore seems reasonable.

Table 19.14 Previous hand injuries in 609 men with DD, by affected hand

Affected hand	n	Injured hands	%
Right	156	20	12.8
Left	86	22	25.6
Both	367	101	27.3
Total	609	143	23.8

As could be expected, hand injuries were most frequently sustained by those involved in heavy labour. When those with previous hand injuries were excluded from Table 19.14, the relationship of DD to heavy work is reduced but not eliminated.

THE NEED FOR SURGICAL TREATMENT

In all, 38 of the 647 men (5.7%) and 8 of the 254 women (3.1%) with DD had been operated on because of their disease. One-third were completely free of bands and nodules when examined. Today, most surgeons do not recommend operation for incipient stages. When the contracture of one or more fingers has reached stage 3 (total contracture of at least 45°), many surgeons will operate. If the numbers of those operated on were added to these figures, approximately 30% of men and 12% of women would be candidates for an operation.

KNUCKLE PADS

The diagnosis of knuckle pads was based upon the following criterion: subcutaneous thickening over the dorsal aspect of the proximal interphalangeal joint, adherent to the skin but mobile over the joint capsule. During a period of 3 weeks 752 men and 1119 women were examined to determine whether knuckle pads were present.

Typical knuckle pads were encountered in slightly less than 10% of the normal population in both sexes; the frequency was higher in those over 30 years of age. A total of 48.6% of men and 33.3% of women with DD had knuckle pads. In both sexes the frequency was higher in patients with bilateral DD, or with involvement of the left hand only. There was no significant difference in the mean stage of contracture in those with and those without knuckle pads. Of 36 men operated on for DD 16 (45%) had knuckle pads. Of 5 women, 9 (62%) had knuckle pads.

HEREDITY

All patients with DD were asked about the occurrence of the disease in their family; only first-degree relatives were counted. Family history was correlated with age of onset (Table 19.15). Those who developed DD at a young age had a greater incidence of positive family history. Ling (1963) showed that of 50 patients with DD, only 8 were aware of a positive family history, while 34 had relatives with the disease. The numbers in Table 19.15 are therefore probably far too small.

Table 19.15 Positive family history of DD correlated with age of onset

Age of onset (years)	Men			Women		
	Total	Positive family history	%	Total	Positive family history	%
<10	2	0		1	0	
10–19	10	4	40.0	2	0	
20–29	21	11	52.4	1	0	
30–39	73	27	37.0	3	0	
40–49	143	38	26.6	33	11	33.3
50–59	159	34	21.4	42	17	40.5
60–69	94	15	16.0	59	15	25.4
70–79	27	2	8.2	34	7	20.6
80–89	3	0		10	1	10.0
Unknown	115			69		

DISCUSSION

The recognition of the nodule as an early sign of DD is so well documented (Krogius 1922; Skoog 1948; Hueston 1960; Early 1962) that by now it must be quite generally accepted.

The prevalence of DD in the present material is higher than Hellgren (1964) found in Sweden, but lower than Lund (1941) found in brewery workers in Denmark, and it supports the general view of a high prevalence in Scandinavians (Early 1962; Hueston 1963). Egawa (1985) published statistics from Japan which call this view into question, finding almost the same high prevalence in his study as was seen in Scandinavia.

Increasing prevalence with increasing age is given in most statistics. This trend is seen in the present material up to 70–75 years of age in men and 80–85 years in women. After that time there is a sudden break in the curve, and the prevalence decreases. This may be ascribed to one or both of the following factors:

1. A complete regression of the disease.
2. A higher mortality of patients with DD than in the general public.

This problem was not foreseen when the study was planned, and hence relevant data were not recorded. However, a number of elderly persons with DD stated spontaneously that both bands and contracture had diminished appreciably after they had stopped working.

A significant decrease of the ratio of men to women found with increasing age is in line with the results reported by Early (1962) and Hueston (1963). I suspect that the variation seen in many statistical studies is due to a failure to discount the age factor.

A substantial number of subjects were not aware of having DD. Many had low grade disease, and this point raises some uncertainty about the stated age of onset. On the other hand, a number of those who had attended the field study without showing any sign of DD consulted me within the following year with typical Dupuytren's nodules. They were almost exclusively white collar workers, which may imply that this group gives a more accurate age of onset than manual workers who often also have occupational indurations in their hands.

In most cases the disease and started in the right hand; this is reported in most relevant series. It appeared in all ages from childhood to old age, but most frequently in middle age. The literature contains few case reports of DD in children: Bunnell (1944) observed a boy of 17, and Jacubic (1965) a girl of 11 and a boy of 17. Personally I have seen typical Dupuytren's nodules in the soles of children with epilepsy, but never in their hands.

The lower age limit of 16 years in the study was determined by the chest examination, so the occurrence of DD in children is not covered by the present study.

The disease affected most commonly the three ulnar fingers, and the degree of contracture increased towards the ulnar side of the hand. This point was commented on by Dupuytren himself, making observations on the function of the palmar fascia: 'It tends constantly to bring the fingers to a state of demiflexion, which is their state of repose, and it is nothing more than the excess of this function produced by disease, which gives rise to the deformity'. This appearance of the disease has caused much philosophical thought, and attention has been attracted to disorders of the ulnar nerve (Eulenberg 1883; Scolz 1953). This may be true in particular cases, but in general it is of little significance.

The study revealed that the disease was more developed in the right than in the left hand, and it was worse in men than in women with corresponding duration of the disease. The contracture was also worse in those involved in heavy labour. These observations support the view that occupation probably has some influence on the development of the disease.

Singular hand injuries also seemed to be of some importance. Hueston (1968) emphasizes the difficulty of trusting the patients' 'sincere assertion that the injured hand had no nodule before the accident', but he believes in the relationship.

Typical knuckle pads were found in about 10% of the population studied. The frequency in those with DD was considerably higher, and also higher than most statistics published up to now (Lund 1941; Skoog 1948; Early 1962). The extremes are represented by Gosset (personal communication), who found knuckle pads extremely rare in France, and Hueston (1963) who found a frequency of 75% in young patients, with recurrences. Thus, the connection of knuckle pads with a more aggressive disease was not seen in the present study.

A positive family history was also the same in subjects with and without knuckle pads (Mikkelsen 1977). The observation of Garrod (1893), which Clarkson & Pelly (1962) subscribe to, that knuckle pads preceded DD, was not in the scope of the present study. If this theory can be proved, it will offer substantial help in the research of heredity.

A strikingly small number had been operated upon for DD. This is a crucial point to bear in mind when evaluating these statistics. In addition to the finger contracture per se, many other factors will determine the wish to have an operation — age, sex, occupation, social status and standard of living. These parameters may vary appreciably in different areas and in different periods, and thus produce a bias.

The results of this study do not permit conclusive statements concerning the role of heredity in DD. When evaluating the relevant literature, it must be taken into account that DD is rather common. A substantial number of those who have it will give a positive family history simply by chance. The number in the present study is, however, adequate to accept the theory of heredity, at least in younger ages. The higher frequency of positive family history in younger than older age groups indicates two types of DD — one with predominant heredity which mainly affects young persons, and one with no or less hereditary influence, mostly seen in elderly people. Both Hueston (1963) and Kipikasa (1968) have made observations in support of this view. This division into inherited and acquired disease is, after all, seen in many other conditions, such as diabetes mellitus and epilepsy.

This study has added to our understanding of DD. At the same time it has revealed that our knowledge is still imperfect. This is frustrating for the investigator, but it may stimulate readers to extend this research.

R. M. McFarlane, J. S. Botz and H. Cheung

Epidemiology of surgical patients

Much has been written about Dupuytren's disease (DD) and many opinions have been expressed, often on the basis of a single case. Unfounded opinions and anecdotal information pervade the literature. In an attempt to obtain more objective data the committee on DD of the International Federation of Societies for Surgery of the Hand undertook an epidemiological study by seeking patient information from surgeons around the world.

A SURVEY OF SURGICAL PATIENTS

The study population consisted of 1150 patients with DD who consulted a surgeon specifically about the disease in their hands. The goal was to correlate, from these patients, epidemiological and surgical factors which affect outcome. Thus the investigation was an attempt to correct misconceptions as well as to confirm opinions by the presentation of objective data. A questionnaire was designed to collect information on four aspects of DD — the patient; the operation; the result of the operation and the long-term result of treatment in terms of recurrence and extension of disease. Preliminary results of this study have been published (McFarlane 1983, 1985).

Patients with DD who consult a surgeon do not necessarily reflect the features of this disease in the general population where many people have minimal disease, elderly patients often have it without their knowledge, and others are content to accept contracture or have been advised not to have an operation. Brouet (1986) reported that in his series of 1014 patients, 496 were operated upon, of whom 11% were women, whereas 518 were not operated upon, of whom 36% were women. Thus it would appear that women are more inclined to accept contracture or that their contracture is not as severe.

In groups of patients with primary diseases such as diabetes, epilepsy or alcoholism, the related incidence of DD is high but these patients do not necessarily seek surgical intervention for their hand contractures. The following analysis considers only those patients who were seen by a surgeon and in most instances were operated upon. They are representative of the more severe type of disease.

Racial origin and family history

It has been assumed, especially since the study of Ling (1963), that DD is genetically transmitted. By implication Hueston has suggested that it is a disease of the Celtic race, or perhaps originated with the Vikings, because the prevalence of DD coincides with the early migrations of these people. Clearly it is very common in northern Europe, less common in southern Europe (Brouet 1986) and South America (Davis 1965) and rare in Africa. It is said to occur in India but there are no reports in the literature. (However there is one east Indian patient in this study who was operated upon in England.) It is not uncommon in Japan, as documented by Egawa (1985; Egawa et al 1985) and Morinaga et al (1979) and discussed further in Chapter 21. The 12 Chinese patients included in this study were retrieved with difficulty from the records of five large hospitals in five different provinces in China (Wang, personal communication). Chow et al (1984), reporting DD in 3 patients, stated that it was extremely uncommon in the Chinese people. Tui (personal communication) has collected some 30 cases over a period of 20 years in Taiwan. Mennen (1986; Mennen & Grabe 1979) has documented its existence in black Africans; Furnas (1979) reported a single case in a black African.

Table 20.1 shows the country of origin and racial or family origin of 1150 patients, as documented by questionnaire. Most descended from northern European stock, very few from southern Europe. Of special interest is the number of Japanese and Chinese patients. This does not reflect so much the frequency of DD in Orientals as the co-operation of the surgeons in those countries; however it does emphasize that DD is not rare in Orientals. The features of all of these patients as well as the involvement of their hands and the type of operation performed are shown in Profile A at the end of this chapter.

On the assumption that northern Europeans have typical disease, this group was further refined by removing patients who had a previous operation, and thus had recurrent disease. This created a group of 670 patients of northern European descent who had not previously been operated upon. The features of this group are shown in Profile B and form the basis for comparison with other groups. For instance, in Profile C the characteristics of southern European patients are documented. There were only 27 patients so statistical analysis is of doubtful value but there were more males and less bilateral disease. One would expect the extent of hand involvement to be less, yet three or more rays were more often involved and radial side disease (thumb and index finger) was more frequent than in northern Europeans.

ANALYSIS OF PROFILES A AND B

As shown in Profiles A and B the sex ratio of 83 males to 17 females is similar to other surgical series. More women are operated upon as age increases (Fig. 20.1). Most patients had disease in both hands but when the disease was unilateral the right hand was involved almost twice as often as the left. This observation suggests that use of the hand or injury may play a role in the development of disease. Only half of the patients were manual workers, which is at variance with Mikkelson's observation in a general population (1972, 1978; see Chapter 19). The age difference between males and females both at onset of disease and at operation is statistically significant ($p<0.001$★). A family history of 29%, taken by a surgeon on a single visit, is highly suggestive of a familial disease. In Ling's (1963) study the prevalence of family history rose from 16 to 68% when he sought out and examined close family members.

The involvement of other areas is a strong diathesis factor. Knuckle pads are most common but clinically it is often difficult to be certain whether or not they are present so the recorded incidence may be incorrect. Plantar fibromatosis is easy to diagnose. Penile fibromatosis is not often associated with DD. All three areas were involved in only 9 patients.

Associated diseases

The fact that DD is associated with other diseases should suggest some common pathway of aetiology or pathogenesis. To date, this has not been revealed. In the past gout and pulmonary tuberculosis were mentioned but from this study there is no evidence that cardiopulmonary disease and

Table 20.1 Country and family of origin of 1150 surgical patients, as documented by questionnaire

Country of origin	n	Family origin	n	%
Australia	37	Northern Europe	865	83
Belgium	37	Southern Europe	27	3
Canada	294	Japanese	126	12
China	12	Chinese	12	1
France	118	Black American	9	1
Japan	128	Black African	5	0.5
Mexico	2	American Indian	2	0.2
South Africa	12	Indian	1	0.1
Sweden	13			
UK	50			
USA	339			
West Germany	108			

★ Statistical methodology consisted of the two-sample Student's t-test for differences between continuous variables and the chi-squared test for differences between categorical variables (Snedecor & Cochran 1967).

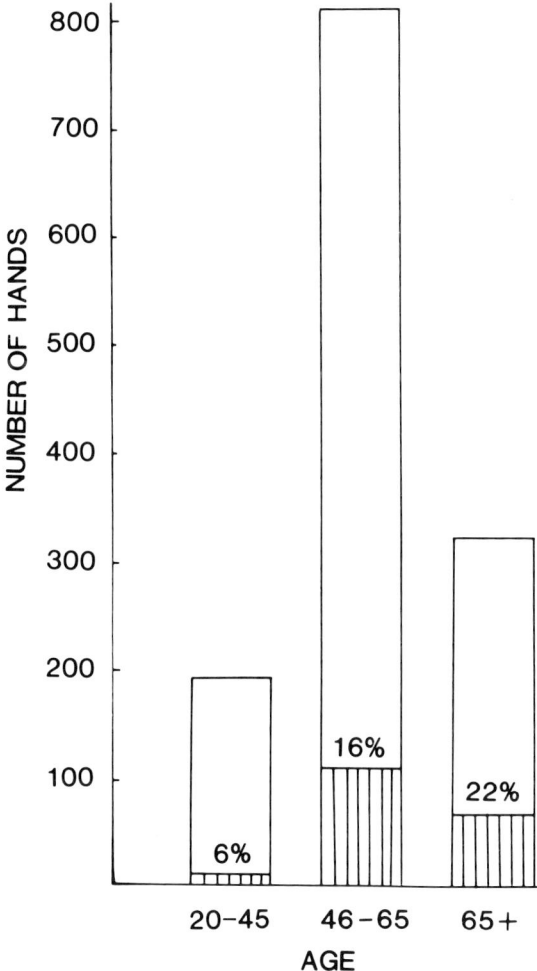

Fig. 20.1 Ratio of males (□) to females (▥) by age at operation. $p < 0.01$.

hypertension or any type of arthritis are related to DD. It is unheard of in leprosy, a disease that destroys collagen and elastin (Enna, personal communication).

The incidence of epilepsy in various countries varies from 0.2 to 0.8% (Laidlaw & Richens 1982). The incidence of epilepsy in these surgical patients was about 3%, or approximately 6 times greater than in the general population (Profiles A and B; Table 20.3). DD was seen in both idiopathic and acquired epilepsy in this study so the association with barbiturate medication is highly suspect, as suggested by Critchley et al (1976). The features of 37 epileptic patients are shown in Profile D. There is more bilateral disease, other areas are more frequently involved, the age at onset and operation is earlier in both males and females and 43% had a previous operation. Also 50% of the epileptic group had three or more rays involved, compared to the non-epileptic group ($p<0.01$) and the incidence of disease on the radial side of the hand was also greater ($p<0.02$). Therefore the type of operation performed in this group was extensive. More skin grafts were used in the palm and more proximal interphalangeal joint procedures were performed. The results of treatment, although not shown, were similar to those in the group as a whole. Clearly the extent of disease is more severe and the course of disease is more aggressive in the epileptic population. This suggests an increased diathesis, discussed in chapter 22. This increased diathesis could be genetic or brought on by barbiturate medication.

Table 20.2 Hand profile by country (percentage)

	USA	Canada	France	Japan	West Germany	UK	Australia
Bilateral	45	78	72	73	82	48	78
Palm only	6	5	5	6	0	4	9
No palm	9	4	0	3	16	4	7
One ray	33	30	36	29	36	50	40
Three or more rays	26	37	33	30	29	16	25
Little finger	70	69	73	75	70	70	67
Ring finger	67	63	56	72	62	36	51
Middle finger	30	34	31	31	41	22	21
Index finger	9	13	20	11	13	2	12
Thumb	18	36	26	12	19	12	35

Concerning diabetes mellitus, quite a different impression is gained if one examines a group of DD patients or a group of diabetic patients. In Profile A and Table 20.3 the prevalence of diabetes is the expected rate for this age group of patients. However in patients attending a diabetic clinic, where the prevalence of DD is higher than in non-diabetics, the duration of the diabetes rather than its severity or insulin dependence is thought to be the contributing factor (Spring et al 1970; Malins 1972; Lawson et al 1983; Crisp & Heathcoate 1984; Noble et al 1984).

The criteria for the diagnosis of diabetes are beyond the scope of this discussion, other than to say that diagnosis cannot be made from a single clinical feature or laboratory test. Likewise, the diagnosis of Dupuytren's disease is uncertain in its early stages; in the diabetic patient limited joint mobility and trigger finger may be mistaken for DD. Because of the margin of error in the diagnosis of both diseases it is difficult to evaluate their association but in Chapter 23 convincing evidence is presented of an association between DD and diabetes. As shown in Profile E, some features of the diabetic patient who comes to operation differ from those of the non-diabetic group. There are proportionally fewer northern Europeans ($p<0.025$) and more Japanese patients ($p<0.005$) with diabetes. This is probably due to the predominance of males in both groups. Diabetes is more common in European females than males, but it is more common in Japanese males. (Rudnick & Anderson 1962; Wada et al 1964; Zimmet 1983; Keen & Ekde 1984). Thus these differences are related more to diabetes than to DD. However, there are more alcoholics in the diabetic group ($p<0.025$) and more bilateral disease ($p<0.05$). These are features of DD which suggest a relationship — albeit tenuous — between the two diseases.

The diagnosis of alcoholism by a surgeon is subjective. A prevalence of 10% in the general population is not high. According to Table 20.3 the prevalence by country varied from 2 to 15%. Bradlow & Mowat (1986) suggest that a daily alcohol intake of 40 g is indicative of a heavy drinker. They reported that 23% of 64 patients operated for DD were heavy drinkers. If an association does exist, the question must be answered whether DD is the result of liver damage caused by increased intake of alcohol, the result of the direct action of alcohol on the fascia, or whether two diseases are genetically related.

The features of the alcoholic patients listed in Profile F suggest a genetic or some fundamental association between alcoholism and DD. When

Table 20.3 Patient profile by country (percentage)

	USA	Canada	France	Japan	West Germany	UK	Australia
Northern European	89	98	95	0	100	98	100
Male	78	84	89	95	89	84	76
Bilateral	45	78	72	73	82	48	73
Family history	25	34	11	5	39	27	57
Other areas	22	32	32	16	35	30	22
Manual work	47	62	34	63	33	54	40
Epilepsy	3	3	6	2	1	2	0
Diabetes	3	7	3	14	6	4	3
Alcoholism	8	15	12	2	6	6	5
Trauma	17	9	10	15	10	14	27
Age at onset							
Male	54.4	47.4	44.1	5351	39.3	50.3	42.3
Female	60.2	54.3	54.6		54.3	54.0	52.0
Age at surgery							
Male	60.2	57.0	56.0	60.3	53.4	56.2	56.0
Female	63.3	61.4	62.8	63.0	64.3	68.5	59.4

compared with non-alcoholic patients, the alcoholic group has more northern Europeans ($p<0.001$), more family history ($p<0.01$), greater incidence of other areas involved ($p<0.001$), and more bilateral disease ($p<0.001$). The age at onset and at operation, although not significant, is earlier. The alcoholic patient has more extensive disease. Not only is there more bilateral disease ($p<0.001$) but there is also a greater incidence of three or more rays involved ($p<0.001$) and more radial side disease ($p<0.001$). These are the features of 'Dupuytren's diathesis'. The corollary is that alcoholism is probably a factor contributing to increased diathesis to DD.

In the context of this study trauma has been considered to be a disease. The prevalence of 14% in Profile A includes a single injury to the hand as well as the repetitive trauma of occupation. The prevalence is the same in patients of northern and southern European and Japanese origin suggesting that there is no association with race. The prevalence ranged from 9% in Canadians to 27% in Australians suggesting a certain bias in reporting. Trauma was more commonly reported in males and patients under 45 years of age as well as in epileptics and alcoholics. It was common in unilateral disease and patients with only one ray involved. A more detailed discussion of the association of DD with occupation and with a single injury to the hand is given in Chapter 23 and 24.

Extent of disease

In the profiles (at the end of this chapter) the types of hand involvement and operations performed are listed. In the northern European group the disease was limited to the palm in 6%. In 4% the palm was not involved. There was an almost equal distribution of one, two and three or more rays involved and the little and ring fingers were most frequently involved. The pattern of hand involvement in Profile B is considered to be 'typical'. Variations would then be more or less severe. Less severe disease would include more unilateral disease, more palm only or finger only or more one ray involvement. More severe disease would show more bilateral disease, more rays involved and, in particular, more radial side involvement of the thumb and index finger.

Types of operation

The many types of operation have been condensed here into four groups. A *local* operation included an open or closed fasciotomy, with or without a skin graft or the fasciectomy of Gonzales (1971), in which the fascia and perhaps some skin is excised locally and a full thickness skin graft is applied. A *regional fasciectomy* is one in which only the obviously diseased fascia is removed. An *extensive fasciectomy* is an operation in which not only the diseased fascia but also the normal or potentially diseased fascia is removed. A *dermofasciectomy*, which removes diseased fascia as well as overlying skin (which is replaced by a full thickness skin graft) is included in this latter group. It is interesting that amputations comprised only 1% of 1339 operations and all of these were of the little finger because of recurrent disease. The commonest operation in the palm as well as all but the little finger was a regional fasciectomy. An extensive fasciectomy was most common in the little finger, which reflects the extensive disease encountered in this finger as well as the difficulties of correcting the flexion contracture.

Most wounds were closed primarily by suture. In the palm 17% of wounds were left open after the method of McCash (1964). Almost 10% of wounds in the palm, fingers and thumb were skin grafted. A dermofasciectomy is often used in the treatment of recurrent disease but it is also the treatment of choice of some surgeons for primary disease.

Regional and general anaesthesia were used equally. Most patients received some kind of postoperative therapy although only 38% were splinted. Accessory procedures at the proximal interphalangeal joint to overcome flexion contracture after the fascia had been removed were uncommon. The overall complication rate was 17%.

Results of treatment

The result of treatment of a certain group were determined at 1 year ($\pm$ 6 months) after operation on the assumption that the full benefit of operation and postoperative therapy would have been attained by that time, but recurrence would not have affected the initial result. The pre- and postopera-

Table 20.4 The distance of the fingertip to the distal crease of the palm before and after operation

	Little finger	Ring finger	Middle finger	Index finger
Patients with full flexion				
	n = 501	n = 497	n = 492	n = 413
Preoperatively	92%	93%	96%	97%
Postoperatively	83%	88%	90%	92%
Patients with full flexion pre- but not postoperatively				
	n = 52	n = 34	n = 33	n = 29
Postoperatively	2.1 ± 1.4 cm	2.5 ± 1.7 cm	2.5 ± 1.6 cm	2.3 ± 1.3 cm
Patients with limited flexion preoperatively				
	n = 42	n = 37	n = 20	n = 14
Preoperatively	1.6 ± 1.1 cm	1.8 ± 1.3 cm	2.0 ± 1.6 cm	2.0 ± 1.1 cm
Postoperatively	1.1 ± 1.1 cm	1.4 ± 1.6 cm	1.3 ± 1.5 cm	1.6 ± 1.4 cm
Full flexion postoperatively	39%	35%	31%	15%

tive angles for each joint of each digit are presented as the mean and standard deviation. In addition to joint measurements the results were also considered by outcome — perfect if the postoperative angle was 0°, improved if the angle was less than the preoperative angle, and worse if the postoperative angle was the same or greater. These outcome groups have proved to be the most sensitive index of a result*. In addition, data on pre- and postoperative flexion of the finger are recorded by measurements of the distance from the fingertip to the distal crease of the palm (Table 20.4). Most patients not only had full flexion preoperatively but also regained full flexion by 1 year. In patients who do not recover full flexion after operation the average distal crease of the palm is about 2 cm. Patients who had limited flexion before operation were not made worse by operation; in fact, some 30% of them attained full flexion after operation.

Two observations stand out clearly. The results at the metacarpophalangeal joint are much better than those at the proximal interphalangeal joint; the results in the little finger at the latter joint are poor. Although 75% of patients gained some improvement by operation for contracture at the proximal interphalangeal joint of the little finger, only 20% obtained a perfect result and 25% of patients became worse. The results in the ring and middle fingers are similar.

As shown in Profile B, in each finger at both the metacarpophalangeal and proximal interphalangeal joint the preoperative angle was lowest in the group with the worst outcome. In most joints where the outcome was worse the preoperative angle was less than 30°. The reason for the poor result is not clear but the observation suggests that joint contractures of less than 30° are best not operated upon. In a previous publication (Legge & McFarlane 1980) it was suggested that the degree of metacarpophalangeal joint contracture influenced the proximal interphalangeal joint result. This observation was tested with our current data in the little and ring fingers, as shown in Table 20.5 and 20.6. The average preoperative metacarpophalangeal and distal interphalangeal joint angle of the three outcome groups was similar in each finger, whereas there was a significant difference at the proximal interphalangeal joint, so it is concluded that the degree of contracture at these joints had no bearing upon the outcome at the proximal interphalangeal joint. It may be that with contractures of less than 30° the diseased fascia is not as apparent. A well developed cord may not be present and the surgeon may not remove sufficient tissue. As a result the contracture is not

---

*Preliminary exploratory analysis revealed that prediction of the outcome of surgery is complex and involves many factors such as pattern of disease, diathesis factors and surgical characteristics. No single general model of prediction is satisfactory for the many different presentations. An in-depth description of the various statistical procedures and methodology employed and the results obtained is beyond the scope of the present discussion.

Table 20.5 The relationship of the outcome in the little finger at the proximal interphalangeal joint (PIPJ) to the preoperative angles at the metacarpophalangeal joint (MPJ) and distal interphalangeal joint (DIPJ)

PIPJ outcome	n	MPJ		PIPJ		DIPJ	
		Pre	Post	Pre	Post	Pre	Post
Perfect	51	32.7 ± 29.3	0.2 ± 1.4	46.5 ± 23.8*	0	6.8 ± 16.7	1.6 ± 5.8
Improved	145	27.6 ± 30.8	1.3 ± 4.5	63.3 ± 21.3*	28.8 ± 17.5	4.8 ± 12.1	2.7 ± 8.5
Worse	66	31.7 ± 30.7	4.2 ± 17.2	34.9 ± 22.7*	44.9 ± 23.3	5.1 ± 12.2	4.1 ± 10.2

*There was a significant difference between each of the three groups at the PIPJ ($p<0.01$).

Table 20.6 The relationship of the outcome in the ring finger at the proximal interphalangeal joint (PIPJ) to the preoperative angles at the metacarpophalangeal joint (MPJ) and distal interphalangeal joint (DIPJ)

PIPJ outcome	n	MPJ		PIPJ		DIPJ	
		Pre	Post	Pre	Post	Pre	Post
Perfect	62	34.1 ± 27.2	4.4 ± 13.1	41.7 ± 24.1*	0	4.7 ± 15.9	1.9 ± 10.6
Improved	58	25.7 ± 27.2	2.8 ± 9.8	64.3 ± 22.8*	29.0 ± 18.2	6.4 ± 18.1	1.2 ± 6.5
Worse	18	35.6 ± 21.7	7.1 ± 12.9	28.2 ± 19.8*	36.2 ± 22.7	3.3 ± 12.1	2.9 ± 6.1

*There was a significant difference between each of the three groups at the PIPJ ($p<0.01$).

corrected and the residual disease, augmented by the postoperative scarring, causes further joint contracture.

The long-term results of treatment have been evaluated according to the prevalence of extension and recurrence of disease. Extension refers to the appearance or progress of disease outside the area of operation, whereas recurrence means the appearance of disease within the area of operation.

As discussed above, the initial result of operation has been evaluated at 1 year. From 2 years onward the patients have been evaluated for extension and/or recurrence of disease. As shown in Figures 20.2 and 20.3, about 20% of hands examined at yearly intervals present with extension and/or recurrence. However, less than 10% of hands, or less than one-half of patients with extension or recurrence, required a second operation.

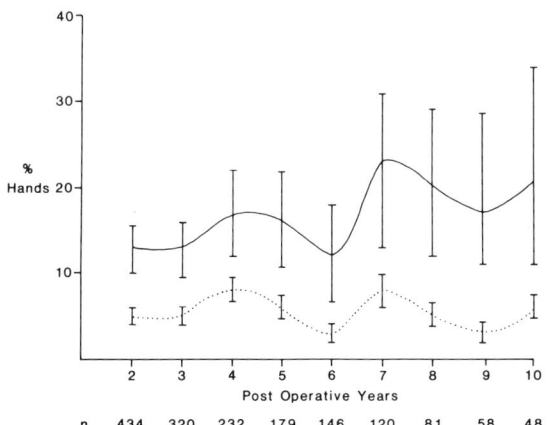

Fig. 20.2 Rate of recurrence of disease. ———
Recurrence; . . . . . recurrence requiring operation. Rate of recurrence within 95% confidence interval.

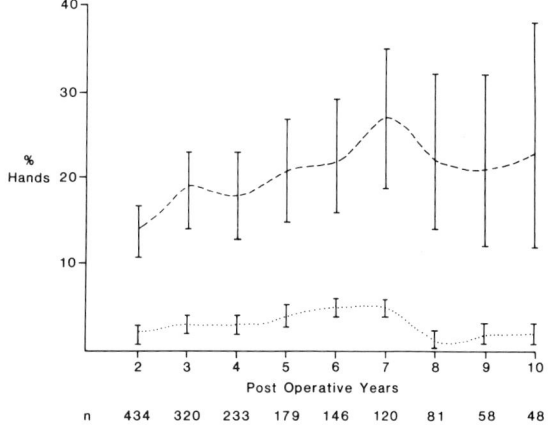

Fig. 20.3 Rate of extension of disease. — — —
Extension; . . . . . extension requiring operation. Rate of extension within 95% confidence interval.

Progression of disease

Figure 20.4 shows that about 20% of patients either developed new disease or showed progression of existing disease in the other hand after they had had an operation. But very few of these patients had an operation on the second hand. Of the patients represented in 20.4, 80% had bilateral disease.

Perhaps of more interest are those patients who originally presented with unilateral disease but eventually had bilateral disease. (Fig. 20.5). This figure shows that about 55% of unilateral patients were affected bilaterally within 5 years of operation. Not many of them required an operation on the second hand. The number of patients in the series followed for longer than 5 years is too small for analysis but it must be assumed that more patients had bilateral involvement with time. Nevertheless, a certain number of patients continued to have unilateral involvement, with less severe Dupuytren's disease. The data in Table 20.7 shows that the average angle recorded at 1 year does not change significantly after several years. The contraction does not continue in the area from which the fascia has been removed. This lends support to the view that the fascia is diseased rather than simply responding to biomechanical forces; the scar tissue that forms as a result of the operation does not respond to biomechanical forces in such a way as to produce continuing joint contraction.

VARIATIONS BY COUNTRY

In Profiles G–M the patient, hand, and operation profiles, and the results of treatment in various countries with sufficient data for analysis are given in descending order of the number of patients provided. The data for individual countries may prove of value in further studies but only some differences will be discussed, as shown in Tables 20.2, 20.3 and 20.8. The proportion of males operated upon in Japan is high although the sex ratio in Japan, as reported by Egawa et al (1985),

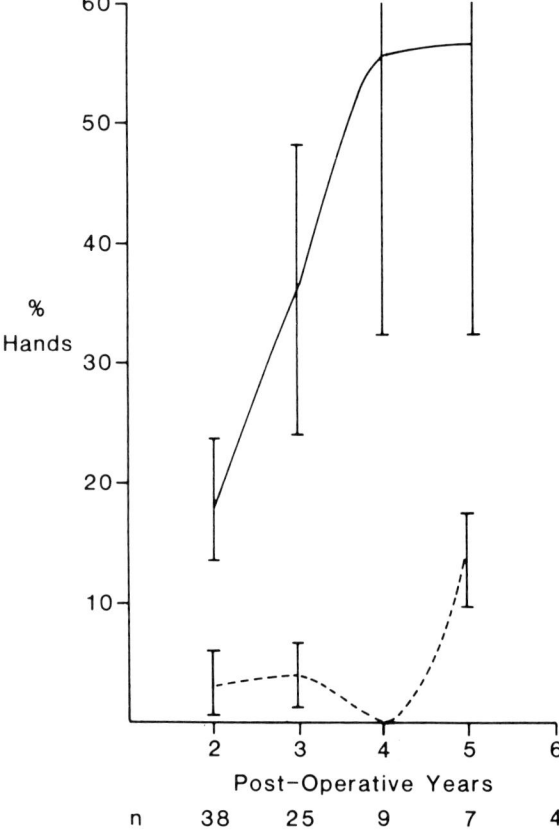

Fig. 20.5 Rate of appearance of disease in other hand of patients operated upon with unilateral disease. ———— Other hand involved; — — — other hand requiring operation. Rate of appearance within 95% confidence interval.

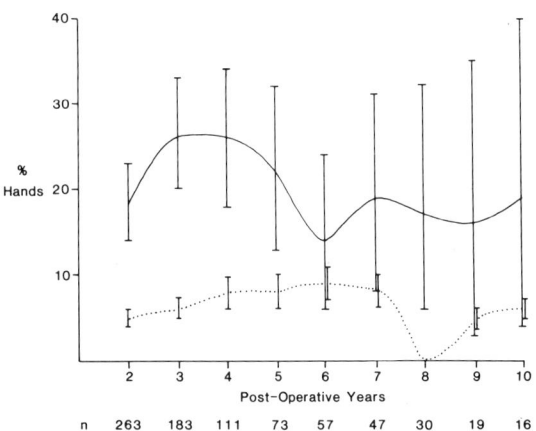

Fig. 20.4 Rate of appearance or progression of disease in the other hand after operation. ———— Other hand involved; . . . . . . other hand requiring operation. Rate of appearance within 95% confidence interval.

Table 20.7 The correction of flexion contracture over time (Northern Europeans with no previous surgery)

Finger	n	Pre operative Degrees	n	Post operative 1 Year (degrees)	n	2 Years (degrees)	n	3 Years (degrees)	n	4 Years (degrees)	n	5 Years (degrees)
LITTLE												
MPJ	164	42.7±24.4	164	3.4±12.3	33	1.6± 5.1	30	2.5±10.2	14	0	4	13.7±27.5
PIPJ	162	50.6±25.5	162	24.9±21.5	37	32.4±25.1	32	29.7±24.4	15	41.0±21.2	3	26.7±30.6
DIPJ	29	30.3±16.6	29	7.6±12.7	8	8.7±12.5	5	11.0±16.0	5	16.2±18.9	0	
RING												
MPJ	163	36.5±18.6	163	1.7± 7.4	42	1.4± 5.7	30	2.8± 7.8	17	2.1± 8.5	5	12.0±26.8
PIPJ	188	50.2±26.6	188	14.0±19.3	18	11.3±16.7	10	2.5± 5.4	7	21.4±25.4	2	45.0±63.6
DIPJ	10	30.5±28.5	10	4.5±14.2	2	0	1	0				
MIDDLE												
MPJ	82	29.0±16.2	82	1.3± 5.7	18	0.3± 1.2	12	4.6±10.8	6	0	2	0
PIPJ	18	33.6±19.2	18	15.6±18.5					2	17.5± 3.5		
DIPJ	3	26.7±20.8	3	16.7±28.9								

MPJ = metacarpophalangeal joint; PIPJ = proximal interphalangeal joint; DIPJ = distal interphalangeal joint.
Notes:
Only hands for which at least 1 years' postoperative data are available are included in this table.
There was no significant change in postoperative angles with time.

Table 20.8 Percentage of Surgical procedures in the palm, by country

	USA	Canada	France	Japan	West Germany	UK	Australia
Local	16	7	0	17	1	2	3
Regional	58	81	49	53	14	90	56
Extensive	26	12	51	30	85	8	42

is similar to that in northern Europeans. The prevalence of bilateral disease is low in patients in both the USA and the UK. Some of this difference may be accounted for by a misunderstanding of the question, but also these two groups of patients had somewhat less severe disease. There were fewer hands with three or more rays involved, less radial side disease and less recurrent disease. Concerning family history, the low prevalence in Japan is consistent with previous reports from that country (Morinaga et al 1979; Egawa et al 1985) and is an indication of the mild expression of the disease in Orientals. None of the 6 black Africans reported by Mennen (1986) or the 12 Chinese reported by Wang (personal communication) had a positive family history. Is this an indication of decreased genetic penetration or does it suggest that factors other than heredity can initiate the disease?

The prevalence in France is not consistent with other features of the French profile, which indicates severe disease, and so presumably is a reporting error. The low figure of 16% for other areas involved in Japanese patients is consistent with the view that the disease is less severe in Orientals.

The ratio of manual to non-manual workers varies considerably, from 63% in Japan to 33% in West Germany. These differences probably reflect a different interpretation of manual and non-manual work.

The prevalence of epilepsy and diabetes is similar in various countries. As mentioned previously there is considerable bias involved in the reporting of alcoholism and trauma and this could account for the variations recorded. Age at onset provides questionable data because the patient's recollection of when the disease first appeared could be incorrect by 5 or even 10 years. Nevertheless, age at onset is always significantly older in females than in males. The age at operation provides reliable data and shows less variation between countries. Again the average age when females are operated upon is significantly greater than for males.

The differences by country are not striking, other than in Japan where more males are operated upon, there is an infrequent family history, other areas are less often involved, diabetes is more common and alcoholism is less common. However, the last two features are representative of the Japanese population in general.

In Table 20.2 the same countries are compared regarding hand involvement. Disease in the palm only is indicative of either early or mild disease. Disease in the thumb and index finger, that is, radial side disease, is indicative of severe disease. The figures are predictably low in Japan but surprisingly low in the USA, West Germany and the UK. Again, there are no apparent trends other than that the Japanese have less severe hand involvement.

In Tables 20.8 and 20.9 the frequency of the type of operation performed in each country is listed; in Table 20.10 the overall operative procedure is compared. There are very obvious differences in methods of treatment. In West Germany an extensive operation is usually performed in the palm but a regional fasciectomy is done in the finger, whereas in Canada the reverse is true. These differences are compared in Table 20.11, related to the results of treatment. A significantly better correction of flexion contracture was obtained in West Germany at the proximal interphalangeal joint by a regional fasciectomy, and the outcome at the proximal interphalangeal joint of the little finger was better. The return of flexion after operation was similar in both countries. There was less recurrence or extension of disease in the Canadian patients in whom an extensive fasciectomy was performed in the finger.

Table 20.9 Percentage of surgical procedures in the fingers, by country

	USA	Canada	France	Japan	West Germany	UK	Australia
Local	13	4	4	8	8	3	7
Regional	53	13	56	61	83	90	17
Extensive	33	82	40	31	5	7	76
Amputation	1	1	0	0	4	0	0

Table 20.10 Operation profile by country (given in percentages)

	USA	Canada	France	Japan	West Germany	UK	Australia
Extensive operation							
Palm	26	12	51	30	85	8	42
Finger	33	82	40	31	5	7	76
PIPJ procedure	14	10	20	8	12	12	5
Palm closure							
Suture	81	66	41	72	98	57	89
Open	10	28	11	13	1	43	0
Graft	9	6	48	15	1	0	11
Finger closure							
Suture	88	92	57	86	93	95	51
Graft	8	7	41	8	6	2	49
General anaesthesia	43	60	82	33	1	60	0
Therapy	77	62	75	91	99	98	74
Splinting	46	59	36	60	16	44	33
Complications	14	17	36	11	16	16	19

PIPJ = proximal interphalangeal joint.

Table 20.11 Comparison of the results of treatment in Canada and West Germany in the little finger

	Canada		West Germany		p
	Pre	Post	Pre	Post	
MPJ	48°	4°	39°	5°	
PIPJ	46°	37°	56°	23°	<0.05
DCP (0°)	91%	82%	83%	76%	
Outcome					
Perfect		9%	15%		
Improved		47%	77%		<0.001
Worse		44%	8%		
Recurrence of extension		40%	66%		<0.001

MPJ = metacarpophalangeal joint; PIPJ = proximal interphalangeal joint; DCP = distal crease of the palm.

In France and Australia skin grafts are used frequently in the palm and fingers, that is, a dermofasciectomy is often performed. In both the UK and Canada the palm is often left open, after the method of McCash (1964). These procedures reflect different concepts of treatment rather than the management of different types of disease.

Correction of the flexion contracture at the proximal interphalangeal joint of the little finger is a good indication of the effectiveness of treatment because this joint is the most difficult to correct. Under all circumstances the worst results of treatment are seen at this joint. Therefore the results at this joint are used throughout this study to test the effect of variables upon treatment (Table 20.12). The best results were obtained in Japan, West Germany and Australia and the worst results in Canada. In Japan and West Germany regional fasciectomy was most often used in the finger whereas extensive fasciectomy was most common in Canada. In Australia and France dermofasciectomy was used frequently in both the palm and the finger; the results shown in Table 20.12 support the value of this procedure.

Regardless of the method of treatment the results at the metacarpophalangeal joint are consistently good. At the proximal interphalangeal joint the best results were obtained either by a regional fasciectomy, which is a conservative operation, or by a dermofasciectomy, a radical procedure. An extensive fasciectomy — a radical operation in which the skin is retained — produced the worst results.

TYPES OF DUPUYTREN'S DISEASE

Sex differences

In Profiles N and O male and female patients are compared and the significant differences are summarized in Table 20.13. It is well known that the disease is not only more common in males but also appears earlier and males are operated upon earlier. Females more often have a positive family history but one wonders if they simply know more about their relatives than do males. A history of trauma and manual work is more common in males but this is unlikely to be related to DD as much as to sex. The severity of disease is somewhat greater in the male. As a result more extensive operations are performed in males. The overall complications rate is no different between

Table 20.12 Results of treatment at the proximal interphalangeal joint of the little finger

	USA	Canada	France	Japan	West Germany	UK	Australia
Perfect	29	9	19	22	15	11	27
Improved	52	47	67	61	77	56	73
Worse	19	44	14	17	8	33	0

Table 20.13 Sex differences

Family history — more females	$p<0.008$
Sympathetic dystrophy — more females	$p<0.02$
Manual labour — more males	$p<0.001$
Trauma — more males	$p<0.001$
Age at onset — earlier in males	$p<0.001$
Age at operation — earlier in males	$p<0.001$
More than two rays involved in males	$p<0.05$
More extensive operation in palm in males	$p<0.01$
Results of operation — similar	
Recurrence and extension — similar	

the sexes, but sympathetic dystrophy occurs twice as frequently in females (7%) as in males (3.5%; $p<0.025$). The preoperative joint contractures were similar and the postoperative angles, although slightly better in males, were not significantly different. There was no difference in the incidence of recurrence and extension of disease.

Thus, differences between the sexes in patients with DD are not great. Presumably the disease is similar in the sexes but with a different genetic expression.

Severity of disease

About two-thirds of patients present with bilateral disease. The disease is usually more severe in one hand; in fact, only 26% of patients with bilateral disease have both hands operated on. Profiles P and Q permit comparison of patients with bilateral and unilateral disease. There is no difference in family origin or sex but the diathesis factors of family history, other areas, alcoholism, and recurrent disease are all less frequent in unilateral disease ($p<0.001$). Trauma is more frequent in unilateral disease but not significantly so. The involvement of the hand operated upon is less in the unilateral group. Fewer rays are involved ($p<0.001$) and there is less radial side disease. Also there are more patients with palm only and no palm disease. As a result the operation in the fingers is less extensive in unilateral disease ($p<0.001$) and complications are fewer ($p<0.005$). Preoperative and postoperative angles are not different but the chance of recurrence or extension is less with unilateral disease ($p<0.02$).

In a further attempt to identify types of disease, patients with one ray or three or more rays involved are compared in Profiles R and S. In the one ray group there are more northern Europeans and fewer Japanese ($p<0.005$). This trend is inconsistent with the view that disease in Orientals is less severe. However these data pertain to patients seeking an operation. It may be that northern Europeans are operated upon earlier than Japanese.

When only one ray is involved there is less bilateral disease ($p<0.001$), less family history ($p<0.05$), fewer other areas involved ($p<0.001$) and less alcoholism ($p<0.05$). There is more trauma ($p<0.005$). When only a single ray is involved the little finger is most often involved. A less extensive operation is performed in both the palm and digit when only one ray is involved and complications are less frequent ($p<0.005$).

Table 20.14 shows that there is no difference in the preoperative and postoperative angles but one ray is more likely to obtain a perfect result and less likely to obtain a worse result.

DD involving only one ray shows a significant decrease in diathesis factors and, like unilateral disease, is a mild expression of disease.

Early onset of disease

Profile T provides data on those patients who developed DD before the age of 45. When compared to patients with a late onset, there are more northern Europeans ($p<0.005$), more males ($p<0.001$), more other areas involved ($p<0.001$)

Table 20.14 Comparison of one ray and three or more rays, using results of treatment at the proximal interphalangeal joint of the little finger

	n	Pre	Post
One ray	97	54.4 ± 23.4	26.8 ± 22.8
Three or more rays	85	49.6 ± 26.7	31.7 ± 24.1

No significant difference in the pre or postoperative angles
Outcome group (%)

	Perfect	Improved	Worse
One Ray	18%	60%	22%
Three or more rays	14%	53%	33%

One ray has a significantly better outcome ($p<0.001$)

and more recurrent disease ($p<0.001$). These are all factors contributing to a stronger diathesis. In addition, these patients have more bilateral disease ($p<0.01$), more often three or more rays involved ($p<0.02$), more radial side disease ($p<0.001$) and the preoperative joint contracture is greater ($p<0.05$). Concerning treatment of this group, extensive fasciectomy was used more often in both the palm and fingers and grafts were more frequently used for closure ($p<0.001$).

The results of treatment were not significantly different from the older group but both recurrence and extension of disease were more frequent. In all, 36% of these patients had already had an operation for DD compared to 16% of patients over 45 years of age ($p<0.005$). Also 5 years after this younger group had been operated upon, 31% showed either recurrence or extension of disease, compared to only 14% of the older patients ($p<0.001$). Clearly, this group represents very severe disease.

Previous operation

In Profile U the data on patients who had previously been operated upon are presented. This group had significantly more family history, other areas involved, and the age at onset of the disease was earlier in both sexes ($p<0.001$). The incidence of bilateral disease, three or more rays involved and radial side disease was all greater ($p<0.001$). More extensive operations were performed, with more frequent use of skin grafts and proximal interphalangeal joint procedures ($p<0.001$).

CONCLUSIONS

This epidemiological study of surgical patients shows that the severity and extent of disease varies amongst subgroups of patients.

Typical disease presents to the surgeon in a white male of northern European origin who is about 57 years of age and has had DD for about 10 years. The disease is bilateral but one hand is more severely involved, with no relation to hand dominance. The patient is unlikely to admit to any diathesis factors such as a family history or recurrent disease, or have other areas involved. He is equally likely to have one, two, or three rays involved in the hand to be operated upon. The type of operation he receives will depend more on the surgeon than on the severity of disease. The operation will be successful but if the proximal interphalangeal joint of the little finger was flexed before operation, it is likely to have a residual flexion contracture. He may show progression of disease in both hands but is unlikely to have a second operation.

Females have later onset and less severe disease.

Japanese have later onset, fewer diathesis factors and less extensive disease.

Unilateral disease is less severe. In most patients this represents the early stage of bilateral disease but in some the disease remains unilateral.

Epilepsy and alcoholism are associated with more severe disease but trauma with less severe disease.

The data support a genetic origin of DD with variable expression by race and sex. The disease is seen in its most severe form in northern Europe and is less severe in Japan. There are insufficient data to consider the severity in the black African.

The results of treatment will be discussed in Section V, but clearly contracture was corrected readily at the metacarpophalangeal joint but not at the proximal interphalangeal joint.

Sufficient data were collected to record the incidence of recurrence and extension as well as the appearance and progression of disease in the other hand. In each case the incidence was about 20% and about half of the patients required an operation. This is evidence of the slow but progressive nature of the disease.

Profile A 1150 Patients; 1339 operations

Family origin		**Sex**		**Hand dominance**		**Hand involved**	
Northern European	83%	Male	84%	Right	94%	Right	23%
Japanese	3%	Female	16%	Left	5%	Left	13%
Southern European	3%					Both	65%
Chinese	1%	**Other areas involved**	26%*				
Black American	1%					**Associated diseases**	
Black African	0.5%	**Family history**	27%			Epilepsy	3%
American Indian	0.2%					Diabetes	7%
Asian	0.1%	**Previous operation**	24%			Alcoholism	10%
						Trauma	14%

		Occupation	
		Manual	51%
		Non-manual	49%
		Age at onset (years)	
		Male	48.3±14.5
		Female	57.6±14.2
		Age at operation (years)	
		Male	57.5±12.0
		Female	62.7±11.4

Hand profile	
Palm only	5%
No palm	6%
One ray	33%
Two rays	31%
Three or more rays	31%
Thumb and thumb web	24%
Index finger	12%
Middle finger	32%
Ring finger	63%
Little finger	70%

Operation profile

	Palm	Fingers	Thumb
Operation			
Local	9%	9%	12%
Regional	61%	49%	70%
Extensive	30%	40%	18%
Amputation	0%		
Incision			
Longitudinal	74%	92%	86%
Transverse	26%	8%	14%
Closure			
Suture	74%	86%	87%
Open	14%	2%	4%
Graft	12%	12%	9%

Anaesthesia	
Local	5%
Regional	51%
General	44%
Procedure at PIP joint	12%
Complications	17%
Therapy	76%
Splinting	42%

*Knuckle pads = 20%; foot = 10%; penis = 2%.

Profile A contd.

	Little finger			Ring finger			Middle finger			Index finger			Thumb	
	n	Pre	Post	n	Pre	Post	n	Pre	Post	n	Pre	Post	Pre	Post
MP joint	258	44.1±24.8	3.2±11.1	251	36.3±20.0	2.5± 8.4	126	28.1±16.3	2.3± 7.5	27	23.3±15.2	4.6± 9.3	19.6±11.6	8.8±17.2
Outcome														
Perfect	84%	42.8±24.1	0	86%	34.3±18.9	0	87%	27.9±15.9	0	78%	21.1±12.2	0	21.5±11.2	0
Improved	13%	54.9±25.3	14.3±11.2	12%	52.5±20.4	15.3±14.0	10%	31.1±20.8	14.8± 8.1	11%	45.0±26.0	20.0±10.0	35.0	30.0
Same/worse	3%	31.4±31.5	46.4±35.9	2%	22.0±16.8	29.0±21.3	3%	25.0±17.3	27.5±20.6	11%	16.7± 5.8	21.7± 2.9	10.4± 7.1	27.5±24.0
PIP joint	263	52.9±25.2	27.2±23.0	138	49.5±26.5	16.9±21.0	42	39.6±21.6	20.8±21.5					
Outcome														
Perfect	19%	46.5±23.8	0	45%	41.7±24.1	0	36%	30.3±14.3	0					
Improved	56%	63.2±21.3	28.8±17.4	42%	64.3±22.8	29.0±18.2	43%	50.4±20.7	26.4±13.4					
Same/worse	25.	34.9±22.7	44.9±23.3	13%	28.2±19.8	36.2±22.7	21%	33.7±25.6	44.2±22.1					
DIP joint	52	26.9±17.0	8.8±11.9	23	32.8±28.1	4.0±10.5	6	18.3±16.0	9.2±20.1					
Outcome														
Perfect	56%	20.9±15.2	0	82%	29.5±23.8	0	66%	12.5± 5.0	0					
Improved	33%	38.6±15.4	16.6± 7.7	9%	87.0± 4.2	32.5±17.7	17%	10.0	5.0					
Same/worse	11%	23.0±13.7	29.7± 8.9	9%	10.0± 7.1	14.0± 1.4	17%	50.0	50.0					

Mean ± standard deviation.
Perfect = the flexion contracture was completely corrected; improved = the flexion contracture was less, but not completely corrected; same/worse = there was no correction or the flexion contracture was worse.

Profile B 670 Northern European patients; 779 operations: no previous operations

Family origin		Sex		Hand dominance		Hand involved		Occupation	
Northern European	100%	Male	83%	Right	96%	Right	24%	Manual	50%
		Female	17%	Left	4%	Left	13%	Non-manual	50%
						Both	63%		
		Other areas involved*			24%	Associated diseases		Age at onset (years)	
						Epilepsy	3%	Male	48.4±12.1
		Family history			29%	Diabetes	6%	Female	57.9±10.3
						Alcoholism	11%	Age at operation (years)	
		Previous operation			0%	Trauma	12%	Male	58.12±11.80
								Female	63.91±10.76

Hand profile

Palm only	6%				
No palm	4%				
One ray	35%				
Two rays	32%				
Three or more rays	28%				
Thumb and thumb web	22%				
Index finger	9%				
Middle finger	31%				
Ring finger	63%				
Little finger	67%				

Operation profile

	Palm	Fingers	Thumb		
Operation					
Local	7%	8%	10%	Anaesthesia	
Regional	63%	48%	74%	Local	7%
Extensive	30%	44%	16%	Regional	49%
Amputation	0%	0%	0%	General	44%
Incision				Procedure at	
Longitudinal	74%	92%	82%	PIP joint	8%
Transverse	26%	8%	18%	Complications	17%
Closure					
Suture	75%	89%	86%	Therapy	75%
Open	16%	2%	5%	Splinting	38%
Graft	9%	9%	9%		

*Knuckle pads = 20%; foot 7%; penis 1%.

Profile B contd.

	Little finger			Ring finger			Middle finger			Index finger			Thumb		
	n	Pre	Post	n	Pre	Post	n	Pre	Post	n	Pre	Post	n	Pre	Post
MP joint	164	42.7±24.4	3.4±12.3	82	36.5±18.6	1.7± 7.4		29.0±16.2	1.3± 5.7	17	22.1±11.7	2.4± 6.6	8	22.0±12.3	0±0
Outcome Perfect	85%	41.2±23.7	0± 0	93%	35.2±17.7	0± 0		28.9±15.9	0± 0	88%	23.0±12.1	0± 0	100%	22.0±12.3	0±0
Improved	11%	58.1±21.7	12.5± 7.3	4%	53.5±21.9	14.6±13.1		41.7±20.2	16.7± 7.6	0					
Same/worse	4%	31.4±31.4	46.4±35.9	4%	21.7±16.1	31.7±25.7		20.0±17.3	20.0±17.3	12%	15.0± 7.1	20.0± 0			
PIP joint	62	50.6±25.5	24.9±21.5	18	50.2±26.6	14.0±19.3		33.6±19.2	15.6±18.5	6	33.3±19.1	7.5±12.5	1	25.0	0±0
Outcome Perfect	20%	48.5±25.0	0± 0	50%	44.3±25.0	0± 0		33.3±16.9	0± 0	67%	31.3±22.1	0± 0	100%	25.0	0±0
Improved	55%	60.3±20.9	26.6±15.4	28%	62.6±23.0	27.5±17.8		47.0±22.2	29.0±15.6	16%	50.0	15.0			
Same/worse	25%	30.7±23.5	41.6±23.5	22%	17.1±14.4	27.1±25.9		17.5± 5.0	33.8±12.5	16%	25.0	30.0			
DIP joint	29	30.0±16.6	7.6± 2.7	3	30.5±28.5	4.5±14.2		26.7±20.8	16.7±28.9	1	35.0± –	0			
Outcome Perfect	66%	20.5±16.0	0± 0	66%	23.9±20.6	0± 0		15.0± 7.1	0± 0	100%	35.0	0			
Improved	20%	38.3±13.7	15.0± 8.9		90.0±–	45.0									
Same/worse	14%	26.3±14.9	32.5± 8.6	33%	50.0			50.0	50.0						

Mean ± standard deviation.
Outcome as in Profile A.

Profile C 27 Southern European patients; 38 Operations

Family origin		Sex		Hand dominance		Hand involved		Occupation	
Southern European	100%	Male	96%	Right	84%	Right	30%	Manual	52%
		Female	4%	Left	16%	Left	22%	Non-manual	48%
						Both	48%		
		Other areas involved			19%	Associated diseases		Age at onset (years)	
						Epilepsy	0%	Male	48.9 ± 12.9
		Family history			24%	Diabetes	7%	Female	—
						Alcoholism	7%	Age at operation (years)	
		Previous operation			26%	Trauma	11%	Male	58.2 ± 10.3
								Female	54

Operation profile

Hand profile			Palm	Fingers	Thumb	Anaesthesia	
Palm only	5%	*Operation*					
No palm	5%	Local	14%	11%	0%	Local	5%
		Regional	69%	47%	86%	Regional	36%
One ray	18%	Extensive	17%	42%	14%	General	59%
Two rays	32%	Amputation	0%	0%	0%		
Three or more rays	45%						
		Incision				Procedure at	
Thumb and thumb web	34%	Longitudinal	17%	73%	67%	PIP joint	10%
Index finger	16%	Transverse	83%	27%	33%		
Middle finger	34%					Complications	18%
Ring finger	60%	*Closure*					
Little finger	68%	Suture	75%	75%	71%	Therapy	82%
		Open	6%	0%	0%		
		Graft	19%	25%	29%	Splinting	55%

Profile D 37 Epileptic patients; 42 operations

Family origin		Sex		Hand dominance		Hand involved		Occupation	
Northern European	88%	Male	81%	Right	100%	Right	16%	Manual	73%
Japanese	6%	Female	19%	Left	0%	Left	14%	Non-manual	27%
Black African	6%					Both	70%		
		Other areas involved	35%			Associated diseases		Age at onset (years)	
						Epilepsy	100%	Male	40.8 ± 13.1
		Family history	24%			Diabetes	3%	Female	44.5 ± 2.1
						Alcoholism	8%	Age at operation (years)	
		Previous operation	43%			Trauma	19%	Male	51.0 ± 11.1
								Female	55.2 ± 9.8

Operation profile

Hand profile			Palm	Fingers	Thumb		Anaesthesia	
Palm only	0%	*Operation*					Local	2%
No palm	2%	Local	5%	8%	13%		Regional	30%
		Regional	70%	57%	75%		General	68%
One ray	31%	Extensive	25%	33%	12%			
Two rays	19%	Amputation	0%	2%	0%		Procedure at	
Three or more rays	50%	*Incision*					PIP joint	14%
Thumb and thumb web	41%	Longitudinal	78%	89%	67%			
Index finger	17%	Transverse	22%	11%	33%		Complications	17%
Middle finger	31%	*Closure*						
Ring finger	64%	Suture	68%	87%	78%		Therapy	76%
Little finger	81%	Open	15%	3%	11%			
		Graft	17%	10%	11%		Splinting	33%

Profile E 83 Diabetic patients; 96 operations

Family origin		Sex		Hand dominance		Hand involved		Occupation	
Northern European	66%	Male	84%	Right	93%	Right	18%	Manual	46%
Japanese	24%	Female	16%	Left	7%	Left	7%	Non-manual	54%
Southern European	6%					Both	75%		
Black American	4%	Other areas involved	28%			Associated diseases		Age at onset (years)	
				Family history	26%	Epilepsy	1%	Male	52.2 ± 11.8
						Diabetes	100%	Female	55.5 ± 12.6
				Previous operation	17%	Alcoholism	17%	Age at operation (years)	
						Trauma	12%	Male	58.7 ± 9.6
								Female	64.0 ± 18.6

Operation profile

Hand profile			Palm	Fingers	Thumb	Anaesthesia	
Palm only	6%	*Operation*				Local	5%
No palm	6%	Local	8%	3%	6%	Regional	48%
		Regional	64%	54%	81%	General	47%
One ray	26%	Extensive	28%	43%	13%		
Two rays	29%	Amputation	0%	0%	0%		
Three or more rays	39%					Procedure at PIP joint	28%
		Incision					
Thumb and thumb web	28%	Longitudinal	71%	88%	63%	Complications	28%
Index finger	17%	Transverse	29%	12%	37%		
Middle finger	36%						
Ring finger	69%	*Closure*				Therapy	79%
Little finger	72%	Suture	75%	87%	100%		
		Open	20%	4%	0%	Splinting	51%
		Graft	5%	9%	0%		

Profile F 111 Alcoholic patients; 149 operations

Family origin		**Sex**		**Hand dominance**		**Hand involved**	
Northern European	93%	Male	90%	Right	94%	Right	10%
Japanese	3%	Female	10%	Left	6%	Left	9%
Southern European	2%					Both	81%
Black American	1%						
American Indian	1%	Other areas involved			44%	**Associated diseases**	
						Epilepsy	3%
		Family history			38%	Diabetes	7%
						Alcoholism	100%
		Previous operation			28%	Trauma	20%

		Occupation	
		Manual	76%
		Non-manual	24%
		Age at onset (years)	
		Male	45.4 ± 15.5
		Female	54.6 ± 8.6
		Age at operation (years)	
		Male	55.2 ± 8.2
		Female	61.3 ± 7.5

Operation profile

Hand profile			Palm	Fingers	Thumb	Anaesthesia	
Palm only	3%	*Operation*					
No palm	2%	Local	7%	8%	9%	Local	5%
		Regional	72%	37%	77%	Regional	39%
One ray	26%	Extensive	21%	54%	14%	General	56%
Two rays	28%	Amputation	0%	1%	0%		
Three or more rays	43%					**Procedure at**	
		Incision				**PIP joint**	15%
Thumb and thumb web	36%	Longitudinal	72%	93%	90%		
Index finger	14%	Transverse	28%	7%	10%	Complications	21%
Middle finger	41%						
Ring finger	69%	*Closure*				Therapy	76%
Little finger	78%	Suture	65%	86%	82%		
		Open	24%	4%	5%	Splinting	48%
		Graft	11%	10%	13%		

Profile G 339 American patients; 373 operations

Family origin		Sex		Hand dominance		Hand involved		Occupation	
Northern European	89%	Male	78%	Right	93%	Right	33%	Manual	47%
Southern European	6%	Female	22%	Left	7%	Left	22%	Non-manual	53%
Black American	4%					Both	45%		
		Other areas involved	22%			Associated diseases		Age at onset (years)	
						Epilepsy	3%	Male	54.4±15.6
		Family history	25%			Diabetes	3%	Female	60.2±15.1
						Alcoholism	8%	Age at operation (years)	
		Previous operation	19%			Trauma	17%	Male	60.2±12.2
								Female	63.3±12.2

Operation profile

Hand profile			Palm	Fingers	Thumb	Anaesthesia	
Palm only	6%	*Operation*				Local	6%
No palm	9%	Local	16%	13%	21%	Regional	51%
		Regional	58%	53%	61%	General	43%
One ray	33%	Extensive	26%	33%	18%		
Two rays	35%	Amputation	0%	1%	0%	Procedure at PIP joint	14%
Three or more rays	26%						
		Incision					
Thumb and thumb web	18%	Longitudinal	75%	85%	78%	Complications	14%
Index finger	9%	Transverse	25%	15%	22%		
Middle finger	30%						
Ring finger	67%	*Closure*				Therapy	77%
Little finger	70%	Suture	81%	88%	81%		
		Open	10%	4%	14%	Splinting	46%
		Graft	9%	8%	5%		

Profile G contd. The results of operation by digit and joint recorded 1 year ± 6 months after operation

	Little finger			Ring finger			Middle finger			Index finger			Thumb		
	n	Pre	Post	n	Pre	Post	n	Pre	Post	n	Pre	Post	n	Pre	Post
D MP joint Outcome	65	43.8±22.5	3.8±12.2	69	34.4±18.7	1.9± 4.9	29	29.4±19.3	1.2± 3.7	6	15.0± 1.8	3.3±8.2	2	23.0±4.2	0±0
Perfect	78%	43.4±22.5	0± 0	83%	31.9±16.0	0± 0	90%	28.7±18.7	± 0	83%	16.0±12.9	0±0	100%	23.0±4.2	0±0
Improved	17%	53.6±19.1	11.3± 6.0	16%	52.5±24.6	9.5± 5.0	7	47.5±24.71	2.5± 3.5						
Same/worse	5%	15.0± 5.0	40.0±43.6	1%	15.0	25.0	3%	10.0	10.0	17%	10.0	20.0			
PIP joint Outcome	56	47.5±26.6	19.5±18.9	40	43.7±26.4	10.4±14.2	6	23.8±15.4	8.3±10.3	1	97.0	5.0	0		
Perfect	29%	44.4±23.1	0± 0	52%	42.7±28.5	0± 0	50%	28.3±18.9	0± 0						
Improved	52%	58.6±24.4	26.6±14.9	38%	54.2±19.7	21.3±13.5	33%	25.0± 7.1	17.5±10.6	100%	97.0	5.0			
Same/worse	19%	22.7±19.8	29.1±22.2	10	17.5±16.6	21.5±14.9	17%	5.0	15.0						
DIP joint Outcome	12	23.3±19.1	2.5± 8.7	7	21.4±20.7	0± 0	1	10.0	0	0					
Perfect	92%	22.6±19.9	0± 0	100%	21.4±20.7	0± 0	100%	10.0	0						
Improved															
Same/worse	8%	30.0	30.0												

Profile H 294 Canadian patients; 345 operations

Family origin		**Sex**		**Hand dominance**	**Hand involved**	**Occupation**
Northern European	98%	Male	84%	Right 94%	Right 15%	Manual 62%
Southern European	2%	Female	16%	Left 6%	Left 7%	Non-manual 38%
					Both 78%	
		Other areas involved	32%			**Age at onset (years)**
					Associated diseases	Male 47.4±11.9
		Family history	34%		Epilepsy 3%	Female 54.3±14.3
					Diabetes 7%	
		Previous operation	30%		Alcoholism 15%	**Age at operation (years)**
					Trauma 9%	Male 57.0±11.6
						Female 61.4±11.0

Operation profile

Hand profile			Palm	Fingers	Thumb	Anaesthesia	
Palm only	5%	*Operation*					
No palm	4%	Local	7%	4%	7%	Local	6%
		Regional	81%	13%	74%	Regional	34%
One ray	30%	Extensive	12%	82%	19%	General	60%
Two rays	28%	Amputation	0%	1%	0%		
Three or more rays	37%					Procedure at	
		Incision				PIP joint	10%
Thumb and thumb web	36%	Longitudinal	53%	99%	98%		
Index finger	13%	Transverse	47%	1%	2%	Complications	17%
Middle finger	34%						
Ring finger	63%	*Closure*				Therapy	62%
Little finger	69%	Suture	66%	92%	98%		
		Open	28%	1%	2%	Splinting	59%
		Graft	6%	7%	0%		

Profile H contd. The results of operation by digit and joint recorded 1 year ± 6 months after operation

	Little finger			Ring finger			Middle finger			Index finger			Thumb		
	n	Pre	Post	n	Pre	Post	n	Pre	Post	n	Pre	Post	n	Pre	Post
MP joint	48	48.0±25.3	3.5±15.5	63	35.8±16.0	1.3±7.2	32	31.1±14.6	1.6±7.2	9	28.9±8.2	3.3±6.1			
Outcome															
Perfect	90%	47.9±24.4	0±0	93%	35.8±15.2	0±0	94%	31.2±14.8	0±0	78%	32.1±5.7	0±0			
Improved	4%	45.0±35.4	7.5±3.5	5%	43.3±28.4	25.0±25.9	3%	20.0	10.0	11%	15.0	10.0			
Same/worse	6%	51.7±43.1	51.7±43.1	2%	10.0	10.0	3%	40.0	40.0	11%	20.0	20.0			
PIP joint	55	46.2±21.6	36.6±20.8	28	55.9±23.7	15.9±15.8	8	33.8±14.3	18.8±18.7	2	52.5±3.5	7.5±10.6			
Outcome															
Perfect	9%	35.0±15.0	0±0	41%	47.7±20.5	0±0	37%	48.3±10.4	0±0	50%	55.0	0±0			
Improved	47%	58.1±19.0	32.4±16.1	56%	63.3±24.4	26.0±10.6	25%	32.5±3.5	17.5±3.5	50%	50.0	15.0±0			
Same/worse	44%	35.7±19.0	48.8±16.4	3%	25.0	40.0	37%	20.0±0	38.3±10.4						
DIP joint	9	19.4±12.1	12.2±16.9	1	14.0	0				1	35.0	0			
Outcome															
Perfect	56%	14.0±6.5	0±0	100%	14.0	0				100%	35.0	0			
Improved	11%	30.0	10.0												
Same/worse	33%	25.0±18.0	33.3±10.4												

Profile I 128 Japanese patients; 118 operations

Family origin		Sex		Hand dominance		Hand involved		Occupation	
Japanese	100%	Male	95%	Right	97%	Right	17%	Manual	63%
		Female	5%	Left	3%	Left	10%	Non-manual	37%
						Both	73%		
		Other areas involved	16%			Associated diseases		Age at onset (years)	
						Epilepsy	2%	Male	53.1 ± 12.1
		Family history	5%			Diabetes	14%	Female	43.0
						Alcoholism	2%	Age at operation (years)	
		Previous operation	10%			Trauma	15%	Male	60.3 ± 11.6
								Female	63.0 ± 1.4

Hand profile		Operation profile		Palm	Fingers	Thumb	Anaesthesia	
Palm only	6%	*Operation*					Local	5%
No palm	3%	Local	17%	8%	50%		Regional	62%
		Regional	53%	61%	50%		General	33%
One ray	29%	Extensive	30%	31%	0%			
Two rays	35%	Amputation	0%	0%	0%		Procedure at	
Three or more rays	30%						PIP Joint	8%
		Incision						
Thumb and thumb web	12%	Longitudinal	70%	89%	100%		Complications	11%
Index finger	11%	Transverse	30%	11%				
Middle finger	31%	*Closure*					Therapy	91%
Ring finger	72%	Suture	72%	87%	100%		Splinting	60%
Little finger	75%	Open	13%	5%				
		Graft	15%	8%				

Profile I contd. The results of operation by digit and joint recorded 1 year ± 6 months after operation

	Little finger			Ring finger			Middle finger			Index finger			Thumb		
	n	Pre	Post	n	Pre	Post	n	Pre	Post	n	Pre	Post	n	Pre	Post
MP joint	28	48.8 ± 28.7	1.7 ± 4.0	23	35.4 ± 24.2	3.0 ± 6.2	12	22.2 ± 13.5	4.0 ± 8.9	3	17.7 ± 7.5	0 ± 0	2	23.5 ± 16.3	45.0 ± 21.2
Outcome															
Perfect	82%	48.6 ± 27.2	0 ± 0	74%	29.8 ± 23.9	0 ± 0	75%	20.3 ± 9.8	0 ± 0	100%	17.7 ± 7.5	0 ± 0	50%	35.0	30.0
Improved	18%	55.4 ± 37.4	9.4 ± 3.8	26%	51.3 ± 18.2	11.7 ± 7.1	25%	27.7 ± 23.7	16.0 ± 12.1				50%	12.0	60.0
Same/worse															
PIP joint	22	56.7 ± 29.8	22.8 ± 20.4	13	33.8 ± 30.4	14.5 ± 17.9	1	43.0	43.0	0	0	0	0		
Outcome															
Perfect	19%	30.0 ± 8.2	0 ± 0	46%	17.5 ± 6.1	0 ± 0									
Improved	67%	72.4 ± 21.8	29.0 ± 17.7	23%	75.3 ± 35.0	20.7 ± 5.1									
Same/worse	14%	15.0 ± 17.3	24.0 ± 28.7	31%	27.0 ± 22.4	31.5 ± 20.4	100%	43.0	43.0						
DIP joint	8	20.3 ± 14.7	7.5 ± 8.9	3	33.0 ± 44.2	11.0 ± 10.1	0			0					
Outcome															
Perfect	50%	14.3 ± 11.1	0 ± 0	33%	10.0	0									
Improved	38%	32.3 ± 14.3	14.0 ± 6.9	33%	84.0	20.0									
Same/worse	12%	8.0	18.0	33%	5.0	13.0									

EPIDEMIOLOGY OF SURGICAL PATIENTS

Profile J 118 French patients; 132 operations

Family origin		Sex		Hand dominance		Hand involved		Occupation	
Northern European	95%	Male	89%	Right	95%	Right	21%	Manual	34%
Southern European	5%	Female	11%	Left	5%	Left	7%	Non-manual	66%
						Both	72%		
		Other areas involved	32%			Associated diseases		Age at onset (years)	
						Epilepsy	6%	Male	44.1 ± 13.1
		Family history	11%			Diabetes	3%	Female	54.6 ± 11.6
		Previous operation	22%			Alcoholism	12%	Age at operation (years)	
						Trauma	10%	Male	56.0 ± 9.8
								Female	62.8 ± 10.4

Operation profile

Hand profile			Palm	Fingers	Thumb		Anaesthesia	
Palm only	5%	*Operation*					Local	13%
No palm	0%	Local	0%	4%	0%		Regional	5%
		Regional	49%	56%	55%		General	82%
One ray	36%	Extensive	51%	40%	45%			
Two rays	26%	Amputation	0%	0%	0%		Procedure at PIP joint	20%
Three or more rays	33%	*Incision*						
Thumb and thumb web	26%	Longitudinal	67%	93%	57%		Complications	36%
Index finger	20%	Transverse	33%	7%	43%			
Middle finger	31%	*Closure*					Therapy	75%
Ring finger	56%	Suture	41%	57%	22%			
Little finger	73%	Open	11%	2%	0%		Splinting	36%
		Graft	48%	41%	78%			

Profile J contd. The results of operation by digit and joint recorded 1 year ±6 months after operation

		Little finger			Ring finger			Middle finger			Index finger			Thumb	
	n	Pre	Post	n	Pre	Post	n	Pre	Post	n	Pre	Post	n	Pre	Post
MP joint	19	43.9 ± 20.9	1.3 ± 5.7	14	40.0 ± 19.5	2.5 ± 6.4	7	29.3 ± 17.9	3.6 ± 9.4	0			4	27.5 ± 15.0	0 ± 0
Outcome															
Perfect	95%	42.2 ± 21.4	0 ± 0	86%	38.3 ± 20.6	0 ± 0	86%	29.2 ± 19.6	0 ± 0				100%	27.5 ± 15.0	0 ± 0
Improved	5%	75.0	25.0	14%	50.0 ± 7.1	17.5 ± 3.5	14%	30.0	25.0						
Same/worse															
PIP joint	18	44.2 ± 22.1	15.8 ± 12.6	6	59.2 ± 12.4	12.5 ± 15.1	1	35.0	0	2	35.0 ± 14.1	0 ± 0	1	25.0	0 ± 0
Outcome															
Perfect	22%	45.0 ± 17.8	0 ± 0	50%	58.3 ± 12.6	0 ± 0	100%	35.0	0	100%	35.0 ± 14.1	0 ± 0	100%	25.0	0 ± 0
Improved	61%	53.2 ± 17.1	18.6 ± 9.0	50%	60.0 ± 15.0	25.0 ± 10.0									
Same/worse	17%	10.0 ± 5.0	26.7 ± 15.3												
DIP joint	3	28.3 ± 7.6	5.0 ± 8.7	0			0			0					
Outcome															
Perfect	67%	27.5 ± 10.6	0 ± 0												
Improved	33%	30.0	15.0												
Same/worse															

Profile K 108 West German patients; 171 operations

Family origin		**Sex**		**Hand dominance**		**Hand involved**	
Northern European	100%	Male	89%	Right	89%	Right	12%
		Female	11%	Left	11%	Left	6%
						Both	82%
		Other areas involved	35%	Family history	39%	Associated diseases	
						Epilepsy	1%
						Diabetes	6%
		Previous operation	37%			Alcoholism	6%
						Trauma	10%

			Operation profile			
				Palm	Fingers	Thumb
Hand profile						
Palm only	0%	**Operation**				
No palm	16%	Local	1%	8%	8%
		Regional	14%	83%	92%
One ray	36%	Extensive	85%	5%	0%
Two rays	35%	Amputation	0%	4%	0%
Three or more rays	29%	**Incision**				
Thumb and thumb web	19%	Longitudinal	97%	95%	83%
Index finger	13%	Transverse	3%	5%	17%
Middle finger	41%	**Closure**				
Ring finger	62%	Suture	98%	93%	100%
Little finger	70%	Open	1%	1%	0%
		Graft	1%	6%	0%

Occupation		
Manual	33%	
Non-manual	67%	
Age at onset (years)		
Male	39.3 ± 12.0	
Female	54.3 ± 8.2	
Age at operation (years)		
Male	53.4 ± 10.8	
Female	64.3 ± 6.5	
Anaesthesia		
Local	0%	
Regional	99%	
General	1%	
Procedure at PIP joint	12%	
Complications	16%	
Therapy	99%	
Splinting	16%	

Profile K contd. The results of operation by digit and joint recorded 1 Year ± 6 months after operation

		Little finger			Ring finger			Middle finger			Index finger			Thumb	
		n	Pre	Post	n	Pre	Post	n	Pre	Post	n	Pre	Post	n	Pre	Post
MP joint		14	39.3 ± 26.2	5.0 ± 13.4	18	38.6 ± 16.9	3.6 ± 14.1	13	21.9 ± 11.1	0.8 ± 2.8	4	11.3 ± 6.3	0 ± 0	2	15.0 ±	0 ± 0
Outcome	Perfect	79%	36.8 ± 26.5	0 ± 0	89%	37.8 ± 17.7	0 ± 0	92%	22.9 ± 10.9	0 ± 0	100%	11.3 ± 6.3	0 ± 0	100%	15.0 ± 0	0 ± 0
	Improved	14%	62.5 ± 17.7	10.0 ± 0	5%	50.0	5.0	8%	10.0	10.0						
	Same/worse	7%	20.0 ± 0	50.0	5%	40.0	60.0									
PIP joint		13	56.2 ± 20.4	22.7 ± 20.9	6	49.5 ± 36.2	42.5 ± 43.4	4	43.8 ± 31.9	26.3 ± 22.9	1	15.0	0			
Outcome	Perfect	15%	52.5 ± 31.8	0 ± 0	33%	27.5 ± 10.6	0 ± 0	25%	25.0	0	100%	15.0	0			
	Improved	77%	55.5 ± 20.5	21.5 ± 10.0	33%	93.5 ± 4.9	82.5 ± 10.6	50%	70.0 ± 14.1	42.5 ± 17.7						
	Same/worse	8%	70.0	80.0	33%	27.5 ± 24.7	45.0 ± 49.5	25%	10.0	20.0						
DIP joint		3	38.3 ± 20.8	8.3 ± 10.4	1	50.0	0 ± 0	2	35.0 ± 21.1	25.0 ± 35.3						
Outcome	Perfect	33%	15.0	0	100%	50.0	0 ± 0	50%	20.0	0						
	Improved	67%	50.0 ± 7.1	12.5 ± 10.6				50%	50.0	50.0						
	Same/worse															

Profile L 50 British patients; 50 operations

Family origin		Sex		Hand dominance		Hand involved		Occupation	
Northern European	98%	Male	84%	Right	97%	Right	36%	Manual	54%
Asian	2%	Female	16%	Left	3%	Left	16%	Non-manual	46%
						Both	48%		
		Other areas involved	30%			Associated diseases		Age at onset (years)	
		Family history	27%			Epilepsy	2%	Male	50.3 ± 16.3
						Diabetes	4%	Female	54.0 ± 14.8
		Previous operation	6%			Alcoholism	6%	Age at operation (years)	
						Trauma	14%	Male	56.2 ± 10.0
								Female	68.5 ± 10.5

Operation profile

Hand profile			Palm	Fingers	Thumb	Anaesthesia	
Palm only	4%	Operation				Local	0%
No palm	4%	Local	2%	3%	0%	Regional	40%
One ray	50%	Regional	90%	90%	100%	General	60%
Two rays	30%	Extensive	8%	7%	0%		
Three or more rays	16%	Amputation	0%	0%	0%	Procedure at PIP joint	12%
Thumb and thumb web	12%	Incision				Complications	16%
Index finger	2%	Longitudinal	12%	59%	33%		
Middle finger	22%	Transverse	88%	41%	67%	Therapy	98%
Ring finger	36%	Closure				Splinting	44%
Little finger	70%	Suture	57%	95%	100%		
		Open	43%	3%	0%		
		Graft	0%	2%	0%		

Profile L contd. The results of operation by digit and joint recorded 1 Year ± 6 months after operation

	Little finger			Ring finger			Middle finger			Index finger			Thumb		
	n	Pre	Post	n	Pre	Post	n	Pre	Post	n	Pre	Post	n	Pre	Post
MP joint	11	27.3 ± 13.7	0 ± 0	7	30.0 ± 15.5	0 ± 0	5	28.0 ± 14.4	0 ± 0	0			0		
Outcome															
Perfect	100%	27.3 ± 13.7	0 ± 0	100%	30.0 ± 15.5	0 ± 0	100%	28.0 ± 14.4	0 ± 0						
Improved															
Same/worse															
PIP joint	9	47.2 ± 34.3	18.3 ± 11.5	6	43.8 ± 36.3	10.8 ± 15.6	0			0			0		
Outcome															
Perfect	11%	25.0	0	50%	24.3 ± 4.0	0									
Improved	56%	74.0 ± 17.1	25.0 ± 10.0	33%	90.0 ± 0	25.0 ± 21.2									
Same/worse	33%	10.0	13.3	17%	10.0	15.0									
DIP joint	0			0			0			0					
Outcome															
Perfect															
Improved															
Same/worse															

Profile M 37 Australian patients; 43 operations

Family origin			Sex			Hand dominance			Hand involved		
Northern European		100%	Male		76%	Right		97%	Right		22%
			Female		24%	Left		3%	Left		5%
									Both		73%
			Other areas involved		22%				Associated diseases		
			Family history		57%				Epilepsy		0%
									Diabetes		3%
			Previous operation		30%				Alcoholism		5%
									Trauma		27%

			Operation profile					
Hand profile				Palm	Fingers	Thumb		
Palm only		9%	Operation					
No palm		7%	Local	3%	7%	0%		
			Regional	56%	17%	57%		
One ray		40%	Extensive	42%	76%	43%		
Two rays		26%	Amputation	0%	0%	0%		
Three or more rays		25%						
			Incision					
Thumb and thumb web		35%	Longitudinal	71%	95%	86%		
Index finger		12%	Transverse	29%	5%	14%		
Middle finger		21%						
Ring finger		51%	Closure					
Little finger		67%	Suture	89%	51%	100%		
			Open	0%	0%	0%		
			Graft	11%	49%	0%		

Occupation		
Manual		40%
Non-manual		60%
Age at onset (years)		
Male		42.3 ± 11.4
Female		52.0 ± 2.9
Age at operation (years)		
Male		56.0 ± 13.0
Female		59.4 ± 8.1
Anaesthesia		
Local		5%
Regional		95%
General		0%
Procedure at PIP joint		5%
Complications		19%
Therapy		74%
Splinting		33%

Profile M contd. The results of operation by digit and joint recorded 1 year ± 6 months after operation

		Little finger		Ring finger			Middle finger			Index finger			Thumb		
	n	Pre	Post	n	Pre	Post	n	Pre	Post	n	Pre	Post	n	Pre	Post
MP joint	12	28.8 ± 20.9	1.3 ± 3.1	8	24.4 ± 17.6	0 ± 0	1	15.0	0 ± 0	0			1	10.0	0 ± 0
Outcome															
Perfect	83%	25.0 ± 14.3	0 ± 0	100%	24.4 ± 17.6	0 ± 0	100%	15.0	0				100%	10.0	0 ± 0
Improved	17	47.5 ± 45.9	7.5 ± 3.5												
Same/worse															
PIP joint	11	57.7 ± 20.4	18.2 ± 15.9	3	38.3 ± 25.7	11.7 ± 10.4	1	10.0	0	2	17.5 ± 10.6	15.0 ± 21.2	0		
Outcome															
Perfect	27%	43.3 ± 33.3	0 ± 0	33%	10.0	0 ± 0	100%	10.0	0	50%	10.0	0			
Improved	73%	63.1 ± 12.5	25.0 ± 12.8	67%	52.5 ± 10.6	17.5 ± 3.5				50%	25.0	30.0			
Same/worse															
DIP joint	1	20.0	10.0	0			0			0					
Outcome															
Perfect	100%	20.0	10.0												
Improved															
Same/worse															

EPIDEMIOLOGY OF SURGICAL PATIENTS 231

Profile N 969 Male patients; 1145 operations

Family origin		Sex		Hand dominance		Hand involved		Occupation	
Northern European	79%	Male	100%	Right	94%	Right	22%	Manual	55%
Southern European	3%	Female	0%	Left	6%	Left	12%	Non-manual	45%
Japanese	13%					Both	66%		
Chinese	1%	Other areas involved	27%			Age at onset (years)		Male	48.3 ± 14.5
Black American	1%					Associated diseases			
		Family history	26%			Epilepsy	3%	Age at operation (years)	
						Diabetes	7%	Male	57.5 ± 12.0
		Previous operation	24%			Alcoholism	10%		
						Trauma	15%	Anaesthesia	
				Operation profile				Local	6%
Hand profile				Palm	Fingers	Thumb		Regional	52%
Palm only	5%	Operation						General	42%
No palm	6%	Local	8%	8%	10%				
		Regional	60%	53%	71%			Procedure at	
One ray	32%	Extensive	32%	38%	19%			PIP joint	11%
Two rays	31%	Amputation	0%	1%	0%				
Three or more rays	31%							Complications	16%
		Incision							
Thumb and thumb web	24%	Longitudinal	74%	89%	87%			Therapy	76%
Index finger	13%	Transverse	26%	11%	13%				
Middle finger	33%							Splinting	41%
Ring finger	65%	Closure							
Little finger	71%	Suture	73%	86%	86%				
		Open	15%	3%	5%				
		Graft	12%	11%	9%				

Profile N contd. The results of operation by digit and joint recorded 1 year ± 6 months after operation

		Little finger			Ring finger			Middle finger			Index finger			Thumb	
	n	Pre	Post	n	Pre	Post	n	Pre	Post	n	Pre	Post	n	Pre	Post
MP joint	179	44.2 ± 24.4	2.9 ± 11.3	173	36.4 ± 19.3	1.6 ± 5.9	88	28.5 ± 15.6	1.7 ± 6.3	17	21.6 ± 10.2	1.8 ± 5.3	10	21.7 ± 12.1	9.0 ± 20.2
Outcome															
Perfect	85%	43.0 ± 23.5	0	88%	35.1 ± 18.4	0	91%	28.0 ± 15.3	0	88%	22.2 ± 10.7	0	80%	21.2 ± 12.2	0
Improved	12%	56.0 ± 25.0	11.8 ± 7.2	10%	50.2 ± 21.3	13.4 ± 11.9	8%	32.6 ± 20.1	15.4 ± 8.6	6%	15.0 ± 0	10.0 ± 0	10%	35.0 ± 0	30.0 ± 0
Same/worse	3%	33.3 ± 34.0	45.8 ± 39.3	1%	12.5 ± 3.5	17.5 ± 10.6	1%	40.0 ± 0	40.0 ± 0	6%	20.0 ± 0	20.0 ± 0	10%	12.0 ± 0	60.0 ± 0
PIP joint	157	50.3 ± 26.3	23.9 ± 21.1	89	47.3 ± 26.2	13.7 ± 18.0	18	34.1 ± 19.1	18.5 ± 18.8	6	42.8 ± 31.0	5.8 ± 12.0	1	25.0 ± 0	0
Outcome															
Perfect	22%	41.6 ± 21.9	0	49%	40.1 ± 24.2	0	39%	35.0 ± 17.8	0	67%	33.7 ± 20.2	0	100%	25.0 ± 0	0
Improved	55%	62.8 ± 22.2	27.4 ± 16.3	42%	60.8 ± 23.4	25.6 ± 14.2	33%	42.5 ± 22.7	25.8 ± 15.9	17%	97.0 ± 0	5.0 ± 0			
Same/worse	22%	27.9 ± 21.4	39.0 ± 22.8	9%	25.0 ± 18.3	34.5 ± 24.6	28%	22.6 ± 12.2	35.6 ± 11.6	17%	25.0 ± 0	30.0 ± 0			
DIP joint	32	25.8 ± 16.3	8.4 ± 12.5	12	38.2 ± 35.3	6.5 ± 13.8	3	26.7 ± 20.8	16.7 ± 28.9	0					
Outcome															
Perfect	59%	21.4 ± 15.9	0	75%	31.1 ± 30.4	0	67%	15.0 ± 2.1	0						
Improved	25%	38.4 ± 12.6	15.2 ± 8.2	17%	87.0 ± 4.2	32.5 ± 17.7									
Same/worse	16%	22.6 ± 15.3	29.6 ± 9.9	8%	5.0 ± 0	13.0 ± 0	33%	50.0	50.0						

Profile O 181 Female patients; 194 operations

Family origin		Sex		Hand dominance		Hand involved		Occupation	
Northern European	94%	Male	0%	Right	94%	Right	28%	Manual	32%
Japanese	4%	Female	100%	Left	6%	Left	13%	Non-manual	68%
Black American	2%					Both	59%		
		Other areas involved	23%			Associated diseases		Age at onset (years)	
						Epilepsy	4%	Female	57.6 ± 14.2
		Family history	35%			Diabetes	7%		
		Previous operation	24%			Alcoholism	6%	Age at operation (years)	
						Trauma	8%	Female	62.7 ± 11.4

Operation profile

Hand profile			Palm	Fingers	Thumb		Anaesthesia	
Palm only	9%	Operation					Local	6%
No palm	8%	Local	14%	20%	25%		Regional	44%
One ray	39%	Regional	65%	45%	63%		General	50%
Two rays	28%	Extensive	21%	34%	12%			
Three or more rays	24%	Amputation	0%	1%	0%		Procedure at PIP joint	15%
Thumb and thumb web	22%	Incision						
Index finger	10%	Longitudinal	73%	92%	73%		Complications	19%
Middle finger	29%	Transverse	27%	8%	27%			
Ring finger	48%	Closure					Therapy	75%
Little finger	67%	Suture	78%	88%	93%			
		Open	10%	1%	0%		Splinting	47%
		Graft	12%	11%	7%			

Profile O cont'd. The results of operation by digit and joint recorded 1 year ± 6 months after operation

	Little finger			Ring finger			Middle finger			Index finger			Thumb		
	n	Pre	Post	n	Pre	Post	n	Pre	Post	n	Pre	Post	n	Pre	Post
MP joint	27	41.9 ± 27.4	3.0 ± 9.0	31	33.1 ± 17.0	3.2 ± 11.1	13	23.8 ± 16.5	1.5 ± 3.8	5	16.0 ± 14.7	4.0 ± 8.9	1	26.0 ± 0	0
Outcome															
Perfect	85%	41.2 ± 27.1	0	84%	29.8 ± 15.0	0	85%	26.4 ± 16.7	0	80%	17.5 ± 16.6	0	100%	26.0 ± 0	0
Improved	11%	55.0 ± 35.0	10.0 ± 0	13%	52.5 ± 20.2	9.5 ± 4.2	15%	10.0 ± 0	10.0 ± 0	20%	10.0 ± 0	20.0 ± 0			
Same/worse	4%	20.0 ± 0	50.0 ± 0	3%	40.0 ± 0	60.0 ± 0									
PIP joint	36	53.3 ± 23.6	28.4 ± 22.4	16	52.5 ± 33.0	17.2 ± 23.9	3	20.0 ± 18.0	5.0 ± 8.7	2	32.5 ± 24.7	7.5 ± 10.6	0		
Outcome															
Perfect	14%	74.8 ± 13.9	0	37%	48.3 ± 30.6	0	67%	27.5 ± 17.7	0	50%	15.0 ± 0	0			
Improved	56%	57.1 ± 17.5	26.2 ± 13.6	37%	80.3 ± 14.2	32.5 ± 30.6	33%	5.0 ± 0	15.0 ± 0	50%	50.0 ± 0	15.0 ± 0			
Same/worse	31%	36.5 ± 26.8	45.2 ± 26.1	25%	17.0 ± 16.5	20.0 ± 14.7									
DIP joint	5	12.0 ± 7.6	2.0 ± 4.5	2	17.5 ± 3.5	0	0			1	35.0 ± 0	0			
Outcome															
Perfect	80%	10.0 ± 7.1	0	100%	17.5 ± 3.5	0				100%	35.0 ± 0	0			
Improved	20%	20.0 ± 0	10.0 ± 0												
Same/worse															

Profile P 744 bilateral patients; 939 operations

Family origin		**Sex**		**Hand dominance**		**Hand involved**
Northern European	83%	Male	86%	Right	94%	Right	0%
Southern European	2%	Female	14%	Left	6%	Left	0%
Japanese	13%					Both	100%
Black American	1%	**Other areas involved**	30%			
Chinese	1%					**Associated diseases**
		Family history	30%			Epilepsy	3%
						Diabetes	8%
		Previous operation	26%			Alcoholism	12%
						Trauma	13%

				Occupation	
				Manual	53%
				Non-manual	47%
				Age at onset (years)	
				Male	47.9 ± 14.5
				Female	55.8 ± 14.0
				Age at operation (years)	
				Male	58.5 ± 11.6
				Female	62.3 ± 11.7

Operation profile

Hand profile			Palm	Fingers	Thumb		Anaesthesia	
Palm only	4%	*Operation*					Local	5%
No palm	5%	Local	8%	9%	10%		Regional	50%
		Regional	60%	48%	72%		General	45%
One ray	27%	Extensive	32%	42%	18%			
Two rays	31%	Amputation	0%	1%	0%		**Procedure at PIP joint**	12%
Three or more rays	38%	*Incision*						
Thumb and thumb web	29%	Longitudinal	73%	92%	85%		**Complications.**	18%
Index finger	15%	Transverse	27%	8%	15%			
Middle finger	37%	*Closure*					**Therapy**	75%
Ring finger	66%	Suture	73%	87%	88%			
Little finger	74%	Open	16%	1%	3%		**Splinting**	43%
		Graft	11%	12%	9%			

Profile P contd. The results of operation by digit and joint recorded 1 year ± 6 months after operation

		Little finger			Ring finger			Middle finger			Index finger			Thumb	
	n	Pre	Post	n	Pre	Post	n	Pre	Post	n	Pre	Post	n	Pre	Post
MP joint	142	44.0 ± 25.9	2.1 ± 7.7	149	36.7 ± 19.3	1.9 ± 7.6	76	27.9 ± 14.9	2.0 ± 6.7	19	21.5 ± 11.2	2.6 ± 6.5	11	22.1 ± 11.5	8.2 ± 19.4
Outcome															
Perfect	86%		0	88%		0	88%		0	84%		0	82%		0
Improved	11%	43.0 ± 24.9	11.2 ± 7.2	11%	35.2 ± 18.6	13.6 ± 12.6	8%	28.3 ± 14.9	15.5 ± 9.5	5%	22.7 ± 11.7	10.0 ± 0	9%	21.8 ± 11.5	30.0 ± 0
Same/worse	3%	56.5 ± 30.2	31.2 ± 27.8	1%	49.9 ± 19.8	35.0 ± 35.4	4%	27.2 ± 15.4	20.0 ± 17.3	11%	15.0 ± 0	20.0 ± 0	9%	35.0 ± 0	60.0 ± 0
		23.7 ± 25.0			25.0 ± 21.2			20.0 ± 17.3			15.0 ± 0			12.0 ± 0	
PIP joint	132	49.7 ± 25.3	25.2 ± 21.5	71	49.4 ± 28.0	16.4 ± 21.1	16	33.6 ± 21.0	18.3 ± 19.8	7	32.1 ± 17.8	6.4 ± 11.8	1	25.0 ± 0	0
Outcome															
Perfect	20%		0	45%		0	44%		0	71%		0	100%	25.0 ± 0	0
Improved	56%	44.5 ± 25.8	27.6 ± 16.1	42%	39.3 ± 23.8	28.8 ± 19.0	25%	32.1 ± 19.3	30.0 ± 17.8	14%	30.0 ± 19.4	15.0 ± 0			
Same/worse	23%	60.1 ± 20.8	41.4 ± 23.1	13%	67.7 ± 22.8	32.9 ± 25.1	31%	51.2 ± 23.2	30.0 ± 17.8	14%	50.0 ± 0	30.0 ± 0			
		29.4 ± 21.2			24.4 ± 19.8			21.6 ± 13.6	34.6 ± 13.4		25.0 ± 0				
DIP joint	27	22.7 ± 13.9	8.0 ± 11.2	9	34.3 ± 32.8	8.7 ± 15.5	3	26.7 ± 20.8	16.7 ± 28.9	1	35.0 ± 0	0			
Outcome															
Perfect	59%		0	67%		0	67%	15.0 ± 7.1	0	100%		0			
Improved	26%	17.3 ± 8.7	16.0 ± 8.6	22%	21.7 ± 15.7	32.5 ± 17.7	33%	50.0 ± 0	50.0 ± 0		35.0 ± 0				
Same/worse	15%	38.3 ± 14.7	25.7 ± 5.7	11%	87.0 ± 4.2	13.0 ± 0									
		17.0 ± 10.1			5.0 ± 0										

Profile Q 406 unilateral patients; 400 operation

Family origin		Sex		Hand dominance		Hand involved	
Northern European	84%	Male	82%	Right	93%	Right	64%
Southern European	4%	Female	18%	Left	7%	Left	36%
Japanese	10%					Both	0%
Black American	1%	Other areas involved	19%			Associated diseases	
Chinese	1%	Family history	21%			Epilepsy	3%
		Previous operation	19%			Diabetes	3%
						Alcoholism	5%
						Trauma	17%

		Occupation	
		Manual	48%
		Non-manual	52%
		Age at onset (years)	
		Male	49.3 ± 14.6
		Female	59.8 ± 14.3
		Age at operation (years)	
		Male	55.5 ± 12.6
		Female	63.3 ± 10.9

Operation profile

Hand profile			Palm	Fingers	Thumb
Palm only	8%		11%	14%	21%
No palm	10%	Operation			
		Local	63%	55%	58%
One ray	49%	Regional	26%	31%	21%
Two rays	30%	Extensive	0%	0%	0%
Three or more rays	14%	Amputation			
Thumb and thumb web	11%	Incision			
Index finger	6%	Longitudinal	76%	80%	89%
Middle finger	21%	Transverse	24%	20%	11%
Ring finger	55%	Closure			
Little finger	62%	Suture	77%	86%	85%
		Open	11%	5%	10%
		Graft	12%	9%	5%

Anaesthesia	
Local	7%
Regional	52%
General	41%
Procedure at PIP joint	11%
Complications	12%
Therapy	78%
Splinting	40%

Profile Q contd. The results of operation by digit and joint recorded 1 year ± 6 months after operation

	Little finger			Ring finger			Middle finger			Index finger			Thumb		
	n	Pre	Post	n	Pre	Post	n	Pre	Post	n	Pre	Post	n	Pre	Post
MP joint	64	43.8 ± 22.1	4.6 ± 16.3	55	33.9 ± 18.1	1.6 ± 4.8	25	28.1 ± 18.4	0.6 ± 3.0	13	13.3 ± 10.4	0	0		
Outcome															
Perfect	83%	42.2 ± 21.8	0	87%	32.0 ± 15.9	0	96%	26.5 ± 17.1	0	100%	13.3 ± 10.4	0			
Improved	12%	54.7 ± 13.4	12.1 ± 6.2	11%	52.5 ± 24.8	10.5 ± 3.9	4%	65.0 ± 0	15.0 ± 0						
Same/worse	5%	41.7 ± 41.9	66.7 ± 40.0	2%	15.0 ± 0	25.0 ± 0									
PIP joint	61	53.4 ± 26.8	23.6 ± 21.1	34	45.4 ± 25.8	9.9 ± 12.4	5	27.0 ± 12.0	11.0 ± 11.4	1	97.0 ± 0	5.0 ± 0	0		
Outcome															
Perfect	21%	48.4 ± 19.3	0	53%	44.2 ± 27.1	0	40%	37.5 ± 3.5	0	100%	97.0 ± 0	5.0 ± 0			
Improved	54%	65.5 ± 22.5	26.1 ± 15.2	38%	53.8 ± 22.1	21.3 ± 10.3	40%	25.0 ± 7.1	17.5 ± 10.6						
Same/worse	25%	31.1 ± 26.6	38.5 ± 24.8	9%	16.0 ± 5.3	20.0 ± 5.0	20%	10.0 ± 0	20.0 ± 0						
DIP joint	10	27.3 ± 21.5	6.5 ± 14.2	5	37.0 ± 38.2	0	0			0					
Outcome															
Perfect	70%	24.1 ± 25.0	0	100%	37.0 ± 38.2	0									
Improved	20%	29.5 ± 0.7	10.0 ± 0												
Same/worse	10%	45.0 ± 0	45.0 ± 0												

EPIDEMIOLOGY OF SURGICAL PATIENTS

Profile R 349 patients with one ray involved; 447 operations

Family origin		Sex		Hand dominance		Hand involved		Occupation	
Northern European	90%	Male	82%	Right	93%	Right	32%	Manual	49%
Southern European	4%	Female	18%	Left	7%	Left	20%	Non-manual	51%
Japanese	4%					Both	48%		
Black African	2%	Other areas involved	20%			Associated diseases		Age at onset (years)	
						Epilepsy	3%	Male	48.9 ± 14.8
		Family history	25%			Diabetes	5%	Female	56.9 ± 15.3
		Previous operation	22%			Alcoholism	8%	Age at operation (years)	
						Trauma	18%	Male	57.1 ± 12.2
								Female	63.9 ± 11.7

Operation profile

Hand profile			Palm	Fingers	Thumb	Anaesthesia	
Palm only	0%	Operation				Local	7%
No palm	9%	Local	9%	10%	60%	Regional	50%
		Regional	65%	51%	10%	General	43%
One ray	100%	Extensive	26%	39%	30%		
Two rays	0%	Amputation	0%	0%	0%	Procedure at	
Three or more rays	0%					PIP joint	10%
		Incision					
Thumb and thumb web	3%	Longitudinal	80%	94%	89%	Complications	13%
Index finger	1%	Transverse	20%	6%	11%		
Middle finger	7%					Therapy	69%
Ring finger	34%	Closure				Splinting	41%
Little finger	55%	Suture	81%	81%	90%		
		Open	8%	3%	10%		
		Graft	11%	6%	0%		

Profile R contd. The results of operation by digit and joint recorded 1 year ± 6 months after operation

	Little finger			Ring finger			Middle finger			Index finger			Thumb		
	n	Pre	Post	n	Pre	Post	n	Pre	Post	n	Pre	Post	n	Pre	Post
MP joint	69	43.6 ± 26.6	3.6 ± 15.4	47	33.7 ± 20.2	1.8 ± 6.8	16	27.4 ± 13.5	0.6 ± 2.5	0			4	17.8 ± 6.8	0
Outcome															
Perfect	88%			89%			94%						100%	17.8 ± 6.8	0
Improved	8%	43.9 ± 26.3	0	9%	30.7 ± 19.3	0	6%	27.4 ± 13.8	0						
		42.0 ± 26.1	11.0 ± 6.5		61.3 ± 9.5	11.3 ± 7.5		20.01	0						
Same/worse	4%	40.0 ± 43.3	63.3 ± 46.2	2%	40.0	40.0									
PIP joint	97	54.4 ± 23.4	26.8 ± 22.8	28	53.0 ± 27.4	9.6 ± 13.5	7	40.3 ± 31.4	18.6 ± 14.9						
Outcome															
Perfect	18%	45.1 ± 18.2	0	51%	46.5 ± 28.0	0	28%	32.5 ± 10.6	0						
Improved	60%	61.8 ± 21.6	26.9 ± 17.5	43%	61.7 ± 24.9	22.5 ± 11.6	42%	67.3 ± 25.8	31.7 ± 7.6						
Same/worse	22%	41.9 ± 24.9	49.2 ± 21.3				28%	7.5 ± 3.5	17.5 ± 3.5						
DIP joint	22	30.8 ± 17.9	11.4 ± 8.6	2	52.5 ± 53.0	0	0								
Outcome															
Perfect	45%	22.2 ± 15.4	0	100%	52.5 ± 53.0	0									
Improved	45%	38.5 ± 18.4	7.5 ± 8.9												
Same/worse	10%	35.0 ± 14.1	37.5 ± 10.6												

Profile S 412 Patients with three or more rays involved; 409 operations

Family origin		Sex		Hand dominance		Hand involved		Occupation	
Northern European	81%	Male	86%	Right	95%	Right	13%	Manual	55%
Southern European	2%	Female	14%	Left	5%	Left	7%	Non-manual	45%
Japanese	15%					Both	80%		
Black American	1%	Other areas involved	33%			Associated diseases		Age at onset (years)	
Chinese	1%	Family history	32%			Epilepsy	5%	Male	46.6 ± 13.5
						Diabetes	9%	Female	57.5 ± 14.8
		Previous operation	31%			Alcoholism	14%	Age at operation (years)	
						Trauma	11%	Male	58.0 ± 11.7
								Female	62.7 ± 13.1

Operation profile

Hand profile			Palm	Fingers	Thumb	Anaesthesia	
Palm only	0%	Operation				Local	3%
No palm	4%	Local	9%	9%	9%	Regional	52%
One ray	0%	Regional	56%	43%	73%	General	45%
Two rays	0%	Extensive	35%	47%	18%		
Three or more rays	100%	Amputation	0%	1%	0%	Procedure at PIP joint	15%
Thumb and thumb web	56%	Incision				Complications	22%
Index finger	32%	Longitudinal	62%	90%	81%		
Middle finger	77%	Transverse	38%	10%	19%	Therapy	76%
Ring finger	91%	Closure				Splinting	47%
Little finger	92%	Suture	62%	85%	85%		
		Open	24%	3%	6%		
		Graft	14%	12%	9%		

Profile S contd. The results of operation by digit and joint recorded 1 year ± 6 months after operation

		Little finger			Ring finger			Middle finger			Index finger			Thumb	
	n	Pre	Post	n	Pre	Post	n	Pre	Post	n	Pre	Post	n	Pre	Post
MP joint	102	44.3 ± 24.9	2.9 ± 9.2	107	39.2 ± 20.6	3.3 ± 10.5	71	28.6 ± 15.5	3.4 ± 9.5	24	24.5 ± 15.1	5.2 ± 9.7	5	26.7 ± 15.4	12.5 ± 14.7
Outcome															
Perfect	85%	41.4 ± 23.4	0	84%	38.4 ± 20.2	0	85%	28.2 ± 15.0	0	76%	22.4 ± 11.7	0	60%	33.3 ± 15.3	0
Improved	13%	56.3 ± 26.9	14.0 ± 7.5	14%	50.7 ± 21.5	18.7 ± 16.9	10%	35.7 ± 19.7	18.3 ± 8.9	12%	45.0 ± 26.0	20.0 ± 10.0	40%	12.5 ± 10.6	22.5 ± 10.6
Same/worse	2%	40.0 ± 28.3	55.0 ± 7.1	2%	22.5 ± 24.7	35.0 ± 35.4	5%	25.0 ± 17.3	27.5 ± 20.6	12%	16.7 ± 5.8	21.7 ± 2.9			
PIP joint	85	49.6 ± 26.7	31.7 ± 24.1	56	47.9 ± 27.0	21.7 ± 26.0	23	41.0 ± 21.7	25.3 ± 25.0	18	22.4 ± 11.7	0			
Outcome															
Perfect	14%	42.5 ± 24.5	0	43%	41.5 ± 21.7	0	30%	22.9 ± 9.9	0	100%	22.4 ± 11.7	0			
Improved	53%	59.8 ± 22.0	32.1 ± 18.8	39%	65.9 ± 24.2	37.0 ± 22.8	44%	49.5 ± 20.6	35.0 ± 15.8						
Same/worse	33%	31.1 ± 22.6	44.4 ± 24.8	18%	29.5 ± 22.1	40.1 ± 26.9	26%	44.7 ± 24.3	55.0 ± 17.4						
DIP joint	15	21.3 ± 12.7	9.9 ± 11.5	13	29.3 ± 25.5	5.6 ± 12.9	6	18.3 ± 16.0	9.2 ± 20.1	0					
Outcome															
Perfect	46%	12.9 ± 6.9	0	76%	29.0 ± 20.0	0	66%	12.5 ± 5	0						
Improved	27%	36.0 ± 7.8	11.3 ± 4.8	8%	90.0	45.0									
Same/worse	27%	17.0 ± 10.1	27.8 ± 5.7	16%	10.0 ± 7.1	14.0 ± 1.4									

Profile T 276 Patients with onset of disease at 45 years or less; 544 operations

Family origin		Sex		Hand dominance		Hand involved		Occupation	
Northern European	87%	Male	95%	Right	92%	Right	28%	Manual	53%
Japanese	8%	Female	5%	Left	8%	Left	4%	Non-manual	47%
Southern European	3%					Both	72%		
Chinese	1%	Other areas involved	41%			Associated diseases		Age at onset (years)	
						Epilepsy	5%	Male	35.9 ± 7.8
		Family history	31%			Diabetes	4%	Female	37.4 ± 7.8
		Previous operation	36%			Alcoholism	12%	Age at operation (years)	
						Trauma	18%	Male	49.7 ± 10.2
								Female	53.3 ± 11.7

Operation profile

Hand profile			Palm	Fingers	Thumb		Anaesthesia	
Palm only	3%	Operation					Local	3%
No palm	7%	Local	5%	7%	9%		Regional	51%
		Regional	58%	48%	81%		General	46%
One ray	33%	Extensive	37%	44%	10%			
Two rays	30%	Amputation	0%	1%	0%		Procedure at PIP joint	13%
Three or more rays	34%	Incision						
Thumb and thumb web	27%	Longitudinal	74%	94%	87%		Complications	19%
Index finger	16%	Transverse	26%	6%	13%			
Middle finger	33%	Closure					Therapy	80%
Ring finger	64%	Suture	71%	82%	84%		Splinting	43%
Little finger	71%	Open	14%	11%	1%			
		Graft	15%	17%	15%			

Profile T cont'd. The results of operation by digit and joint recorded 1 year ± 6 months after operation

		Little finger			Ring finger			Middle finger			Index finger			Thumb	
	n	Pre	Post	n	Pre	Post	n	Pre	Post	n	Pre	Post	n	Pre	Post
MP joint	93	42.5 ± 26.4	3.0 ± 8.9	108	35.5 ± 21.5	3.2 ± 9.4	48	28.1 ± 15.5	2.2 ± 7.9	11	29.4 ± 18.7	4.5 ± 10.4	9	22.8 ± 13.7	8.3 ± 13.2
Outcome															
Perfect	83%			82%			88%			82%			67%		
Improved	15%	40.5 ± 25.3	0	13%	32.9 ± 20.6	0	10%	27.9 ± 14.0	0		22.6 ± 12.4	0		24.1 ± 14.3	0
		51.1 ± 26.0	18.2 ± 15.1		56.6 ± 15.4	18.6 ± 15.8		29.7 ± 24.1	11.0 ± 5.5	18%	60.0 ± 0	25.0 ± 7.1			
Same/worse	2%	10.0 ± 7.1	12.5 ± 10.6	4%	17.5 ± 15.5	21.3 ± 14.3	2%	40.0	50.0						
PIP joint	107	57.4 ± 23.7	30.4 ± 26.4	59	52.6 ± 27.2	20.1 ± 22.2	26	40.3 ± 23.5	23.5 ± 22.4						
Outcome															
Perfect	22%			36%			31%								
Improved	54%	46.6 ± 23.4	30.7 ± 18.5	49%	40.7 ± 23.3	0	46%	26.9 ± 16.0	0						
		63.3 ± 21.8	59.0 ± 22.0		69.0 ± 21.8	27.7 ± 17.4		52.7 ± 20.3	27.5 ± 13.2						
Same/worse	23%	48.1 ± 21.1		5%	32.0 ± 20.2	42.8 ± 25.8	23%	33.3 ± 27.9	46.7 ± 23.6						
DIP joint	26	30.4 ± 17.7	7.9 ± 10.6	14	33.3 ± 28.4	4.6 ± 12.8	5	20.0 ± 17.3	11.0 ± 21.9						
Outcome															
Perfect	58%			86%			60%								
Improved	38%	22.3 ± 12.9	0	14%	26.3 ± 19.9	0		13.3 ± 5.8	0						
		44.8 ± 16.4	17.7 ± 6.9		87.0 ± 4.2	32.5 ± 17.7									
Same/worse	4%	10.0	30.0												

Profile U 246 Patients with previous operation; 323 operations

Family origin		Sex		Hand dominance		Hand involved		Occupation	
Northern European	90%	Male	85%	Right	95%	Right	14%	Manual	52%
Japanese	5%	Female	15%	Left	5%	Left	11%	Non-manual	48%
Southern European	3%					Both	75%		
Chinese	2%	Other areas involved			40%	Associated diseases		Age at onset (years)	
						Epilepsy	5%	Male	41.8 ± 14.0
		Family history			36%	Diabetes	5%	Female	51.1 ± 16.1
		Previous operation			100%	Alcoholism	12%	Age at operation (years)	
						Trauma	18%	Male	54.9 ± 11.5
								Female	61.9 ± 11.0

Hand profile		Operation profile					
			Palm	Fingers	Thumb		
Palm only	3%	Operation				Anaesthesia	
No palm	13%	Local	10%	8%	9%	Local	3%
One ray	31%	Regional	57%	46%	71%	Regional	51%
Two rays	27%	Extensive	33%	43%	20%	General	46%
Three or more rays	39%	Amputation	0%	3%	0%		
		Incision				Procedure at	
Thumb and thumb web	36%	Longitudinal	76%	94%	93%	PIP joint	22%
Index finger	20%	Transverse	24%	6%	7%	Complications	16%
Middle finger	36%	Closure					
Ring finger	55%	Suture	70%	77%	92%	Therapy	73%
Little finger	79%	Open	9%	1%	0%	Splinting	45%
		Graft	21%	22%	8%		

Profile U contd. The results of operation by digit and joint recorded 1 year ± 6 months after operation

		Little finger			Ring finger			Middle finger			Index finger			Thumb	
	n	Pre	Post	n	Pre	Post	n	Pre	Post	n	Pre	Post	n	Pre	Post
MP joint	53	46.5 ± 26.8	4.3 ± 11.2	49	40.0 ± 24.0	5.1 ± 12.9	26	28.3 ± 18.7	4.8 ± 11.5	5	36.0 ± 24.3	15.0 ± 14.1	5	14.0 ± 10.8	10.0 ± 12.7
Outcome															
Perfect	80%	42.7 ± 25.5	0 ± 0	78%	34.3 ± 23.3	0 ± 0	76%	28.2 ± 18.3	0 ± 0	40%	20.0 ± 21.2	0 ± 0	40%	20.0 ± 14.1	0 ± 0
Improved	20%	52.2 ± 27.4	21.5 ± 16.7	18%	60.0 ± 19.6	23.1 ± 19.6	20%	29.0 ± 24.0	14.0 ± 8.2	40%	60.0 ± 0	25.0 ± 7.1	60%	10.0 ± 8.7	16.7 ± 12.6
Same/worse				4%	22.5 ± 24.7	25.0 ± 21.2	4%	40.0 ± 0	50.0 ± 0	20%	20.0 ± 0	25.0 ± 0			
PIP joint	75	60.2 ± 23.3	34.2 ± 25.8	34	52.5 ± 24.8	25.2 ± 25.1	22	47.8 ± 21.3	25.0 ± 24.1	11	34.1 ± 18.0	22.3 ± 14.2	1	70.0	10.0
Outcome															
Perfect	15%	49.1 ± 25.1	0 ± 0	36%	44.6 ± 21.6	0 ± 0	29%	25.8 ± 8.6	0 ± 0	9%	25.0	0			
Improved	52%	67.3 ± 20.6	33.1 ± 20.8	45%	66.6 ± 21.9	35.9 ± 20.2	57%	54.3 ± 19.4	26.7 ± 12.7	55%	46.7 ± 14.7	24.2 ± 11.1	100%	70.0	10.0
Same/worse	27%	46.3 ± 18.5	55.1 ± 20.1	18%	40.0 ± 20.2	49.2 ± 18.8	14%	61.7 ± 20.8	68.3 ± 14.4	36%	17.5 f	2.9			
DIP joint	17	33.8 ± 16.6	11.7 ± 12.2	10	27.0 ± 18.3	1.7 ± 5.0	3	10.0 ± 0	1.7 ± 2.9	1	20.0	35.0			
Outcome															
Perfect	40%	26.7 ± 14.7	0 ± 0	89%	30.6 ± 18.8	0 ± 0	66%	10.0 ± 0	0 ± 0						
Improved	53%	41.3 ± 18.1	18.8 ± 7.4				33%	10.0	5.0	100%	20.0	35.0			
Same/worse	7%	25.0	30.0	11%	15.0	15.0									

T. Egawa, H. Senrui, A. Horiki and M. Egawa

21

Epidemiology of the oriental patient

INTRODUCTION

As Hill (1985) has described, Dupuytren's disease (DD) is most prevalent in peoples of Scandinavian or Celtic descent and is extremely rare in Mediterranean and semitic populations. This disease had been believed to be uncommon in Asian populations. In reviewing the literature, detailed analysis of the prevalence of DD was reported by Hueston (1960, 1962, 1963) of Australia, by Early (1962) of England, by Ling (1963) of Scotland, by Mikkelsen (1972) of Norway, and by Rafter (1980) of Ireland. In Japan, the current authors (Egawa et al 1974), Maeda et al (1974) and Morinaga et al (1979) have reported on the prevalence of Dupuytren's disease.

Most of the literature concerns pathology, surgical technique or case reports. It is strange that the incidence of DD is still unclear in most countries of the modern world (Fig. 21.1).

The authors have performed studies to determine the prevalence of this disease in Japan. A preliminary survey was made in 1972 and the result was interesting enough for us to undertake another survey. A population study was performed by examining people aged 60 years or older in old people's homes in the Osaka and Kobe area three times from 1973 to 1986. Another survey was

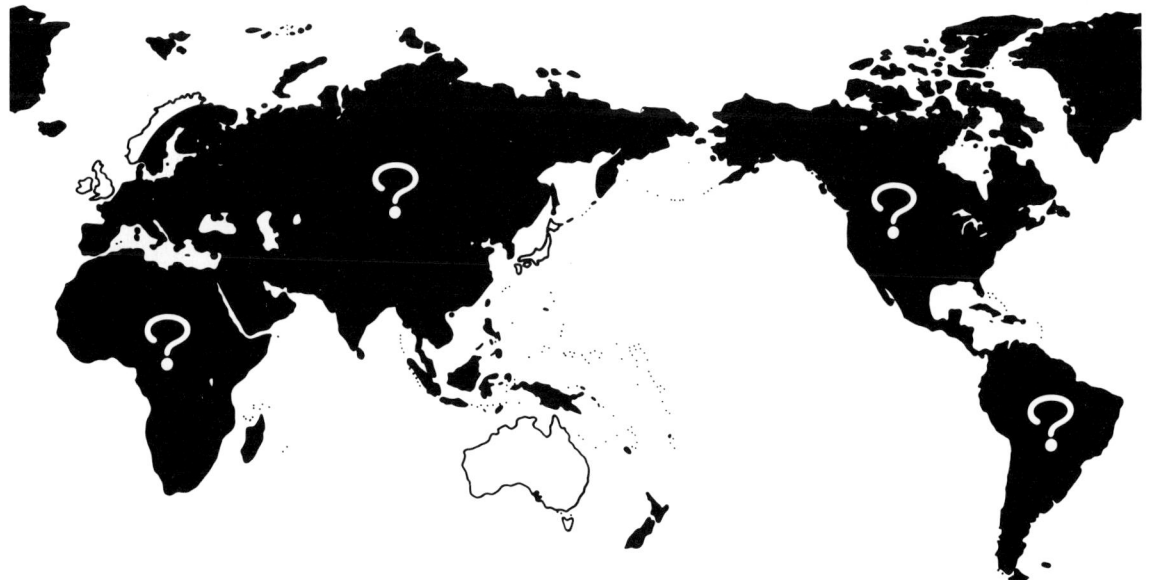

Fig. 21.1 Map of the 'dark continents' where the prevalence of DD is unknown; prevalence has only been reported from Australia, the UK, Ireland, Norway and Japan.

made by examining patients who visited the authors' surgery not only for DD but also for any kind of orthopaedic disorders.

Analysis of the results obtained suggests that the incidence of DD in Japan is comparable to that in British, Norwegian and Australian populations.

MATERIALS, METHODS AND RESULTS

Diagnostic criteria

The diagnostic criteria may be defined as follows: a thickening in the palm fixed to the palmar fascia as a nodule, band or plaque without flexion contracture of the finger was accepted as stage 0. Those cases with flexion contracture were classified by Iselin as:

Stage 1 — flexion of the metacarpophalangeal joint.
Stage 2 — flexion of the proximal interphalangeal joint.
Stage 3 — flexion of the distal interphalangeal joint.
Stage 4 — hyperextension of the distal interphalangeal joint.

The method is simple and convenient when examining many subjects in a limited period of time as it does not require joint angle measurement with a goniometer.

Preliminary survey

In 1972, the authors examined 411 residents over 30 years of age in the Tonda district, 150 km south of Osaka. In this group, 15 individuals, all over 60, were found to have DD, 5 of these had typical flexion contracture of the fingers. The series examined was not large enough to present as a prevalence study, but the figures obtained were sufficient to encourage us to proceed with the survey.

Visit to old people's homes

In the second stage of the study, a survey was performed by examining people aged 60 years or older in old people's homes in the Osaka and Kobe areas (Fig. 21.2). The first series of visits was carried out from 1973 to 1975, followed by a second (in 1979) and third series (in 1986). The aims of these visits were:

1. To reveal the prevalence of DD.
2. To determine the incidence in the same place after an interval of several years.
3. To observe the change in clinical features in the same individuals over three visits.

Enquiries were made with the doctors of the homes and the residents themselves regarding the association of chronic disease or occupation.

Our first series of visits was started in 1973 and continued until 1975. In these visits, 1370 residents, aged 60 years or older, living in 10 old people's homes were examined. Among these subjects, 21.5% of males and 9.8% of females had DD (Tables 21.1 and 21.2).

The second series was carried out in 1979; 1015 residents of six old people's homes were examined. The prevalence of the disease was 25.2% in males and 10.5% in females (Tables 21.3 and 21.4).

In the third series, performed in 1986, in which 1154 subjects were examined in eight homes, 19.7% of males and 9.0% of females had Dupuytren's disease (Tables 21.5 and 21.6).

In four homes visited three times in the first,

Table 21.1 Age and sex distribution of 1370 people at 10 old people's homes in the Osaka and Kobe areas, from 1973 to 1975

Age	Total population	Dupuytren's disease	
		n	%
60–69 years			
Male	97	14	14.4
Female	123	10	8.1
70–79 years			
Male	293	74	25.3
Female	449	46	10.2
80–89 years			
Male	110	22	20.2
Female	265	28	10.6
90 years and over			
Male	11	0	0
Female	22	0	0
Total	1370	194	14.2
Male	511	110	21.5
Female	859	84	9.8

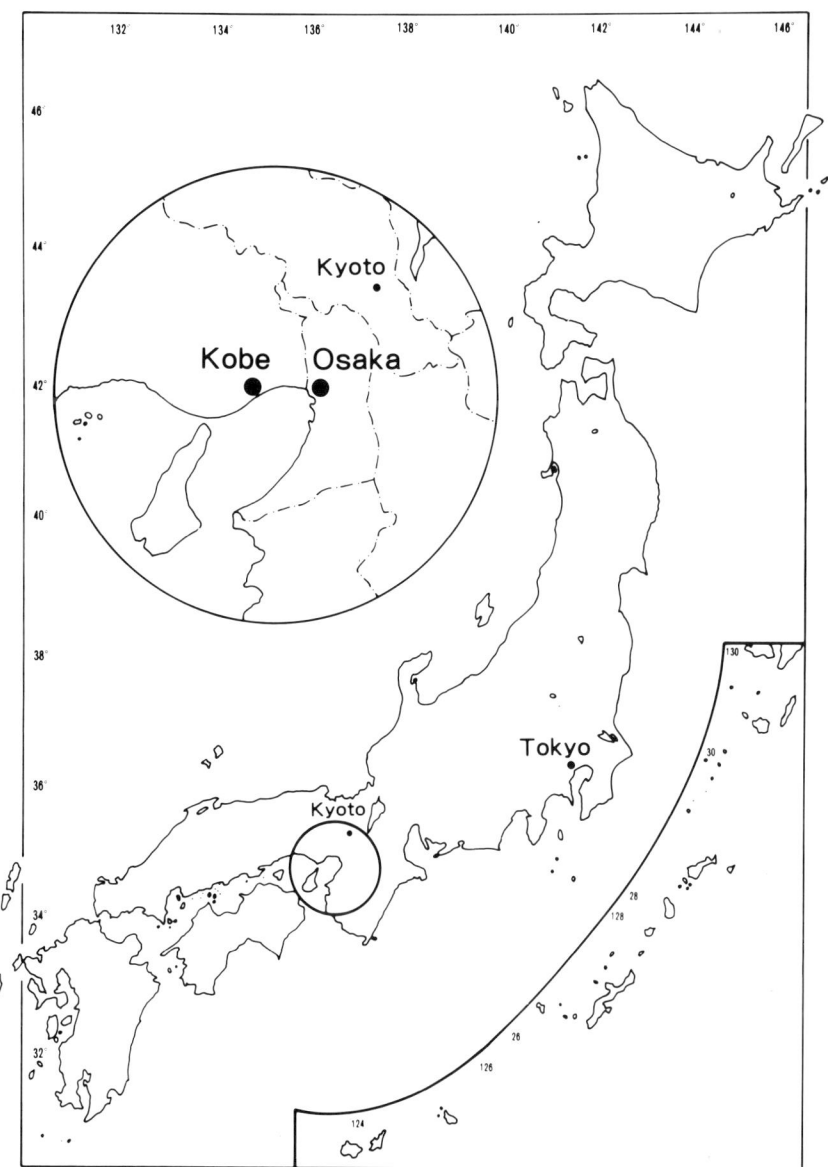

Fig. 21.2 Map of Japan, indicating the location of the Osaka and Kobe areas where the surveys were carried out.

second and third series, 120 residents were still living in same home and were examined at all three visits. Of these 120, 95 subjects had disease which remained in the same stage; 93 were normal, 1 had stage 0 and 1 had stage disease. Eight subjects were less affected; all of these changed from stage 0 to normal. Progression of the disease was seen in 19 cases — 18 went from normal to stage 0 and 1 went from normal to stage 1. Those changes differed according to sex: advancement of disease was more likely to be found in males than in females and most females remained in an uninvolved state (Fig. 21.3).

Outpatient analysis

All patients above 20 years of age who visited the authors' surgery for any reason from May 1980 to

Table 21.2 Number of contractures in each stage and hands involved in the study carried out between 1973 and 1975

	n	%
Stage 0	176	90.7
Stage 1	15	7.8
Stage 2	2	1.0
Stage 3	1	0.5
Total	194	100
Right	62	32.0
Left	25	12.9
Bilateral	107	55.1
Total	194	100

Table 21.3 Age and sex distribution of 1015 people at six old people's homes in the Osaka and Kobe areas in 1979

Age	Total population	Dupuytren's disease	
		n	%
60–69 years			
Male	72	15	20.6
Female	69	6	8.7
70–79 years			
Male	193	52	26.9
Female	302	32	10.6
80–89 years			
Male	116	32	27.6
Female	230	25	10.9
90 years and over			
Male	7	0	0
Female	25	3	12.0
Total	1015	165	16.3
Male	389	99	25.2
Female	626	66	10.5

Table 21.4 Number of contractures in each stage and hands involved in the study carried out in 1979

	n	%
Stage 0	149	90.3
Stage 1	13	7.9
Stage 2	2	1.2
Stage 3	1	0.6
Total	165	100
Right	61	37.0
Left	15	9.1
Bilateral	89	53.9
Total	165	100

Table 21.5 Age and sex distribution of 1154 people at eight old people's homes in the Osaka and Kobe areas in 1986

Age	Total population	Dupuytren's disease	
		n	%
60–69 years			
Male	66	12	18.2
Female	59	7	11.9
70–79 years			
Male	159	30	18.9
Female	284	16	5.6
80–89 years			
Male	142	33	23.2
Female	339	40	11.7
90 years and over			
Male	28	3	10.7
Female	77	5	6.5
Total	1154	146	12.7
Male	395	78	19.7
Female	759	68	9.0

Table 21.6 Number of contractures in each stage and hands involved in the study carried out in 1986

	n	%
Stage 0	139	95.2
Stage 1	6	4.1
Stage 2	1	0.7
Stage 3	0	0
Total	146	100
Right	67	45.9
Left	24	16.4
Bilateral	55	37.7
Total	146	100

December 1983 had their hands examined. The purpose of this was to assess the incidence of Dupuytren's disease in the under 60 age group, as well as to compare the clinical features of the disease in those aged 60 or over in different situations, such as old people's homes or usual daily activity. In all, 3852 subjects were examined; the age range was 20–95 years, average 62.7 years. Some 2.9% of males and 0.9% of females were found to have DD. When subjects were 60 or over, the incidence was 15.4% in males and 3.2% in females (Tables 21.7 and 21.8).

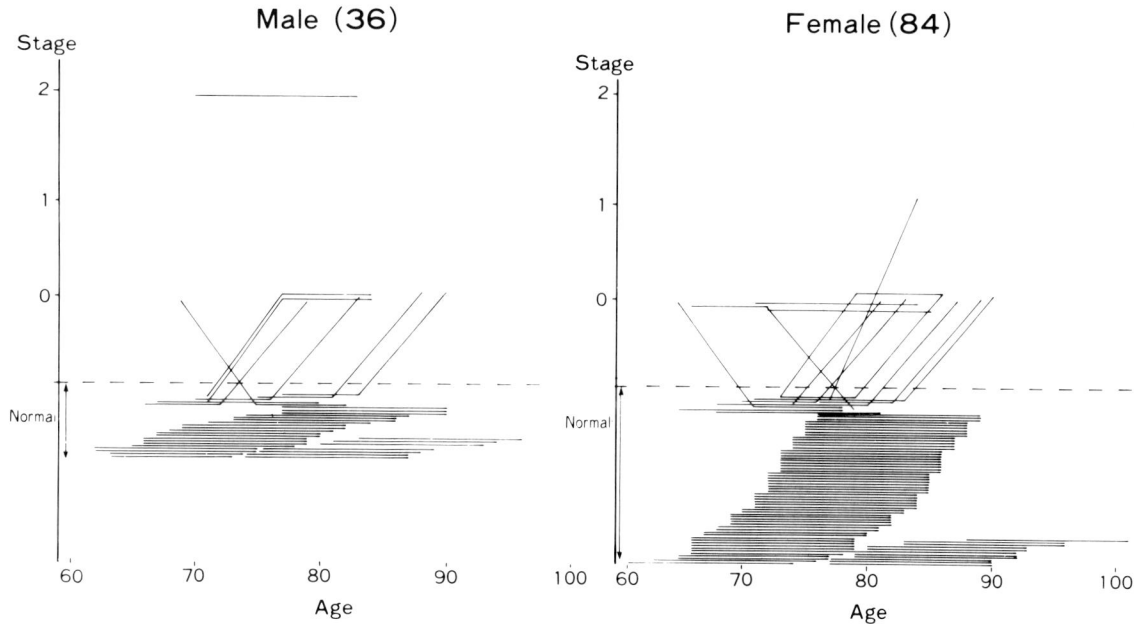

Fig. 21.3 Progression of DD in 120 subjects examined at all three visits. Each line indicates one subject. Lines start at the subject's age at the first examination and end at the third. Progression of the disease is seen to occur after the age of 70.

Summary of results

At the conclusion of these surveys the following results were obtained. The incidence of DD in subjects over 60 years of age was 16–25% in males and 3–10% in females. The incidence was highest in those aged 80 and above. Males were 2–3 times more likely to be affected than females; 90% had disease graded as stage 0. The incidence was highest in the ring finger, followed by the middle and small finger. Involvement of the digits of the right hand was almost twice as common as that of the left. Concerning the past history, including medical, social and occupational histories, no statistically significant relationship between any particular disease or social condition and DD could be observed.

DISCUSSION

In considering the aetiology of DD, racial differences constitute a significant factor in incidence. The literature concerning surgical treatment of the contracture is abundant, while reports about incidence are few, with the exception of those by Hueston, Early, Ling and Mikkelsen. These authors results vary somewhat, but for all authors the range of incidence in males was 16–28.5% and in females 7–19.7%, depending on age. Our findings in Japan also fall within this range (Table 21.9). This similarity of results implies that this disease is just as prevalent in Japanese people as in Australian, English, Scottish, Irish and Norwegian populations. Yost (1955), Su (1970), Zaworski (1979) and Haeseker (1981) reported cases of DD in black patients, however none of these authors gave details of incidence. It is strange that the incidence of DD is still unclear in most countries of the world.

Some chronic diseases have been considered to be causative factors of the disease, but in our study no statistically significant relationship was found between Dupuytren's disease and conditions such as diabetes mellitus, heart disease, hypertension, liver disease, bronchial asthma, cervical spondylosis, alcoholism or epilepsy. A genetic factor is also believed to be associated with the disease, but

Table 21.7 Age and sex distribution of 3852 people who visited the authors' surgery between 1980 and 1983

Age	Total population	Dupuytren's disease n	%
20–29 years			
Male	381	0	0
Female	564	0	0
30–39 years			
Male	534	0	0
Female	319	0	0
40–49 years			
Male	456	4	0.9
Female	345	2	0.6
50–59 years			
Male	382	15	3.9
Female	402	7	1.7
60–69 years			
Male	181	22	12.2
Female	153	5	3.3
70–79 years			
Male	63	14	22.2
Female	52	1	1.9
80–89 years			
Male	8	3	37.5
Female	10	0	0
90 years and over			
Male	1	0	0
Female	1	1	100
Total	3852	74	1.9
Male	2006	58	2.9
Female	1846	16	0.9
Total age 60 years and over	469	48	10.3
Male	253	39	15.4
Female	216	7	3.2

Table 21.8 Number of contractures in each stage and hands involved in the study carried out between 1980 and 1983

	n	%
Stage 0	66	89.2
Stage 1	3	4.1
Stage 2	2	2.7
Stage 3	3	4.1
Total	74	100
Right	24	32.4
Left	13	17.6
Bilateral	37	50.0
Total	74	100

Table 21.9 Prevalence of DD, according to various authors

Author	Age of subject	Sex	
		Male	Female
Hueston 1960 Australia	>60 years	22.8	22.5
Hueston 1962 Australia	>60 years	27.6	17.5
Hueston 1963 Australia	>60 years	28.5	19.7
Early 1962 England	>65 years	20.0	10.0
Ling 1963 Scotland	>65 years	28.5	7.0
Mikkelsen 1972 Norway	>60 years	27.6	9.5
Rafter 1980 Ireland	>50 years	30.0	
Maeda et al 1974 Japan	>60 years	6.0	1.8
Morinaga et al 1979 Japan	>60 years	14.2	8.6
Egawa First visit	>60 years	21.5	9.8
Egawa Second visit	>60 years	25.2	10.5
Egawa Third visit	>60 years	19.7	9.0
Egawa Out patients	>60 years	15.4	3.2

no patients in our series had a positive family history. It may be difficult for elderly people to remember the appearance of their parents' hands if they had not had severe deformity.

Manual work is also believed to have a significant relationship to the disease. We found it extremely difficult to evaluate work. It is only possible in a limited field such as Early's (1962) survey of locomotive workers. Our results showed that those involved in heavy manual work, such as farmers and carpenters, had a higher prevalence than those doing light manual work, such as office workers.

The prevalence of DD in the present study includes stage 0 cases; stage 0 is considered to be the beginning of the disease. These cases could be accepted as giving a true index of the incidence, as Hueston (1963) has indicated. But when examining old people, thickening of the palmar skin in labourers and of the ulnar margin of the palmar fascia in the thin female hand are confusing in making a correct diagnosis.

Only Early (1962) mentioned the proportion of patients with flexion contracture. About 90% of his patients did not have flexion contracture of the fingers. This figure is surprisingly similar to ours, but the average ages are different: Early's are 54, 57 and 57 years, in different groups, while the average age in the authors' study was 77 years. This suggests either that the progression of the disease is slower in Japanese than in English people, or that the disease has a later onset in the Japanese population.

Surgical treatment depends on the severity of the disease. We prefer a regional fasciectomy with or without skin graft and a subcutaneous fasciotomy with or without digital fasciectomy.

J. T. Hueston

Dupuytren diathesis

Recognition of the existence and importance of the diathesis to Dupuytren's disease (DD) in all patients and their relatives, has in recent years changed the surgical advice offered. No longer is an individual finger assessed and treated — it has become clear that total assessment of the patient is imperative if proper advice is to be proffered.

Derived from the Greek root to dispose or distribute, the word *diathesis* can be seen to give a guide to the disposition of what the Oxford English Dictionary terms 'a permanent condition of the body which renders it liable to a special disease'. This permanence has been demonstrated to depend on an inherited genetic pattern or 'disposition' of the chromosomal material responsible for the development of DD. Therefore it should be clear that it is impossible for a patient with DD to have no diathesis.

It would appear that there has been some difficulty in appreciating this concept of DD, McFarlane (1985) expressed surprise when a computer study of 1000 operated patients confirmed not only the existence of a diathesis but its importance in the assessment of the natural history of DD.

Of the utmost importance in counselling patients with DD is the expected outcome of treatment. It can safely be stated that unsatisfactory results fall into two categories — early and late. The early or postoperative complications of hematoma, infection and skin necrosis are due to the surgeon. The late appearance of new Dupuytren's tissue, either in recurrence or extension, is due to the patient. In particular it is due to the strength of the diathesis of the patient to the production of this palmar fibroplastic tissue.

It is therefore manifestly important to assess as well as possible the factors indicating the strength of the diathesis, and advise the patient on the likelihood or not of further development of the fibroplastic tissue of Dupuytren's disease, either in the operatively cleared zone (recurrence) or beyond the area of operation (extension). To be precise, the radical procedure of skin replacement (dermofasciectomy) will be advised if recurrence is deemed probable, but it will not be advised if recurrence is regarded as unlikely.

What then are the features to be considered in assessing the strength of diathesis and hence the risk of recurrence in any particular patient?

RACE

Despite the extremely rare and patently incontestable reports of DD in isolated Africans (Furnas 1979; Mennen 1983), DD has not been seen in non-Europeans until the recent reports in Japanese by Egawa et al (1985). These will be placed in perspective presently.

Even within Europe there is wide variation not only in incidence but also in the strength of manifestation. Thus it is difficult — indeed impossible — to compare objectively the clinical manifestations of the condition and its treatment, even within Europe itself. The condition treated in Vienna by Millesi is clearly at a lower level of penetration in the population than that treated in Ireland by Varian. Hence the need for skin replacement, because recurrence is higher in the UK than in central Europe.

The incidence in Scandinavia, the Netherlands,

Scotland, England and Ireland is higher than in the Mediterranean basin. In Italy there is a far higher incidence in the north than below Naples; this is consistent with the introduction of genetic predisposition in the north-west from French invasions and in the north-east from Austro-Hungarian invasions. Despite the fact that Australia has the highest Greek population outside Greece, I have seen only one Greek male with very mild DD, — palmar nodule only — and on questioning he revealed that his mother was Irish!

An explanation of this north-west European dominance of DD has been that it was in the genetic spectrum of the Celts. More likely, in view of their wide raiding patterns, it could be regarded as a Viking disease. Indeed the occasion of finding DD in a Sicilian with blue eyes is likely to be due to the Norman invasion of Sicily in 1066 by the brother of William the conqueror, who invaded England in the same year.

A neat study by Brouet (1986) in Toulon has noted a striking difference in the incidence of DD in the dark-eyed Mediterraneans of local stock and that in the blue-eyed Nordic stock, comprising sailors who for generations have settled in the milder climate of this French coast and have manifestly brought their genetic pool with them. A far stronger diathesis is noted in the Toulonese of Nordic than of local Mediterranean stock.

But what of the recent reports from Japan? There is no historical evidence of Celtic or Viking invasion there. While naval visits from American and European ships may possibly have seeded a few cases, another possibility exists. It is to be noted that the diathesis of the Japanese patients is very low. Very few progress to surgery for correction of deformity. The demography of the condition in Japan has not yet been established but it is well known that the tall, paler Hokkaido population are already genetically distinguished from the shorter, darker southern Japanese. In a study of the linguistic patterns of the northern people of Europe and Asia, Collinder (1957) has demonstrated that a group of linguistically related peoples at the northern region of the Urals, before the Vikings dispersed both east and westwards along the line of the Arctic Circle, passed through Mongolia to the eastern littoral. It is certainly not impossible that this basically northern European strain was thus introduced in a very diluted form into some areas of Japan.

The absence of any genetically pure Negro in the USA after four centuries of cohabitation makes DD in a black patient of no interest in this racial consideration. Conversely the high incidence in Canada, where kilts are commoner than in Scotland itself, supports the known Viking excursions through Iceland and Greenland to the mainland of Canada — not to mention the subsequent millenium of migration from the British Isles. The same Scottish and Irish predominance in the early white settlers of Australia explains, by this distillation of the genetic pool, the high incidence in this country and in the white settlers of New Zealand.

This racial factor is by far the most important single element determining the incidence of DD. The patient's universal enquiry: 'Why do I have this condition?' can truthfully be answered: 'You were born to get it'.

AGGRAVATING FACTORS

The strength of the diathesis can be increased by genetically related epilepsy or diabetes mellitus. In a genetically predisposed population other factors seem to dispose the clinical manifestation of the condition to appear earlier or more commonly than in their absence. These factors include chronic pulmonary disease, cirrhosis and alcoholism, all of which have classically been associated with other changes in the connective tissues of the hands, such as clubbing of the fingers and 'liver palms'. The difficulty in grasping the concept of a diathesis has been failure to realize that all these predisposed populations have a diathesis of some degree, but the clinical manifestation may remain latent. It is only in the presence of some added factor that DD may appear or progress in these special disease groups.

The simplest of these factors is disuse. The onset or aggravation of DD in patients rendered inactive by a major injury, such as major fracture of the legs or back, has been seen to be followed within weeks by the onset or progress of DD often bilaterally.

Injury

In the absence of a racial predisposition to Dupuytren's disease, any amount of injury to the hand will fail to produce DD. However, where the diathesis is racially disposed the appearance or progression of DD has been noted to follow almost any injury to the limb associated with a period of swelling and disuse of the hand. These injuries range from radical mastectomy through proximal limb ruptures, dislocations of shoulder or elbow joints, forearm fractures, superficial burns of the hand, to direct local tissue disruption with hematoma or open wounds and fractures in the hand itself. That all these different identities will act through some final common pathway on the palmar connective tissue between the dermis and the palmar aponeurosis, without necessarily injuring this well defined connective tissue compartment, indicates that a basic balance of tissue turnover or entropy has been disturbed in this compartment. Whatever the basic mechanism of the metabolic change — and changes in the fat as a possible mediating element have been identified (Rabinowitz et al 1983) — it is of paramount importance to note that the palm itself does not have to be the site of the injury. Plewes' (1956) observed that every patient with Sudek's atrophy showed the palmar proliferation of DD, despite a multiplicity of causes of the Sudek's atrophy. This points to the importance of a change in the general vasomotor status of the hand as a pathogenetic pathway.

The persistent proposal of partisan theories based on rupture of the longitudinal fibres of the palmar aponeurosis fails to explain the phenomenon of onset without local injury apart from disuse and local oedema. The evidence supporting the extra-aponeurotic origin of the primary Dupuytren's nodule — apart from the observation that the primary nodule is on the palmar and never the dorsal aspect of the palmar aponeurosis — has been confirmed by the author's observation of retraction induced in the digital extensor apparatus by a dorsal plaque of DD (Hueston 1982a). Iselin (personal communication) noted a similar phenomenon. Finally, the hypothesis of pathogenesis with intrinsic rupture of longitudinal aponeurotic fibres fails to explain the phenomenon of recurrence.

Every fasciectomy must be recognized as a specific local injury to the volar compartments of the palm and fingers. It is biologically inevitable that swelling and disuse, however temporary, will follow this surgical injury. The longitudinal fibres still cited by some reactionaries as the site of origin of DD are no longer present after fasciectomy. Yet the incidence of recurrence within the operative area is now recognized as being between 40 and 60% in an Anglo-Saxon community (Hueston 1963; Rank & Chang 1978 Tonkin et al 1984; Niebauer; personal communication). The tissue where the recurrent tissue forms — very frequently within a few weeks — is the tissue of the replaced flaps of volar skin elevated for exposure. This is the tissue in which the original change leading to the primary nodule had arisen, possibly aggravated by the vasodilatation (Bauer et al 1985) and oedema (Plewes 1956) of a specific episode of regional injury and disuse (Hueston 1982b). Only by the sacrifice of the subcutaneous tissue and its overlying skin, along with the fascia, has it been found that recurrence can be avoided. This locally more radical procedure is usually reserved for the digits rather than the palm.

Occupational factors

In the absence of a specific injury to the hand or the proximal limb leading to swelling and temporary disuse, there is no evidence that manual labour initiates or aggravates DD (see Chapters 19, 24 and 25). Indeed the opposite is the case; progress of the disease is often observed when the maximum physiological use of the hand in heavy labour is replaced by a more sedentary job involving supervising or writing with, of course, the ulnar digits flexed and unused.

That the diathesis over-rules any claimed local hand activity is confirmed by:

1. The fact that there is no relation between the disease and handedness.
2. The fact that the workers are often aged 50 or older when DD is first noticed; this is normal in the natural history of the disease.
3. There may be racial groups in a job, such as Dutch or German stock in a brewery business or migrant labourers from Scotland

and Ireland in Australia. Vibrating tools have no relation to DD (Hunter et al 1944).

There is no doubt that most work in Third World nations is heavily manual and yet DD is not seen there, for the simple reason that no diathesis exists in the absence of an inherited genetic predisposition.

CLINICAL ASSESSMENT

The first clinical examination of every patient with DD must involve removal of the patient's shoes. The author's practice is to do this before noting the details of the hands. The clinician must record whether one or both soles has nodules and how extensive they are. This observation is checked at subsequent annual visits.

The presence and distribution of knuckle pads over the proximal interphalangeal joints is also noted. Knuckle pads may also be over the metacarpophalangeal joint or, most commonly, on the thumb at the interphalangeal joint. It should be recognized that depression over the joint as a result of early adhesion of the dermis to the paratenon may be present before the much commoner single or multiple nodular mass is seen (Hueston 1984). Regular annual recording will often show that these knuckle pads occur on new digits or, rarely the knuckle pads may be noted to shrink or disappear from one or more digits. The palm may appear clear of nodules or bands in a patient with knuckle pads but it is inevitable that palmar lesions will ultimately appear.

The justification for taking these ectopic deposits of identical fibroplastic tissue masses as an index of the strength of the diathesis is that a far higher incidence of recurrence has been found in patients with knuckle pads. What is more, those patients with knuckle pads are generally younger than those without, so it is important to identify young patients with knuckle pads as having a stronger diathesis and greater likelihood of recurrence than those patients who are elderly when the condition appears and in whom no knuckle pads are present. In such elderly patients recurrence is unlikely and less radical surgery can usually be advised.

The mode and rate of onset of the palmar changes may indicate a stronger diathesis. If the disease is rapid in onset and progress and particularly if it follows soon after a specific local injury or previous surgery, the risk of recurrence after further surgery is greater; it is inevitable if the patient is young and has ectopic deposits.

Skin involvement is difficult to assess as a prognostic factor in diathesis but if it is extensive then the field of palmar extra-aponeurotic fibroplasia is manifestly more widespread and reflects a greater tendency to the production of this tissue before — and therefore very likely after — the injury of fasciectomy.

Previous surgery should always be presumed to have been well done. Derogatory statements that the recurrence is due to the previous surgeon's poor technique show an ignorance of the fact that it is the patient who is producing the recurrence because of the strength of the diathesis. Further surgery must be directed towards prevention of recurrence by replacing the skin, otherwise the early appearance of a further recurrence will leave the critical surgeon red-faced.

Of least practical importance in assessing the strength of the diathesis is the absence of a family history. While a positive family history of one or several close blood relations with DD supports the assessment of a stronger diathesis, the absence of a family history should not lead the surgeon into presuming a low penetration of the disposition. The classical study of Ling (1963) confirmed what we find very often, namely that the patient who on the first visit denied any family history later reveals one or more relatives involved. A negative family history is the most unreliable of all the factors outlined above in the assessment of the strength of the diathesis.

The strength of the diathesis determines the treatment. Attempts to grade numerically the degree of diathesis have not yet appeared in the literature, but should be regarded with a healthy scepticism in this essentially clinical process of individual assessment.

Discussion

John Hueston has provided an eloquent account of his original concept of Dupuytren's diathesis. I would, however, take issue with his closing comment that attempts to grade numerically the degree of diathesis should be regarded with scepticism. Lord Kelvin said:

When you can measure what you are talking about and express it in numbers, you should know something about it; but when you cannot measure it, when you cannot express it in numbers, your knowledge is of a meagre and unsatisfactory kind: it may be the beginning of knowledge, but you have scarcely, in your thoughts, advanced to the stage of a science.

The goal of the statistical analysis reported here was to determine which factors, if any, contributed to an increased incidence of recurrence or extension of disease following appropriate operation; that is, to show that under certain circumstances the disease is more aggressive and to evaluate the causative factors. Five factors were found to affect appreciably the course of the disease but, as shown in Figure 22.1 only two of these factors, 'other areas involved' and 'early onset of disease', had a statistically significant effect. Clinically this would mean that either factor, when present alone, should alert the surgeon that there was a very good chance of recurrence and extension of disease and that more extensive surgery such as extensive fasciectomy or dermofasciectomy was indicated. The other factors, 'bilateral disease', 'family history' or 'more than two rays involved', acting alone would not have an effect upon the course of the disease. However, the presence of two or three factors would probably cause aggressive disease. As shown in Figure 22.1, when all five factors are present there is a profound difference in the rate of recurrence and extension. These interrelation-

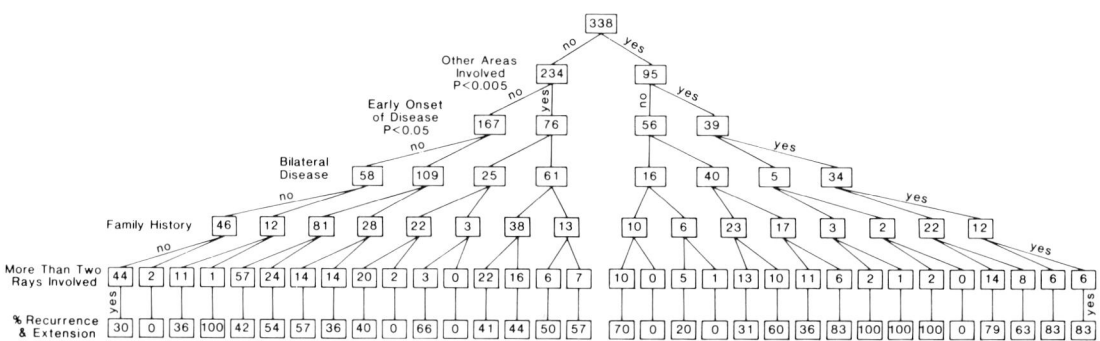

Fig. 22.1 Rate of recurrence and extension of disease according to the factors contributing to an increased diathesis. The group consists of 338 patients who had had no previous operation and who were examined 2 years or more after operation. If all five factors are present the rate of recurrence or extension is 83%. If none of the factors are present the rate is 30%. Acting alone, only the factors 'other areas involved' and 'early onset of disease' have a statistically significant effect upon recurrence and extension. Acting in combination, these five factors have a profound effect.

Table 22.1 Knuckle pads and plantar nodules: 50 Patients; 67 Hands

Family origin		Sex		Hand dominance		Hand involved		Occupation	
Northern European	92%	Male	84%	Right	86%	Right	10%	Manual	49%
		Female	16%	Left	14%	Left	10%	Non-manual	51%
						Both	80%		
		Other areas involved			100%	Associated diseases		Age at onset (years)	
						Epilepsy	16%	Male	40.2 ± 13.0
		Family history			46%	Diabetes	6%	Female	46.4 ± 13.5
		Previous operation			46%	Alcoholism	18%	Age at operation (years)	
						Trauma	18%	Male	53.5 ± 10.5
								Female	58.5 ± 12.2

Operation profile

Hand profile			Palm	Little finger	Thumb		Anaesthesia	
Palm only	3%	Operation					Local	2%
No palm	3%	Local	8%	8%	6%		Regional	45%
		Regional	60%	32%	65%		General	53%
One ray	33%	Extensive	32%	59%	29%			
Two rays	22%	Amputation		1%			Procedure at	
Three or more rays	42%						PIP joint	19%
		Incision						
Thumb and thumb web	40%	Longitudinal	76%	99%	100%		Complications	24%
Index finger	36%	Transverse	24%	1%				
Middle finger	37%							
Ring finger	52%	Closure					Therapy	79%
Little finger	66%	Suture	70%	83%	76%			
		Open	14%	0%	0%			
		Graft	16%	17%	24%		Splinting	42%

ships and trends are illustrated in Figure 22.2. The percentage of hands involved increases directly with the number of rays involved for factors associated with aggressive disease.

Because 'other areas involved' is such a strong diathesis factor, a patient profile was prepared and is shown in Table 22.1. Knuckle pads occurred in 20% of surgical patients and plantar nodules in 7%. Only 50 patients (4%) had both knuckle pads and plantar nodules. Penile involvement was not included because this would eliminate females.

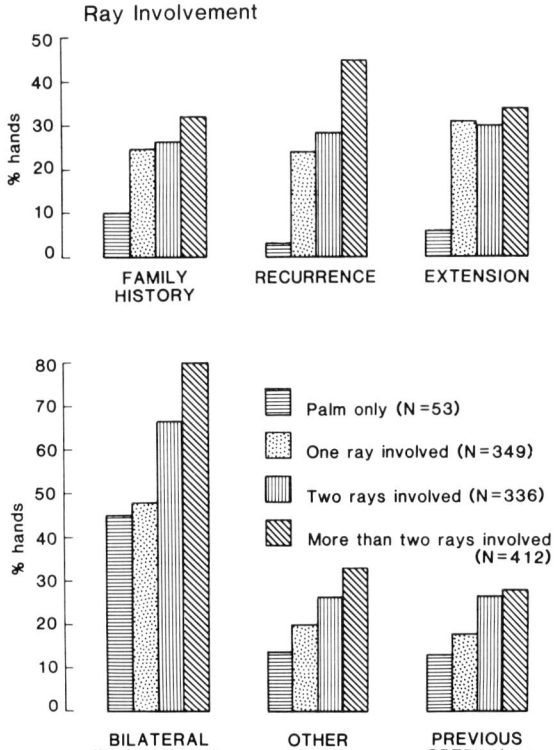

Fig. 22.2 Positive relationship and increasing trend of various diathesis factors with increasing ray involvement in the hand.

Predictably the combination of knuckle pads and plantar nodules influenced many factors in Table 22.1. Note the increased prevalence of family origin, bilateral disease, family history, previous operation, epilepsy, and alcoholism and perhaps trauma, and the marked reduction in the age at onset and operation in both sexes. There were more rays involved and more radial side disease. Skin grafts were used more frequently in the palm and fingers. There were more procedures upon the proximal interphalangeal joint and more complications, indicating that more extensive operations were performed.

Our conclusions are similar to those of Hueston but with statistical support. The most important factors are 'other areas involved' and 'early onset of disease'. These two factors stand alone and are not sex-related. Racial origin is not a strong factor simply because most of the patients studied were of northern European origin. For the same reason, bilateral involvement is not a strong factor because most patients have bilateral disease. Family history would be a significant factor if a 'proper' family history was obtained. However from a practical point of view only 25–30% patients seen by a surgeon will know of a close relative having the disease. This information is of no value in predicting the course of disease. Epileptics and alcoholics have severe and aggressive disease. It is not known whether this is genetic or drug-induced. Diabetics have mild disease; in fact, the majority do not require treatment. Concerning trauma the data are conflicting because the disease appears in younger males. However the disease is less extensive and less aggressive so trauma would not appear to be a diathesis factor.

The term 'Dupuytren's diathesis' has been in common usage for many years without being clearly understood. We have presented here some scientific evidence in support of this concept.

L. C. Hurst and M. Badalamente

23 Associated diseases

INTRODUCTION

The association of Dupuytren's disease (DD) with other diseases, especially alcoholism, diabetes, and epilepsy, has been recognized for many years (Hueston 1960; McFarlane 1985). The first extensive study relating alcoholism and DD was done in 1956 (Wolfe et al 1956) but these authors pointed out that Skoog had cited an alcohol related case in 1948. In 14 patients with DD, Fere & Francillon (1902) reported that there was only 1 patient with known alcoholism. The suggestion of an association between diabetes and DD was made as early as 1883 independently by Cayla and Viger. In 1902 Fere & Francillon mentioned only 14 patients out of 226 (6.2%) with DD and epilepsy. The first complete review of the association of DD with epilepsy was done by Lund (1941). This study clearly established the presence of a higher incidence of DD in epilepsy patients than in the general population.

DD AND ALCOHOLISM

Possibly stimulated by the reports of Wolfe et al (1956) and Skoog (1948), who noted an occasional alcoholic case in patients with DD contemporary hand surgeons often express the clinical impression that alcoholics are more likely to have DD, and to have it more severely, than healthy patients (Su & Patek 1970).

Since 1956 numerous clinical studies have attempted to assess scientifically the association between DD and alcoholism. The question has been approached in two different ways. Some investigators have studied the incidence of alcoholism in populations composed of patients with known DD (Wegmann & Geiser 1964; Rafter et al 1980; Houghton et al 1983; Bradlow & Mowat 1986). Others have studied the incidence of DD in populations composed of alcoholics (Wolfe et al 1956; Hueston 1960; Summerskill et al 1960; Nazari 1966; Su & Patek 1970; Pojer et al 1972; Aron 1977; Bertrand et al 1977; Bulfoni 1980). In most of these studies, the diagnosis of DD has been made by surgeons based on the presence of Dupuytren's nodules, cords, positive table top tests, and/or the presence of contractures.

The diagnostic basis for alcoholism was more variable. Two studies simply recorded the medical history of alcoholism on a yes/no basis (McFarlane 1985; Hurst et al 1986). Others assessed alcohol intake by questions about number of daily drinks and equated this to the number of grams of alcohol consumption (Su & Patek 1970; Houghton et al 1983; Bradlow & Mowat 1986). Liver function was assessed by enzyme levels (Pojer & Javickova 1970; Pojer et al 1972; Houghton et al 1983; Bradlow & Mowat 1986) or by liver biopsy (Summerskill et al 1960; Nazari 1966; Su & Patek 1970; Houghton et al 1983). Still others picked their alcoholic population by the presence of patients in acute alcoholic detoxification units or alcoholic rehabilitation units (Wolfe et al 1956; Hueston 1960).

In those studies of alcoholism in DD populations, the average incidence of alcoholism was 39% (range 8.6 to 78%; Wegmann & Geiser 1964; Rafter et al 1980; Houghton et al 1983; Bradlow & Mowat 1986). The controls (those who did not have DD) in these studies had an average incidence of alcoholism of 23% (range 1 to 65%). Two studies also noted the incidence of cirrhosis in DD populations (Wegmann & Geiser 1964; Rafter et al 1980). One had 11.5% and the other 38.7% incidence of cirrhosis. Only the second study noted the incidence of cirrhosis in the control group (12.5%).

Two studies (Rafter et al 1980; Houghton et al 1983) claimed that there was no significant difference in the percentage of alcoholics in their Dupuytren's population versus their control 'normal' populations. Houghton's group found an 8.6% alcoholism rate in the Dupuytren's group versus 3.6% in their control group. The Rafter study found 78% alcoholism in the Dupuytren's group and 65% in their control group. The Houghton study did statistically analyse the data but relied on patient reporting of alcohol abuse and defined an alcoholic as one who takes in greater than 80 grams of alcohol per day. Half this amount was used to identify alcohol abuse in other studies. Further, no attempt was made to define alcoholism by total life time consumption. The Rafter study gave no definition of alcoholism and presented no statistical data despite the 13% difference between their Dupuytren's group and their control group.

In those studies of the incidence of DD in alcoholic and cirrhotic populations (Wolfe et al 1956; Hueston 1960; Summerskill et al 1960; Nazari 1966; Su & Patek 1970; Pojer et al 1972; Aron 1977; Bertrand et al 1977; Bulfoni 1980), the average incidence of DD was 26% (range 10 to 40%) in alcoholics and 40% (range 18 to 66%) in alcoholics with cirrhosis. In the studies which used controls, the average incidence of DD in the controls was 12% (Wolfe et al 1956; Hueston 1960; Su & Patek 1970; Bertrand et al 1977; Bulfoni 1980). In five of these studies of alcoholic populations (Wolfe et al 1956; Hueston 1960; Su & Patek 1970; Bertrand et al 1977; Bulfoni 1980) the incidence of DD at different ages was also investigated (Fig. 23.1). The incidence of DD was higher than expected in all age groups of the alcoholic population in these studies. Despite the fact that the composite age-related data show that alcoholism with cirrhosis clearly leads to a higher incidence of DD especially after age 50, the studies reviewed here were equally divided on the

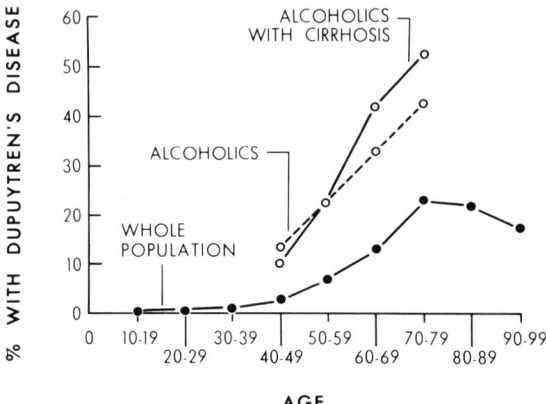

Fig. 23.1 Incidence (%) of DD versus age in three groups: alcoholics with cirrhosis, alcoholics without cirrhosis (data from multiple authors; see text), and the whole (normal) population. The normal population statistics are a combination of Mikkelsen's male and female data (Mikkelsen 1972).

true effect of cirrhosis (Wolfe et al 1956; Hueston 1960; Summerskill et al 1960; Nazari 1966; Su & Patek 1970; Aron 1977; Bertrand et al 1977; Bulfoni 1980). Four studies stated that cirrhosis increased the incidence and severity of DD while the remaining four stated that chronic alcohol intake alone was the cause of its higher incidence.

Why does alcohol increase the incidence of DD? The answer to this question is unknown. Several investigators have suggested that the appearance of clinically evident DD is facilitated in genetically predisposed individuals by metabolic disorders such as alcoholism (Summerskill et al 1960; Bertrand et al 1977; Bradlow & Mowat 1986). The mechanism of this relationship is uncertain but alcohol may trigger local neurovascular changes in these individuals (Su & Patek 1970). Microvascular occlusions have been shown in Dupuytren's tissue (Kischer & Speer 1984). Others (Rabinowitz et al 1983) have described altered palmar fat composition in DD which may be secondary to hypoxia. Their hypothesis states that the altered fat acts as an irritant which can precipitate a fibrotic repair response. Possibly, in addition to hypoxia, the palmar fat may be metabolically altered by chronic alcoholism and predisposes to DD by an effect on the fatty acid cascade and subsequent prostaglandin metabolism.

Prostaglandin F2 has been shown in vitro to induce Dupuytren's myofibroblasts to contract (Hurst et al 1986). Prostaglandin E2 has been shown to induce Dupuytren's myofibroblasts to relax in vitro. Interestingly, the prostaglandin literature (Pennington et al 1979; Horrobin 1980; Hall & Behrmann 1982) has documented that prostaglandin E is decreased in both animals and humans in response to chronic ethanol. Therefore, relaxation of myofibroblasts in DD (associated with alcoholism) may be inhibited by decreased prostaglandin E2 levels while these cells are stimultaneously influenced by the constrictive ability of prostaglandin F2.

DUPUYTREN'S DISEASE AND DIABETES MELLITUS

As previously noted, the French suggested an association between DD and diabetes mellitus before the turn of the century (Cayla 1883; Viger 1883). Despite the early recognition of this association, many surgeons have remained sceptical about this connection. One large surgical series which based its diagnosis of diabetes mellitus on a positive history for clinical diabetes mellitus found an unexciting 8% incidence (McFarlane 1985). At first glance this surgical scepticism seems to be supported by the incredible range (1.6–42%) in the incidence of DD in cases of diabetes mellitus previously reported in the medical literature (Spring et al 1970; Heathcote et al 1981; Noble et al 1984). However, this variation — and particularly the reports of a low incidence of DD in diabetes mellitus — has been based on studies with flaws in their methodology.

First, some studies have been done on surgical cases where the diagnosis of diabetes mellitus was based on a positive history for clinical diabetes mellitus only. These studies failed to recognize and correct for the fact that diabetics with DD rarely need surgery (Davis & Finesilver 1932; Fossati et al 1975; Noble et al 1984). Secondly, studies of diabetic populations which did not have qualified hand surgeons to make the diagnosis of DD have probably underestimated the incidence of DD (Noble et al 1984). Thus, the true incidence of DD in diabetes mellitus probably does approach 40%, as reported by Noble et al. Surgeons who have only looked for clinically evident diabetes in their surgical patients have probably made accurate observations but drawn scientifically unsound conclusions.

The incidence of DD in diabetic populations appears to be positively influenced by two factors: the duration of the diabetes and the age of the patients (Fig. 23.2; Cammarn & Weckesser 1961; Schneider 1964; Montenero et al 1965; Ravid et al 1977; Noble et al 1984; Larkin & Frier 1986). Some investigators disagree that duration of the diabetes mellitus is a factor (Ipbuker & Erkurt 1965; Spring et al 1970). However, all studies do agree that the type of therapy used for the diabetes is not a factor. The incidence of DD is no greater in insulin-dependent diabetics than in diet-controlled diabetics (Ipbuker & Erkurt 1965; Spring et al 1970; Ravid et al 1977; Noble et al 1984). DD may even appear before the diabetes manifests itself (Paeslack 1962). Further, the quality of diabetic control may not be a factor, but obese diabetics appear to have more DD (Ipbuker & Erkurt 1965). The sexual differences in the incidence of DD, which are well known in normal populations (Mikkelsen 1972), are not as striking in diabetics with DD. This was especially noted in studies which carefully assessed diabetic patients for mild DD (Montenero et al 1965; Fossati et al 1975; Noble et al 1984).

In addition, the severity and location of DD in the diabetic hand is atypical. Especially in women,

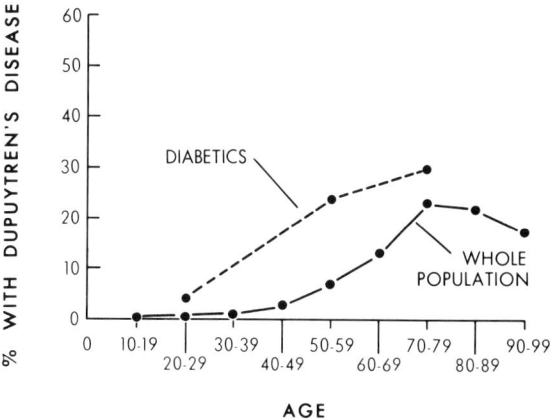

Fig. 23.2 Incidence (%) of DD versus age in diabetic population — data from several authors (see text) — and a whole (normal) population (Mikkelsen 1972).

knuckle pads, nodules and tethering without contracture are much more common in diabetic DD (Fig. 23.3); Paeslack 1962; Noble et al 1984). Also the DD is more radial in diabetic hands. The third and fourth digits are predominantly involved instead of the fifth (Fossati et al 1975; Noble et al 1984; Larkin & Frier 1986; Fig. 23.4). Sometimes palmar erythema precedes clinical DD in diabetics (Schneider 1964). Like early DD in the non-diabetic population, and diabetic retinopathy in diabetic populations, diabetic DD can undergo spontaneous regression and progression (Schneider 1964).

In some DD surgical series the incidence of diabetes is very low (Spring et al 1970; Noble et al 1984). However, in those series that looked

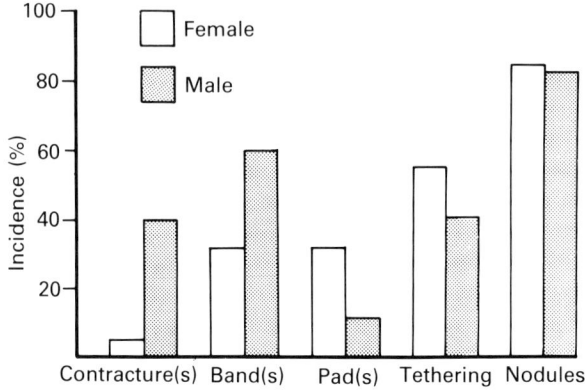

Fig. 23.3 Most diabetic patients, particularly women, do not have contractures and do not require surgical treatment. From Noble et al (1984) with permission.

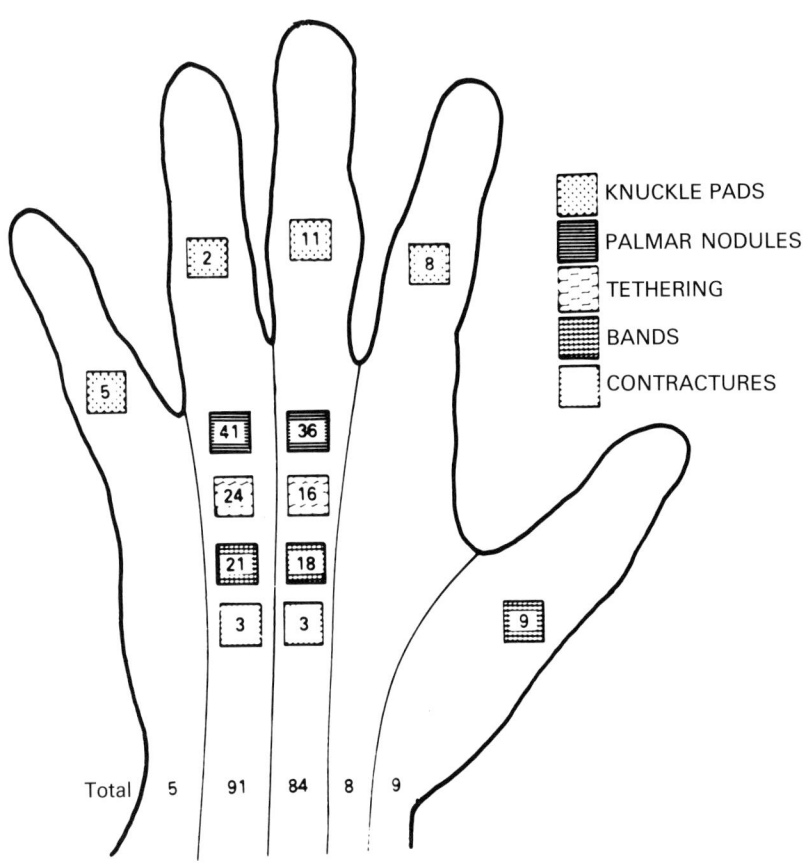

Fig. 23.4 There is minimal involvement of the fifth digit (2.5 %) in diabetic DD. From Noble et al (1984) with permission.

carefully for chemical (latent) diabetes mellitus, a remarkably high incidence of diabetes was found in presumably normal patients with DD (Paeslack 1962; Rhomberg 1967; Spring et al 1970). Using a rapid intravenous glucose tolerance test, Spring et al showed a statistically significant difference in the rate of glucose utilization in presumably non-diabetic patients with DD versus controls. In 100 patients Rhomberg used a tolbutamide test to define chemical diabetes and found only 19 patients with normal results. The other 81 patients either had overt diabetes or the tolbutamide test results suggested chemical diabetes. In his non-diabetic patients with DD, Paeslack noted an abnormal glucose tolerance test in one-third of the men and half of the women. More recently, Nardoni et al (1981) found an abnormal glucose tolerance test in 93% of 368 patients with DD. They felt that impaired glucose metabolism was an important factor in the pathogenesis of DD.

Why is there a higher incidence of DD particularly the milder, more radial type, in diabetic patients? As with the association of DD with alcoholism, the exact answer is unknown. Perhaps diabetic DD is a different disease from the non-diabetic one. This appears unlikely, because no one has shown a difference in the histology of DD in diabetics from that seen in non-diabetics. It is possible that the metabolic and biochemical changes of diabetes or chemical diabetes mellitus cause or promote the onset of DD. It may be that individuals are born with a genetic predisposition which simultaneously causes DD and diabetes (Paeslack 1962; Kay & Slater 1981; Noble et al 1984). Alternatively, the microangiopathy of diabetes mellitus may be the important inciting factor. Combined diabetic vascular disease and DD have been noted and an increased incidence of DD has been related to the vascular complications of diabetes (Montenero et al 1965). Also, microangiopathy has been demonstrated in DD (Kischer & Speer 1984) and in diabetes mellitus microvascular changes have been related to myofibroblast differentiation and proliferation (Kay & Slater 1981). Despite these observations earlier work exists which, at least on the light microscopic level, was unable to identify microangiopathy in diabetic Dupuytren's tissue (Cammarn & Weckesser 1961).

Others have suggested that diabetic peripheral neuropathy causes the increased incidence of DD in diabetics (Ipbuker & Erkurt 1965; Spring et al 1970; Jung et al 1971). Spring et al found evidence of early neuropathy in 24 of 25 non-diabetic patients with DD but were unable to explain why this should increase the incidence of DD in diabetes or how the neuropathy related to the aetiology of the DD even in their non-diabetic patients.

The best hints regarding the cause of the increased frequency of DD in diabetes and possibly the cause of diabetic DD itself come from studies on a related disorder, limited joint mobility in diabetic hands. Patients with limited joint mobility have a positive table top test in at least one finger bilaterally, not because of contracted palmar aponeurotic tissues, but because of metacarpophalangeal joint or interphalangeal joint stiffness (Fig. 23.5; Knowles 1981; Rosenbloom et al 1981; Kennedy et al 1982; Lawson et al 1983). Patients with limited joint mobility have associated thick tight waxy skin and a significant increased risk for microvascular complications such as retinopathy. It has also been shown that limited joint mobility and DD can coexist in diabetic patients (Lawson et al 1983).

Skin biopsy studies from patients with limited joint mobility have shown increased dermal thickness, increased connective tissue, and increased non-enzymatic glycosylation compared to controls (Buckingham et al 1981; Knowles 1981). Non-enzymatic glycosylation of collagen might explain the scleroderma-like skin and possibly the limited joint mobility. However, more recent studies have shown that the tissue glycosylation is equally increased in skin from diabetic patients with and without limited joint mobility (Lyons & Kennedy 1985). Because of this finding, Larkin & Frier (1986) have suggested that limited joint mobility may be a 'vascular related phenomenon of aging'. Interestingly, others have shown that fibroblast cultures from diabetics show characteristics of accelerated ageing, and particularly in cells from juvenile diabetics, these fibroblasts synthesize more collagen than fibroblasts from non-diabetics

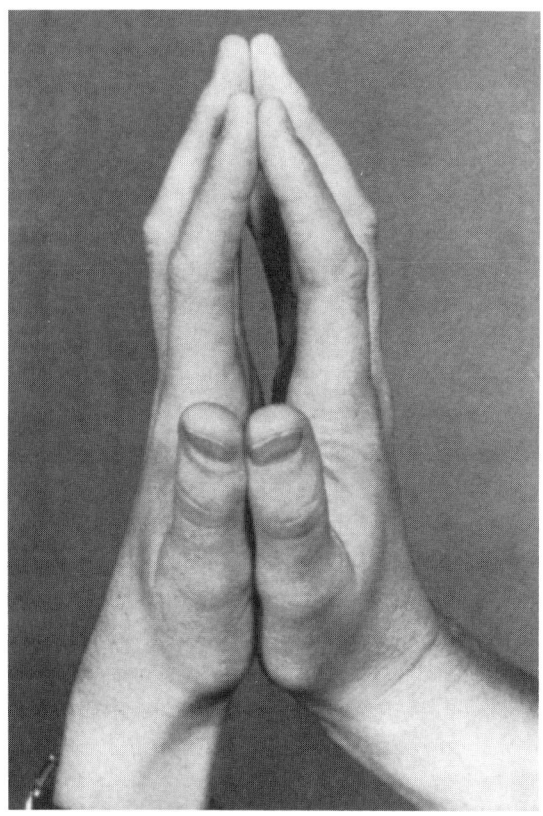

Fig. 23.5 Limited joint mobility in a child with juvenile diabetes mellitus. Note the fixed bilateral proximal interphalangeal joint contractures and absence of DD. From Kennedy et al (1982) with permission.

34% (range 8 to 57%; Lund 1941; Skoog 1948; Arieff & Bell 1956; Hueston 1960; Early 1962; Pojer et al 1972; Critchley et al 1976; James 1985). Early reported the 8% incidence but also noted that his epileptic population was unusually young. Further, in severe epilepsy, he found that DD was five times more frequent in epileptic males and eight times more frequent in epileptic females than in the general population.

Few DD populations have been investigated with regards to the incidence of epilepsy (James 1985; McFarlane 1985). In 1969 Thieme (as reported by James 1985) found an 8.6% incidence of epilepsy in 371 patients with DD, when the expected incidence was 1.86%, assuming a 0.5% incidence of epilepsy in the general population. He also found a high incidence of DD in the relatives of his epileptic patients. McFarlane (1985) reported a 3% incidence in a large co-operative study of surgical patients with DD.

These studies have all shown that the incidence of DD in epileptic populations increases with age and duration of epilepsy (Fig. 23.6). The incidence of DD in epileptic patients does not correlate with the frequency or severity of the seizures, age of onset of epilepsy, type of seizures, type of electroencephalogram changes (focal versus non-focal) or the type of drug therapy (Lund 1941;

(Rowe et al 1977). Perhaps accelerated ageing or glycosylation of collagen in the palmar aponeurosis causes the increased incidence of DD in diabetes mellitus. The exact cause remains unknown but future investigations on both DD and limited joint mobility may be enlightening.

DD AND EPILEPSY

Despite a 1902 report (Fere & Francillon 1902) which purported to disprove any connection between DD and epilepsy, an association was demonstrated by Lund (1941) and Skoog (1948). These studies and those that followed account for 2828 epileptic patients examined for signs of DD. In these studies the average incidence of DD was

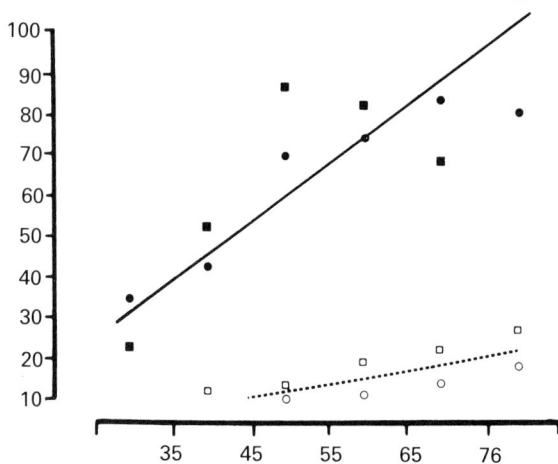

Fig. 23.6 Incidence (%) of DD versus age in a population with epilepsy (unbroken line) and a general (normal) population for comparison (dashed line). From Critchley et al (1976) with permission.

Skoog 1948; Arieff & Bell 1956; Hueston 1960; Early 1962; Critchley et al 1976). Epileptic patients do have a very high incidence of associated knuckle pads, plantar nodules and Peyronie's disease (Lund 1941; Skoog 1948; Early 1962; Critchley et al 1976). An interesting finding in a series of Dupuytren's patients has also been demonstrated by Zachariae et al (1970) who found a significant increase in abnormal electroencephalogram findings in age-matched non-epileptic Dupuytren's patients versus controls.

The typical Dupuytren's hand in epilepsy, according to Skoog (1948), does not deviate from the common picture but both he and Stuhler & Stankovic (1977) report that the ring finger is the predominantly involved digit. Early (1962) has noted that DD in epileptic populations is often bilateral, symmetrical and steadily progressive.

Why is there an increased frequency of DD in epileptic patients? Like the relationship of DD to alcoholism and diabetes, the exact answer to this question is unknown. There are two hypotheses. The first suggests that there is a genetic link between DD and epilepsy (Lund 1941; Early 1962; Stuhler & Stankovic 1977; Hueston 1985; James 1985). The second hypothesis suggests that the cause of increased DD in epilepsy is secondary to the drugs used to treat epilepsy, especially phenobarbitone (Lund 1941; Skoog 1948; Critchley et al 1976; Froscher & Hoffman 1983).

The first hypothesis is supported by Stuhler & Stankovic's (1977) observation that DD is more frequent in idiopathic than in traumatic epilepsy. Further, Thieme (as reported by James 1985) found a high incidence of DD in the relatives of his epileptic patients with DD. He felt that the incidence was high enough to suggest an autosomal dominant genetic link between DD and epilepsy. Neither Thieme nor Arieff & Bell (1956) could find a link between drug therapy and the incidence of DD.

The second hypothesis is supported by several observations. In 1902 Fere & Francillon examined 226 patients and found only 14 patients with DD (6.2%). This finding is significant because none of the drugs (specifically phenobarbitone) currently used for treating epilepsy had been introduced in 1902. Studies done after the introduction of phenobarbitone strongly suggest that this drug causes the increased incidence of DD in epilepsy (Lund 1941; Skoog 1948; Critchley et al 1976; Froscher & Hoffman 1983; Schmidt 1983). Lund was unsure whether phenobarbitone (Luminal) was important but he noted less DD in epileptics treated with bromide and in epileptics who had received Luminal for a shorter period of time. Skoog found a comparable incidence of DD in his traumatic and idiopathic epileptics. All his patients were treated with phenobarbitone. Critchley et al were unable to relate the increased incidence of DD in their epileptic patients to a particular type of drug but felt that phenobarbitone was causative since only 2 of 21 patients who did not receive phenobarbitone had DD.

More recently, Froscher & Hoffman (1983) noted DD in their small series of epileptic patients treated with phenobarbitone. The degree of contracture appeared to vary with the drug dosage. Further, they found that in half of these patients, the fascial abnormalities diminished or disappeared when the phenobarbitone was discontinued. In 80% of these patients, the size of the knuckle pads diminished when the drug was stopped. Finally, Schmidt (1983) has shown DD and Lederhose's syndrome in a female non-epileptic patient who received phenobarbitone for migraine headaches. When the phenobarbitone was discontinued, she improved. Why phenobarbitone should effect changes in the fascia of the palm is uncertain. Critchley et al (1976) have suggested that it may cause release of peripheral growth factors which may affect the myofibroblast.

CONCLUSIONS

1. There is a higher incidence of DD in alcoholics than in the general population. The link between DD and alcoholism may be related to the metabolic effect of alcohol on fat and prostaglandin metabolism.
2. There is a higher incidence of DD in diabetics than in the general population. Diabetics with DD have a milder, often non-surgical and more radially located DD. Non-diabetics with DD have a high incidence of chemical diabetes mellitus. The

metabolic link between DD and diabetes may relate to glycosylation or to advanced fibroblast ageing.

3. There is an increased incidence of DD in epileptic populations. The link is probably an altered tissue metabolism secondary to drug therapy. Non-epileptics with DD often have electroencephalogram changes that are not entirely explained by age.

4. When studying associations between DD and other diseases, surgeons should be aware that those patients who require surgical treatment for DD represent a small percentage of the Dupuytren's population.

S. W. Meagher

24 Manual work and industrial injury: a personal commentary

To determine the current opinion concerning the relationship of manual work and industrial injury to Dupuytren's disease (DD), statements related to this topic were submitted to the current delegates to the International Federation of Societies for Surgery of the Hand and to one member of the American Society for Surgery of the Hand in each one of the United States of America.

DD MAY BE WORK-RELATED AND SOMETIMES QUALIFIES FOR COMPENSATION

Twenty-eight respondents agreed with this statement, an equal number disagreed and 2 expressed no opinion.

In the Commonwealth of Massachusetts the administrative judges of the Industrial Accident Board rely on the opinion expressed by the medical experts for the plaintiff and defendant insurer and, on occasion, the opinion expressed by an impartial physician to determine whether or not the plaintiff is eligible for compensation. Therefore, it is important for involved physicians to be familiar with the investigations and opinions expressed in contemporary literature to assist the administrative judges in making a just decision in each case.

DD CAN BE CAUSED BY THE TRAUMA OF WORK

Nine respondents indicated that DD could be caused by the trauma of work; 2 of these individuals qualified their assent by stipulating the presence of a predilection for the disease. A total of 46 respondents felt that it could not be caused by the trauma of work and 3 held no opinion on the matter.

There is no absolute evidence to prove that DD can be caused by the trauma of work. Mikkelsen (1978) found a higher prevalence of DD disease and more severe contractures in people doing hard manual work than in those doing light or nonmanual work. An opposing view was expressed by Hueston (1960) who suggested that decreased hand activity might be a factor determining the appearance of contracture in chronic invalids. Neither Herzog (1951) nor Fisk (1985) found that occupation had an effect upon the disease process. Roberts (1981) cited vibration as an exogenous factor in 2 cases of DD involving grinding wheel use. Neither case had a familial history. In Skoog's (1957) cases 44% of his 300 patients had a familial history. Are we to conclude that the remainder of his cases were due to trauma despite the problems involved in obtaining accurate familial information? His findings of microtears and haemorrhages would seem to spotlight the presence of trauma.

If a traumatic element exists and aggravates the condition, the claimant should not be deprived of compensation. De la Caffinière (1985) imposed the qualification that a history of prolonged hard manual work should be present to consider DD as a compensatable condition.

PROLONGED FORCEFUL USE OF TOOL HANDLES CAN AGGRAVATE DD

The majority of those surveyed believe that prolonged use of tool handles can aggravate DD.

A total of 31 respondents agreed with this statement and 24 disagreed. Three expressed no opinion.

There is a logical basis for endorsing this statement. The longitudinal bands of the palmar aponeurosis lie superficial to the flexor tendons. This location places these bands of fascia prominently in the palm and exposes them to pressure from outside in a manner which would not exist if they were located between the rays of the hand. Because of their density, the rigid unyielding flexor tendons and metacarpals beneath do not significantly cushion or absorb pressure from tool handles and the hard angular edges of stock which increase as grasping pressure increases. This permits considerable compression on the radially arranged elements of the palmar fascia.

However, a wide variety of tool handle shapes would not produce the high incidence of involvement in the ring and small finger rays of the hand that is familiar to all. Ring and plier-type handles which are commonly in use for stripping, holding, crimping and cutting tools do not even come into contact with the central and distal palm of the hand. They are manipulated by the digits, thenar muscles and the thumb.

It is true that skin and subcutaneous fat absorb and dampen the transmission of energy to underlying structures from hand tools and the effect of torque from rotary movement but this ameliorating effect varies according to the thickness of skin and underlying fat. At skin creases subcutaneous fat is non-existent, making these areas more susceptible to injury. Hueston (1963) provides an illustration of an inked hand that has grasped a hammer. This shows that the areas of skin creases are protected by a shielding compression of segmental fat pads in the palm and digits during flexion. The implication is that the skin creases are not directly exposed to contact pressure or torque from tool handles. The conclusion is somewhat misleading because the presence or absence of skin crease contact on a tool handle depends upon the type and diameter of the tool handle. Large handles encountered on pick and axe handles and plier-type handles force the fingers into greater extension, exposing the skin adjacent to the creases to direct trauma from compressive forces.

Pistol-grip pneumatic tools commonly cause trigger fingers in the automotive industry. It is reasonable to believe that the constant compression of the palm by pistol grips, with the added factors of vibration and torque, have an aggravating effect upon established contractures.

Tools made from flat bar stock such as files without handles may traumatize the skin and palmar fascia significantly. Poorly maintained tools with scarred and chipped plastic handles can also have a traumatic effect. One can find scrapers with square handles that present four points of pressure upon narrow areas of skin and fascia, preventing diffusion of force over a broad area. Deep and widely fluted handles pinch off areas of skin and fascia and add an injurious torquing to the tissues supplementary to the basic compressive force when making rotary movements with screwdrivers. Tool handles with a low coefficient of friction, e.g. untextured metal, polished plastic and gloss urethane, require the application of excessive force for tool retention, increasing blanching of the skin and fascia which may result in periods of relative hypoxia when such a tool is used extensively throughout the work day. This may be a cause of the hypoxia cited by Yodaiken (1979) which he believes is related to the thickening of the basal laminae of vessels. Kischer & Speer (1984) consistently found occluded microvessels in Dupuytren's contracture bands and nodules due to the large number of concentric lamina layers.

The slender hand, lightly muscled with thin subcutaneous padding, is more susceptible to microtrauma from extensive use of narrow and angular tool handles. DD is infrequently seen in very obese people which may have some relevance. Striking tools with handles which have low shock absorbance permit a high transmission of energy into the palmar tissues. An unclad metal hammer handle permits the full force of each blow to enter into the hand as well as into the work piece.

The foregoing theories and findings may support Skoog's (1957) belief that manual labor may result in trauma to the palmar fascia resulting in microtears and haemorrhages. Clarkson (1961) and Larsen (1975) believe that DD can be precipitated by trauma in individuals.

Hunter & Ogdon (1975) express the concept of fibre (and fibril) orientations of connective tissues being a living 'diagram of the forces' reflecting the longitudinal thickening in response to the lines of stress such as those encountered in sustained forceful repetitive digital extensions in manual work. They believe that when the disease process spreads to join the dermis to aponeurosis, the strains produced in the tissue by normal hand movements act on the Dupuytren's tissue, resulting in remodelling.

REPETITIVE TRAUMA SUCH AS POUNDING WITH THE HAND, HOLDING A STENOGRAPHIC PAD OR A HAND TOOL CAN PRODUCE DD AT THE POINT OR POINTS OF CONTACT WITH THE HAND

Seven respondents agreed with this statement; 45 disagreed and 6 expressed no opinion.

Skoog presented his findings of iron pigment at the centre of new connective tissue, which he felt provided evidence of microtrauma resulting in small haemorrhages in the aponeurosis. He further reported that microscopic examination of surgical specimens also revealed recent partial ruptures in the fascia and various stages of scar formation from fibroblastic activity to mature scar formation. This lends credence to the importance of repetitive microtrauma to the palmar fascia by pounding with the hand on tight assembly parts, the forceful use of hand tools with scarred or angular handle shapes and the handling of very sharp-edged stock repetitively.

Skoog also offers an interesting theory to explain the appearance of knuckle pads. He believes that the large range of movement in the proximal interphalangeal joints contributes to the development of ruptures of the fibrils of the fascia overlying the joint, which would result in the same sequence of events of scar formation at the sites of microscopic tears with a subsequent enlargement of the knuckle pad.

DISCUSSION

Skoog (1967) found that the transverse fibres of the palmar aponeurosis were not involved in 300 hands examined at operation. He pointed out that this ligament is intimately related to the paratendinous septa which together form a well defined tunnel system in the rays of the palm. Flexion and extension movements do not stress the transverse elements of the palmar aponeurosis. The paratendinous septae are likewise spared from the distribution of stress in flexion and extension in the hand. One can speculate upon the genetic specificity of the Dupuytren's process which involves the longitudinal portion of the palmar aponeurosis and spares the transverse ligament beneath. This would lead us to consider the importance of repetitive flexion and extension of the longitudinal fibres as one factor producing the fascial ruptures described by Skoog.

Is the sparing of certain aponeurotic elements due to genetics or stress lines? The reports of Skoog, Brody et al (1981), and Hunter & Ogdon (1975) command us to give weight to the effect of repetitive movements in the development of Dupuytren's contracture, whether or not one believes that predisposition is a prerequisite.

Meagher (1971) has postulated that the tissues of each individual have a threshold of resistance to pathological change. When that threshold is crossed by too many units of work in a unit of time over a period of time, a pathological change in the tissues will result. The use of incorrect work performance movements, defectively designed hand tools or work stations may accelerate the onset of pathological change in the tissues. There is no basis for believing that the tissues involved in DD are immune to this process, at least to the extent of aggravation if not causation.

CONCLUSIONS

The author believes that an acceptance of a genetic predisposition in most cases is warranted. It would appear to be premature to state that in every case a genetic link is an essential factor. Certainly the histological findings of Skoog and Kischer & Speer (1984) and the theories expressed by Brody et al (1981), Hunter & Ogdon (1975) and Skoog indicate that microtrauma and repetitive digital flexion and extension may play a definite role in the formation of contractures and knuckle pads.

The tissues of DD are no less susceptible to the aggravating effects of heavy manual work and selected hand tool designs than other soft tissues. The presence of tenderness in an established contracture should be considered a physical sign of aggravation when combined with an appropriate history of proximate cause. Patients with such a finding should not be deprived of compensation in jurisdictions which consider aggravation of a pre-existing condition a complaint worthy of compensation.

25 A single injury to the hand

In Chapters 19 and 24 Mikkelsen and Meagher associate Dupuytren's disease (DD) with manual work. The former author found an increased prevalence of DD in heavy manual workers. The significant differences between manual and non-manual workers did not appear until after 60 years of age, that is, until after a lifetime of work and at an age when DD is most common. It is difficult to evaluate work patterns from epidemiological studies because workers change jobs and jobs change with time. Sedentary workers often abuse their hands in their hobbies or sporting activities. However, Mikkelsen's results suggest that manual work is not associated with the early appearance or the rapid progress of disease.

Meagher has made a case to associate DD with manual work on the basis that Dupuytren's tissues are no less susceptible to the aggravating effects of manual labour and hand tool designs than other soft tissues. Unlike trigger finger and carpal tunnel syndrome there are no work patterns — other than heavy manual labour — associated with DD. Further, there is no report in the literature of a series or even a case report of DD related to a sporting activity. Professional golfers, racquet, baseball and cricket players as well as professional musicians apply prolonged and repetitive stresses to their hands. They often develop soft tissue injury at the wrist, elbow and shoulder, but are not prone to DD.

Thus it is doubtful whether the onset of DD is associated with use or abuse of the hands and there is no evidence that the course of the disease is influenced by activity or inactivity of the hands. However, many cases have been reported of DD appearing after a single injury. Clarkson (1961) reported only 2 cases of his own but discussed several cases provided by his authoritative colleagues. His paper is most supportive of a single injury causing DD. Hueston (1962) reported 11 cases of forearm fracture, forearm infection, and elbow and shoulder dislocation in which the onset or progress of DD occurred within months of injury. He attributed this phenomenon to immobilization of the hand with swelling and vascular changes. In the same study Hueston included 21 patients with 'acute invalidism' due to myocardial infarction, lower limb injury, eye surgery, abdominal surgery, pulmonary tuberculosis, and diabetic crisis. These patients also developed DD, presumably because of enforced bedrest. There are no similar reports, although Hueston stated that Plewes (1956) had noted DD in patients with Sudek's atrophy.

AN EPIDEMIOLOGICAL ANALYSIS

As part of the survey reported in Chapter 20, one of the questions asked was of a history of a single injury associated with the onset of DD. The significant variables compared to those patients who did not have a single injury are listed in Table 25.1. Race was not a factor. The prevalence in northern European and Japanese people was the same. More males, and also more males of less than 45 years of age were involved. Most patients were manual labourers. The disease was less severe: more frequently it was unilateral and only one ray was involved.

This analysis identifies a group of young male labourers in whom a single injury to the hand may

Table 25.1 Variables associated with patients who related a single injury to the onset of disease

Variable	Injury (n = 106)	No injury (n = 1114)	p Value
Northern European origin	81%	83%	NS
Japanese origin	12%	10%	NS
Male	91%	76%	<0.02
Age at onset if Male < 45 years	18%	12%	<0.02
Manual labour	58%	42%	<0.002
Unilateral disease	47%	32%	<0.02
One ray involved	46%	35%	<0.05
Outcome at PIPJ V			
Perfect	29%	18%	<0.05
Improved	63%	55%	NS
Worse	8%	27%	<0.05
Recurrence and extension	17%	23%	NS

PIPJ V = fifth proximal interphalangeal joint.
NS = not significant.

have precipitated the appearance of rather mild disease. It is noteworthy that racial origin and the diathesis factors, except age, had no significant influence.

ANALYSIS OF A PERSONAL SERIES

A total of 309 fully documented cases were reviewed in order to select those patients in whom a close relationship between a single injury and the onset of DD was likely. The following guidelines were used to select the patients:

1. History of a single injury to the hand.
2. Objective evidence of tissue damage, such as scarring or healed fracture.
3. DD in the area of injury.

According to these guidelines 18 patients (6%) of the series qualified. These patients had a palpable nodule or cord in the area of the injury, with the exception of 1 patient with a Colles' fracture. She was included because she was the only patient in the series with a close association in time between Colles' fracture and DD. The other 17 patients were male labourers.

Sixteen of the patients were right hand dominant. Only 2 patients were left-handed and contracture was seen in the left hand alone in only 1 patient (who was right-handed). Bilateral disease was noted in 9 patients.

The extent of disease was minimal in most patients and consisted of a palpable nodule or cord in the area of injury (Fig. 25.1). All but 2 patients were operated upon and they were reviewed 1–18 years later. The preoperative diagnosis in each case was DD but on review of the pathological specimens (by DTS), the tissue of 9 patients was considered to be scar tissue and not fibromatosis.

Histological features of DD and scar tissue

Microscopically, distinguishing between scar tissue resulting from trauma and DD may be difficult. This is true when examining specimens of the residual stage of DD when the fibroblastic proliferation has completely subsided and the cellular nodule is replaced by acellular tendon-like collagenous tissue. Similarly, a recent hyperplastic scar can mimic the proliferative stage of DD so that cases of flexion contracture following trauma could be mistaken for DD resulting in trauma being credited as the causal and aetiological factor. The presence of a cellular nodule is necessary to confirm the diagnosis of DD.

It is therefore important to be critical about the histological diagnosis of DD especially in patients with a history of previous trauma. Criteria for differentiating between DD scar tissue are listed in Table 25.2.

Lesions of DD are best delineated from adjacent fibroconnective tissue under lower power examination. The proliferating fibroblastic nodules (Luck 1959) are angiocentric and cellular (Fig. 25.2), whereas in the involutional and residual stages, the tissues tend to be less cellular or fibrous cord-like, and on cross-section may appear nodular but relatively acellular (Fig. 25.3).

Cleft-like spaces which are tissue artefacts from sectioning are frequently encountered in DD lesions. There artefactitious spaces may reflect the non-infiltrative nature and the lack of adhesions between the Dupuytren's lesions and adjacent tissue. Clefting artefacts are seldom noticed in scar tissue. While clefts are peculiar to DD, hyaline change of collagen is almost pathognomonic of

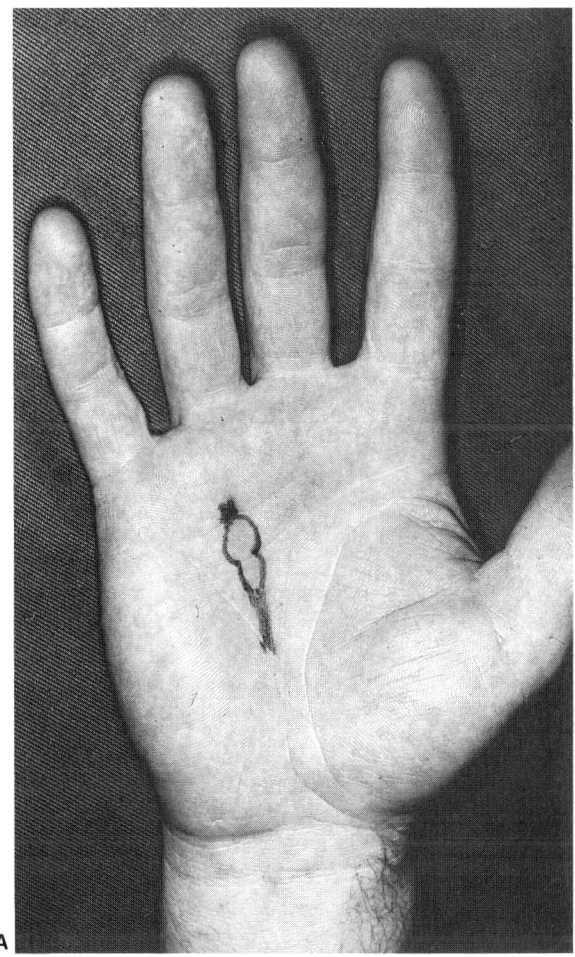
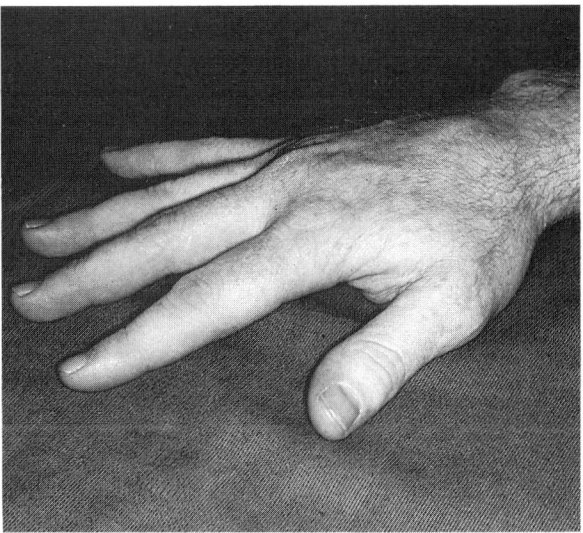

Fig. 25.1 SG suffered a severe crush injury to the right hand at age 17. There were no fractures and only a minor laceration of the index finger but the hand remained swollen for about 2 months. He first noted thickening of the palm at age 22. **A** The hand at 28 years of age. There is a nodule and cord in the fourth ray. **B** He cannot lay the hand flat. Metacarpophalangeal joint contracture is progressive.

Table 25.2 Histopathological differences between DD and scar tissue due to trauma

Dupuytren's disease	Scar tissue due to trauma
Lesions tend to be nodular in configuration in the proliferative stage; nodular or cord-like during involutional and residual stages	Irregular in shape and configuration related to type of trauma
Non-encapsulated but usually well demarcated from surrounding tissue; may have clefting artefact (Fig. 25.1)	Infiltrative boundary and merges with surrounding tissue; no fixation artefact (Fig. 25.2)
Predominantly subcutaneous in location with fibrous cord-like extensions to overlying dermis	Predominantly dermal or deep dermal in location
No epidermal reaction	Epidermal reaction, i.e. atrophy or hypertrophy may be present; focal loss of dermal elastic fibres and adnexal structures
Fibroblasts in proliferative lesions tend to be uniform and angiocentric	More pleomorphic fibroblasts, spindle or stellate-shaped; haphazardly arranged
No hyaline change	Hyaline change of collagen is the hallmark of keloid or hypertrophic scar.
Minimal inflammation	Inflammation may be marked; may have foreign body-type granulomatous inflammation.

hyperplastic scar tissue. Hyalinization describes a morphological change of collagen characterized by intense eosinophilia. The collagen fibres become widened, homogenized, and assume a pinky-red and almost refractile property (Fig. 25.4). Such a change has never been described in Dupuytren's tissue.

Under higher magnification, fibroblastic proliferation in scar tissue tends to be more disorganized and the fibroblasts are usually more

268 DUPUYTREN'S DISEASE

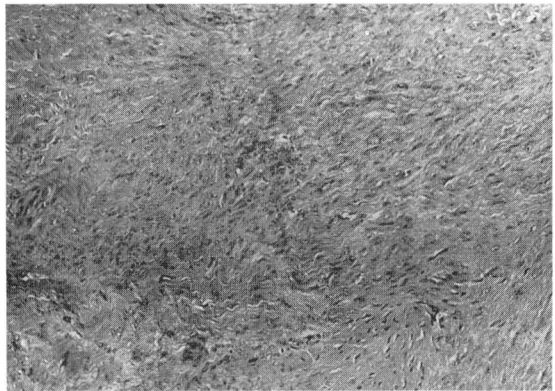

Fig. 25.2 Proliferating fibrous nodule of DD. Note the cellularity and lack of hyaline change of the collagen. Haematoxylin-eosin stained; × 100 original magnification.

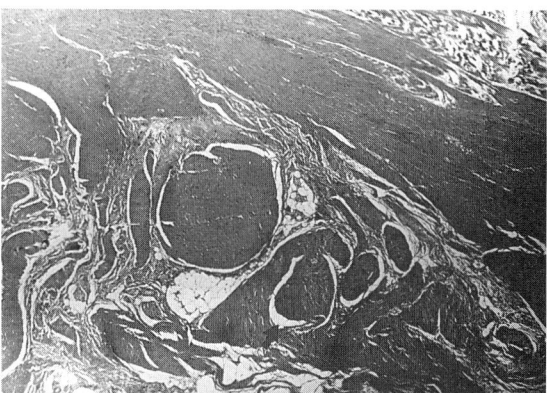

Fig. 25.3 Cord-like and nodular profile of residual tissue of DD. Arrow shows cleft-like space which is tissue artefact commonly observed in this type of lesion. Haematoxylin-eosin stained; × 25 original magnification.

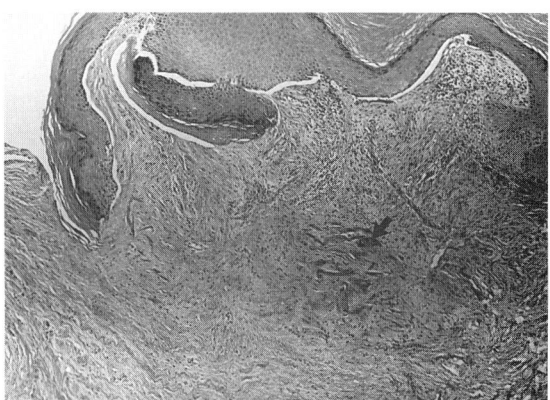

Fig. 25.4 Skin showing hyperplastic scar in dermis. Arrow shows hyaline change of collagen pathognomonic of scar. Haematoxylin-eosin stained; × 40 original magnification.

pleomorphic cytologically with their cell bodies varying from spindle to stellate-shaped. Although haemorrhage and haemosiderin pigment deposition may be seen in both lesions, the finding of more intense inflammation or foreign body-type granulomatous reaction would definitely favour the diagnosis of scar due to trauma.

Differential diagnosis of DD and scar

On the basis of the clinical assessment of the nature and course of the disease, but particularly on the pathological report, the 18 patients were placed into three groups, as shown in Table 25.3.

Seven patients were thought to have DD associated with a single injury. Each was injured and noticed DD before age 30. Four of the 7 patients had a severe laceration (perhaps with an element of crush injury; (Figs 25.5 and 25.6). All had both scar tissue and Dupuytren's tissue removed at operation and 2 needed skin grafting. That is, these patients had both scar contracture and Dupuytren's contracture. Three patients in this group had bilateral disease. The disease in the uninjured hand appeared later and was operated upon after the age of 45 in 2 patients.

Two patients were considered to have DD unrelated to their injury. This judgement was made primarily because the age at injury and onset of disease was in the sixth decade, when DD most often appears. Also both patients had 'typical' bilateral disease and there was no appreciable time interval between the onset of disease in the injured and uninjured hand. Nine had fractures of metacarpal IV and V; JP, who was the only female in the series, had a Colles' fracture.

Nine of the patients who were diagnosed as having DD did not have histological evidence of the disease. In 4 of these patients, the nodule disappeared (Fig. 25.7). In the other 5 patients, the surgical specimens revealed scar tissue rather than fibromatosis. Two of these 9 patients were thought to have bilateral DD. In JF the nodule disappeared on the injured side but a nodule remains on the uninjured side 14 years later without progression. In TR the cord removed from the little finger was scar tissue (Fig. 25.8). A palpable cord in the other hand is unlikely to be DD because he had similar injuries to that hand.

Table 25.3 The relationship of injury to DD

Patient	Site of disease	Age at injury - Injury	Age at injury - Disease	Operation	Type of injury	Extent of disease	Type of operation operation	Disease in other hand	Reason for category
Dupuytren's disease related to injury									
SG	Right	17	22	—	Crush	Nodule	None	None	Early onset
RH	Bilateral	29	29	35	Crush	Severe	Dermofasciectomy	Severe	Early onset
AG	Bilateral	29	29	35	Laceration	Nodule and cord	Dermofasciectomy	Nodule	Early onset
RP	Bilateral	20	21	40	Laceration	Nodule and cord	Fasciectomy	Progressive	Early onset
JO	Right	10	?	39	Laceration	Nodule and cord	Fasciectomy	None	Early onset
RDd	Right	10	?	51	Laceration	Nodule and cord	Dermofasciectomy	None	Early onset
TM	Right	24	24	26	Fracture	Nodule and cord	Fasciectomy	None	Early onset
Dupuytren's disease not related to injury									
LG	Bilateral	52	55	61	Fracture	Nodule	Fasciectomy	Nodule	Typical disease
JP	Bilateral	56	56	59	Fracture	Severe	Fasciectomy	Progressive	Typical disease
Not Dupuytren's disease									
JE	Right	53	53	53	Crush	Nodule	Correct scar contr.	None	Nodule disappeared
DB	Right	45	45	45	Crush	Nodule	Correct scar contr.	None	Pathology
RK	Right	51	51	56	Crush	Nodule	Excise nodule	None	Pathology
RD	Right	34	34	34	Crush	Nodule	Correct scar contr.	None	Nodule disappeared
JF	Bilateral	40	41	—	Crush	Nodule	None	Nodule	Nodule disappeared
JL	Right	25	25	34	Puncture	Nodule	Fasciectomy	None	Pathology
TR	Bilateral	28	28	28	Fracture	Cord	Fasciectomy	Cord	Pathology
FP	Left	34	34	34	Electric burn	Cord	Correct scar contr.	None	Pathology
RDo	Right	61	61	61	Infection	Cord	Fasciectomy	None	Pathology

It is likely that all patients who develop DD, including those with a single injury, have a genetic predisposition to the disease (Hueston 1987). Of the 7 patients in Table 25.3 whose disease was related to injury, 3 had bilateral disease and 2 others had a positive family history. The absence of a family history in the remaining 2 patients is meaningless because it is well known that most patients with DD do not know the correct status of even close relatives.

Both series reveal that age is a factor in relating DD to a single injury. The average age of onset is 48.3±14.5 years in men and 57.6±14.2 years in women (Chapter 20). In the large series, a single injury was associated with young men with minimal disease. In my personal series all 7 patients whose DD was related to a single injury were under 30 years of age when the disease appeared.

Perhaps a single injury could precipitate DD in an older person, but there is no evidence from these studies to support such a theory. If DD appears within the expected age group, it would not be possible to assign a causal relationship to a single injury.

Age is an important factor when assigning a causal relationship between DD and a single injury. But age is also a feature of an increased diathesis in which the patient develops early and aggressive disease. The diathesis factors associated with severe disease are discussed in Chapter 22. Before accepting and rejecting a causal relationship, the other diathesis factors must be considered:

1. *Race*. Most people with DD are of northern European origin, although the disease is not

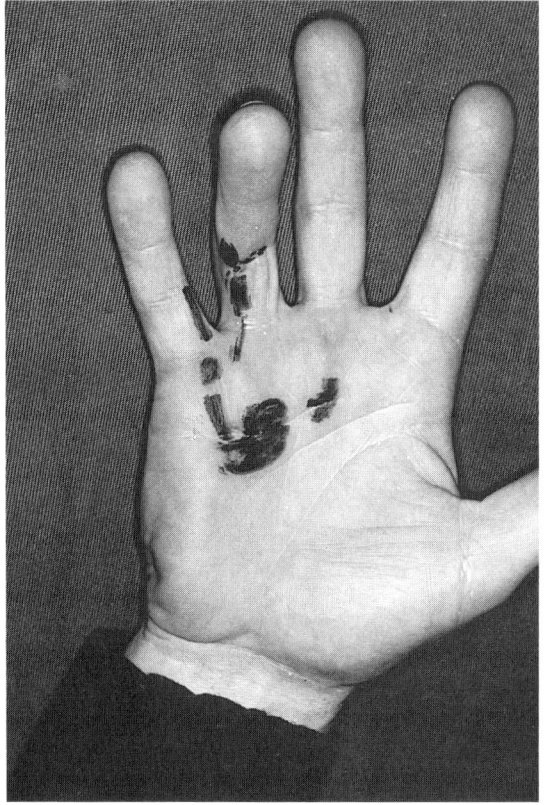 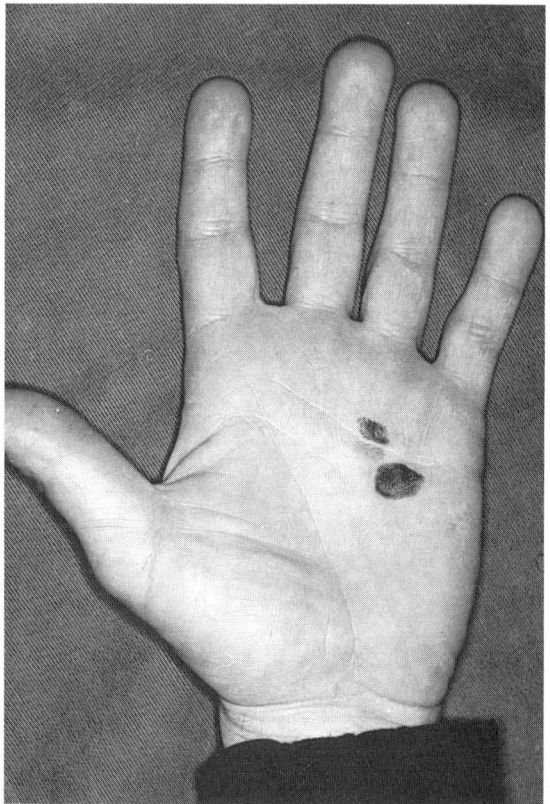

Fig. 25.5 Patient AG: a 35-year-old labourer who had a severe laceration of the right ring finger at age 29. This healed with a flexion contracture of the finger and shortly after he noticed thickening in the palm and finger. **A** Appearance of the right hand with scarring in in the finger and DD in the palm. He was treated by excision of DD and correction of the scar contracture. A full thickness skin graft was applied to the finger. He has remained free of disease for 8 years. **B** There are two nodules in the palm of the left hand which were discovered at examination at age 35. It is assumed that this patient's right hand disease appeared early because of the injury but also because of a predisposition to disease.

uncommon in the Orient and India and has been reported in black Africans. In the large series (Chapter 20), the prevalence of a single injury was the same in Japanese and northern Europeans. Thus, racial origin is not a factor which would determine whether DD is associated with a single injury.

2. *Epilepsy and diabetes mellitus*. The prevalence of both these diseases is increased in patients with DD. If the patient had either of these diseases, it would not be possible to establish a causal relationship with a single injury.
3. *Bilateral disease*. Most patients have bilateral disease when first seen, but bilateral disease in a young person is evidence of a strong diathesis. If a person had bilateral disease within 2 or 3 years of injury, it would be unreasonable to assume any causal relationship between the injury and disease.
4. *Knuckle pads and plantar nodules*. Because ectopic deposits are evidence of an increased diathesis to disease, a causal relationship could not be accepted if either was present.

Thus, to qualify for consideration of an association between a single injury and the onset of DD, the individual must be younger than the usual age of onset (less than 40 years old), be free of epilepsy or diabetes, have unilateral disease and have no ectopic deposits.

The types of injuries considered were crush injuries, lacerations and fractures (Table 25.3). It

A SINGLE INJURY TO THE HAND   271

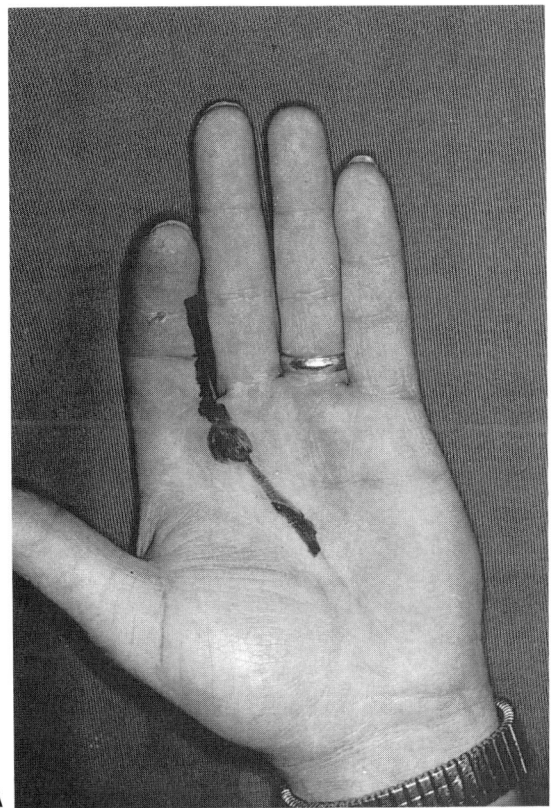

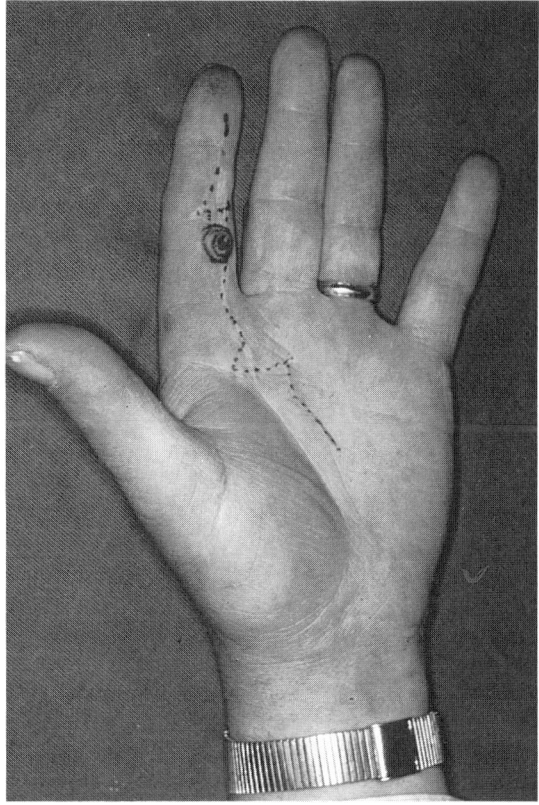

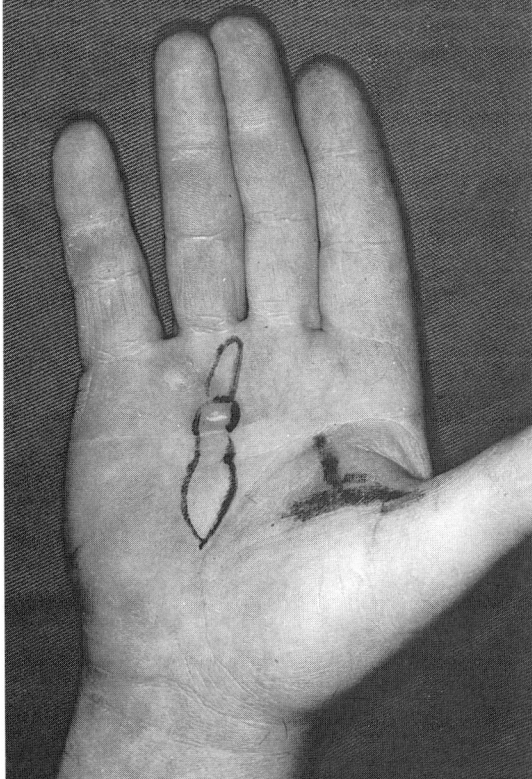

Fig. 25.6 Patient RP: a 40-year-old farmer who cut his left hand with a chain saw at age 20. There has been gradual contraction since then. **A** Note the unusual pattern of disease which corresponds to the skin scar. There is 55° contracture at the proximal interphalangeal joint of the index finger. **B** Appearance of his hand 5 years after fasciectomy. He has full flexion and extension but has a recurrent nodule over the proximal phalanx. This has now been removed. **C** The disease in his right hand. There is a causative relationship between injury and disease in the left hand but also a predisposition to disease.

would be expected that most damage would occur from crush injuries and fractures, but lacerations produced the most convincing evidence of an association between DD and injury. These 4 patients had severe lacerations, perhaps associated with an element of crush. The lacerations themselves produced flexion contracture and this was compounded by Dupuytren's contracture. Both scar and DD were confirmed histologically.

The mechanism by which DD is precipitated by injury is not explained by our studies, although it might be due to the tethering effect of scar tissue

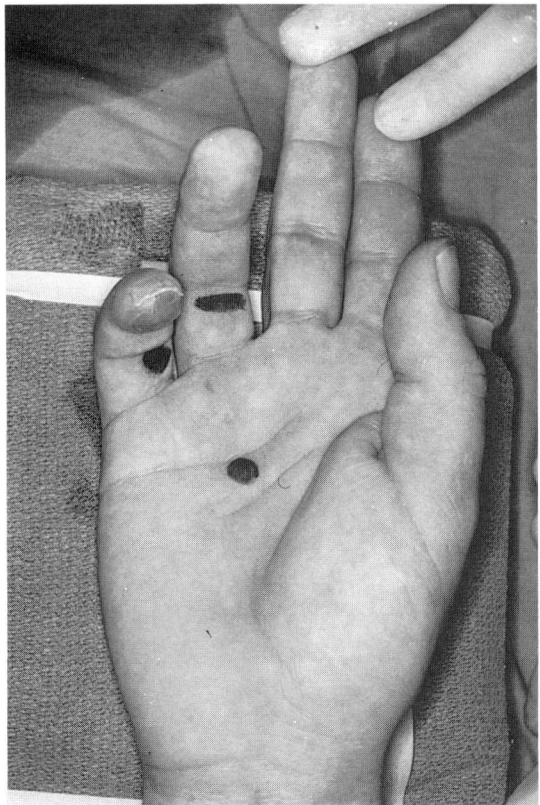

Fig. 25.7 Patient DB: a 45-year-old diesel mechanic. He had avulsed the tip of his right little finger in a drive shaft 3 months before. A split thickness skin graft was applied; this was slow to heal. He was unable to return to work because of extreme pain in the fingertip and flexion contracture of the finger. Appearance of the hand 6 months after injury when a cross-finger flap is to be applied to the fingertip. Three supposed Dupuytren's nodules are marked. The nodule within the little finger was removed and histologically found to be scar tissue. Three months later the remaining two nodules had disappeared.

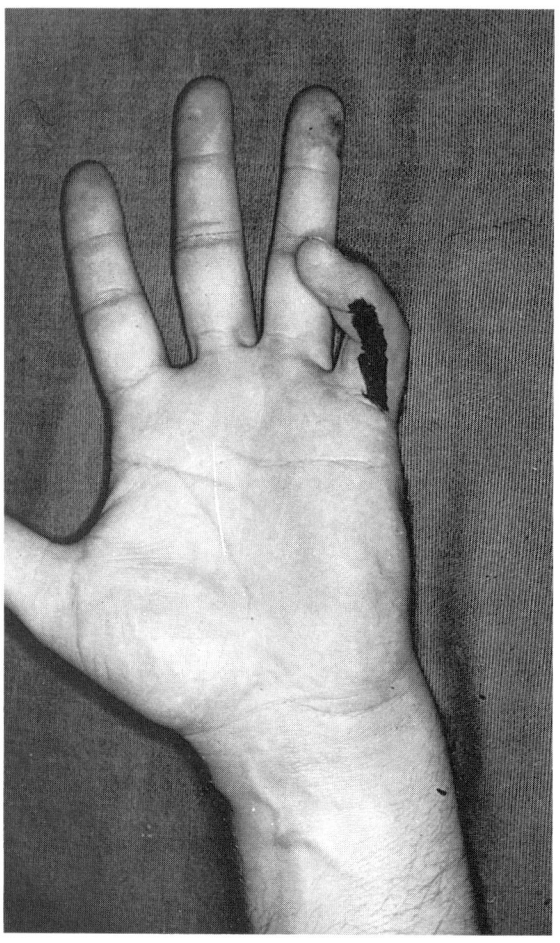

Fig. 25.8 Patient TR: a 28-year-old farmer who hit a wall with his fist, suffering a fracture of the fifth metacarpal. The finger was immobilized in flexion for three weeks. A palpable cord was present but there was no nodule. Note the slight hyperextension at the metacarpophalangeal joint. The tissue removed at operation was scar tissue.

on the fascia involved in DD. This would occur with lacerations and perhaps crush injuries. The alteration in the biomechanics at the site of injury could hasten the onset of DD in the genetically susceptable fascia. It is unlikely that swelling and immobilization of the hand were the causal agents. Both are common after severe injury, especially fractures and particularly following Colles' fracture. More permanent scarring resulting from tissue disruption is the likely cause.

The single patient with Colles' fracture (JP) in our series of 309 patients reflects the experience of Stewart et al (1985) who noted only 2 patients with joint contracture due to DD in 235 patients after Colles' fracture. On further questioning, it was found that JP had DD before her injury. Thickening of the palmar fascia following injury such as Colles' fracture is not uncommon. It is also seen in patients with reflex sympathetic dystrophy as well as after an operation for DD. This type of thickening is transient.

Only three metacarpal V fractures were selected

for this study even though many other patients in the series gave a history of a previous fracture in the hand or finger. Malunion of a fracture of metacarpal V frequently results in a compensatory flexion contracture at proximal interphalangeal joint V. A fibrous band often develops on the ulnar side of the finger originating near the tendon of insertion of the abductor digiti minimi muscle and extending distally to be attached to the skin. This band is the result rather than the cause of the flexion contracture. It is also seen in other states of flexion contracture such as malunion of the proximal phalanx, camptodactyly, and burns, and simply represents foreshortening of the normal fascia. TM, TR, and FP are examples of patients with this condition. A lateral cord is frequent in patients with DD but invariably a palpable nodule is also present.

There was no example of a hyperextension injury leading to DD although there may have been an element of hyperextension in some of the crush injuries. Gordon & Anderson (1961) presented a well documented case report supported by histological evidence of DD and Hueston (1962) reported 6 cases. Hyperextension with forceful tearing of a contracting cord can also overcome joint contracture as reported by Grace et al (1984) and many years ago by Adams (1878). It seems that hyperextension can cause or cure the disease.

A nodule in the palm or finger is thought to be a pathognomonic sign of DD, and yet in 9 of our patients the nodule either disappeared spontaneously or histologically was not DD. The Dupuytren's nodule does not disappear although it becomes less obvious as the disease progresses to joint contracture and the cords become more prominent. Thus, the disappearance of thickened fascia or discrete nodules indicates that the process was not DD.

CONCLUSIONS

Although the vast majority of injuries to the hand do not result in DD or even thickening of the palmer aponeurosis, we have shown that occasionally a single injury can precipitate the onset of DD. Presumably this occurs in genetically susceptible individuals and our studies suggest that a causal relationship can only be established in young people.

Thickening in the palm, nodule formation, or a palpable cord does not necessarily constitute DD. If a definite decision is to be made that a specific injury has precipitated its onset, a histological diagnosis of the tissue should be obtained. In this regard, it would be helpful to compensation agencies and fairer to workers and employers if criteria were established to serve as guidelines when establishing a relationship between a single injury and the onset of DD. The following are suggested:

1. The appearance of DD before age 40 in men and 50 in women suggests a causal relationship unless the individual expresses a strong diathesis such as the presence of epilepsy, diabetes, bilateral disease or ectopic deposits.
2. If the DD is bilateral, the disease in the uninjured hand should have appeared after age 40 in men and age 50 in women.
3. The injury was within the hand.
4. There is objective evidence of injury.
5. DD is in the area of the injury in the hand.
6. DD appeared within 2 years of injury.
7. Histological proof of fibromatosis is needed to make a definite diagnosis of DD.

SECTION 4

Aetiology and pathogenesis

An insight into the Italian literature on aetiology and treatment

INTRODUCTION

As can be seen from the 100 or so papers in the literature, Italian researchers have made a substantial contribution towards the aetiology and treatment of Dupuytren's Disease (DD). One of the earliest and most complete monographs on DD was written by an Italian. This 400-page treatise by Ferrarini (1941) offers a wealth of original research on the normal and pathological palmar fascia. Its publication during the Second World War, however, and the untimely death of the author in action have resulted in its being virtually unknown, especially abroad. Many of Ferrarini's intuitions and many aspects of DD that he had already covered at length were thus denied to those who came after him.

THE PAST

Pathology

Ferrarini (1941) made a detailed study of the palmar fascia in DD. He carried out a thorough histological examination of all the palmar tissues from the hands of 5 cadavers with Dupuytren's disease. His findings were clear evidence that DD is fibrotic in nature and that only the palmar lesion alone is primary disease, compared with the damage observed in the skin, vessels and surrounding tissues.

He also undertook an extensive investigation, covering both clinical cases and the literature, and especially medicolegal sources, of the relation between injury and the onset of the contracture. He did find a certain relationship between trauma and DD. Even so, he asserted that the view that injury is responsible for all forms of DD could not be accepted.

Butturini (1950) observed avitaminosis E in DD patients and proposed that the disease should be treated medically through the protracted administration of high doses of vitamin E.

Next came a set of studies on vascular alterations in the palms of DD patients, using oscillography and photoplethysmography (Pietrogrande & Maiotti 1955: Sanmartino 1957), oscillography, rheography and arteriography (Parrini & Brunelli 1959) and arteriography and plethysmography (Becchi et al 1972). Similar work was also done by Verga et al (1972). All these investigations stated that *vascular alterations are secondary to contracture of the palmar fascia.*

Mention must be made of the important histological investigations of the structure of the normal fascia carried out by Candiollo (1956), an anatomist in Turin.

Histochemical studies by Tessari & Parrini (1959) revealed a fall in total nitrogen and water and an increase in hexosamines and sulphuric fractions in the fascia mucopolysaccharides in DD. Further investigations of the mucopolysaccharides led Spina & Tessari (1960) to suggest that DD might be the local expression of collagenosis. In view of the greater frequency of DD in central nervous system patients, Ballettico & Campailla (1972) collected electroencephalograms from a group of DD subjects. They reported that alterations were not infrequent, but were apparently devoid of any specific meaning.

Treatment

The surgical management of DD attracted the attention of Italian surgeons at the beginning of the 20th century and the first reports of experience gained with the recently introduced techniques soon appeared (Salaghi 1902; Tricomi 1907).

Some workers proposed various kinds of personal incisions. A few of these incisions subsequently found favour, though proposed by other writers and obviously bearing different names. It was after the Second World War, however, that a true surgical philosophy towards this disease was adopted, especially by orthopaedic and plastic surgeons. Owing to the influence exerted by the French school on Italian hand surgery, the earliest papers were on the technique of Iselin & Dickemann and that of Tubiana.

The approaches to the two main questions raised by the surgical management of DD — the type of incision and extent of fasciectomy — reveal the following preferences: split Z incision (Parrini & Brunelli 1959; Marsonano 1965; Mantero et al 1966); the transverse according to McIndoe (Calati & Morelli 1960); Tubiana's sinusoid incision (Vigliani & Rodighiero 1964: Chiandussi et al 1979).

Operti (1979) and Luppino et all (1974) carried out an extensive study of all the possible access routes and described a large number of them.

Parrini & Brunelli (1959), Vigliani & Rodighiero (1964), Gasperini & Paparoni (1969) and Mollica et al (1980) declared themselves in favour of total fasciectomy, whereas subtotal or selective fasciectomy found favour with Mantero et al (1966), Tasca et al (1969), Santoni-Rugiu (1969) and Losapio et all (1978).

De Negri (1972) proposed a personal method for the treatment of DD namely total fasciectomy via multiple transverse incisions in both the palm and the fingers. In cases where the process extended to the skin, he resorted to a bipedicled flap.

The problem of treating recurrences was addressed by Lauro & Verga (1970), Rinaldi & Orso (1974) and Morelli (1982). Conservative radiotherapy was the subject of papers by Marsico (1963) and Pastremoli (1968).

Increasing diffusion of scientific news has also led to the extension of newly emerging techniques in Italy. Salvi (1973) introduced McCash's 'open palm' technique. Another illustration of this trend is the introduction of selective aponeurectomy according to Skoog by Corrado et al (1979) and Panciera et al (1980).

THE PRESENT

The watershed year was 1982: DD was the main subject of the Italian Hand Surgery Society's national congress at Turin. This resulted in a thorough overview of the Italian approach to the pathology of and treatment of the disease.

Pathology

An extensive statistical study by Corvella (1982) covering the entire population of Piemonte reached the interesting conclusion that there is a higher incidence of DD among subjects with pale eyes and straight hair. This is in line with the lower predisposition to DD among Mediterranean people.

Sadun & Ronconi (1982) reported the confirmation of previous histochemical and ultrastructural findings with regard to the palmar fascia in DD. Work by Caroli et all (1982) has helped to show the existence of both arterial and venous vascular alterations. These, however, are secondary to mechanical compression on the part of the contracted tissues.

Tajana et all (1982) have carried out research on the presence and characteristics of myofibroblasts in the pathological tissue of DD. A paper by Moschella et al (1982) examines the thermographic features of affected hands.

Treatment

The papers presented at the Turin congress showed that four techniques are currently in favour among Italian hand surgeons:

1. Iselin & Dieckmann's technique (Brunelli 1982).
2. Tubiana's technique (Messina 1982; Mollica et al 1982).

3. Skoog's technique (Bocchi et al 1982; Fonzone Caccese & Soldati 1982; Santoni-Rugiu 1982). The 'open palm' technique according to McCash (Salvi & Porrino 1982; Valpato et al 1982).

4. Fongo (1982) described Bocca's experience with total fasciectomy using a long, sinusoid digitopalmar incision, opening of the carpal tunnel and 'open' treatment of the wound.

27 Is Dupuytren's disease an inherited disorder?

Many studies have noted Dupuytren's disease (DD) in several members of a family, but the exact nature of the relationship remains unclear. Goyrand (1833) described a severe bilateral contracture in M. Chaine, bursar of his hospital; M. Chaine believed his contracture to be hereditary because his father had also been afflicted.

Present opinion is based on surprisingly few studies. Skoog (1948) reviewed two valuable contributions published in the German language literature by Stackebrandt (1932) and Schroder (1934) who investigated the relatives of DD cases. Stackebrandt suggested that there were two forms of DD — a hereditary (dominant) form and a sporadic form, the latter also being influenced by a hereditary tendency. Schroder considered that he could establish dominant hereditary in 10 of his 30 cases. Studies in twins (Jentsch 1937; Couch 1938; Then Bergh 1939) have shown a similar distribution of DD in twins but it might be argued that all DD has a similar distribution in the hand.

The most detailed analysis available is that of Ling (1963) who examined 832 relatives of 50 patients. He was well aware of the limitations of such investigations.

Firstly, he noted that the number of affected relatives rose from 16% on history taking to 68% after examination of relatives, thus demonstrating that little statistical value can be placed on the familial incidence as suggested by history alone. This is hardly surprising in a non-lethal condition which often has an onset in later life and when many — perhaps most — do not seek treatment. The patient is often unaware of early signs and it would be surprising if relatives were more sensitive to the patient's state. Therefore all information obtained from history alone is of limited value.

Secondly, Ling was aware of the difficulty in establishing the prevalence of a condition with an onset in middle age — the younger generations, although apparently unaffected, may develop it later when the older generation may have passed on. Correction factors were introduced for this. He concluded that a single gene, behaving as a mendelian dominant, was likely to be involved but that DD may not be a homogeneous condition from the pathogenic standpoint.

Thieme (1989) has discussed four possible modes of genetic transmission — sex-linked, polygenic, autosomal dominant and autosomal recessive. He has rejected the sex-linked hypothesis as the ratio of affected male and female first-degree relatives was unchanged in his study group, whether the index patient was male or female (female:male = 0.67). The approximately equal frequency of Dupuytren's disease among parents (84%, age-corrected), siblings (65%) and children (63%) makes a polygenic mechanism extremely unlikely. Thieme compared simple dominant and recessive modes of inheritance for DD. The observed numbers in his study did not differ significantly from those expected for the dominant hypothesis; therefore he concluded that DD is an inherited disease with an autosomal dominant mode of transmission.

Both Ling and Thieme, however, performed their studies in Edinburgh, a high incidence area. It must be asked what is the mode of transmission in Japan (Chapter 21) and in geographical areas with a low incidence. Bocanegra et al (1981) have noted a virtual absence of DD in black patients in Florida despite diabetes, epilepsy or alcoholism. Mennen (1986) has documented six rare cases from South Africa.

Nyberg et al (1982) have recorded the familial transmission of Peyronie's disease as an autosomal trait in three pedigrees. DD was noted in 7 of 9 affected individuals, suggesting that both of these disorders are pleiotropic effects of the same gene in these families.

There appears to be a need for a population study in DD with repeated assessment of families over many years to clarify the question of inheritance.

M. H. Flint and D. A. McGrouther

28 Is Dupuytren's disease a connective tissue response?

In our view Dupuytren's is not so much a disease as a sequence of connective tissue responses. Whilst recognizing the possible influence of exogenous factors such as diabetes, epilepsy and alcoholism in its pathogenesis we believe that ultimately the local responsiveness of palmar connective tissues is of paramount importance. If any of these exogenous factors are relevant it is possible that they operate by causing changes in the physical compliance or biomechanical properties of one or other constituents of the palmar connective tissue continuum. In this way we can regard DD as the common fibroplastic endpoint of a wide variety of exacerbating factors — physical, physicochemical and metabolic — rather than a single disease process.

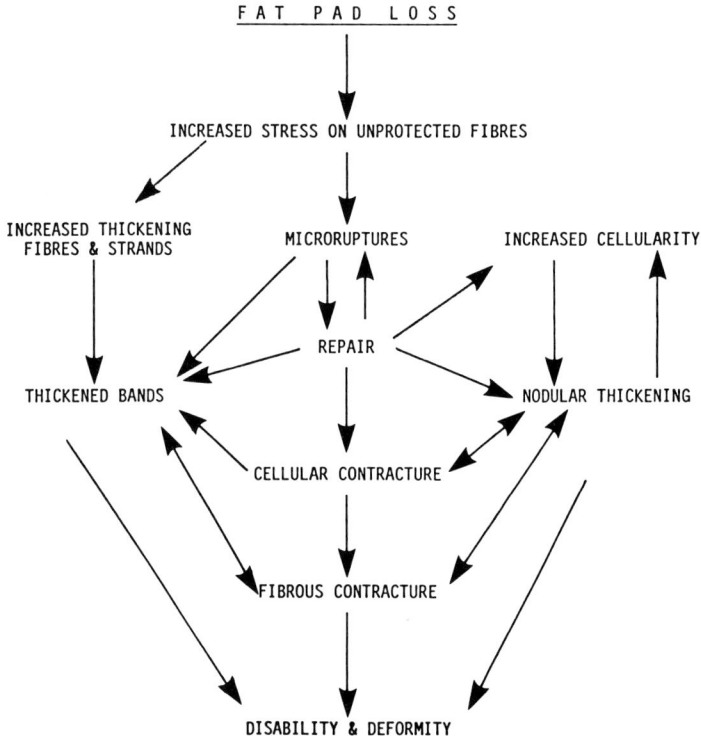

Fig. 28.1 A concept of pathogenesis.

EXTRINSIC AND INTRINSIC CONCEPTS OF PATHOGENESIS (Fig. 28.1)

In several of his writings Hueston developed the concept of the extrinsic and intrinsic theories of the pathogenesis of DD (Hueston 1977, 1985, 1987). He considered that the intrinsic theory stemmed from the demonstration by Skoog (1948) of microruptures within fascial bands and from Millesi (1959, 1965, 1985), who felt that changes in the compliance of the collagen and elastic fibres of the superficial palm, was an initiating factor in the pathogenesis of the disease.

Hueston (MacCallum & Hueston 1962; Hueston 1975, 1977, 1985) based his concept of the extrinsic theory on his observations that primary nodules develop within the subcutaneous space on the anterior aspect of the palmar aponeurosis. However, the work of Millesi (reviewed in Millesi 1985), McGrouther (1982) and Flint et al (1982) in recent times and even the original writings of Dupuytren (1834) and Madelung (1876) indicate that this subcutaneous layer is in reality an integral part of the palmar 'connective tissue continuum' (see Chapter 2). When viewed in this way it is apparent that Hueston's concept of the primary nodule developing within the hypodermis 'on the anterior aspect of the palmar aponeurosis' (MacCallum & Hueston 1962; Hueston 1985) is entirely in accord with our own observations and those of Meyerding et al (1941) and Millesi (1985). We believe that no distinction between extrinsic and intrinsic pathogenesis should be made since the hypodermal connective tissues are anatomically and functionally inseparable from the palmar fascial continuum.

BIOLOGICAL EVENTS IN DD

If in the light of recent knowledge we analyse the various biological events which occur in the Dupuytren's process, we can identify the primary thickening of the superficial palmar fascia, especially the superficial longitudinal bands; the development of intrafascial cellular lesions; secondary fascial thickening; contraction and contracture (Table 28.1). Histochemical and biochemical analysis of the nodular areas reveals a

Table 28.1 Biological events in DD

Primary thickening of superficial palmar fascia, especially superficial longitudinal bands

Matting of longitudinal vertical and oblique fibres and loss of compliance

Loss of hyaluronate from fascial fibres?

Development of intrafascial cellular lesions

Secondary fascial thickening

Contraction — cellular and extracellular

Contracture — connective tissue remodelling

strong similarity between the changes occurring in the nodule and those occurring in hypertrophic scarring (Gabbiani & Majno 1972; Bailey et al 1977; Brickley-Parsons et al 1981; Ehrlich et al 1982; Flint et al 1982). From a biological point of view it appears that the new tissue within the nodular area is most likely to represent a prolonged intrafascial reparative reaction. Histological examination of longitudinal pretendinous fascial bands taken from hands clinically uninvolved by the Dupuytren's process have shown evidence of collagen fibre rupture, endotenon perivascular reaction and cellular proliferation between the fascial bundles and into the zone of fibre dehiscence. The transverse fibres are invariably unaffected. These observations strongly indicate that the lesions in the intrafascial nodular areas are indistinguishable from a wound healing response within the longitudinal fascial strands.

As we have already indicated (see Chapter 13), we believe that the causes of the intrafascial fibre ruptures which lead to the development of the nodular areas are due to changes in the compliance and stress resistance of the longitudinal fascial fibres within the palmar fascial continuum. In young subjects these superficial longitudinal fibre bundles are enclosed within their own paratenon-like sheaths and therefore are able to glide over a short traverse within the sheath in response to changing load. In the young child, these fibres and their gliding sheaths run between compartmentalized fibrofatty loculi which appear to serve the double purpose of insulating the fibres from compressional shock as well as providing a compliant bed through which the fascial fibres can move and adapt to variations in hand flexion and posturing. However, our histological studies have indicated that by early adolescence the fascial fibres have frequently become coalesced and furthermore that the protecting fibrofatty loculi have been lost or replaced by dense collagenous fibrosis. The matting together of the palmar connective tissue continuum during adolescence and growth, and the proportional decrease in intrafascial hyaluronic acid, cannot but severely influence the compliance and adaptability of the longitudinal fascial fibre bundles (McGrouther 1982; Evans 1986). Whereas in the ideal situation in youth they are perfectly designed to transmit tensional loading, the development of the superficial fibrosis and the loss of the free transverse space around the fibres limits their mobility and gives rise to stress concentrations within the longitudinally running collagen fibres.

Although collagen fibres are extremely strong in transmitting or withstanding tensional forces, they are notoriously weak when subjected to compressive or shearing stress. It is probably for this reason that collagen fibres in cartilage are embedded in a proteoglycan-rich matrix which absorbs or dissipates the compressive loads (Rosenberg & Buckwalter 1986). If the longitudinally running collagen fibres in the superficial pretendinous bands are deprived of their protective surrounding fibrofatty pads, and free mobility, they will become vulnerable to compressive and shearing loads and in consequence more liable to viscoelastic failure.

It is important to appreciate that compression or shear loading applied to the palm will result in increased tension loading of the longitudinally running structures. Initially, whilst the protective insulation of the fibrofatty loculi is intact and the longitudinal fascial fibres are still relatively mobile, either compression or shear loading of the palm will lead to increased tensional loading and compensatory thickening and hypertrophy of the longitudinally running fascial fibres. However, if the compressive absorptive capacity of the fat pads has been lost by increasing fibrosis, and particularly if fascial fibre excursion is limited, the collagen fibres of the superficial longitudinal bundles will be less compliant and less able to slide to accommodate the applied stress. These factors would subject regions of longitudinal fascial fibres to greatly increased stress concentrations, especially in zones of greatest anteroposterior mobility such as the fourth and fifth rays of the palm (Bruner 1970; Littler 1977). We feel that the combination of the loss of connective tissue compliance with fibre matting and adherence of the longitudinal fibrous elements of the palmar connective tissue continuum is an extremely important factor in the pathogenesis of DD.

We believe that the cumulative effect of these circumstances provides the basis for the development of intrafascial ruptures. We realize that these changes do not necessarily, or universally, occur in all stressed collagen fibres and that the susceptibility to intrafascial rupture or dehiscence may also be related to genetic differences in the collagen structure or slight differences in glycosaminoglycan content affecting their compliance.

However, the frequency with which regions of intrafascial dehiscence or cellular response in longitudinal pretendinous bands have been observed in our histological and electron microscope studies of uninvolved hands, encourages the belief that it is not an unusual occurrence. The fact that we have not observed these changes in the transverse fibres of Skoog from the uninvolved palms strengthens our belief that the longitudinal fibres may be subject to greater stress than their transverse counterparts.

The identification of cellular reaction even within very minute areas of fibril dehiscence supports our concept that there is a causal relationship between fibre dehiscence, cellular infiltration and nodular development.

We have purposely used the phrase 'intrafascial dehiscence' or 'interfascial rupture' rather than 'fascial rupture' in this and other chapters to emphasize our belief that the primary event frequently occurs within the core of the fascial fibre bundles leaving a rim of intact peripheral fibres. As we have explained elsewhere (Chapter 13), the central core rupture produces a self-perpetuating cellular reparative reaction which does not subside or consolidate in the manner of a repair of a completely divided tendon. As a result the internal lesion tends to spread, extend and progress, producing more fibril damage and a greater cellular reaction. The phenomenon of central core rupture and dehiscence is also observed within the tendoachilles and in the long head of biceps. A series of experimental studies clearly demonstrated the different effects of tension and pressure on tendon morphology and connective tissue cell metabolism (Gillard et al 1977, 1979; Flint et al 1980; Merrilees & Flint 1980) and provided the clue to the interpretation of histological and biochemical data obtained from Dupuytren's and tendoachilles specimens.

We believe that this concept of central core rupture and repair explains the nature and behaviour of the nodular lesion in DD. The lack of unidirectional tensional information to cells in the damaged area leads to the perpetuation of the reparative response, just as it does in dermal hypertrophic scarring where the damage to the deep dermis appears to interfere with the transmission of uniaxial tensional information to the reparative cells in the dermis.

It is our belief that this lack of unidirectional tensional signal to the cells in the reparative area is the cause of perpetuation of their whorl-like disposition, their 'chondroid' morphology, and their increased chondroitin sulphate and type III collagen synthesis, all of which are hallmarks of lack of directional control in wound repair (Flint 1981).

The perpetuation of the intrafascial reparative reaction and the accumulation of chondroitin sulphate leads to further fibre dehiscence and cellular extension along the established longitudinal fibre pathways after the primary cellular nodules have become established.

Unfortunately, the concept that Dupuytren's nodular lesions could arise from intrafascial ruptures has been repeatedly criticized, but without any firm scientific rebuttal (Hueston 1975, 1985, 1987). Appraisal of experimental plantar fascial lesions, which closely mimicked DD (Larsen et al 1960) cannot be lightly dismissed because 'monkeys don't develop DD' (Hueston 1975, 1985, 1987).

The success of full thickness skin replacement in preventing recurrence is often quoted as evidence of the determining role of the palmar dermis, rather than the underlying fascia, in influencing the progress of the disease (Hueston 1962, 1977, 1984, 1985, Gonzales 1971). However, the success of full thickness skin grafting does not necessarily indicate that the palm skin is the source of the primary lesion. The excision of involved skin and its replacement by skin graft not only removes the longitudinal fibres of the palmar fascial continuum but also introduces a dermal collagen network of a different pattern with less longitudinal fibre orientation and hence with less potential for compensatory fibre hypertrophy or stress rupture of the collagen network.

It is our belief that there has been some resistance to the acknowledgement of the role of intrafibrillar rupture in the pathogenesis of the Dupuytren's process for fear that if a causal relationship between trauma and DD was established and recognized, there would be a plethora of legal claims attempting to prove that DD has been caused by damage to the hands at work. However, we feel that whereas a few cases may show an undoubted causal relationship to the type of work, in many instances the pathogenesis of the fibre damage has a multifactorial basis over a prolonged period of time in which everyday living, sporting activities as well as hereditary genetic factors all play a part. In these circumstances, it would be almost impossible to apportion any degree of industrial liability. We feel that the term 'trauma' can, in this instance, be used to include all forms of physical and physicochemical perturbation which could result in changes in the physical characteristics of the fibre organization of the palmar connective tissue continuum.

In this regard, we believe it is very important to look beyond the described occupation of individuals with the disease and enquire about their out-of-work-hours activity. Often patients who have non-labouring types of jobs have softer palms, the connective tissues of which may be easily damaged by incidental or occasional trauma. However, no epidemiological study has yet been precise enough to separate and define the roles of age, inheritance, and hand usage in the pathogenesis of DD.

The fact that fibre rupture has frequently been observed in palms which are clinically uninvolved by the Dupuytren's process indicates that these initial changes may occur before the onset of the nodular cellular response. However, observations of specimens taken from clinically involved hands undoubtedly demonstrate that the process may be perpetuated by further rupture and cellular extension along the fibrils after the primary cellular nodules have become established. These later or secondary ruptures are facilitated by weakening of the extracellular matrix of nodules and cellular bands, particularly by the increase of proteoglycans and the inclusion of water, both of which tend to disturb the fibril integrity further and render them more liable to disruption.

The consequential effects of contraction, contracture and connective tissue remodelling have been discussed at length in Chapter 10. These secondary phenomena are all a natural progression — and an inevitable consequence — of extension of the cellular response into other longitudinal and obliquely running fibre bundles. Without the pre-existing anatomical fascial framework the contractural process would be much less significant. In fact, the pathogenesis of the disease itself is largely determined by the distribution and biomechanical properties of the fibrofatty palmar connective tissue continuum.

Perhaps some patients' fascial fibres are better able to withstand usage than others. This may be due to a subtle genetic difference in the collagen quaternary structure, in the character of the proteoglycans or glycosaminoglycans or elastin, or in the efficacy of the hydroelastic supporting system of the hypodermal fibrofatty loculi.

Although, as yet, no studies have been undertaken to investigate the viscoelastic properties of the hypodermal fat pads in different metabolic conditions, there is some evidence to suggest that the fatty acid composition of these subdermal fat pads is altered in alcoholics (Rabinowitz et al 1983; Bradlow & Mowat 1986). It is conceivable that these changes in fatty acid composition in the palmar hypodermal fat pads could lead to changes in their viscoelastic properties and hence to changes in pressure absorption, thereby increasing the chances of fascial collagen fibril damage.

Similarly, changes in collagen glycosylation and cross-linking which may be associated with diseases such as diabetes (Noble et al 1984; Pal & Griffiths 1987) could also lead to changes in collagen fibre compliance. It is also conceivable that the supposed links with such conditions as epilepsy, if substantiated, will be shown to be associated with genetically linked defects in the biomechanical properties of connective tissues.

NEOPLASM OR REPAIR?

The proliferation of fibroblasts in Dupuytren's nodules (Kocher 1887) led to the belief that DD might be a benign mesenchymal tumour. This idea was developed by Luck (1959), but he recognized that it was difficult to distinguish between neoplasia and dysplasia. More recently biologists using newly developed cytoskeletal recognition techniques (Bhawan et al 1979; Bartal et al 1987) and tissue culture cytological studies (Lagace 1980; Lipper et al 1980; Seemayer et al 1981) have again noted the similarity between the behaviour and morphology of Dupuytren's cells and sarcomata and other neoplastic conditions. However, it must be remembered that fibroblasts of wound healing and reparative situations may exhibit some of the morphological characteristics and behaviour patterns of rapidly growing tumour cells. This, however, is a reflection of their post-mitotic activity rather than their tumorogenic potential. We are therefore not surprised that the very active post-mitotic cells of the Dupuytren's nodule exhibit some features of sarcomata and feel that this is in keeping with their frustrated reparative role.

TISSUE ANOXIA

Recent studies have again raised the question of tissue anoxia as being a prime factor in the disease process (Kischer et al 1982). Ward Kischer has produced evidence of blood vessel occlusion caused by endothelial proliferation (Kischer et al 1982; Kischer & Speer 1984) while changes in palmar fatty acid metabolism (Rabinowitz et al 1983) have been ascribed to palmar connective tissue hypoxia. However, our studies indicate that these hypoxic changes are probably secondary manifestations of the progressive fibrosis which we have observed in many samples of apparently normal palm skin. In fact, our histological observations indicate that the very earliest stages of the fibrous replacement are preceded by and associated with a markedly *increased* vascularity of the hypodermal fatty tissue (see Chapter 13) and that this hypervascularity is associated with cellular proliferation and a creeping fibrosis. The fibroplastic stimulating effect of fibrin and fibrin breakdown products may be of consequence in this regard (Merlo et al 1986, 1987). It is interesting to note that the histological observations of Meyerding et al (1941) and MacCallum & Hueston (1962) also emphasize the increased vascularity of the hypodermal fat in DD.

Whilst we can now begin better to understand the basis of the intrafascial ruptures, the nodular formation, the contraction process, contracture and connective tissue remodelling, we are as yet unable to explain the reasons for the initial increased vascularity, the perivascular reaction, the replacement fibrosis of the fibrofatty loculi, or the differences in susceptibility of some tissues and some individuals. However we are confident that the changes which occur in the palmar connective tissues long before the Dupuytren's process becomes clinically apparent hold the secret to the pathogenesis of the condition (Fig. 28.1).

R. M. McFarlane

Is Dupuytren's disease a neoplasm?

In Chapter 28, my colleagues have explained their theory of pathogenesis as a series of biological events, starting early in life, with intrafibrillar rupture of collagen fibres. They consider the nodule to represent a 'prolonged intrafascial reparative reaction'. The concept of a palmar fascia continuum, as originally described by Millesi (1966), is central to their scheme and should put to rest further discussion of intrinsic and extrinsic theories concerning the site of origin of DD. The disease is clearly located in the superficial components of the palmar fascia comprising the pretendinous bands of the palmar aponeurosis, the natatory ligament and Grayson's ligaments. The finer extensions of these gross fascial structures that pass to the dermis complete the palmar fascia continuum and it is not unreasonable to expect the disease to begin in any component.

Although biomechanical stress upon the collagen may contribute to propagation of the disease, it is difficult to assign a principle aetiological role to this process. Presumably, disruption of fibre bundles is an everyday event, but not every disruption progresses to the formation of a pathological nodule. Everyone uses and abuses their hands and yet few develop DD. Flint & McGrouther assign a minor role to 'genetic differences in the collagen structure' even though DD is thought to be a familial disease and follows an autosomal dominant mode of transmission. Concerning aetiology, I agree with Hueston (1987) who reiterated his view that 'inheritance remains the single most important factor in the production of this condition'.

In the early and active stages of disease, cells are the prominent histological feature. It is our view that determination of the origin and characteristics of these cells will explain the aetiology and pathogenesis of DD. Have these cells appeared as a reparative response, as suggested in Chapter 28? Do they represent a quasi-neoplastic reparative process (Seemayer et al 1980)? Enzinger & Weiss (1983) classify DD as a superficial fibromatosis. In contrast to the deep fibromatoses, DD grows slowly, does not invade other tissues and does not form large tumour masses. However, histologically the superficial and deep fibromatoses are similar. Allan (1977) discusses juvenile and adult types of fibromatosis and subdivides the latter into Dupuytren's type and desmoid type and refers to the whole group as 'nonmetastasizing fibroblastic tumours'.

In general, pathologists assume that DD is a tumour-like condition best classified as a fibromatosis. Present research is directed toward more accurate definition of the cell or cells involved. As described in Chapters 3, 4 and 8, modern techniques of histochemistry provide an insight into the origin and activity of cells. Azzarone et al (1983), from Gabbiani's laboratory, compared the growth characteristics of cultured fibroblasts from DD and fibrosarcoma. They found that five characteristics were similar to those of normal fibroblasts, but six others were similar to those of sarcoma cells. For instance, the level of plasminogen activator, which is a mitogenic agent, was elevated in the Dupuytren's cells compared to normal cells, although not as high as in sarcoma cells. The authors concluded that DD is a benign mesenchymal tumour and the high level of plasminogen activator is a mitogenic stimulus for the formation of the nodule. Thus, the

Dupuytren's nodule is 'a mode of tumour progression in a benign situation'.

Bartal et al (1987) tested diseased palmar fascia with monoclonal antibodies generated from human sarcomata and found that some of the specimens immunostained; that is, some of the cells were similar to sarcoma cells. As an aside, these authors suggest that such immunological probes may better define the variety of clinical patterns of DD. This is consistent with the concept proposed by Flint & McGrouther in Chapter 28; they regard DD as a common fibroblastic endpoint rather than a single disease process.

Cancer cells are characterized by abnormalities of their chromosomes, but little is known about cytogenetics of benign tumors. Cell grown from Dupuytren's nodules have non-random chromosome abnormalities. Bowser-Riley et al (1975) found an abnormal cell line in 4 of 6 specimens of DD tissue. Sergovitch et al (1983) found chromosome abnormalities in 10 of 26 specimens, and in more recent unpublished work in which several cultures were prepared from the same specimen, at least one abnormal cell line was found in every specimen. Wurster-Hill et al (1988) reported chromosome abnormalities in all 8 patients studied. They postulated that fascial tissue in DD suffers DNA damage, and misrepair in the growth process is manifested as chromosome instability. Loss of chromosome 7 and the Y chromosome in males was common, but the most common abnormality was trisomy 8. This abnormality is common in acute and chronic myeloid leukaemia and Burkett's lymphoma, but also in benign salivary gland tumours and Peyronie's disease.

Thus, there is an apparent contradiction between the chromosomally abnormal but non-malignant cells of DD that needs further study. Chromosome abnormalities conincide with the location of known oncogenes such as the human *myc* oncogene on chromosome 8. Growth factors, such as epidermal growth factor, are present in Dupuytren's cells. Oncogenes and growth factors are involved in the pathogenesis of neoplasia, but are also involved in the chronic inflammatory process.

Whether DD is a reactive or neoplastic process, growth factors and oncogenes must be studied in order to understand how the process is controlled. This is a logical and exciting step in the ongoing study of DD. Caster & Cabral (1985) stated: 'when the actions of growth factors in health and disease are precisely defined, genetically engineered competitive inhibitors may offer a wide array of useful therapeutic modalities'.

SECTION 5

Treatment

30 Assessment of the patient for operation

Patients with Dupuytren's disease (DD) are seen for one of three reasons. Some are concerned about the appearance of a lump in the palm; they need reassurance that the lump is not cancer. Others complain of pain associated with palmar thickening; usually these people have only recently noticed the lump. If the nature of the disease and its likely course is explained to these two groups of patients, they usually accept the advice that no treatment is needed at that time.

Most patients have established contractures when first seen. There are few, if any, in this third group who cannot be helped by operation. DD may be a unique surgical condition because it is not a matter of whether or not an operation should be performed, but rather of choosing the operation which is suited for each patient.

THE PATIENT

Age at onset of disease and family history are factors that establish the strength of the diathesis or the aggressiveness of the disease. Unfortunately, often neither factor is reported accurately by the patient. The average age of onset in males is about 48 years and in females about 59 years. Patients in whom the disease appears much earlier, that is in the third or fourth decade, are likely to have aggressive disease that requires extensive operations to control. Those in whom the disease appears in the seventh decade are likely to have localized disease that is easily corrected by minimal operation.

A positive family history, especially one in which more than one close relative and more than one generation is involved, suggests a strong diathesis. However, a negative family history is meaningless because most patients do not know the status of even close family members.

Contrary to a recent report by Zemel et al (1987), sex is not a factor in deciding if the patient should have an operation or what operation should be performed. As reported in Chapters 20 and 36, all parameters of results are similar in males and females. The disease appears later in women and is usually less severe and less aggressive, but the only difference of concern is that the prevalence of reflex sympathetic dystrophy is twice as common in females. However, the prevalence of this complication was only 7% and it is preventable to some extent with proper management. It is unfair, if not unscientific, to treat females differently.

Occupation does not influence the course or severity of disease, but is a factor concerning postoperative management. Sedentary workers often return to work within a few days of operation whereas a manual worker could be off work for 3 or 4 months after the same operation. Seasonal workers usually schedule their operation when they are not working. In Canada retired people often want their operation just before leaving for the south in November. This is unwise because the patients do not reappear until April. Their postoperative status should be satisfactory before they migrate.

Epilepsy, diabetes mellitus, and alcoholism are seen in patients with DD but the results of treatment and the incidence of recurrence and extension of disease are not affected by the presence of these diseases. Patients with long-standing idiopathic epilepsy or chronic alcoholism often have severe bilateral disease but they do surprisingly well with appropriate treatment. DD is common in diabetic patients but few of them develop joint contractures. Those diabetic patients who come to operation have typical DD and their results of treatment are no different from those of other patients

Very few patients with rheumatoid arthritis have DD but if joint contracture is present it can be corrected by minimal operation. Also, few patients with troublesome osteoarthritis in their hands have DD but again treatment can be planned to minimize postoperative joint stiffness. Nissenbaum & Kleinert (1980) reported that patients in whom carpal tunnel release was performed with fasciectomy were at greater risk of developing complications. They recommended that carpal tunnel syndrome should be treated first and fasciectomy performed later. In those patients who have carpal tunnel syndrome and require fasciectomy, I have done both procedures at the same operation and have not had untoward complications. This is also the experience of Watson & Gonzales (1988).

Some patients with trigger finger also have Dupuytren's nodules in the involved ray. These patients may also be diabetic because both DD and trigger finger are common in the middle and ring finger rays of the diabetic (DDT syndrome). Parker (1979) and Burgess & Watson (1987) suggest that the DD can cause the triggering by becoming adherent to the A_1 pulley of the flexor tendon sheath. I have not observed an anatomical relationship between the diseased fascia and the tendon sheath. In fact, such a relationship would be inconsistent with the known anatomy. These patients do not (usually) have metacarpophalangeal joint contracture and the Dupuytren's nodules are small and well proximal to the A_1 pulley. They can be left in situ when the trigger finger is released. If the disease is more advanced it should be removed by regional fasciectomy, as recommended by Burgess & Watson (1987).

Patients in poor health can be helped by adjusting the magnitude of the operation. Anticoagulants need not be stopped. Fasciotomy and limited fasciectomy are well received by patients who might be considered unfit for operation. More and more operations for DD are being performed on outpatients under local anaesthesia in healthy as well as chronically ill patients.

THE HAND

Skin involvement in the palm can occasionally be a factor in deciding upon the type of operation. The patient may have nodular disease in three or four pretendinous bands with pits and infolding of the skin about the distal crease. These patients may not have metacarpophalangeal or proximal interphalangeal joint contracture and yet the palm is contracted and uncomfortable. They should be offered an operation. When the adjacent fingers are held together by disease in the natatory ligament, intertrigo of the web skin develops and should be treated before operation to avoid postoperative wound infection.

Occasionally a single nodule is large enough to interfere with grip. It is reasonable to remove the nodule even in the absence of joint contracture but the surrounding diseased fascia should be removed at the same time by regional fasciectomy.

Most patients with DD have disease in the little or ring finger ray and less severe disease in a second ray. If the disease is more extensive, or if it is also present on the radial side of the hand, it is likely to be aggressive and difficult to control.

The usual indication for operation is joint contracture. As a rule, 30° of contracture at the metacarpophalangeal joint is annoying if not troublesome, so this degree of contracture is useful in advising a patient to have an operation. Metacarpophalangeal joint contracture can always be corrected so an operation can be planned at the patient's convenience. This is not so at the proximal interphalangeal joint. Thirty degrees of contracture may not be troublesome but the patient should know that the longer the contracture is present, the more difficult it is to correct. However, as noted in Chapters 20 and 36, contractures of less than 30° are often not corrected or may be made worse by operation. Thus, the surgeon faces the dilemma of not correcting the contracture by operating early or being unable to correct the contracture by operating late.

In assessing a patient for operation, the surgeon should consider those factors that indicate whether the disease is more or less aggressive as well as the condition of the patient to tolerate an operation. With information from both sources, an operation can be designed to benefit the patient.

D. A. McGrouther

31 An overview of operative treatment

There are many different ways of operating on Dupuytren's disease (DD) and so many individual variations, particularly when one considers the extent of resection, method of haemostasis, open and closed wound techniques and postoperative rehabilitation programme, that perhaps no two surgeons apply an identical treatment plan. It will be seen from the accounts in the following Chapters that most surgeons employ a range of treatment options from which they make a choice for the individual patient. Our authors are well known surgeons from many parts of the world, exposed to different incidences and apparently different severities of DD. Their combined wisdom serves to provide a broad picture of current treatment practice. This chapter seeks to coordinate their opinions and to integrate them with the literature to provide an overall picture of the many different treatment possibilities.

In formulating an individual plan of management one should give consideration to the patient, the physiology of the hand and the distribution of contracture.

In relation to the timing of surgery there is no general agreement, although it is widely recognized that the metacarpophalangeal joint can be readily released at any stage of contracture, whereas release of established proximal interphalangeal joint contracture is more unpredictable. For this reason it is desirable to operate early when the proximal interphalangeal joint is involved; a figure of 30° contracture is widely taken to be an indication for surgery. Certainly the surgeon should formulate an idea of the rate of progression of contraction in the individual patient and intervene before there is severe joint contracture.

Because of the multiplicity of possible operative techniques a framework is required for analysis of the various approaches by considering separately the management of the skin, the fascial structures and the proximal interphalangeal joint (Table 31.1). This classification has a practical value as the surgeon should have in mind a plan for these three problems — management of skin, contracted fascia and contracted proximal interphalangeal joint — before commencing the operation.

MANAGEMENT OF SKIN

Whether the skin is involved in the Dupuytren's process or not the surgeon must cut through it to reach the involved fascia and therefore the pattern of skin incision is significant in relation to recurrence. Skin replacement by graft or flap has been performed for a number of reasons and these will be discussed separately.

Incisions

The simple limited incisions of the early 19th century (see Chapter 1) became more complex, in parallel with more extensive fascial resections, as advances in anaesthesia and wound management made possible more sophisticated surgery. The many different patterns of skin incision which have been described (Fig. 31.1) can be associated with varying degrees of undermining. The choice of whether skin incisions are made in continuity or in separate steps will be influenced by the extent of fascial dissection which is planned. A longitudinal incision will usually be chosen for fas-

Table 31.1 Operations for DD

Management of the skin	Management of contracted fascia	Management of contracted PIPJ
Incisions	Fasciotomy	Release
Longitudinal	Open	Release of tendon sheath
Zig-zag for exposure	Closed	Check-rein ligament release
Linear followed by Z-plasty (for exposure and lengthening)	Fasciotomy and Z-plasty	Volar capsulectomy
	Fasciotomy and graft	
Transverse — open palm		Arthrodesis
	Limited fasciectomy	
Skin replacement	Regional	Arthroplasty
Grafts	Selective	
To replace deficiency resulting from contracture		Osteotomy
	Radical or extensive fasciectomy	
Prophylactically required to interrupt contracture continuity		Accept deformity
	Dermofasciectomy	
If excision of involved skin is necessary		Amputation
Flaps		

PIPJ = proximal interphalangeal joint.

ciectomy in continuity, but McIndoe et al (1958; previously reported by Skoog 1948) performed a fascial resection in continuity by undermining between separate incisions in the palm and digit. Incisions may have a predominantly longitudinal or transverse orientation.

Longitudinal incisions

The guiding rule in planning exposure is to prevent future skin contracture by avoiding continuous straight incisions on potentially concave surfaces. The undesirability of a straight longitudinal midline digital incision of the type used by Kocher (1887; see Fig. 31.1) has long been accepted (Bunnell 1944). A straight mid lateral incision has been used to avoid contracture (Ashley 1953; Tubiana 1964; Carr 1974; Jacobsen & Holst-Nielsen 1977) but access to the entire volar surface requires extensive dissection. Devitalization of skin should be avoided by placing incisions so as to limit undermining.

Zig-zag patterns of incision offer several advantages. They improve access by facilitating the elevation of flaps. Such patterns prevent volar contractures as the small amount of scar contracture, which must inevitably occur along the incision lines, will not restrict joint range. The pattern of Bruner (1951) is popular. The honeycomb technique described by Bedeschi (Chapter 32) combines a zig-zag approach with the benefits of an open wound technique, which will be described later.

In addition to these advantages of zig-zag designs some patterns also offer the possibility of lengthening contracted palmar skin — there is a redistribution of skin in the chronically flexed digit, in addition to the contracture which occurs in the Dupuytren's process. Two techniques of achieving such a lengthening are possible; the Y-to-V advancement and the Z-plasty. A multiple Y-to-V advancement was advocated by Deming (1962), Watson et al (1975), and Baker & Watson (1980). It is not generally appreciated that this Y-to-V technique was previously described by Palmen (1932) and was widely used before the Z-plasty technique.

Use of the Z-plasty for lengthening is a much more recent device and seems to date from the work of Sir Archibald McIndoe et al (1958), who used a single Z in the proximal segment of the digit. A single Z elevated in this way can improve exposure in comparison with a straight incision. Marc Iselin (1955) used multiple Zs in series but François Iselin has now discontinued this method (Chapter 32). McGregor (1967) has advocated a midline incision with multiple Zs centred on the joint creases. Robbins (1981) deferred the Z-plasties until a later operation if they proved to be required.

A disadvantage of zig-zag incisions is that where there is skin involvement by the Dupuytren's process, such an incision will carry the risk of flap tip devascularization. All zig-zag scars tend to straighten during wound healing, due to slight

AN OVERVIEW OF OPERATIVE TREATMENT 297

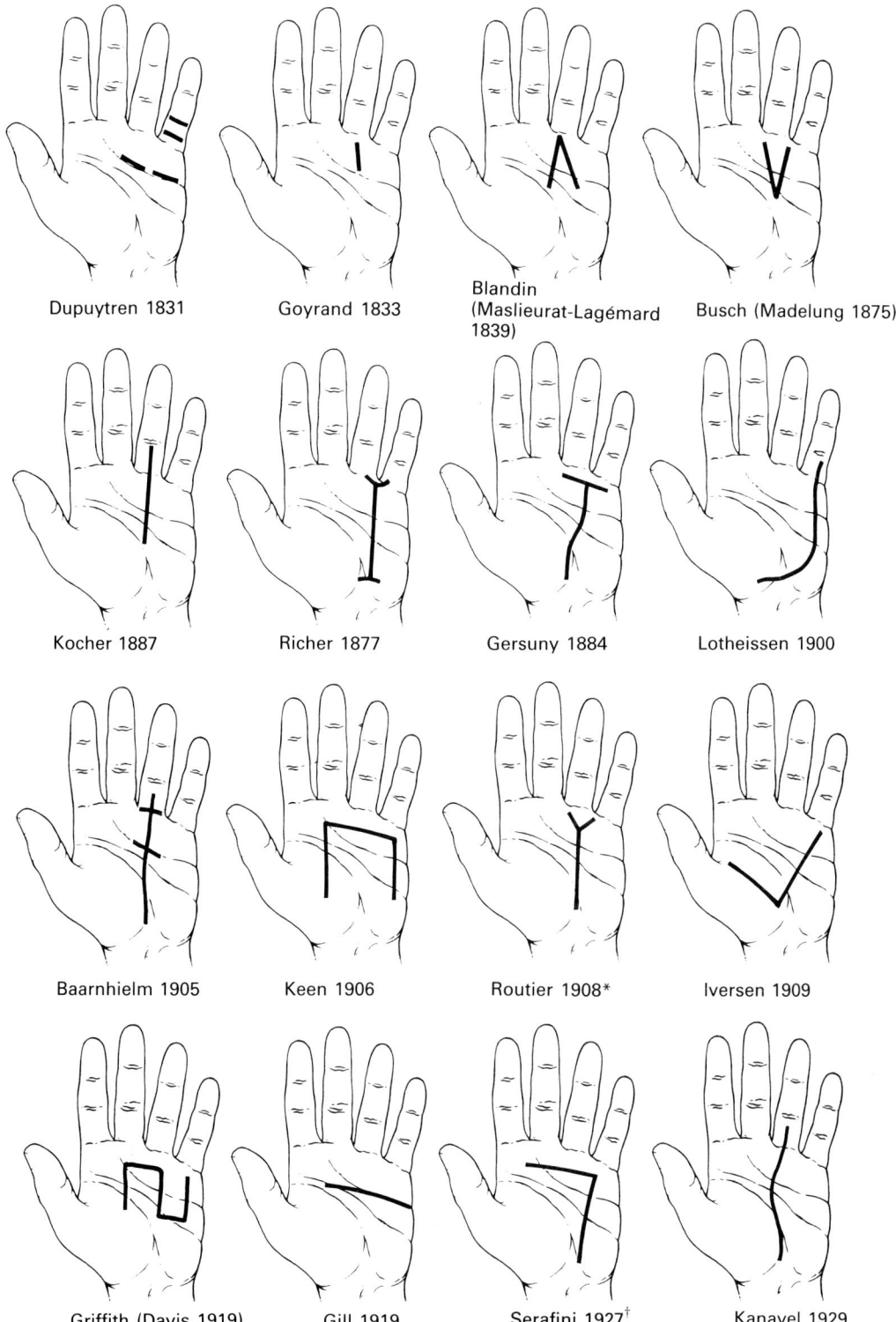

Fig. 31.1 Operative incisions for DD. Charts of this type have been published by Einarsson (1946), Skoog (1948)★, Webster (1957), Parrini & Brunelli (1965)† and Geldmacher (1972)◇ (Cited by author indicated where original source untraced)

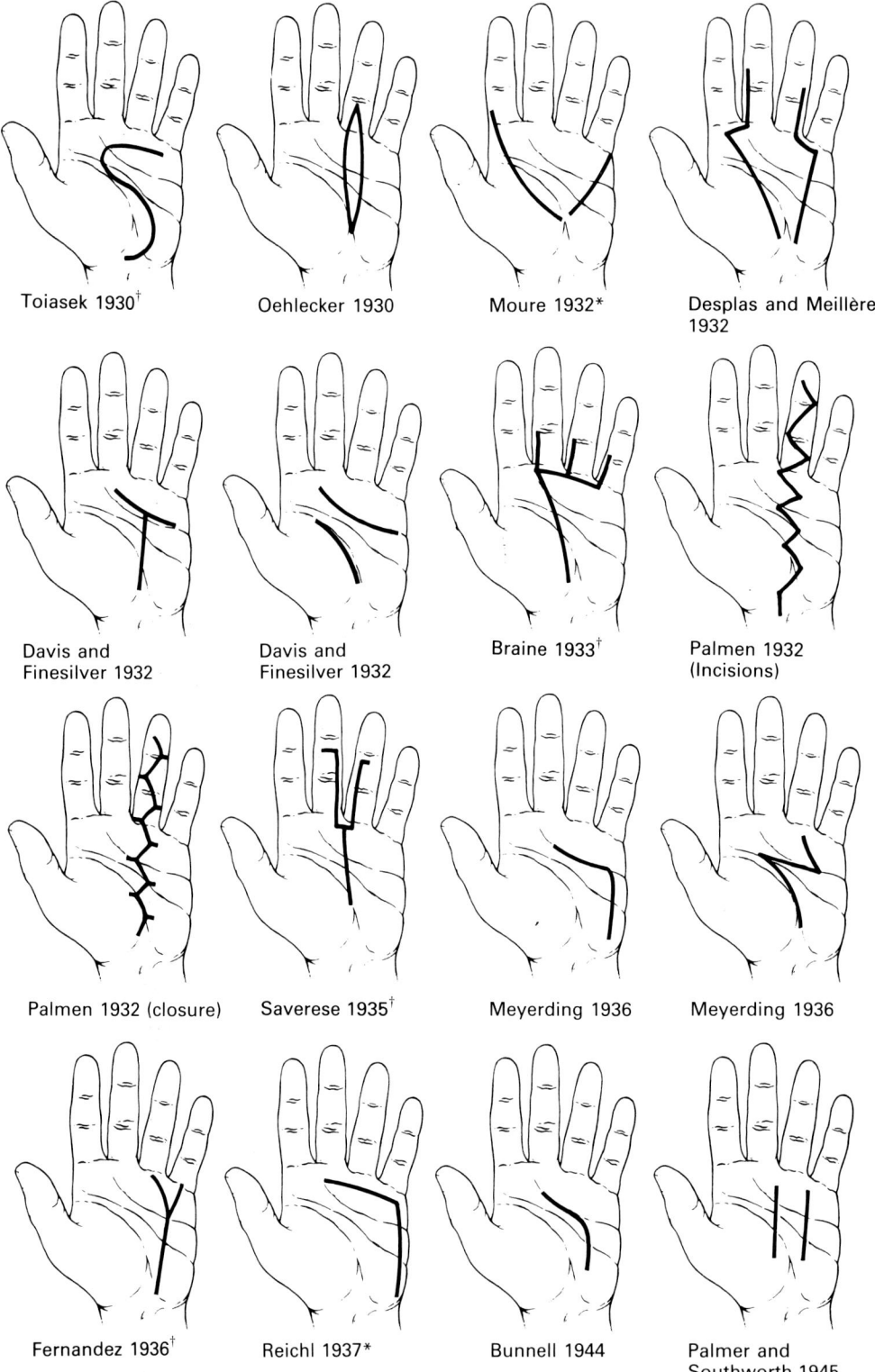

Fig. 31.1 (contd)

AN OVERVIEW OF OPERATIVE TREATMENT 299

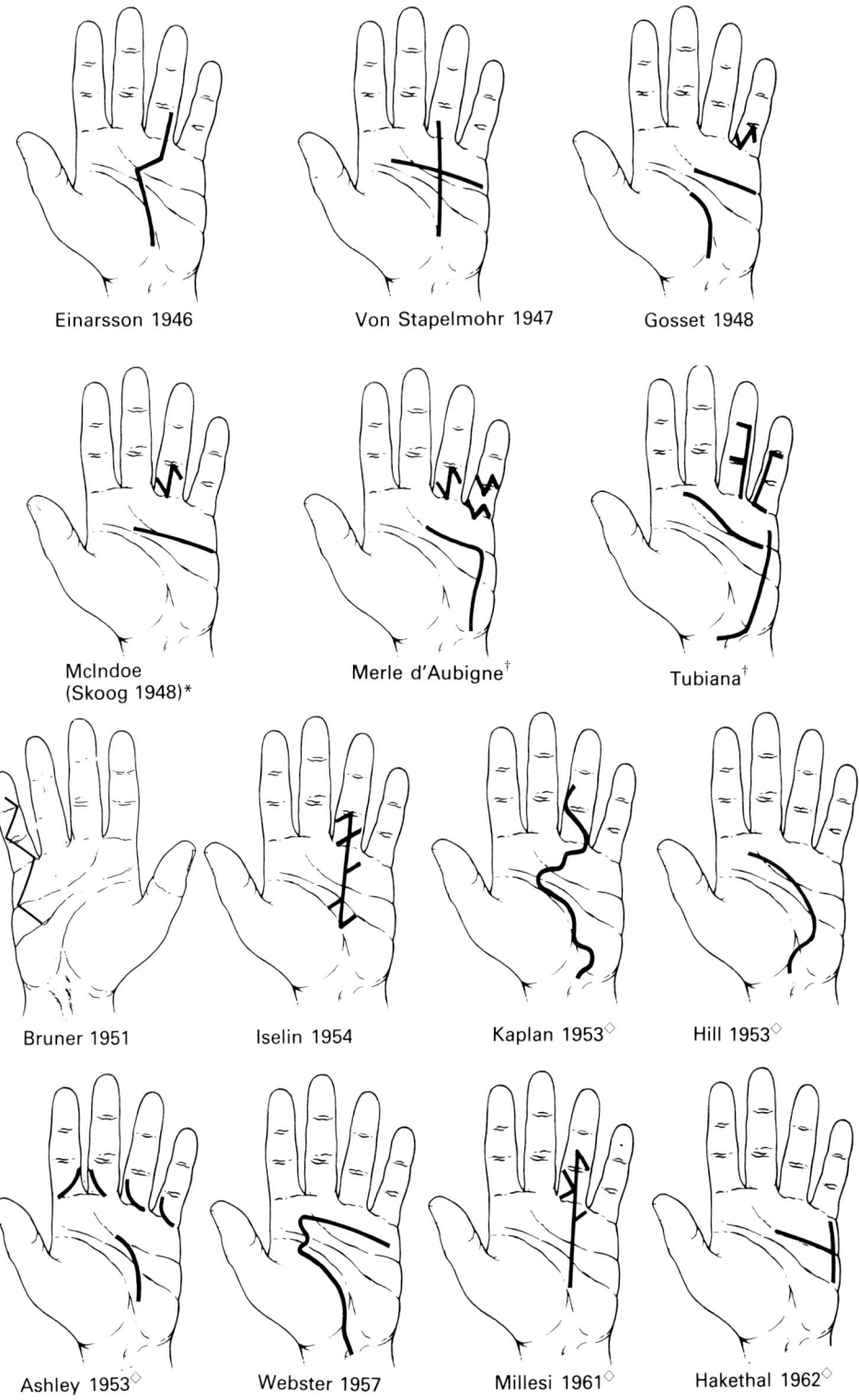

Fig. 31.1 (contd)

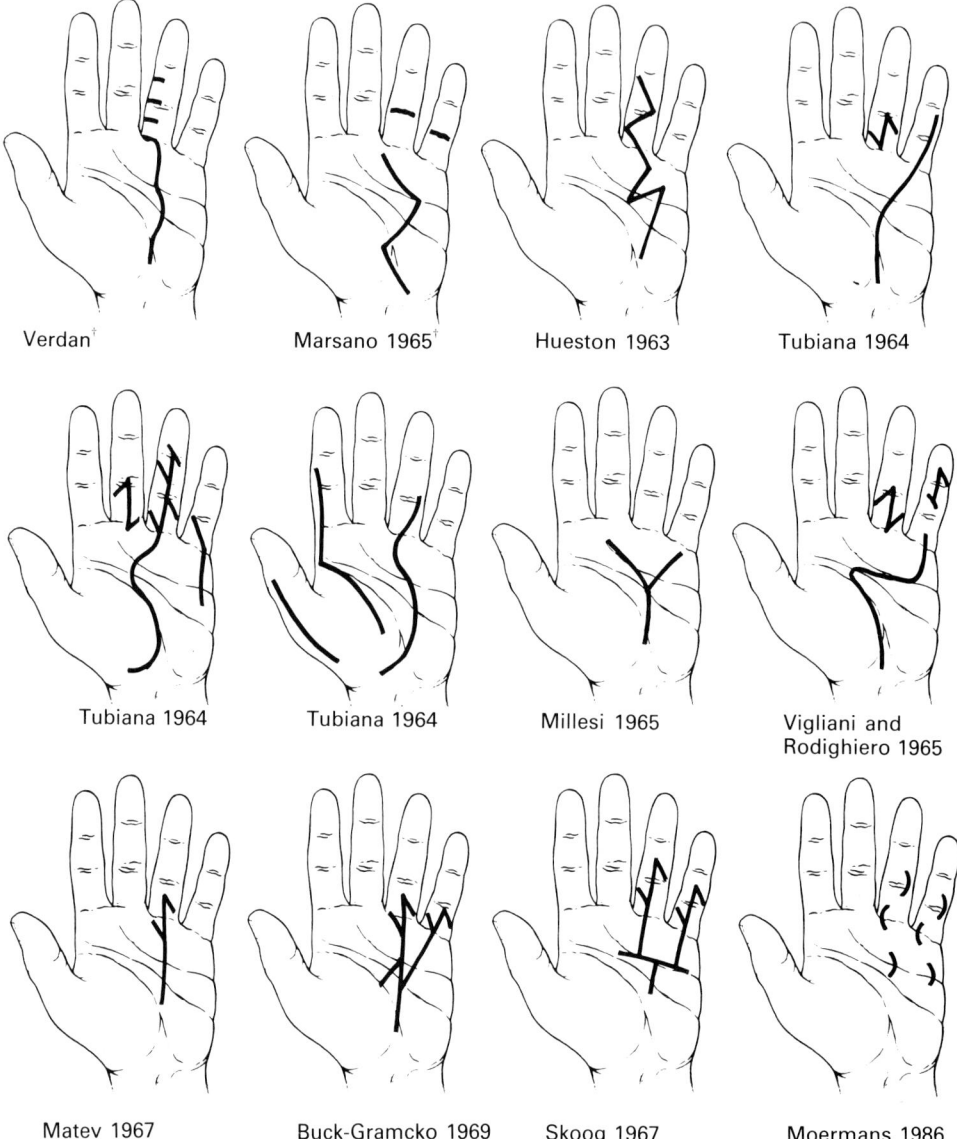

Fig. 31.1 (contd)

wound contracture but subsequent straightening of the scars due to flap tip necrosis may also be more frequent than generally recognized!

When designing a series of Z-plasties it is probably better to make an initial linear incision and design the Zs at a later stage in the operation. In this way the flaps can be elevated to take advantage of vascularization and 'buttonholes'!

In dissecting a single ray contracture, incisions with a predominantly longitudinal orientation are frequently employed as these allow the neurovascular bundles to be progressively displayed without injury in the manner of extensile exposure. Where more than one ray is involved, a transverse distal palmar incision has been advocated by Skoog (1967a and b, 1985) combined with a longitudinal approach to each digit and usually one proximal extension of varying length (Fig. 31.1).

Transverse incisions

Transverse incisions have been used for simple release, limited or more extensive fascial resection. The greater the fascial dissection required, the more extensive the necessary undermining.

If the palm alone is involved, a transverse incision at the distal palmar crease may give enough exposure to excise all the apparently involved fascia.

The use of a series of transverse incisions makes the anatomy much more difficult to visualize, but it leaves unscarred skin segments between each incision which are less likely to be a source of recurrent contracture of the skin than in the case of a longitudinal incision.

The use of transverse incisions in the finger allows only limited fascial resection. Gonzales (Chapter 32) has used such an incision at the base of the finger and Beltran et al (1976) and Burkhalter (Chapter 32) at the proximal interphalangeal crease.

The description of the open palm technique of McCash (1964) surprised the surgical community, but should not have done so as Dupuytren used a similar means of managing the skin and open wound techniques were widely used during the 19th century (reviewed by Adams 1879).

McCash felt that poor graft take in the hand and the need to immobilize the hand after grafting were disadvantages of such techniques and that the impaired vitality of palmar skin made flaps undesirable. He described a total approach, rather than merely a technique of wound care comprising:

1. Incision in the transverse skin creases; no longitudinal incisions were made.
2. By advancing the undermined skin bridges proximally and distally the whole of the skin shortage was 'accepted' by the distal palmar crease incision, which remained wide open.
3. After a week's complete rest a night splint was worn.
4. No physiotherapy was used and the hand was dressed at weekly intervals.

All open wounds now tend to be loosely termed 'the McCash technique', but this pays insufficient respect to this author's total treatment plan. Only the diseased fascia was removed. The open wound caused little discomfort when healing (in marked distinction to Dupuytren's first case) and McCash remarked on the freedom from haematoma or oedema during recovery. The wounds generally closed in 2–5 weeks. In his article, he mentioned that Mr O. T. Mansfield of Birmingham had employed a similar method, but used Z-plasties or grafts in the digits.

McCash's results were supported by Zachariae et al (1970), Salvi (1973), Briedis (1974), Conolly (1974) and Ariyan & Krizek (1976). Noble & Harrison (1976) and Jacobsen & Holst-Nielsen (1977) have combined a mid lateral digital incision with a transverse palmar incision, the latter being left open. Salvi has described his experiences with the open palm technique in Chapter 32.

Borden (1974) and Beltran et al (1976; Beltran 1985) have used an open method in the fingers which healed leaving linear scars. Care was taken to preserve the tendon sheath intact and residual proximal interphalangeal contracture was accepted. Burkhalter (Chapter 32) describes the open method in the digits.

A disadvantage of the open palm technique is that the patients are apprehensive about the appearance of the open wound. Careful counselling is always necessary. Advocates claim that the patient can return to full use of the hand immediately, despite the open wound and frequent dressings (Lubahn et al 1984).

The great merit of the technique is its safety; it is a reliable method of preventing retained haematoma while providing extra skin from unfolding if there are convolutions. It is unnecessary where a limited dissection has been performed with good haemostasis. It should not be used as a substitute for adequate haemostasis.

Gelberman et al (1982) have compared operative incisions. They performed longitudinally oriented incisions (Z-plasty or Bruner techniques) with transverse incisions by the technique of McCash. A higher incidence of early wound complications (flap necrosis, haematoma and infection) was noted with the zig-zag and Z-plasty incisions than with the transverse incisions, but this may reflect the benefits of open wound over closure rather than the incision pattern per se.

Skin grafts

Skin grafts were used by Professor Busch (cited by Madelung 1875) to accelerate the healing of the wound; Busch's operation of fasciotomy was performed through a distally based triangular flap which probably became necrotic on occasions. John Hueston has cited Berger (1892) in the use of grafts and Lexer (1931) combined skin grafting with a radical fasciectomy around 1900. Split skin grafts were used by Baarnhielm (1905) and Orbach (1934); full thickness grafts were used by Davis (1919), Gillies (1945), Grenabo (1946), and Langvad-Nielsen (1946).

There seem to be currently three indications for skin grafting:

1. *Skin grafts to heal a skin deficiency.* Skin deficiency may be due to chronic flexion deformity, scarring of previous operations, or necrosis at or following surgery. Crockett (1980) described a technique of insertion of full thickness skin gussets to augment skin shortage in the palm. The failure of revascularization of a flap is mentioned by McFarlane & Jamieson (1966) who advised the use of a tie-over dressing where skin is thin. Should the skin not survive, skin grafting is advised. When skin is replaced at the time of contracture release a full thickness graft is generally used. For later closure of a defect, split skin graft is usual as the bed is often less favourable.
2. *Skin grafts to separate contracted fascia.* The concept of breaking up the contracture line by a skin graft is implicit in the work of Piulachs & Mir Y Mir (1952), which will be discussed below. Gonzales (Chapter 32) believes that a full thickness skin graft should be inserted in addition to that required to break up the contracture line. He believes that DD should be treated in a similar manner to post burns contracture.

   McGregor (1985) has inserted split skin grafts after adequate division of the fascia. Initially he divided the contracted palmar fascia in the involved rays, but later undertook a more extensive release from the ulnar border of the hand to the radial border along the distal palmar crease. Additional releases were made in the digits, no fascia was excised and split skin grafts were inserted after ensuring that the contracted fascia had retracted. Hueston's (1984) firebreak concept is similar, but a more extensive fascial resection is done.
3. *Elective skin excision.* Piulachs & Mir Y Mir (1952) suggested that recurrence is reduced or eliminated when the involved skin is replaced by skin grafting. Gordon (1957) in reporting a large series of operations mentioned that grafts had been done on 13 hands and these areas remained free of disease.

   The elective excision of skin involved in recurrent Dupuytren's disease was described by Hueston in 1962, and in a primary case in 1964, in the belief that the palmar dermis exerts 'control' on the disease process. Skin was excised over the proximal segment of the digit from one neutral line to the other. The idea was taken up by Tubiana (1963), Gordon (1964), and Rudolph (1979). Further large series presented have been by Tonkin et al (1984) and Iselin (1985).

   Iselin and Hueston have presented their experiences in this book (Chapter 32).

Skin flaps

Local skin flaps may be elevated to facilitate access to the underlying fascia, or they may he moved to reconstruct areas of skin shortage. Anderson (1897) illustrated a flap from the dorsum of the digit (Fig. 31.3). In the palm Griffith transposed two quadrilateral flaps (described by Davis 1919) and Von Siemen (1936) used a large rotation flap extending around the ulnar border from the dorsum. Bruner (1949) used a flap similar to that of Anderson. In the digits, Harrison & Morris (1975) have designed a transposition flap from the dorsal surface to lie transversely across the proximal digital crease, used when the proximal interphalangeal joint is being stabilized, to facilitate movement at

AN OVERVIEW OF OPERATIVE TREATMENT 303

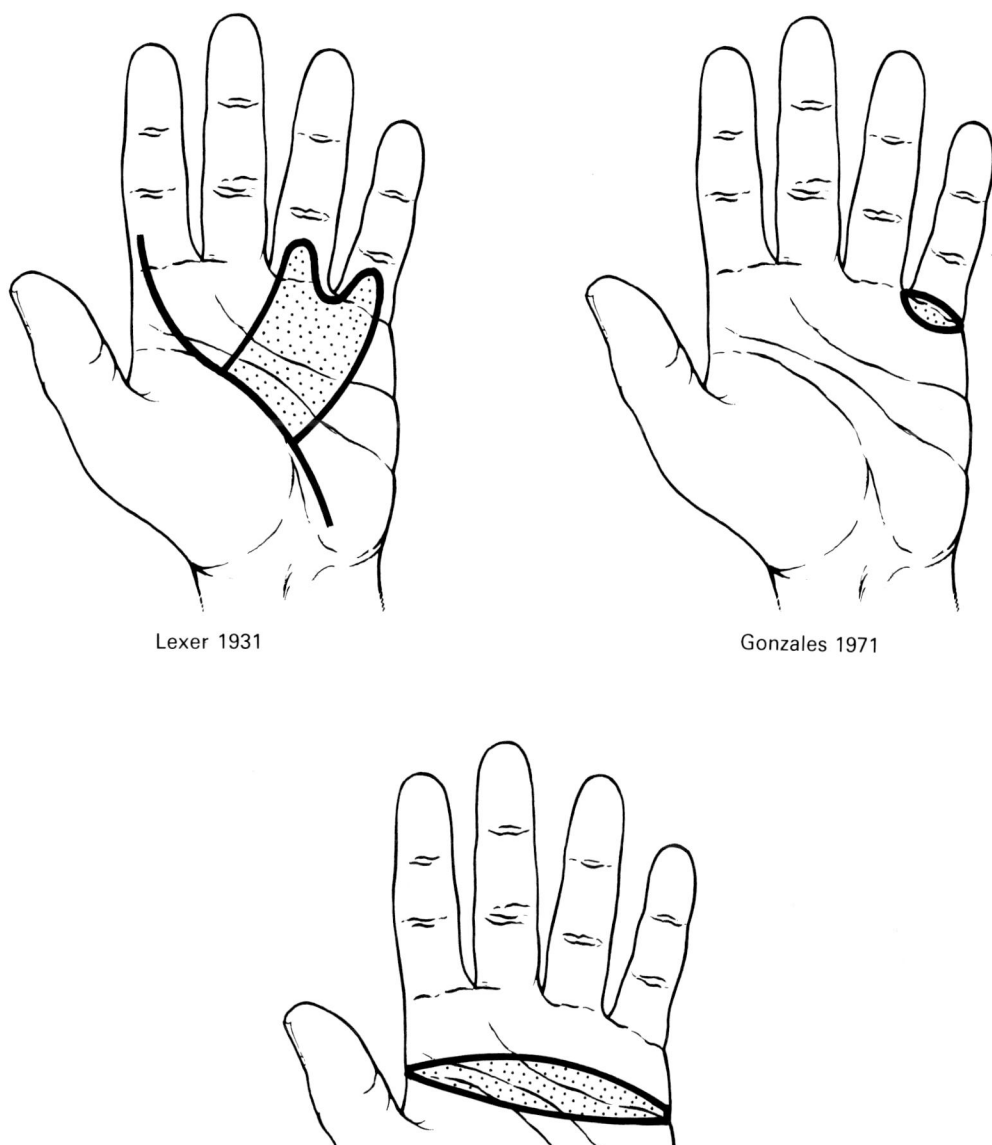

Fig. 31.2 Skin grafting techniques.

the metacarpophalangeal joint. On review, they noted no recurrences beneath the flap.

A particular problem in the digits is the situation where release of the proximal interphalangeal joint necessitates opening of the flexor tendon sheath. On extension of the digit there is found to be a volar skin defect with exposure of the flexor tendons. Hueston has advised care in prevention of this problem. If it does occur, he has used local transposition flaps, using whatever skin is available to cover the defect in the sheath and skin grafts for the remainder.

Gonzales (Chapter 32) seems to avoid the problem by dividing the contracture at the proximal digital crease rather than the proximal interphalangeal joint crease. McGregor (1985) has successfully covered exposed tendons with split skin grafts, provided that the visceral paratenon layer has not been damaged; a gliding layer is re-established. Lane (1981) has described a sliding volar flap which is elevated by making two mid lateral incisions on the digits and joining these by a transverse cut over the middle phalanx. The resulting proximally based flap retreats proximally on extending the digit, leaving a skin defect over the intact flexor tendon sheath in the middle segment, which can be grafted.

Cross-finger flaps have been used; Hueston attributes to Moberg the view that cross-finger flap replacement may prejudice the progression of disease in the donor finger.

Distant flaps from the chest have even been used, in long-standing cases, by Berger (1892), Guinebault (1897) and Fredet (1932). Wagner (1932) used such a technique after skin necrosis. Davis (1919) and Lexer (1931) used abdominal flaps and Oehlecker (1930) a pedicled flap from the scrotum. Clarkson (1966) used thigh flaps in the salvage of digits with severe DD.

Miscellaneous operations on the skin and subcutaneous fat

A number of miscellaneous procedures, now largely discredited, demonstrate the ingenuity of our predecessors in tackling what they viewed as the basic pathological processes. Skinner (1941) and Palmer & Southworth (1945) have advocated placing a skin graft underneath a bridge of contracted fascia after undermining; the diseased tissue is excised at a second stage.

Von Stapelmohr (1947) used a cruciate incision, trimming the palmar skin to the thickness of Wolfe grafts, and used tie-over dressings. By contrast the importance of subcutaneous fat was appreciated by Madelung (1875). Peiser (1917), Gill (1919), and Ramstedt (1933) inserted free fat transplants beneath the skin. Spitzy (1916) recommended vegetable or swine fat, Desplas & Meillere (1932) amniotic membrane, Woolf (1920) fascia lata together with fat, Abbott (1929) fascia lata alone and Reichel (1937) sterile paraffin!

MANAGEMENT OF THE CONTRACTED FASCIA

Fasciotomy

That simple release can result in a prolonged or permanent release of contracture has been demonstrated by the release of the contracture by trauma (Cline 1777; Adams 1879; Grace et al 1984). Historically open and closed wound approaches have been used for fasciotomy.

Open wound release was performed by Dupuytren, (1831), Richet (1873), Hardie (1885), and Abbe (1888). Jobert & Blandin (1846) made a V-shaped incision pointing proximally or distally. They cut beneath the aponeurosis elevating the triangular flap together with the retracted aponeurosis which remained attached to the skin. Lannelongue, according to Durel (1888) closed such a flap in a V-to-Y manner. Madelung (1875) described the technique of Busch in which a skin flap was raised before performing a fasciotomy. Vogt (1881), Koenig (1889) and Merker (1897) favoured this technique, but problems of flap necrosis were recognized by Zimmerman (1898), Lotheissen (1900) and Hutchinson (1917).

Closed fasciotomy was advocated by Sir Astley Cooper (1822) by the subcutaneous division of a band with a pointed bistoury introduced through a small wound in the integument; a splint was applied to maintain this finger in a straight position. Annandale (1865) found that the subcutaneous methods were of less value when the skin was largely adherent to the aponeurosis. William Adams (1879) reviewed the merits of the sub-

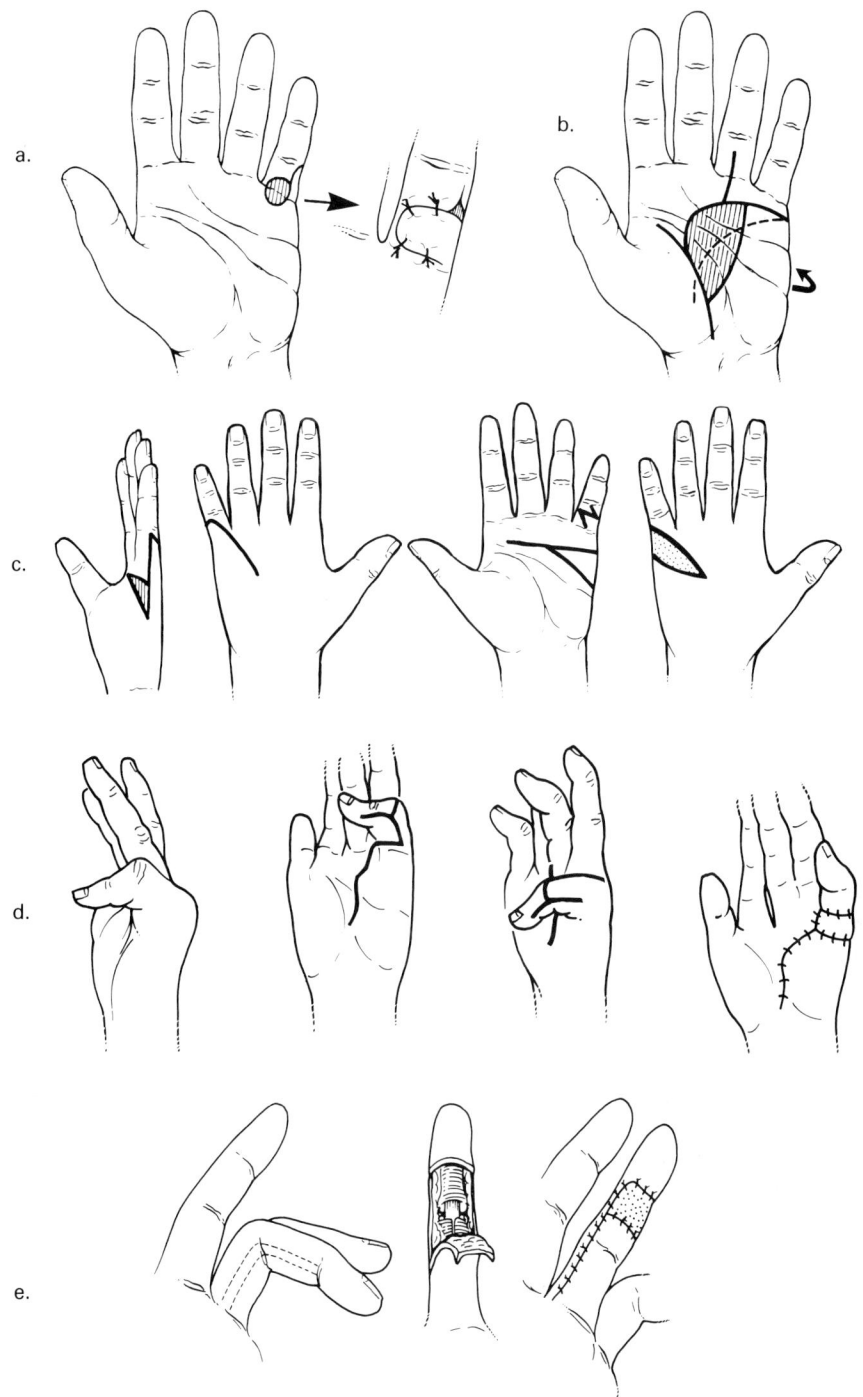

Fig. 31.3 Flaps in Dupuytren's disease. (**a**) Anderson 1897; (**b**) Von Siemen 1936; (**c**) Bruner 1949; (**d**) Harrison and Morris 1975; (**e**) Lane 1981.

cutaneous operation, principally the avoidance of the introduction of infection, substantiating his argument by quoting the theories of John Hunter on the introduction of air. Adams described in detail the operative steps. Smith (1884, 1885) urged the need to ensure maximum separation of the severed parts to prevent re-union. In some cases, he sectioned the cords diagonally to obtain union in a lengthened position.

The possibility of recurrence was becoming apparent. Macready (1890) quoted Adams's (1879) estimated recurrence rate to be 10%. Hedges (1896) reported 9 cases with 6 recurrences. Dickson (1928) found recurrences more likely than with other methods. Davis & Finesilver (1932) described 6 hands which had remained free of recurrence at 1–5 years. It seemed that fasciotomy may be curative but only in certain cases (Fergusson 1846; Fisher 1885; Trelat 1888; Drehmann 1913; Roth 1920, 1928; Hohmann 1936; Meyerding et al 1936).

Bunnell (1944) used subcutaneous fasciotomy in severe cases to lengthen the skin gradually before fasciectomy; Colville (1983) and Nagay (Chapter 32) have supported this view. Skoog (1948) summarized the disadvantages of subcutaneous surgery. Luck (1959) revived fasciotomy as part of a treatment plan tailored to the individual patient. He advised removal of nodules and division of subcutaneous cords. A limited role for fasciotomy has therefore evolved. Careful selection is necessary and various criteria have been described by Howard (1959), Hueston (1964), McFarlane & Jamieson (1966) and Colville (1983). These are clearly described by Colville, and repeated here.

Luck (1959) and Tubiana (1964) have advised against fasciotomy in the digits, but Colville (1983) had 'no hesitation' provided the band was well defined and bow-stringing. Rowley et al (1984) restricted fasciotomy to the division of bands proximal to the distal palmar crease.

Gonzales (Chapter 32) varied his approach to the fascia in the individual digit, advocating either fasciotomy or limited fasciectomy. The operation of fasciotomy and graft (McGregor 1985) requires division without resection of the contracted cords. Management of the skin by these surgeons has already been discussed.

Watson (1984) has broken up the line of contracture by performing fasciotomy and Z-plasty, transferring flaps of the full thickness of skin and subcutaneous palmar fascial ligaments. This operation has been suggested for the early palmar contracture, or the thumb, but is less suitable in the digits because of the difficulty of transposing the rather thick flaps.

Limited fasciectomy

Goyrand (1834) has been credited with the first fasciectomy. Sir William Fergusson (1846) advised removal of part of the palmar fascia. Gersuny (1884), Reeves (1885), Kocher (1887) and Moser (1894) undermined the skin edges and excised the thickened aponeurosis. Ritter (1930) made two incisions across the cord and excised the intervening part. Oehlecker (1930) excised a longitudinal narrow ellipse of skin.

Russ (1908) performed an excision through multiple small incisions. Schmidt (1889) used the V-incision of Busch, and Routier (1908) and Palmer (1933) used similar incisions.

Skoog's verdict of limited fasciectomy in 1948 was that the results were disappointing. The concept of partial fasciectomy was unpopular at that time and was criticized because of the likelihood of recurrence. The publication by Hamlin in 1952 of a report of limited fasciectomy marked a change in management philosophy with a general enthusiasm for limited or partial fasciectomy, which was to last until the present day. Ten years later he presented the follow-up results (Hamlin 1962).

Hueston (1961) emphasized that the poor reputation of operations for DD had largely arisen from complications; the radical palmar clearance which was then in vogue was particularly responsible. He defined his operation, 'limited fasciectomy', as the 'excision of the palpably thickened fascia with a narrow margin of normal aponeurosis'. In 1982 he presented the term 'regional fasciectomy', defined as excision limited to macroscopically involved retracted tissue.

Hueston's approach can be considered as a near-total fasciectomy in the involved ray or rays extending from the mid-palm to the base of the middle phalanx — 'Essentially a dissection of the digital nerves'.

The basic principles of his operative technique

(Hueston 1961) required direct exposure of bands or nodules through individual incisions with avoidance of extensive undermining of palmar skin flaps. Some fat was preserved on the skin flaps. Dissection commenced proximally with display of the superficial palmar vascular arch. The neurovascular bundles were then dissected and displayed into the fingers. For a single pretendinous band it was usual to clear over the two adjacent tendon sheaths. He recommended initiative in the planning of exposure rather than using a preconceived plan. Z-plasties were used to prevent contracture of longitudinal scars.

Hueston's article in a prominent American journal (Plastic and Reconstructive Surgery, 1961) followed by a monograph on DD (1963) and a Hunterian lecture (1964) were to establish the ground rules for the next quarter century.

In short, the advantages perceived by Hueston were of a relatively simpler operation than radical fasciectomy with a smoother and more rapid return to full functional recovery. He found no difference in the rates of recurrence or extension.

Many other workers were moving in a similar direction, away from radical towards the Hamlin/Hueston view. Freehafer & Strong published in 1963 a conservative procedure which they had used since 1952. Cords were exposed through short longitudinal incisions in the palm, and in the digits, either a mid lateral or Z incision was used. The fascia was excised in continuity; after freeing the fascia in the proximal wound, the diseased tissue was mobilized beneath the bridge of skin and pushed into the distal wound. Tubiana (1964), in an article entitled 'Selective Treatment' (not to be confused with selective fasciectomy), supported the philosophy that recovery of function was more necessary than prophylaxis and suggested that surgery should be more extensive only when the surgeon felt that it would not impair wound healing or delay active exercises.

Larsen & Posch (1958) and Shaw & Eastwood (1965) recognized a role for limited fasciectomy, and defined different indications for a radical or selective operation.

McFarlane & Jamieson (1966) attempted to select the correct patient for treatment and then varied the type of operation. In 100 patients, the operations performed were limited excision, radical excision, fasciotomy or amputation.

A further refinement of limited fasciectomy was described by Skoog (1967, 1985) who introduced an anatomically precise and selective operation, the details of which are described in Chapter 32. He first recognized in 1959 that the transverse fibres of the palmar aponeurosis were not involved in the disease.

Zachariae (1967) considered that there was little difference between the so-called 'radical' and the limited fasciectomy for DD and Honner et al (1971) supported this view. Zachariae presents his surgical approach in Chapter 32. The limited fasciectomy method was adopted by Honner et al (1971), Rodrigo et al (1971) and Orlando et al (1974).

Variants of limited fasciectomy (with or without an open palm) have been the most popular choice of surgeons in the English- and French-speaking world for 30 years. Operations of this type have been the 'bread and butter' approach with certain patients being selected for either more limited (fasciotomy) or a more radical (dermofasciectomy) treatment. This type of view is reflected in Chapter 32 by Burkhalter.

Moermans, however, has provided a quite different philosophy — that of segmental aponeurectomy in which the aim is to break up the line of contracted fascia by excising short segments (Chapter 32). This procedure lies between a fasciotomy and a limited fasciectomy, as not all the longitudinal contracture band is removed.

The author's own approach has been to perform a similar limited excision based on the anatomy of the palmar fascia, releasing the metacarpophalangeal and proximal interphalangeal joints separately rather than aiming to excise all Dupuytren's tissue (Chapter 32).

Radical palmar fasciectomy

Radical clearance of the palm emerged at the turn of the 20th century when more extensive operations became technically possible and at the same time there was a realization that recurrence of contraction was a problem after less extensive operations. Adams had certainly been aware of the possibility of recurrence in 1879 when an open wound operation performed elsewhere on a former colleague, a physician practising obstetric medicine, returned 'in an aggravated form' at the proximal interphalangeal joint.

Lexer (about 1900, subsequently published 1931), performed a very radical operation on the palm excising fascia and overlying skin from the involved rays. This extensive procedure was still advocated by May in the USA in 1948. Keen (1906) and Iversen (1909) performed 'total' excision of the palmar aponeurosis by the incisions shown in Figure 31.1. Further reports of radical operations were published by Kanavel et al (1929), Desplas & Meillere (1932), Wagner (1932), Gerritzen (1936), Meyerding et al (1936), Einarsson (1946) and Von Stapelmohr (1947).

Einarsson (1946) believed that an indication for operation was the mild case in early life as a prophylactic procedure. He admitted, however, to 20% poor results. In common with other advocates of these extensive operations, he appreciated that a good outcome could not be guaranteed for the patient. Skoog in 1948, reporting on 50 cases of Sir Archibald McIndoe (40 operated on by McIndoe and 10 by himself), favoured his mentor's radical approach at that time. The technical details were enlarged on by Shaw (1951) and by McIndoe & Beare (1958). This operation comprised a single transverse palmar incision from which the skin was extensively undermined to within 2.5 cm (1 inch) of the wrist crease. Distal undermining extended into the finger. The transverse natatory fibres were included in the block dissection. The fingers were approached by a Z incision centred on the digital midline. The entire palmar fascia was removed in a single block extending into the finger by undermining. Great emphasis was placed on dressings technique to prevent haematoma and oedema. Shaw (1951) recommended performing the first dressing after 2 weeks — a much longer interval than most surgeons would favour today.

As described above, in the English language literature the tide began to turn against the preeminence of radical fasciectomy in the 1950's with attempts to define different indications for extensive and limited operations. Iselin (1954) was aware that an attempt at total removal of fascia did not preclude recurrence, as he felt that any remaining minimal strand might develop into a contracture band — a rather speculative view of recurrence which still persists today. He therefore advocated limited fasciectomy through Z incisions.

Surgeons were looking for a simpler procedure with no greater recurrence rate and fewer complications. Luck's (1959) very conservative approach, although not generally accepted, probably influenced most surgeons to become less radical.

At the same time as Hueston's advocacy of limited fasciectomy, Patrick Clarkson at the Second Hand Club Meeting in 1962 condemned radical fasciectomy, showing a number of serious complications from Dupuytren's operations resulting in stiff scarred hands. In the same year he wrote:

The radical procedure has been supported in the view that it removes the potential sites of further recurrence. This is, of course, not so, as the nodules and bands frequently occur and recur along the proximal digits and in the first web and in the thumb — sites not included in any prophylactic radical fasciectomy.

Another change in philosophy in response to the complications of radical operations was the publication by McCash of his open palm fasciectomy in 1964. This technique has been described above, but it is relevant to note here that McCash advised removal of the diseased fascia alone.

In spite of this general trend towards more limited operations in the UK, the USA, Australia and France, a number of long-term reviews of radical operations were published in the following years (Weckesser 1964; Webb-Jones 1965; Hakstian 1966; Dickie & Hughes 1967) with optimistic results. In the long term, the results reported by Hakstian of Sir Archibald McIndoe's personal cases showed 49% of patients were clear of disease, which is a much more optimistic figure than Hueston's 20%. McIndoe's cases, however, showed a predominance of limited contractures and he performed 10 amputations in 24 cases, perhaps favouring the long-term results by ensuring no recurrence in these digits!

Dickie & Hughes (1967) operated on much more severely involved cases and reported excellent results: two-thirds of their patients were clear of recurrence or extension in 10 years. These good long-term results were largely ignored as opinion had moved towards Hueston and McCash. The reason for the established change probably lies more in the results which were not published than those which were. Although a technically able surgeon can achieve a good result and avoid complications with a radical operation, it is not a safe procedure in the hands of the inexperienced or occasional operator. Perhaps more significantly, the rehabilitation almost certainly requires to be more professional and intensive after such procedures. It may be said that radical fasciectomy was discredited on unscientific grounds, on anecdote and horror story rather than statistic.

Although extensive fasciectomy became unpopular amongst English- and French-speaking surgeons, a radical approach to the palm persisted in much of Europe, particularly in Germany and Austria. The German Speaking Hand Society is much more familiar with English language literature than the converse and the adherence of German surgeons to a radical palmar approach cannot be dismissed as a lack of awareness. It seems rather that they have not experienced the same problems with radical palmar approaches, perhaps due to better rehabilitation. Millesi (1965) used a Y-shaped *Mercedessternformige* (Mercedes-star-shaped) incision to preserve the skin blood supply. Geldmacher (1972) and Buck-Gramcko (personal communication) use a similar method. Careful haemostasis and effective rehabilitation ensure good results. There has therefore been no strong motivation for change.

The wide variety of surgical approaches provides strong evidence that patient motivation, and surgical and therapy skills are much more significant to the final outcome than the amount of tissue excised.

Digital fasciectomy

Skin incision patterns to obtain access to the digit have been described above, but the extent of fasciectomy in the digit and the structures removed have received much less attention than in the palm. This is most unfortunate as it is the degree of digital involvement and proximal interphalangeal joint contracture which is the main prognostic feature.

The report of McFarlane (1974) marked a milestone in describing for the surgeon the structures which were being removed (Chapter 14). He described three types of cords developing along the line of anatomical ligamentous structures. It is possible to identify and remove not only involved cords, but also to remove prophylactically the anatomical bands which may be the site of further disease contracture. Based on this knowledge, McFarlane has advocated an extensive removal of involved and potentially involved digital fascia.

On reviewing other authors it seems that McIndoe & Beare (1958), Iselin (1955), McGregor (1985), Hueston (1961), and McCash (1964) have only removed involved fascial cords rather than performing a prophylactic fasciectomy, although these surgeons have not described the specific structures removed from the digits. Hueston (1982), emphasized fasciectomy as essentially a dissection of the neurovascular bundles and this procedure may encourage the removal of subcutaneous fat in the proximal segment of the digit. Skoog (1967) advised preservation of connective and fatty tissues as a general rule, but did not describe in detail his approach to the digits. Strickland & Bassett (1985) have described an isolated digital cord arising proximally from periosteum over the base of the proximal phalanx and also from the intrinsic tendons. Distally it displaces the neurovascular bundles medially and inserts into the flexor sheath in the middle segment of the digit. They advised complete removal.

MANAGEMENT OF THE CONTRACTED PROXIMAL INTERPHALANGEAL JOINT

Dupuytren (1831) appreciated the difficulty in straightening the proximal interphalangeal joint.

As described above, much of the literature on DD has concentrated on the palm when the major problem is correction of proximal interphalangeal joint contracture and maintenance of this correction.

Orthopaedic correction of the contracture was performed by Ombredanne (described by Nelaton 1908) who resected the interphalangeal joint. Kosinki (1940) also performed a similar procedure and divided the flexor tendons as well. Hutchinson (1917) excised the head of the proximal phalanx and shortened the extensor tendon. Eckstein

(1922) removed 1 or 2 cm from the middle of the proximal phalanx.

In general the preferred operation in the early 20th century was amputation. Hakstian (1966) reported 10 primary amputations in 24 operations.

Amputation at metacarpophalangeal joint level may allow the use of dorsal skin flaps to resurface areas of the palm extensively scarred by DD. Tonkin et al (1984) emphasized this point. Amputation at proximal interphalangeal joint level is also frequently performed and Christ (personal communication) has mobilized the distal pulp on two neurovascular pedicles (after the manner of Littler) to resurface the scarred proximal segment of the digit. This type of amputation maintains the width of the palm and avoids neuroma problems.

Moberg (1973) suggested three ways of avoiding amputation in advanced contractures:

1. Arthrodesis of the proximal interphalangeal joint.
2. Dorsal wedge osteotomy of the proximal phalanx.
3. Proximal interphalangeal joint arthroplasty.

For arthrodesis Moberg used a bone peg from the ulna. Dorsal wedge osteotomy carries the theoretical chance of shifting the available arc of rotation dorsally into a more functional position, but little has been written of its results in practice.

Haimovici (1978) has used a Swanson's replacement arthroplasty at the proximal interphalangeal joint and reports a 40° arc of motion in 90% of his cases, but Tonkin et al (1984) report that extension is rarely maintained postoperatively.

Soft tissue correction of proximal interphalangeal joint contracture is more recent than osteotomy. Curtis (1970) reported an operative capsulectomy as an alternative when amputation of the finger was being considered. He enumerated the reasons for lack of complete extension:

1. Inadequate skin over the volar surface of the finger.
2. Contraction of the fascia within the finger.
3. Contracture of the flexor tendon sheath.
4. Contracted flexor muscles or adherent flexor tendons. (There is, however, no published evidence to indicate that flexor tendons became adherent in the primary Dupuytren's case.)
5. Contracture of the volar plate of the capsular ligament.
6. Adherence of Landsmeer's retinacular ligament to the collateral ligaments or shortening of the retinacular ligament.
7. Adherence of the accessory volar ligament to the neck and condyle of the proximal phalanx.

After adequate fasciectomy Curtis excised a section of the volar plate on either side of the flexor tendon together with a portion of the accessory volar ligament. In a few cases excision of the entire volar plate was necessary. A precise postoperative splintage and therapy programme was required.

Watson et al (1979) adopted a slightly less radical approach than Curtis. They recognized a contracture band, the check-rein ligament passing from the proximal edge of the volar plate to the neck of the proximal phalanx, and recommended its division. Eaton (1971) had previously described the check ligament or its anatomical counterpart at this site in the digit.

In the author's view the fascia in this site is less structured than suggested by Watson et al (1979) or by Bowers (1987). A rather amorphous aggregation of Dupuytren's tissue is often found at this site.

The extensor apparatus is of considerable interest in Dupuytren's disease. Smith (personal communication) has recently tried to shorten the attenuated middle slip by plication.

The prognosis remains poor when proximal interphalangeal joint release is necessary.

Although the various views and techniques of treatment in the following chapter have generally covered a range of options, each contribution highlights areas of special interest. We have therefore placed these contributions according to emphasis on the skin, fascia or joints.

32 Various views and techniques

MANAGEMENT OF THE SKIN
Incisions
    Honeycomb technique *P. Bedeschi*
    Open palm and digit technique *W. E. Burkhalter*
    Open palm technique *V. Salvi*

Skin grafting
    Limited fasciectomy and skin graft *R. I. Gonzalez*
    Dermofasciectomy *J. T. Hueston*
    Fasciectomy and dermofasciectomy *F. Iselin*

MANAGEMENT OF THE FASCIA
Fasciotomy
    Fasciotomy *J. Colville*
    Two-stage operation *B. Nagay*

Limited fasciectomy
    Various techniques *J. Varian*
    Evolution of a surgical technique *L. Zachariae*
    Comments on treatment *E. A. Rosenthal*

Variations
    Segmental aponeurectomy *J. P. Moermans*
    Skoog's selective fasciectomy *D. A. McGrouther*
    Extensive fasciectomy *R. M. McFarlane*
    Distal joint hyperextension and flexion *R. M. McFarlane*

MANAGEMENT OF THE SKIN

INCISIONS

PART 1
HONEYCOMB TECHNIQUE
P. Bedeschi

In the treatment of Dupuytren's disease (DD) the overall complication rate is high — almost 20% (McFarlane 1983). Complications related to closed wound techniques are haematoma, skin necrosis, persistent oedema and incomplete correction of the contracture (Tubiana et al 1967).

The complications of the open palm technique (McCash 1965) are inadequate exposure for an extensive digital fasciectomy with a risk of injury to the neurovascular bundles, and the likelihood of incomplete correction of the digital contracture at the proximal interphalangeal joint. Additionally, in the palm an excessive length of time (4–6 weeks) is required to achieve complete healing of the open wound.

THE HONEYCOMB INCISION

This new surgical procedure for DD has been used in 20 cases operated upon consecutively by the same surgeon with a follow-up at 6–18 months. The pattern of the incision of this surgical approach is suggestive of a honeycomb.

In general, a palmodigital incision is made along the contracted finger (Figs 32.1 and 32.2) but sometimes the palmar incision does not correspond with the digital incision. The incision angles are

312 DUPUYTREN'S DISEASE

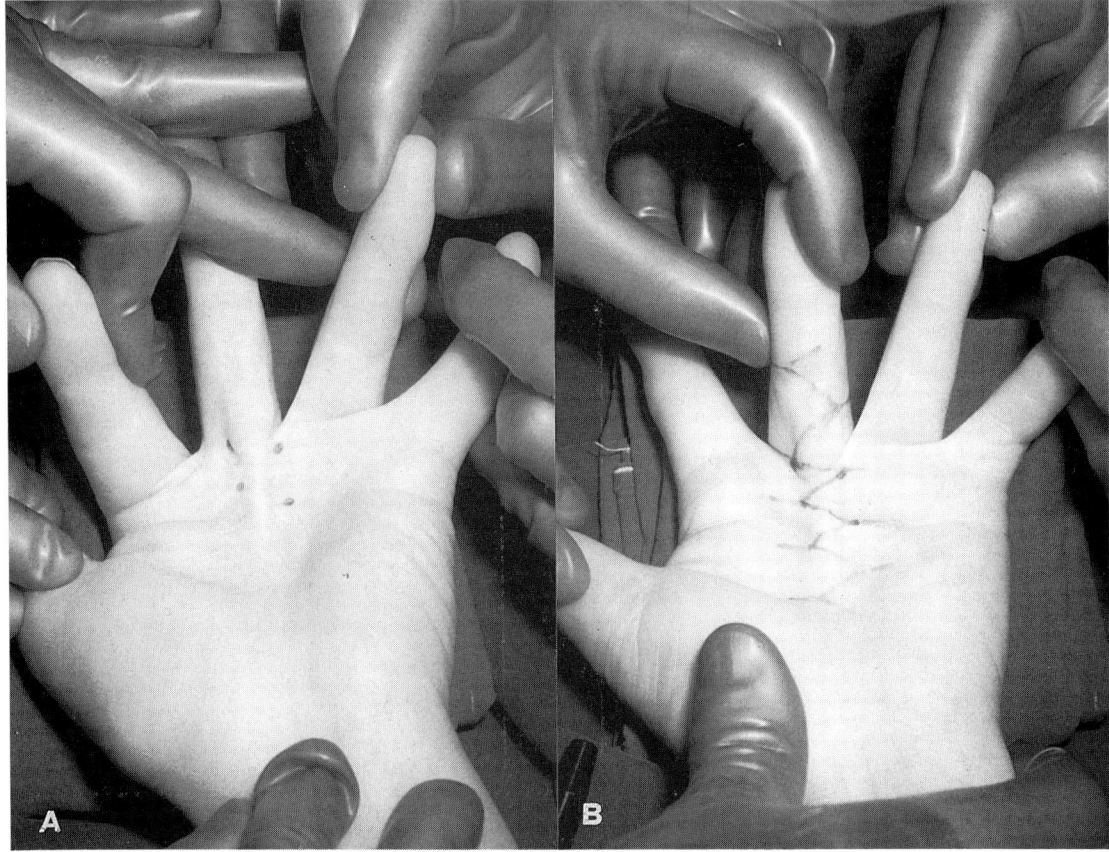

Fig. 32.1 Dupuytren's contracture of the middle finger. **A** First four basic markers for the top angles of the zig-zag incision at the palmodigital level **B** The incision design. **C–D** The wide exposure allowed by this technique enables extensive and safe palmar and digital fasciectomy. **E** At the end of the operation: note the complete correction of contracture; only the zig-zag incision is sutured. Transverse incisions become small open areas avoiding tension of wounds and preventing haematomas. **F** After 14 days.

90–110° according to the greater or lesser severity of the digital contracture and according to the point of maximum contracture whether it is at the metacarpophalangeal or proximal interphalangeal joint. The transverse incisions in the palm must be long enough for an extensive palmar fasciectomy. The digital transverse incision should reach the mid lateral lines both to prevent tension on the sutures and so that an extensive digital fasciectomy may be performed.

In this way complete contracture correction can generally be obtained, even at the proximal interphalangeal joint, without having to perform a capsulotomy.

Figure 32.1A illustrates the first four basic markers for the top angles of the zig-zag incision at the palmodigital level. Two of these are on the ulnar side of the contracture (one at the distal palmar crease and the other 2 or 3 mm proximal to the palmar digital crease).

The other two are on the radial side (one halfway between the two on the ulnar side and the other 2 or 3 mm distal to the palmodigital crease). It is extremely important that the incisions which cross the digital crease both at the metacarpophalangeal and, proximal interphalangeal joint form an angle of less than 45°, bearing in mind that after correction of the contracture the wounds

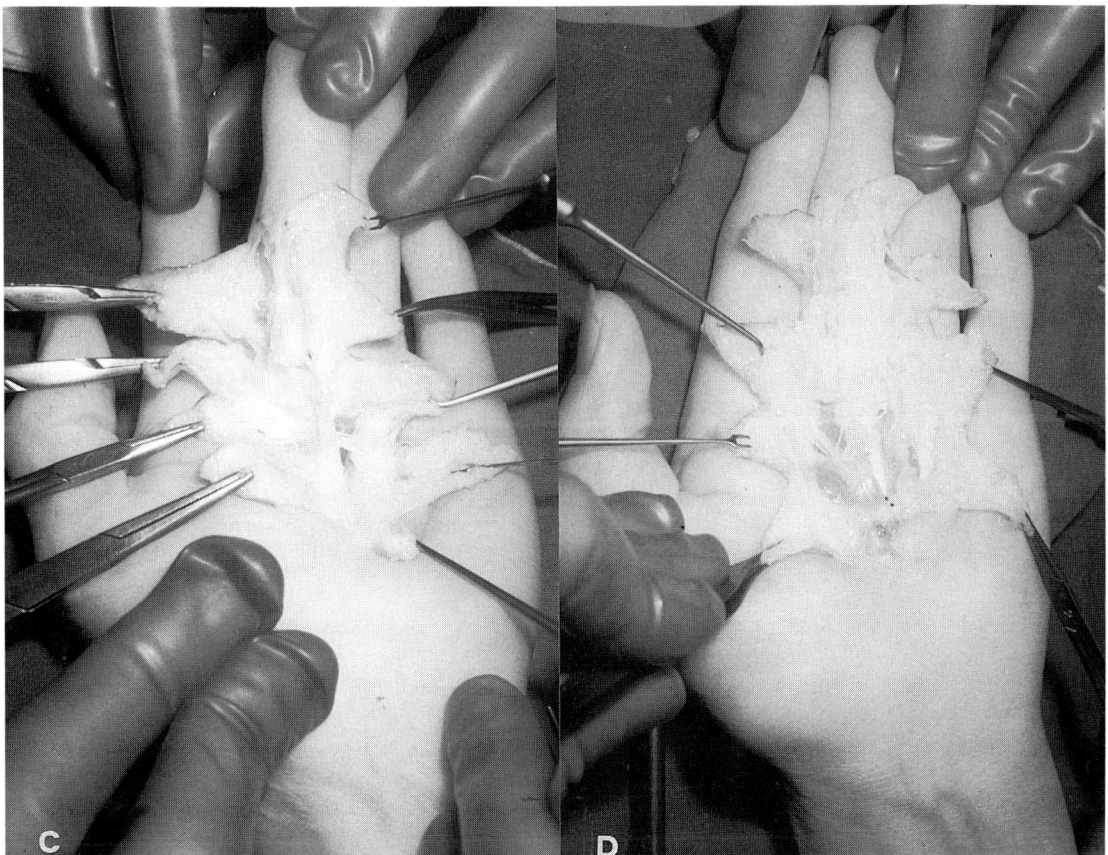

Fig. 32.1 (contd)

will become more longitudinal (Fig. 32.2B–C). The skin flaps provide wide exposure for safe palmar and digital fasciectomy (Fig. 32.1C–D).

Only the zig-zag incision is sutured; the transverse incisions become small open areas that avoid skin tension and prevent haematoma formation (Figs 32.1B and 32.2B). No postoperative splinting is used. Therapy is commenced immediately.

The pattern of the incisions — a zig-zag palmodigital incision and multiple open transverse wounds of this new surgical approach reminds us of a 'honeycomb'.

This surgical procedure has had few postoperative complications (three superficial flap tip necrosis) and the correction of the contracture is well maintained at follow-up in the majority of cases.

ADVANTAGES OF THIS TECHNIQUE

1. It provides wide palmodigital exposure which permits extensive and safe palmar and digital fasciectomy.
2. The many small open areas avoid tension on the wounds and prevent haematoma formation.
3. There is complete contracture correction not only at the metacarpophalangeal but also at the proximal interphalangeal joint.
4. Open wound healing time is 2–3 weeks as against 4–6 weeks for the open palm technique.
5. No longitudinal contracting scar is produced if the incision angles are correct, especially in crossing the digital crease at both

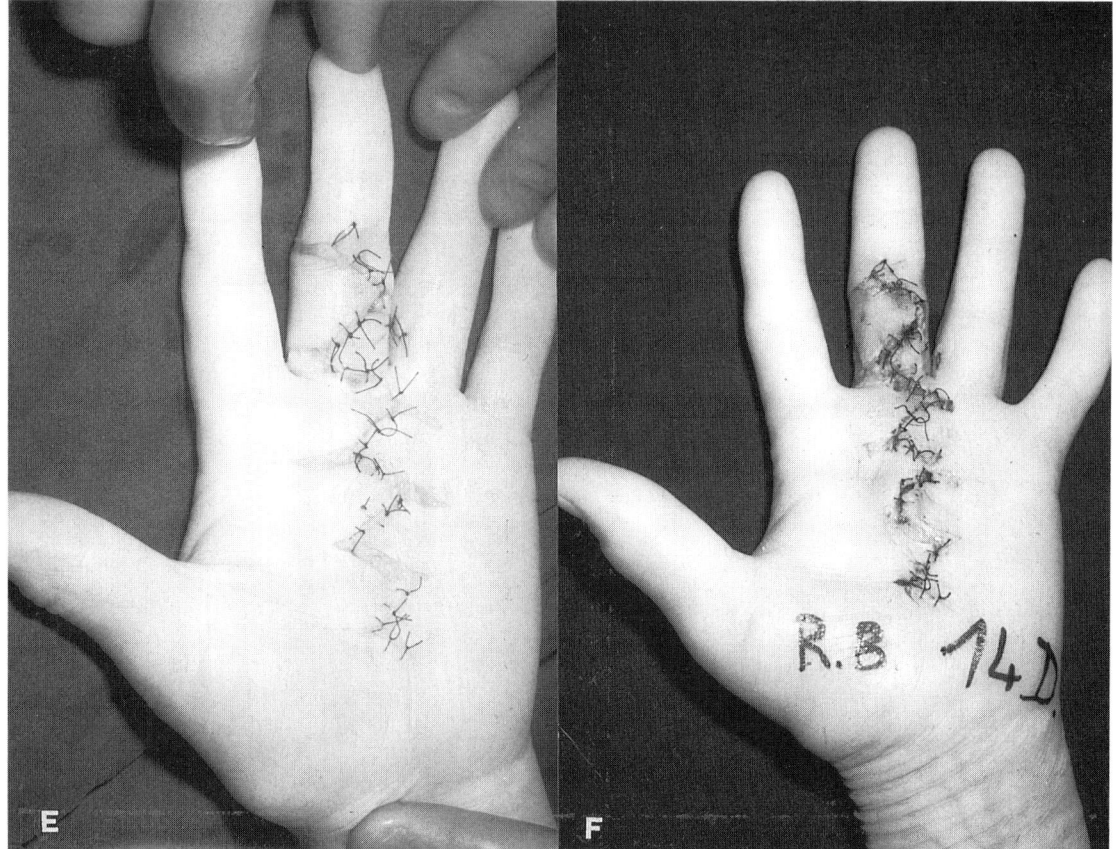

Fig. 32.1 (contd)

metacarpophalangeal and proximal interphalangeal joints.

CONCLUSIONS

The honeycomb technique combines the advantages of the open palm and the digital palmar closed wound techniques without their respective disadvantages.

This surgical approach is particularly indicated for single ray, moderate and severe DD.

PART 2
OPEN PALM AND DIGIT TECHNIQUE
W. E. Burkhalter

What are the advantages and disadvantages of the open palm and digit techniques? The major disadvantages of multiple transverse incisions are relatively limited surgical exposure and the potential danger of loss of these bipedicle flaps.

Fig. 32.2 (right) Dupuytren's contracture of the ring finger. **A** The incision design. **B** After suturing the zig-zag incision: note the small open areas' and the complete correction of contracture. **C–D** After 13 Months. Note excellent functional results.

VARIOUS VIEWS AND TECHNIQUES 315

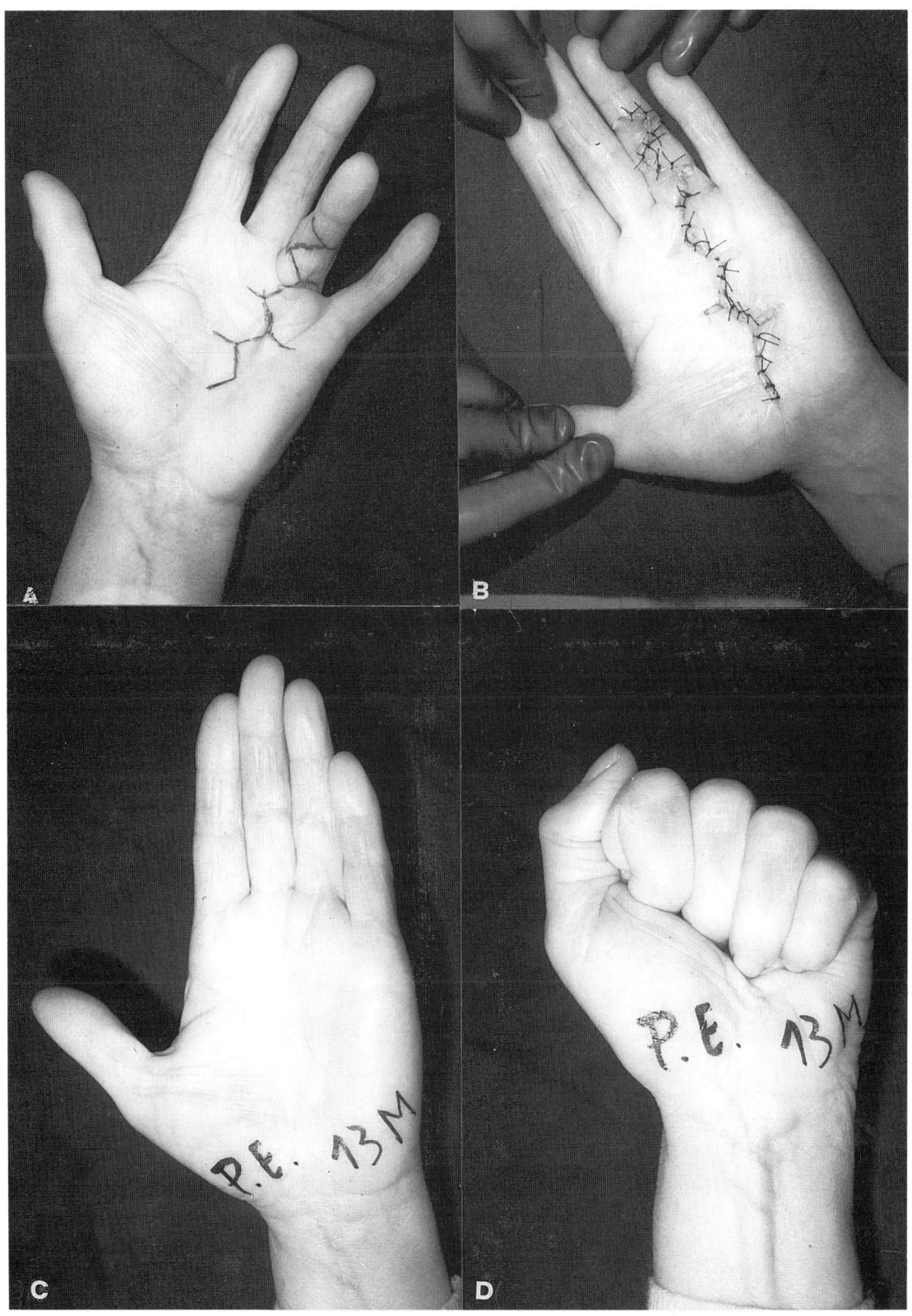

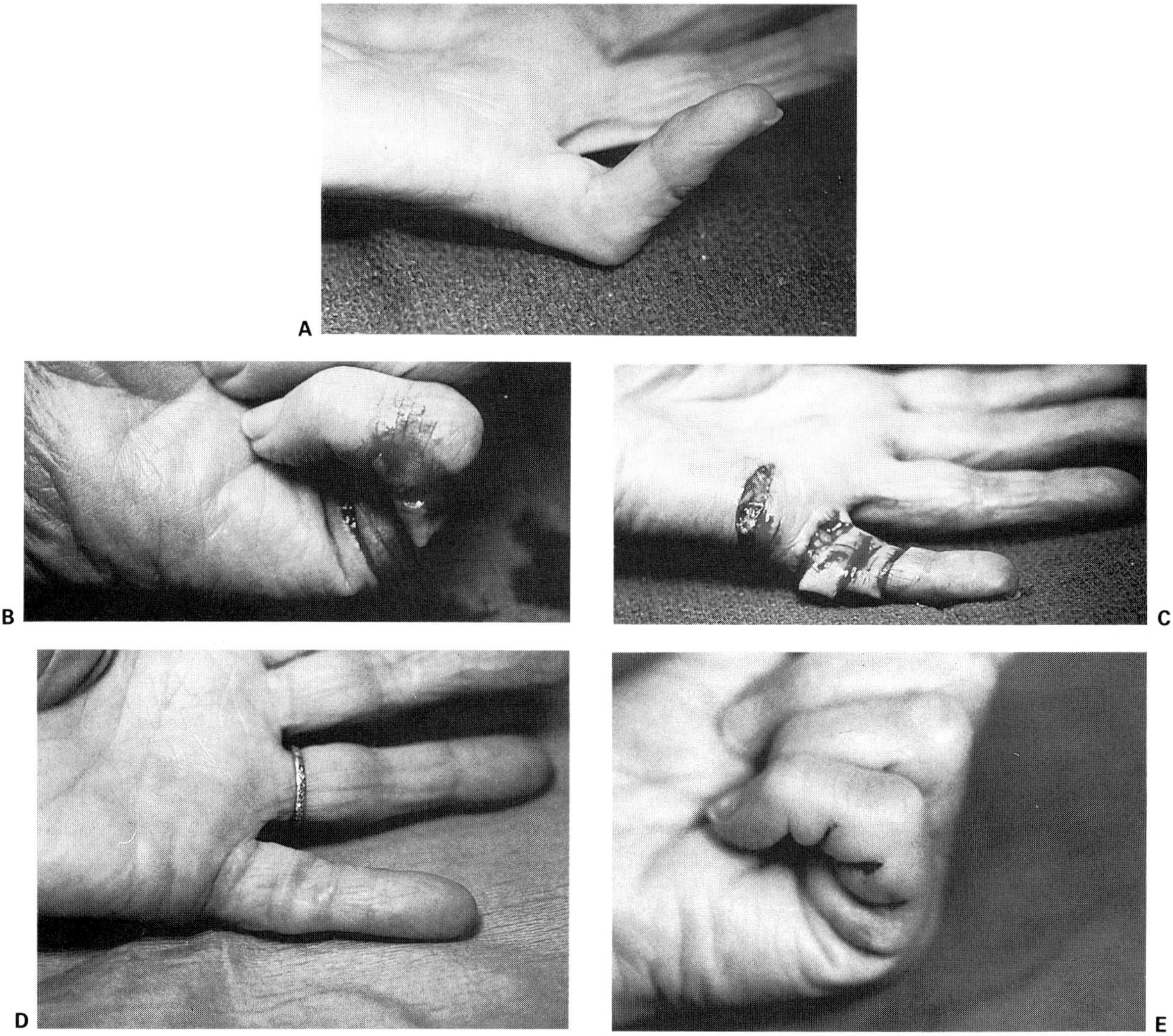

Fig. 32.3 A An isolated proximal interphalangeal joint contracture in a 62-year-old woman. Multiple transverse incisions were used to correct the deformity. Postoperative rehabilitation consisted of active range of motion exercises and splinting in extension at night with local wound care. **B–C** These exercises were begun 24 hours postoperatively. **D–E** At 10 days the wound is healing well with excellent proximal interphalangeal joint motion. At 3 weeks the wound has solidly healed. **F** There was no evidence of recurrent disease at 1 year with barely discernible surgical scars in a wound that was allowed to heal by secondary intension.

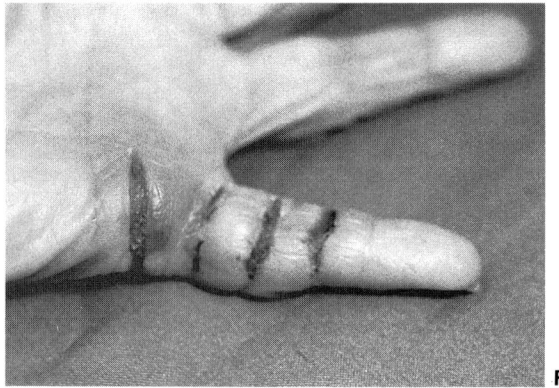

The major area of concern with limited exposure is the base of the finger, not distally in the digit or in the palm. The skin flaps can be elevated easily in the palm through two separate incisions and the contracting fascia divided and excised. With the realization that the diseased fascia need not be excised in a single sheet from palm to distal digit, surgery through transverse incisions is easier. Once the palm is open and the fascia removed there is a gain in digital extension.

A transverse incision is made at the base of the finger, thin flaps are elevated and a search is made for the neurovascular bundles. The incision must extend from mid axial to mid axial line. If the bundles cannot easily be found, an oblique or longitudinal extension is used to connect the palm and base of finger incisions. With this the nerve and vessel can be easily found and protected.

The palmar fascia is divided at this level at mid proximal phalanx and so some extension of the proximal interphalangeal joint flexor contraction is achieved. Another incision is made transversely from mid axial to mid axial line proximal to the middle flexor crease and another of the same length distal to the flexor crease. Then the flaps are elevated.

These long transverse incisions allow us to look behind the contracting bands for the vessel and nerve. With a conventional exposure the digital nerve is usually identified first. With transverse incisions the emphasis is on first identifying the digital vessel because one's approach is from dorsal to volar. When both nerve and vessel can be identified on both sides of the finger, the palmar fascia is incised. This brings about greater extension of the digit.

The transverse wounds are now gaping and more extensive exposure of the nerve and vessel is possible with subsequent excision of the diseased fascia. It is important that diseased fascia should be excised, not simply incised, and that a transverse incision should be made distal to the last contracted joint. Exploration of the retrovascular area about the proximal interphalangeal joint will define involvement of the retinacular ligament which can be excised, further releasing the joint.

The major advantages of the open palm and digit technique are absence of local wound breakdown and haematoma, reduced postoperative pain and less need for skin shifts or advancements.

There is no loss of skin in DD. The skin with its viscoelastic properties has simply conformed itself to the shape demanded of it by external forces. The shortening of the diseased fascia allows the skin likewise to shorten. With open transverse incisions which are allowed to heal by second intention, the dynamic healing wound gradually elongates the contracted skin (Fig 32.3–32.5).

The same viscoelastic properties of the skin that gradually resulted in 'shrinkage' are now utilized

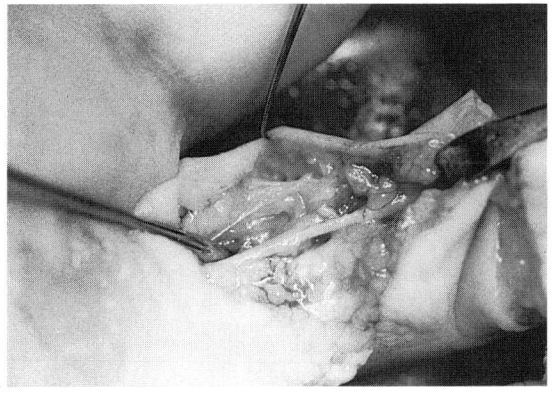
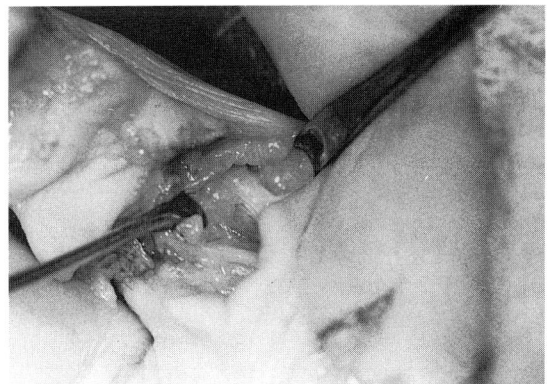

Fig. 32.4 A, B Even though transverse incisions limit exposure of versels and nerves in the palms and fingers, undermining of the flaps and exposure and protection of the neurovascular structures permit adequate exposure of the diseased fascia. Although this surgical exposure takes longer than volar zig-zag or longitudinal incisions, rehabilitation by active motion can be instituted imediately without concern for wound disruption, haematomas or skin slough. Operating time is spent with exposure rather than closure.

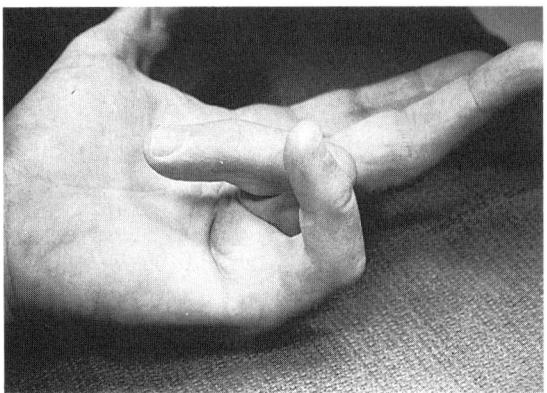
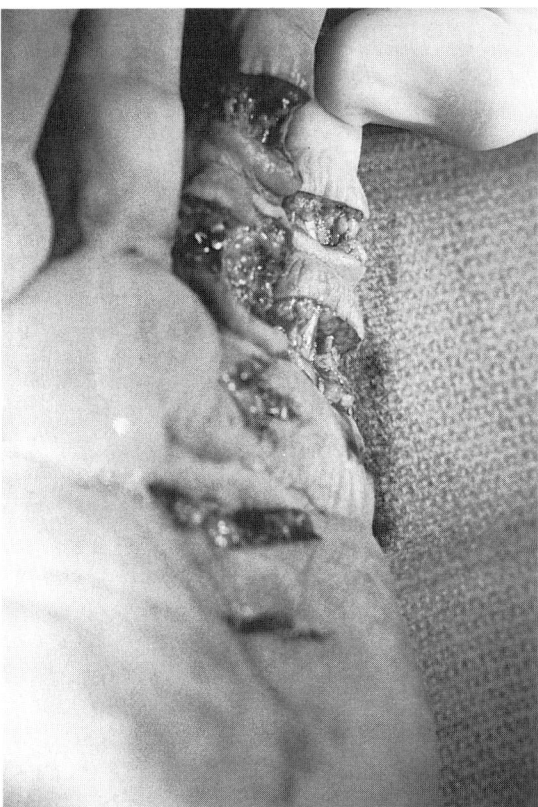
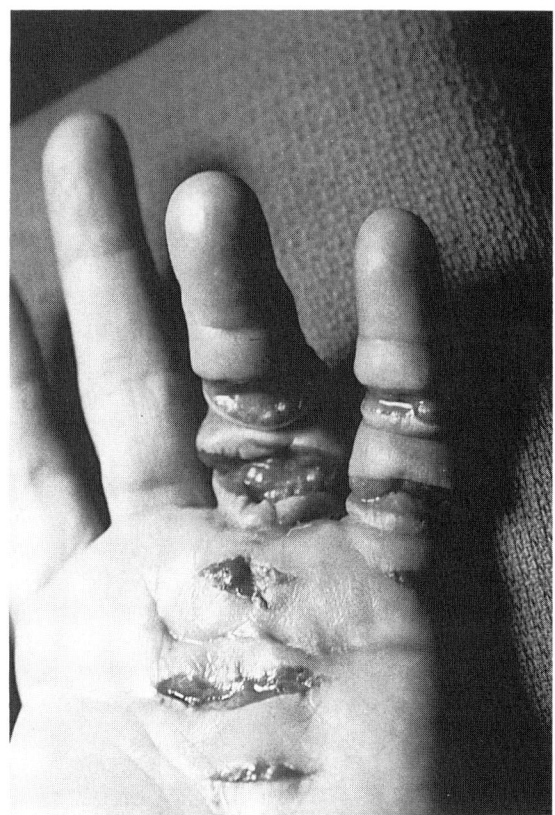

Fig. 32.5 A This patient, a 65-year-old man with long-standing DD, demonstrates severe flexion contractures on the ulnar side of the hand. **B** Multiple transverse incisions were used to correct the defomity. **C** At 3 days the fingers and skin flaps were oedematous, but with prolonged splinting in extension at night and active use of the hand in the day, the wound healed with good flexion at 6 weeks. A persisting extensor lag, however, was present at the proximal interphalangeal joint of the ring finger. There was no contracture, however, because of continued splinting at night. **D–E** At 1 year flexion remained full and extension was completed with absence of lag. In this case the severe deformity resulted in weak extension postoperatively. Extension splinting at night avoided a contracture.

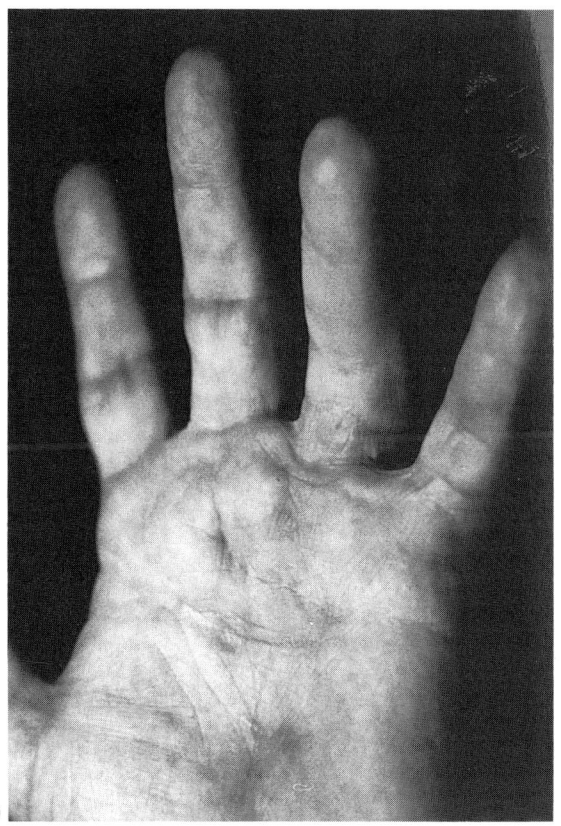
D

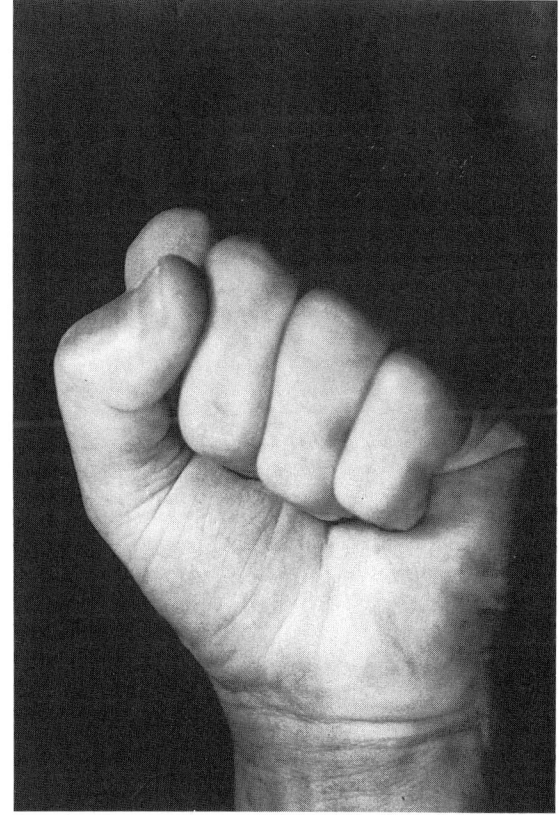
E

to lengthen the contracted skin. One has only to look at these incisions which were allowed to heal by secondary intention after a few months to realize that there is no skin deficit. The incisions heal linearly and are barely visible. Since there is no shortage of skin, Z-plasty and V–Y plasty are not necessary.

Diminished postoperative pain is a real advantage of leaving the surgical incisions open. Sutures in swollen flaps create tension and a feeling of cutting. The patient can always tell you where you placed stitches in an extensive dissection for DD when a portion of the wound was left open. The wound closed with sutures will be far more painful than the one left open. This will be all the more noticeable when the patient begins active motion of the hand.

With open wounds prolonged immobilization postoperatively is not necessary. Motion can begin within 24–48 hours postoperatively. In a condition in which postoperative stiffness is common, early motion is a definite advantage.

Invariably two additional questions are asked concerning the open palm and digit technique. How do the operative times compare between the transverse incisions and longitudinal incisions with Z-plasty? How does one prevent infection with the open wound?

The operative time would seem to be much longer when working under small bipedicle flaps than when the finger is opened widely. This is only partly true. Careful dissection is necessary in both. The time to complete removal of the diseased fascia is shorter with the longitudinal incision. At that point, however, creation of multiple Z-plasties and closure is necessary. With multiple transverse incisions, once the fascia is excised, the operative procedure is complete. Therefore the total operative time is similar with both techniques.

The management of the open wound in the hand is an area of concern. We have been told for years that open wounds in the hand create excess collagen, increased scar, loss of motion and functional impairment. Nothing could be further from the truth. Secondary intention wound healing in the presence of active motion and functional activity will not result in scar deformity or contracture. Initially, relatively large amounts of newly formed collagen will be present in the wound. As the wound contracts with active motion and intermittent splinting in extension, the viscoelastic skin lengthens and the wound closes. Once the wound is healed organization of the newly formed collagen begins. Within a few months the skin is soft and the transverse scars are linear.

How does one manage the wound in the interim? At the completion of the surgical release, xeroform, adaptic or Owen's silk are applied over the wounds. This is followed by a fluff of gauze and the hand is held in extension by means of a Kling-film type dressing. Plaster is applied to maintain the wrist and fingers in extension. The day following operation this bulky dressing is removed and flexion and extension is begun.

Full flexion, including distal interphalangeal joint motion, is stressed in order to obtain differential motion between flexor digitorum superficialis and flexor digitorum profundus. A static splint of thermoplastic material is fabricated to be worn at night. The need for full digital flexion and extension hourly during the day is stressed.

Wound care consists of gentle soap and tap water washing of the wounds and the hand is held under running water or a shower for 5 minutes three times each day. Soaking of the hand should be avoided. Antibiotics are not used. Full digital extension and full distal joint flexion must be stressed always.

Wounds usually heal in 3–4 weeks. Most wound discomfort is gone by 7 days. However, close supervision for the first 2–3 weeks is necessary in order to make certain that the extremes of motion are being achieved during active motion. Splinting at night in the case of proximal interphalangeal joint contractures continues for approximately 3 months and occasionally longer. For metacarpophalangeal joint contractures splinting for 6–8 weeks is usually adequate.

Splinting into full extension is extremely important in the postoperative rehabilitation. Static splinting of the proximal interphalangeal joint into full extension may be difficult to maintain. However, changes from palmar to dorsal splints and even dynamic extensor assists may be used to obtain full proximal interphalangeal joint extension. If, during the operative procedure a formal joint release was necessary in order to regain full extension, splinting of the proximal interphalangeal joint into extension at night may be necessary for up to 6 months postoperatively.

PART 3
OPEN PALM TECHNIQUE
V. Salvi

Since 1968, I have been using the so-called 'open palm' technique described by McCash in 1964. Initially reserved for elderly patients, it has subsequently been adopted on all occasions on account of its excellent results.

This technique employs a transverse distal crease incision according to McIndoe with ample exposure of the aponeurotic tissue contracted in the palm. Total, subtotal or selective fasciectomy can be performed. My preference is for the selective.

In the presence of digital extension of the contracture, a Z incision is made for each affected finger, starting from the distal edge of the palmar incision. In this way, the operator can visualize all the pathological tissue to be removed.

The finger incisions are sutured at the end of the operation, whereas the transverse incision in the palm is left open.

Surgery is performed using a pneumatic tourniquet, though without preceding emptying with an Esmarch's bandage. This detail is of major importance, since it ensures that the small vessels remain fully visible and haemostasis can be immediately achieved if they are cut. On completion of the operation, bandaging is carried out before the tourniquet is removed.

The open wound in the palm is covered with damp gauze. A compressive and elastic bandage allowing flexion and extension of the fingers is applied. This, indeed, is the great advantage of the method: the patient can immediately mobilize the fingers since no pain is felt.

This method avoids oedema of the hand itself and stiffness of the fingers. The bandage is replaced by a very light one on the fifth day. This covers the open area, but allows ample mobility of the fingers. If appreciable bleeding occurs and the bandage becomes soaked with blood (observed only twice in 146 cases), it is best to remove the bandage immediately and arrest the flow from the bleeding vessel. A dressing is performed every 5 days.

Gradual approximation of the edges, which are usually at least 2 cm apart after the incision, proceeds to juxtaposition by the 20th day, followed by direct cicatrization of the borders. Healing is not by second intention with a formation of granulation tissue, but by first delayed intention.

The open palm technique is indicated in any type of DD although not in the treatment of recurrences: I have used it for this purpose on some occasions, but the results have not been satisfactory and I now use the free grafts described by Hueston.

Good results have been achieved with the open palm technique in 77% of the author's 146 cases. The failures cannot be blamed on the technique, but on the appearance of recurrences and extension, obviously dependent on the type of fasciectomy employed.

It must be emphasized that this method is very well accepted by patients, since full recovery of the hand is achieved without pain.

SKIN GRAFTING

PART 4
LIMITED FASCIECTOMY AND SKIN GRAFT
R. I. Gonzalez

Primary treatment of DD should be restricted to those hands that demonstrate flexion contractures, as 50% of early DD without joint contractures do not progress. Once contractures have developed, early release of the joint should be done. This is particularly true if the proximal interphalangeal joint is involved. If this joint is allowed to remain contracted for any length of time, complete release and recovery of full extension may not be possible. I feel that release of a contracted proximal interphalangeal joint is an emergency, contrasted to the metacarpophalangeal joint, which can be released at almost any time. It is equally important to release recurrent contractures of the proximal interphalangeal joint as early as possible. Of course, secondary release may be very difficult if the primary treatment was a digital 'clean-out' without skin replacement. The proximal segment of the finger may be totally replaced with DD scar, and locating and protecting the neurovascular bundles may be very difficult or impossible. The volar joint capsules may also be secondarily shortened and fixed, and capsulotomy may be necessary in order to achieve extension. In my experience, the release following capsulotomy is only temporary, and full permanent extension does not occur. Therefore, it is important that the primary surgery should be done early, and should not produce scar.

Over the past 20 years I have released Dupuytren's contracture as any other soft tissue contracture by dividing the skin and fascial bands at the point of maximal tension, protecting the neurovascular bundles and excising the overlying skin and adherent fascia. It is my feeling that wide resection of the overlying skin largely prevents recurrent contractures, and in those that recur, can be secondarily released easily and by the same method. The recurrence rate is 6% at 2 years and 15% at 5 years.

AUTHOR'S TECHNIQUE

The operative technique which I have used for 30 years is extremely simple (Gonzalez 1969). It is performed with the patient under local anaesthesia and as an outpatient. In a bloodless field, the skin and underlying fascial bands are divided transversely at the point of maximal tension after the neurovascular bundles have been located and protected.

All involved skin and fascial bands are excised.

The blood pressure cuff is released and an ellipse of full thickness skin is removed from a hairless area in the opposite groin. The bottom layer of dermis is left intact and the wound is closed. The graft is then sutured into the denuded area of the digit with interrupted 3-0 silk sutures, which are left long and tied over a bolus of wet cotton.

If a limited palmar fasciectomy is indicated, the hand is re-exsanguinated, the area is infiltrated with local anaesthesia, and a routine limited fasciectomy is performed. If two or three rays are operated on and large flaps are developed, the dermal layer of the flaps is tacked to the underlying fascia of the intrinsic muscles with absorbable sutures in order to eliminate dead space. Any compromised skin can be excised.

The wound closes easily, as the shortness of skin has been released by the distal skin and fascial release. The tourniquet time is always less than 10 minutes for each area of dissection. This may account for the extremely low incidence of postoperative morbidity.

A voluminous dressing is applied, incorporating a volar plaster slab that keeps the wrist in slight dorsiflexion and the involved digits in full extension. This dressing remains in place for 1 week. The wounds are then inspected and the bolus removed. A new short volar plaster splint is applied to the affected digits to keep them in full extension. The distal joints are left free, and flexion of these joints is encouraged. Recovery of flexion is rapid and postoperative complications, such as pain, swelling, haematoma, sympathetic dystrophy, nerve damage, are nil. Multiple digits can be operated on at one sitting; care must be taken to release the tourniquet after each dissection. No tourniquet is necessary while the skin grafts are sutured in place.

Cosmetically, the early depression at the site of the skin graft smooths out in a matter of weeks (Fig. 32.6) If pigmentation of the graft is a problem, the graft should be taken from the instep of the foot. This graft gives perfect colour and texture match. Usually, the foot donor site can be closed; however, if a large graft has been taken, it may be necessary to split-graft this area. Therefore, this is not the common donor site and is recommended only in dark-skinned females. Hueston (1962) achieves good colour and texture match by utilizing the skin from the inner aspect of the arm.

Postoperative care is extremely important. After all sutures have been removed, the patient is told to soak the hand in warm, soapy water for 5 minutes three times a day, actively flexing and spreading the fingers while they are in the water. After each exercise session, the patient dries the hand thoroughly and applies cold cream or light lotion to the operated areas, massaging the incisional area. If 100% take of the grafts has not been achieved, the grafted areas could either be left open to the air, or covered with a dry plaster.

The following week guided active exercises are started. The patient firmly stabilizes the metacarpophalangeal joint with the opposite thumb and index, and then vigorously, actively flexes and extends the distal two joints. It is important for the surgeon to work with the patient to be sure that the exercises are done properly. The patient is instructed to carry out these exercises at home during waking hours.

The next week, if there is any lack of flexion,

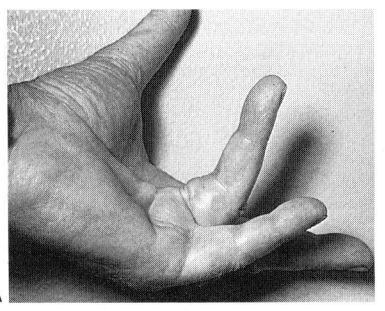
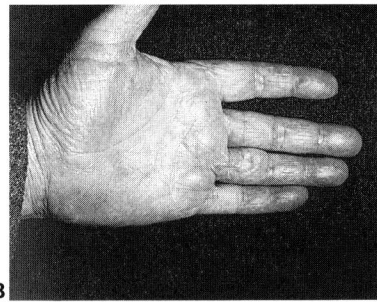
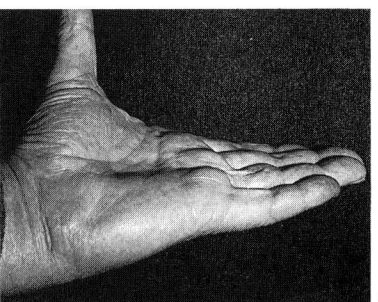

Fig. 32.6A This patient had a contracted ring finger, with the major contracture only at the metacarpophalangeal joint. **B, C** The patient is shown 2 months postoperatively.

the patient is fitted with a simple, adjustable web strap and buckle which is applied across the fingers and the palm in the form of a loop. The patient gently tightens the loop by means of the buckle in order to produce continuous gentle pressure over the middle segments of the finger. If the tension is painful, the strap should be loosened. The strap and buckle should provide continuous gentle pressure over a long period of time.

It is far more common to find a mild recurrence of the preoperative flexion deformity of the proximal interphalangeal joint, particularly of the little finger. This must be counteracted by the use of an adjustable 'safety-pin' splint. The splint should be adjusted so as to put pressure over the proximal interphalangeal joint in a gentle continuous fashion. The strap and buckle also provide a means of adjusting this splint. Splinting may be necessary for several weeks following surgery, particularly if the proximal interphalangeal joint was 'springy' at the time of the original release.

In summary, the postoperative care is just as important, or more important than the primary surgery, and the patients must be seen frequently by the surgeon, who carefully monitors progress. Splinting and exercises should be continued until full extension and flexion have been achieved. Very often such achievement of full flexion and extension is obtained very early, even within 21 days. However, occasionally longer periods of treatment are needed. I emphasize that the splinting and exercises should be carried out, even if the grafts are not completely healed. Usually it is just the superficial areas of the graft that do not heal per primum; the dermis always seems to take well, although epithelialization may take a few weeks.

Although I have been pleased with the results of digital release with the inset of full thickness skin grafts, there are some problems which have not been overcome. The primary one is that of the proximal interphalangeal joint. It has been my finding that if it has been contracted for over 4 years, it may not be possible to release the joint at the time of surgery. If there has been marked shortening of the volar capsule, extension can be achieved only by capsulotomy. Contractures usually recur postoperatively. In my series of 100 operations, I found that 15 proximal interphalangeal joints could not be released completely. Therefore, it is imperative to release the proximal interphalangeal joint, particularly of the little finger, at the earliest possible moment. The metacarpophalangeal joints do not have this problem and surgery can be delayed indefinitely, as full extension is easily achieved.

Apart from this, the results have been very satisfactory. There has been a very low incidence of recurrent contracture in fully released joints — only 6% recurred after 2 years, and 15% after 10 years.

TREATMENT OF RECURRENT CONTRACTURES

The release of recurrent contractures following primary 'clean-out' procedures is very difficult, as the entire digit may be replaced with DD scar. This tissue is entirely different from the original Dupuytren's tissue. There are no definable bands, but instead, there is a mass of undifferentiated scar. The neurovascular bundles are enmeshed in this scar, and are difficult to locate and protect. The skin is almost always involved and must be replaced with a full thickness skin graft. The joint may also have become secondarily contracted and necessitate a capsulotomy. This is done by incising the entire proximal limb of the volar plate and the adjacent check reins. Great care should be taken not to rupture the capsule or allow dislocation of the proximal interphalangeal joint, as this certainly results in a fixed joint.

If multiple attempts have been made to correct recurrent contractures, then salvage procedures must be contemplated (Fig. 32.7). I feel the best salvage procedure is the release of the contracture, replacement of the scarred skin with free full thickness grafts, and fusing the mid-joint in 30–40° of flexion. In my opinion, fusion of the proximal interphalangeal joint is far superior to amputation. In my review of the Canniesburn group, I found that all 18 patients who had undergone amputation were unhappy with their results. They reported continuous pain, accentuated by cold weather, and loss of grip. I have also seen extension of the disease to the previously uninvolved adjacent digits, recreating the same

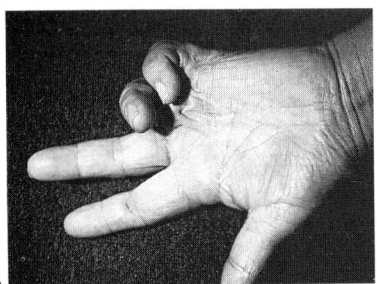 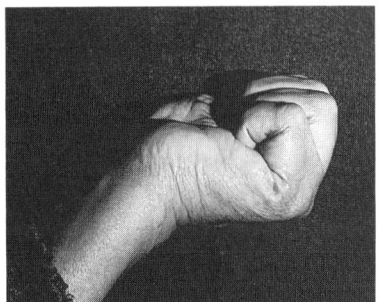 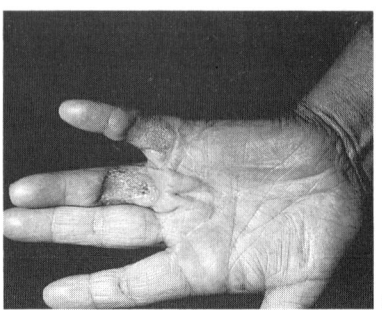

Fig. 32.7 One of the real challenges in the treatment of DD is the treatment of recurrent contractures following multiple surgical procedures. This patient has had four 'clean-out' operations. **A** Preoperatively, it was impossible to determine whether the proximal interphalangeal joints were firmly fixed or if they could be released by simple division of the skin and subcutaneous glands. Intraoperatively, it was found that the joints were mobile and full release was obtained. However, there was extreme shortness of skin, as well as scarring of the skin; all scar tissue was excised and replaced with full thickness skin grafts. **B** Full extension was obtained as well as full recovery of flexion. **C** Cosmetically, the result could have been improved by further excision of the digital skin borders in order to eliminate this ridge.

problem as in the amputated digit. As stated previously, if recurrent contractures occur, following simplified primary surgery (open fasciectomy, plus replacement of overlying skin with full thickness skin graft), secondary release is very simple, as no scar has been produced, and secondary release is no different from the original primary surgery (Fig. 32.8). Fortunately, the recurrence rate following this type of primary release is very low, and so far, no salvage procedures have had to be done.

DISCUSSION

DD is a puzzling condition. Its aetiology and pathology are obscure, and treatment is controversial. If one treats DD as any other scar contracture, it is possible to control the disease by dividing the contracting bands at their point of maximal tension, excising the involved overlying skin, and inserting a full thickness skin graft. The operation, which is done under local anaesthesia as an outpatient procedure, produces little operative or postoperative morbidity. Elderly patients with major systemic diseases can be treated without difficulty. Healing is rapid, and function is recovered early. Recurrent contractures, which in my experience were found in approximately 15% of patients over a 5-year period, can easily be treated by repeating the original, simple surgical procedure. Great emphasis should be placed on the early release of a contracted proximal interphalangeal joint, as secondary shortening of the volar capsule can make full correction of the contracture impossible.

In summary, there is growing evidence that the volar skin of the digits is intrinsic in the development of digital DD. It must be removed if recurrent contractures are to be prevented. Removing the skin simplifies the surgical exposure of nerves and tendons, and this decreases the danger of damage to these important structures. I feel that almost all joint contractures should be primarily released by this method. I do not feel that the procedure should be reserved for those with a strong Dupuytren's diathesis (Hueston 1962), but should be offered to all patients, both young and old. As dissection is minimal and tourniquet time is short, postoperative morbidity is nil. Control with minimal surgical morbidity is the objective of treatment of this incurable disease. Finally, in these days of cost containment, this technique eliminates hospitalization and general anaesthesia, saving thousands of dollars.

PART 5
DERMOFASCIECTOMY
J. T. Hueston

The failures of fasciectomy have already been simply classified as postoperative complications of

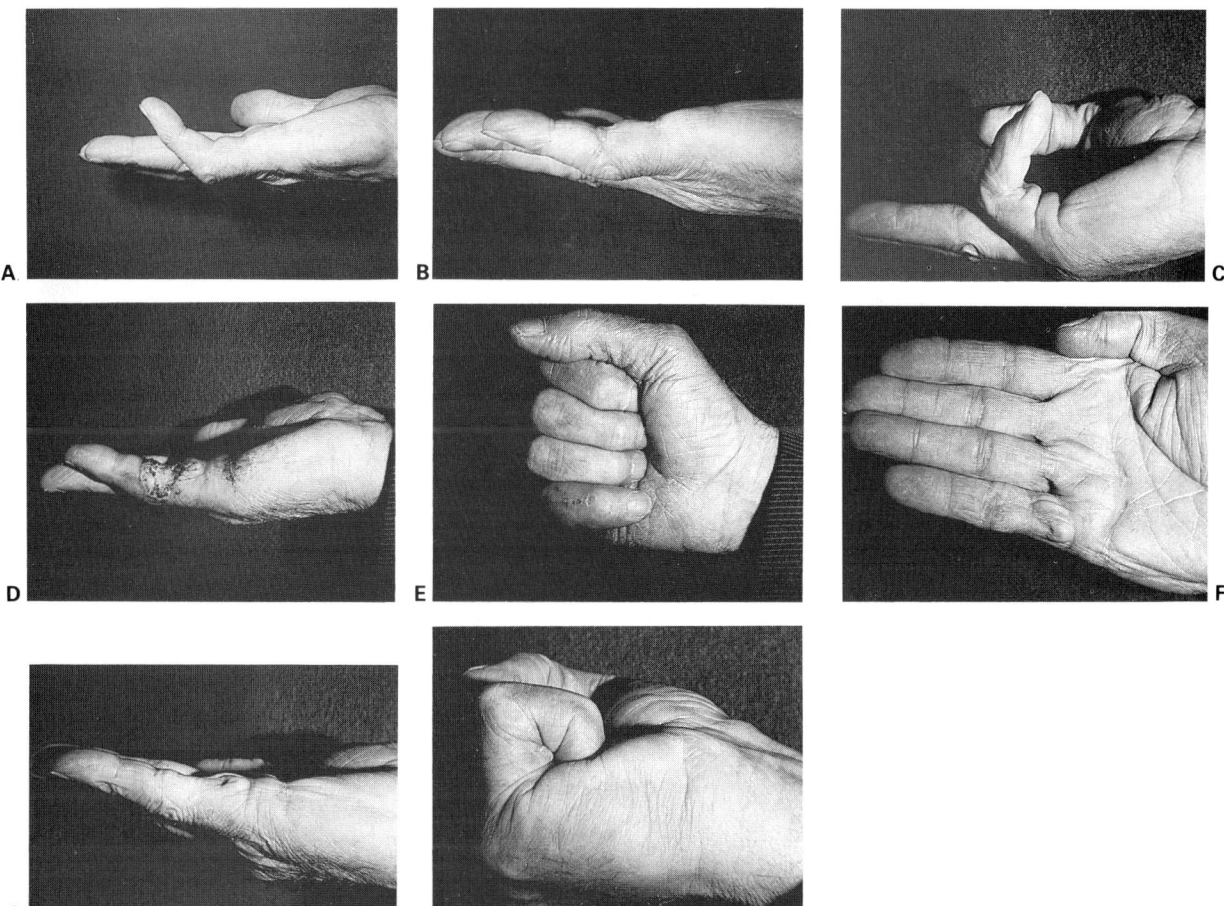

Fig. 32.8 The greatest advantage of the primary use of full thickness skin grafts in releasing contractures is illustrated by this case. The patient had a moderate flexion contracture of the middle joint of his little finger, which was well released by the routine division of the contracting bands and inset of a full thickness skin graft. However, after 5 years the contracture recurred. The skin adjacent to the skin graft was supple, and it was possible to release and add an additional full thickness skin graft. Rapid short- and long-term correction was obtained. **A** Preoperatively. **B** Four months after the first operation. **C** Five years after the initial operation. **D** Eleven days after the second operation. **E** Eleven days after the second operation. **F–H** Five years after the second operation.

wound healing attributable to the surgeon, and progression of the DD process as recurrence, attributable to the patient. In particular, the strength of the diathesis or inherited predisposition to the production of DD is the principal factor responsible for the appearance of recurrent disease.

An important difference in the pathological disposition of the recurrent Dupuytren's tissue is to be noted. A virgin mass can be dissected fairly cleanly from the fibrous flexor tendon sheath and neurovascular bundles, revealing often deeper discrete or diffuse deposits to be dissected off the joint capsule and ligaments. A recurrent mass lacks even the often dismal definition of a virgin mass, arising as it does from the remaining subdermal fibrofatty layer and extending then to involve, not normally pre-existing aponeurotic structures, but in the case of recurrent tissue directly invading the epineurium of the digital nerves, the fibrous flexor sheath and the joint ligaments. It is thus a far more difficult task technically to retain intact these essential anatomical structures during a dissection of recurrent DD than it is in the primary disease when these structures are rarely directly invaded.

Clearly therefore it is from a careful clinical assessment of the diathesis in a particular patient that it may be felt that recurrence is a probability. There is in these patients a place for primary prophylaxis. If so then it is reasonable to try to make the first dissection the last dissection. Certainly if the patient already has a recurrence then it is eminently reasonable to try to make this far more difficult dissection the last dissection.

It has been observed that recurrence does not occur beneath a free skin graft (Hueston 1984a, 1985). If this empirical clinical finding of prevention of recurrence by 'changing the skin' is accepted, then it is reasonable to use 'dermofasciectomy' — the discarding not only of the recurrent Dupuytren's tissue but also of the overlying skin — when operating on a recurrent mass. More ambitious and perhaps radical but equally reasonable is the application of this technique to the primary surgery in patients where an assessment of the diathesis has made it seem probable that recurrence — and hence far more difficult secondary surgery — will occur.

The application of full thickness skin grafts requires a satisfactory bed at the end of the fasciectomy so that a complete take of the graft will occur. An intact fibrous flexor tendon sheath is required although the author has confirmed the claim by Gonzalez (1985) that the skin graft will take on the visceral paratenon of the exposed flexor tendon. Such an added risk, however, of graft failure from flexor tendon movement is best avoided. It is safe to leave a very fine layer of recurrent Dupuytren's tissue over the flexor tendon — the sheath often having been lost in part at least at the primary fasciectomy — and to place the skin graft on to this Dupuytren's tissue. Involution of the active Dupuytren's tissue appears to occur beneath the newly introduced dermis of the skin graft.

It is far more important to retain the digit with a residual proximal interphalangeal joint deformity of up to 45° or 50° but with full flexion to the palm, than to force it by capsulotomy and fibrous sheath rupture to full extension and jeopardize the successful take of the skin graft. A straight but stiff finger is useless. Fusion of the proximal interphalangeal joint eliminates the flexion to the palm on which we depend for the power grip of the digit. In many cases most fingers can be straightened by careful dissection to 45° at the proximal interphalangeal joint, which is about where it would be fused — so why sacrifice flexion by arthrodesis?

If by chance a major defect is left in the fibrous flexor sheath then a local flap of retained skin can be turned in to cover the moving tendons and skin grafts applied proximal and distal to this flap. No recurrence has been seen beneath such a flap, which is occasionally needed.

The use of a cross-finger flap to resurface the volar aspect of a finger after radical skin and fascial resection is to be condemned. If one finger has required this dermofasciectomy because of recurrence or diathesis implying likely recurrence, then that patient is very probably going to develop new Dupuytren's tissue in the adjacent finger. If this occurs and dermofasciectomy is indicated in the adjacent finger, the operation would be extremely hazardous because the dorsal integument through which the venous and tissue fluid return of the dermofasciectomized digit must then flow will have previously been removed in the cross-finger flap. Thus, because dermofasciectomy is frequently needed in more than one digit simultaneously or over the years, the vascular stages of the other fingers should not be jeopardized by previous cross-finger flap transfers. There is rarely any problem in preparing a perfectly safe bed for the graft if dermofasciectomy is performed as the primary procedure.

Thus a perspective of surgical intervention presents itself proportionate to the degree of diathesis:

1. A *low* diathesis, e.g. an elderly patient with no ectopic deposits and no history of recurrence. This calls for a standard fasciectomy by whatever technique the surgeon feels most competent to correct the deformity. No skin replacement is required. The patient is observed for at least 3 years, after which the risk of recurrence is very low indeed although extension in unoperated areas may arise and require separate similar simple surgical correction (Hueston 1965).
2. A *moderate* degree of diathesis, e.g. a young to middle-aged man with fairly diffuse skin involvement in the proximal segment of the

finger and ectopic deposits. Here recurrence is a distinct possibility but total sacrifice of uninvolved volar skin is not necessary. A 'firebreak' skin graft can be inserted in the proximal segment of the finger after discarding say 1 cm of skin, and the finger cleared into the distal ray and proximal palm by the usual longitudinal exposure and local flap rearrangement to prevent scar contracture (Hueston 1984b). This 'firebreak' effectively separates a recurrence in the palm from any recurrence in the digit, thus preventing a linking up of these two contracting hyperplastic cellular masses. Recurrent metacarpophalangeal joint deformity is prevented. Of course, proximal interphhalangeal joint deformity from recurrence in the finger segment beyond the 'immunity' of the recurrent area of the graft would require treatment on its own merits — most likely further dissection and grafting to the distal interphalangeal crease.

3. A *strong* diathesis, e.g. a young man with rapid progress of proximal interphalangeal joint deformity and diffuse deposits in the fingers — often several fingers — and ectopic deposits and a strong family history. Here a total resurfacing of the digit from the distal interphalangeal joint to web space or even the distal palmar crease is indicated.

A longitudinal incision exposes the Dupuytren's tissue distally to the distal interphalangeal joint or pulp level if the latter is flexed and well into the palm, proximal to the distal palmar crease if the metacarpophalangeal joint is flexed. The skin is elevated even if Dupuytren's tissue is retained in it, until the fasciectomy is completed with intact neurovascular bundles and fibrous flexor sheath as a satisfactory bed to support the skin graft. One or all fingers may require this.

The skin flaps are then resected back to the 'stationary' mid axial line along the side of the digit with darts backward at each joint crease and web space, to retain at these points the marginal scarline of the grafted defect at, or slightly behind, the midline axis of the digit. If the scarline junction of the grafted skin is even slightly anterior to this important 'stationary' line there will, by the normal process of scar contracture, longitudinal tension exerted anterior to the axis of the interphalangeal joints and flexion deformity reproduced to some degree. Attention to this detail of 'dressmaking' makes all the difference between a complete correction and a compromise correction.

Full thickness skin grafts can be taken either from the inner aspect of the same arm or the groin, and the donor site may be sutured or even split-skin grafted if necessary.

If there has been extensive palmar dissection with resultant potential dead space, then the junctional wound between the palmar skin and the proximal transverse border of the graft is often left incompletely sutured to prevent any blood running from the extensive palmar wound down beneath the digital graft.

Each digit is bandaged individually to ensure completely adequate yet safe pressure on the graft. The whole hand is immobilized on a plaster volar slab for 5 days with the fingers in extension until the first dressing when, as the graft has taken completely, it can be left open during the day for digital flexion. However, the straight plaster volar slab should be used at night for protection and the prevention of relapse through protective flexion occurring during sleep.

Work can be resumed at 2–3 weeks with a loose cloth glove over protective lanoline or cream until sensation of a protective nature has returned in 6 weeks.

Historically, radical fasciectomy was advocated in the 1940s and 1950s to remove prophylactically the entire palmar aponeurosis. This was discarded because of haematoma risks in the palm and the realization that the palmar aponeurosis need not be entirely blamed or removed. Limited fasciectomy of only the macroscopic deforming nodule band system then allowed more rapid recovery of function, but 40–60% recurrence followed either radical or limited fasciectomy.

Now this locally ultra-radical process of dermofasciectomy of the digit in danger of recurrence is advocated — but only when it is indicated! In areas of the world where, for racial reasons, the diathesis is less strong than in the Scottish–Irish–Australian population, dermofasciectomy will be very rarely required.

The rationale of dermofasciectomy is the freedom from recurrence beneath the full thickness skin graft. Three types of recurrence have been observed in over 500 patients with grafts:

1. Recurrent Dupuytren's tissue along the marginal scars with some recurrent deformity (28 patients). When reoperated, the graft can be left in place as the recurrence is found to be under retained adjacent skin. This is further resected and further graft strips are applied to widen the grafted, and hence immune, area.
2. Proximally along one or both neurovascular bundles for up to 1 cm beneath the graft — the rest of the graft remains free (5 patients). With great care these linear deposits, presumably arising from deep to the neurovascular bundles, have been resected without need for further grafting.
3. A single case of true recurrence over the sheath in the middle phalangeal segment of a young patient with a very strong diathesis who had multiple other grafts without recurrence. The first of the few?

No operation should be performed routinely.

No operation should be performed if it is not indicated for good reasons.

No operation should be avoided if it is adequately indicated — and in the case of dermofasciectomy the alternative is repeated surgery with recurrences and ultimate amputation.

Dermofasciectomy has virtually eliminated amputation in the author's practice.

PART 6
FASCIECTOMY AND DERMOFASCIECTOMY
F. Iselin

Our personal experience, in over 1000 operated cases, has led us to the same conclusions as Hueston (1962) that there are two types of DD — oponeurotic and cutaneous.

In the aponeurotic type only the palmar fascia is retracted; there is no skin or joint involvement. This is the 'standard' DD; it is usually benign, is easy to operate on, and not likely to give postoperative problems. (Fig. 32.9).

The cutaneous type combines fascial retraction and invasion of the overlying skin. It is more severe for two reasons:

1. *Early type:* the invaded skin, whether retained or excised, may be the cause of delayed healing which generally leads to joint stiffness.
2. *Late type:* the invaded skin is responsible for most recurrences of the disease.

This distinction between the two types is not new and has been described by Fasquelle (1928), who added an articular type which is the ultimate evolution of a long-standing contracture with capsular retraction of the proximal interphalangeal joint in flexion, and sometimes of the distal interphalangeal joint in hyperextension.

There are two varieties of both types of contracture — simple and complex.

Simple varieties have palmar contracture of one or two digits, usually on the ulnar side of the hand; radial contractures seem to be more frequently observed now (Tubiana & De Frenne 1976), especially in the first web space.

Complex varieties have severe contractures of many adjacent digits invading the web spaces and the digital joints.

We have also noted that there is a definite difference between patients: 'good' patients are men in their fifth or sixth decade with no associated diseases, while 'bad' patients are alcoholic, epileptic, diabetic, or psychologically depressed people, who are frequently encountered. Women are usually troublesome patients from the point of view of their disease — fortunately they are less frequently involved (15% of our cases). So are young people under 40, who are more likely to develop active fulminating types of disease with a high potential for recurrences and complications.

These young patients are also frequently affected by ectopic 'diathetic' localizations such as knuckle pads, foot nodules and penile lesions.

It is generally observed that 'good' patients will

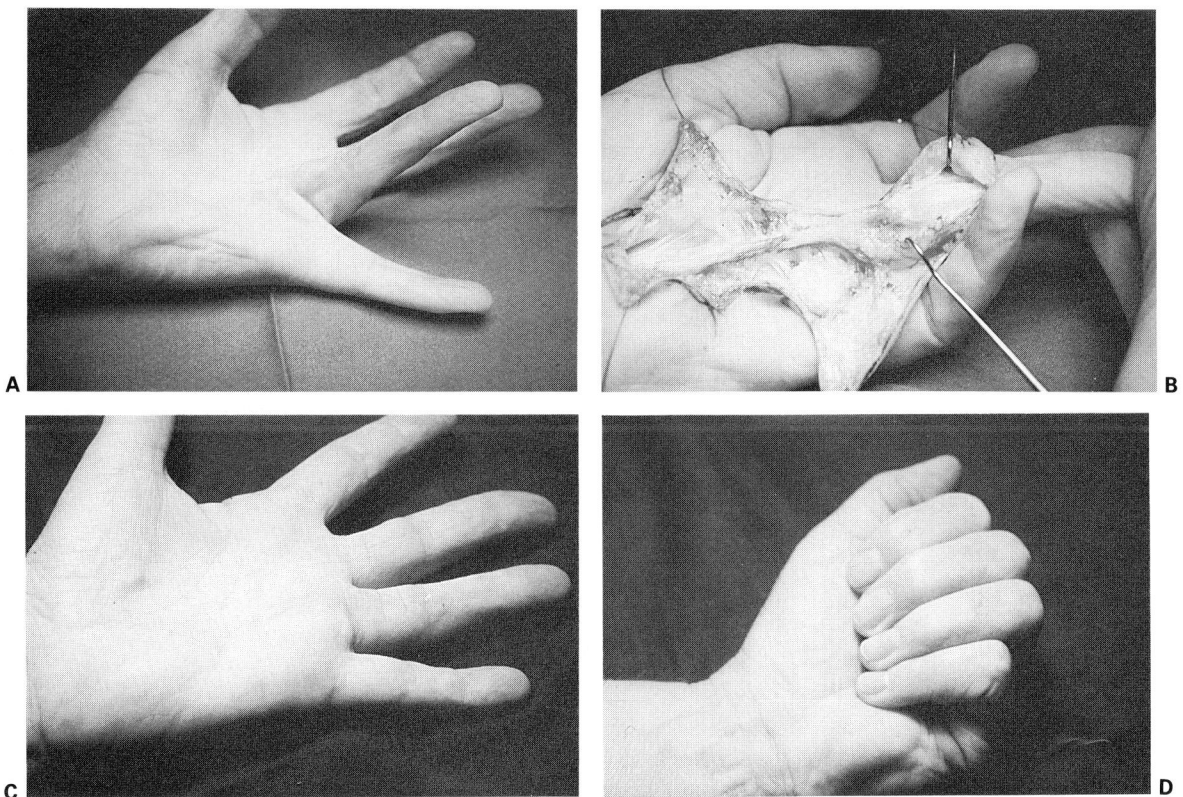

Fig. 32.9A Aponeurotic type of DD preoperatively. B Intraoperative view of pure contracture band before fasciectomy. **C** At 12 months' follow-up: extension; **D** flexion.

develop simple aponeurotic types and that the others mainly suffer complex and cutaneous types.

It is therefore obvious that DD is not a homogeneous condition. There are many different varieties and surgical indications depend not only on the type of contracture but also on the type of patient.

SURGICAL TECHNIQUES

Three techniques can be used in the surgical treatment of DD — fasciotomy, fasciectomy and dermofasciectomy.

Fasciotomy

Subcutaneous fasciotomy is performed in the palm (see Colville, p. 333).

Open fasciotomy is performed in the digits under local anaesthetic using a longitudinal palmar approach directly over the contracting nodule, from palmar crease to palmar crease, sufficient to be able to identify and protect the neurovascular bundles on each side while the retracted fascia is transected.

Skin closure is not usually necessary.

Fasciectomy

We always limit the fasciectomy to the contracted fascia. We do not believe that fasciectomy can always be performed in the same way but techniques must be adapted to the type of contracture. The difference mainly relies on the skin incisions and the following rules apply:

1. Never cross over a flexion crease to prevent contracted scars.
3. The exposure should be large enough to

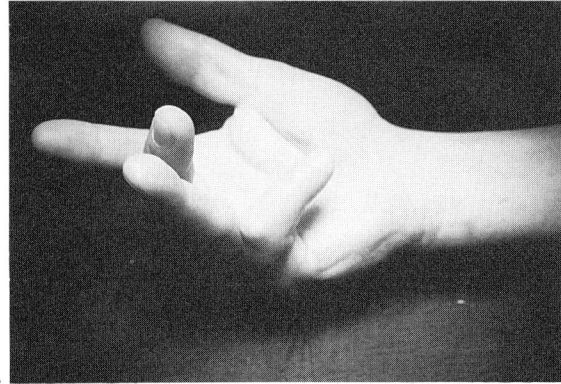
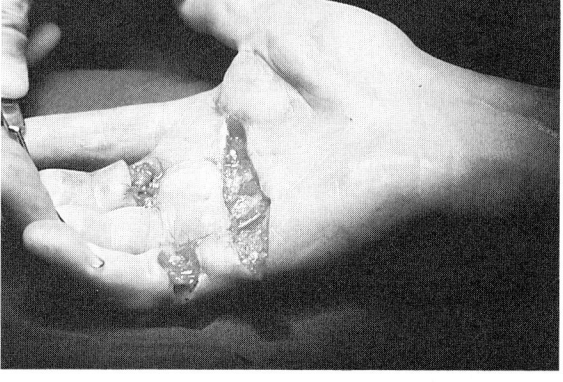
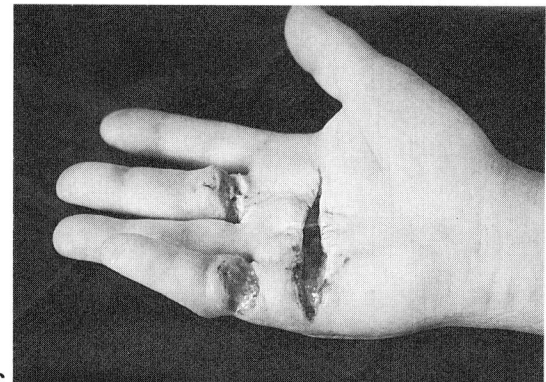
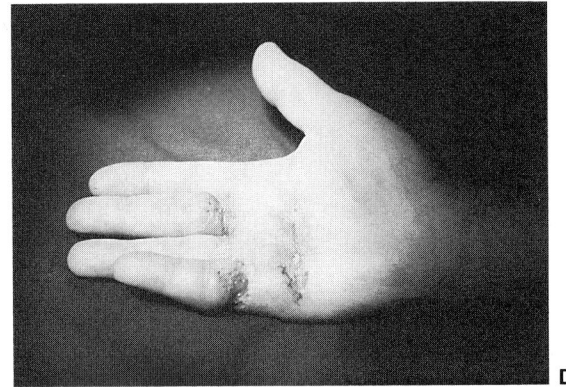
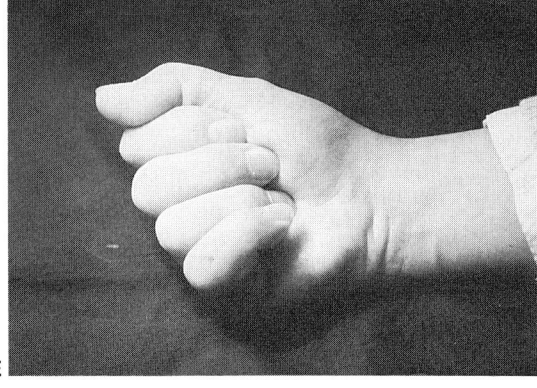

Fig. 32.10 A Juvenile complex disease in an epileptic patient. **B** Fasciectomy; open palm and open fingers. **C** Tenth postoperative day; **D** and **E** 20th postoperative day.

visualize the neurovascular bundles throughout the entire excision of the pathological fascia.
3. Avoid unnecessary skin dissection and give preference to a direct rather than a subcutaneous approach. Therefore always use a continuous palmodigital approach.

When only one digital ray is involved, we favour the zig-zag Bruner (1960) incision. If many digits are retracted, the zig-zag incision is used on each digit. A transverse palmar incision is made with a proximal extension towards the wrist and a distal extension towards the best placed digital incision.

We have virtually stopped doing Z-plasty incisions because of the poor quality of the triangular skin flaps. We nevertheless still use them in very special cases of severe retraction of a single digit with good quality skin over a well localized fascial contracture.

We believe that skin closure is not compulsory after fasciectomy and, especially in the palm, we will leave the skin open if closure appears to be too tight. McCash (1964) has demonstrated that spontaneous healing will occur in about 3 weeks and that this open palm technique prevents formation of subcutaneous haematoma and helps in early mobilization (Fig. 32.10).

Although we do not use this procedure deliberately, we always leave the wound open when skin closure does not appear perfectly safe.

Dermofasciectomy

Hueston (1962) has thus named this procedure, which is as old as Lexer (1931). It consists of the complete removal of the contracted fascia with its overlying skin which will be replaced by a skin graft.

The operation begins like a regular fasciectomy. Unless the skin cannot be separated from the fascia, we advise keeping it intact until the fasciectomy is completed, so that should a neurovascular bundle or a flexor tendon sheath be damaged, its repair could be covered by a skin flap rather than by a skin graft. When the sacrifice of skin is decided, the drawing of the incision should follow the cutaneous functional units so as to avoid secondary scar contractions (Iselin 1983).

Hueston (1985) and Varian (1985) restrict skin grafting to the digit. We do not hesitate to use larger skin grafts over digit and palm. Quite often we leave open the proximal palmar line, as in McCash's procedure, to avoid haematoma.

We have demonstrated in a study of 60 dermofasciectomies (Iselin 1986) that there is no difference in the functional results regarding the type of skin graft (full or split thickness). Our choice is therefore dictated by the surface to be grafted and the desire to leave the least conspicuous donor site (Fig. 32.11).

POSTOPERATIVE CARE

Whatever technique is performed, our postoperative routine is unchanged:

1. Fluffy dressing of hand and wrist with dorsal splint to the tips of the digits to immobilize them for 1 week.
2. Reduced dressing involving only the hand and the digital skin incisions for 1 week.
3. Optional dressing after removal of stitches for the second week.

Active motion is encouraged from the beginning as most of our surgery is performed under local or regional anaesthesia.

Passive extension devices are only indicated when full active flexion has been regained. Therapy is usually necessary daily during the first postoperative month and then reduced, but it is not infrequent to continue until the third month, when we undertake routine postoperative evaluation.

Like many others, we have noted that the results depend more on the patient than on the type of operation performed. This emphasizes the importance of case selection based on surgical indications.

SURGICAL INDICATIONS

Obviously surgery should not be proposed for a patient with no contracture, or even when there is a contracture but no functional complaint. These patients should be re-evaluated every 6 months.

Patients with disabling contracture can be separated into two groups, as described above — 'bad' and 'good' patients.

As previously noted, bad risks include very old and very young, alcoholic, diabetic and neuropathic patients. These patients should benefit from fasciotomy which can be repeated if the contracture recurs, if the patient remains in this category. If the patient becomes a better risk for surgery, fasciotomy can be sometimes considered as the first stage before more radical surgery.

'Good', or rather, 'acceptable' risks are straightforward cases which can be treated by a regular fasciectomy. In recurrences and cutaneous types with fulminating evolution in young patients, constituting a potentially recurrent group, a dermofasciectomy is proposed.

Dermofasciectomy is indicated in two main situations:

1. Unavoidable dermofasciectomy when the skin overlying the contracted fascia cannot be dissected whatever the type of the disease.
2. Deliberate dermofasciectomy when skin sacrifice does not initially appear necessary but is decided upon because of the type of disease, namely actual or potential recurrence.

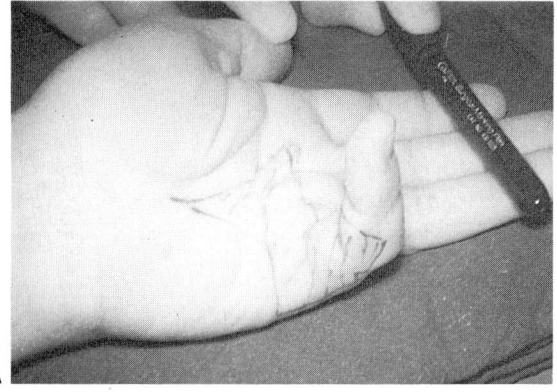
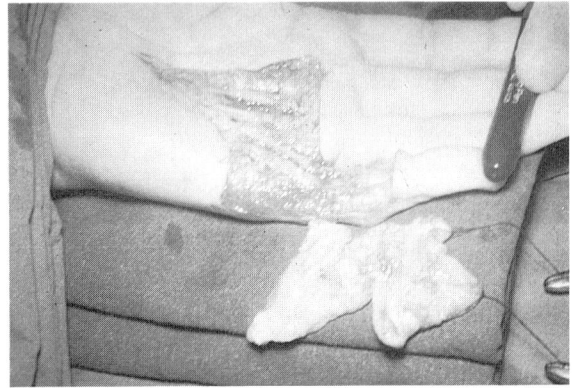
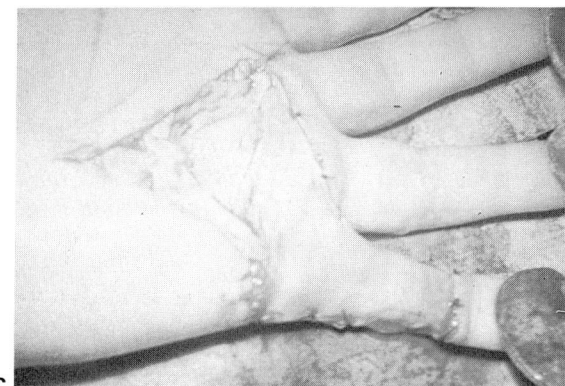
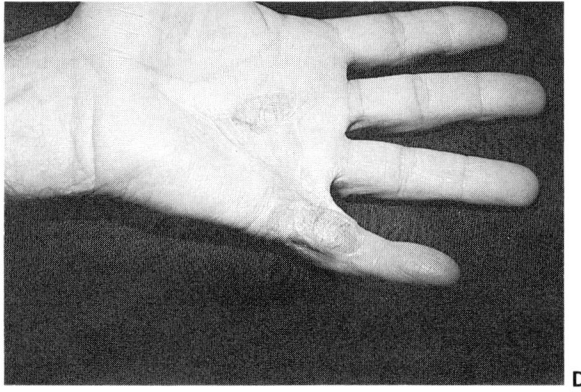
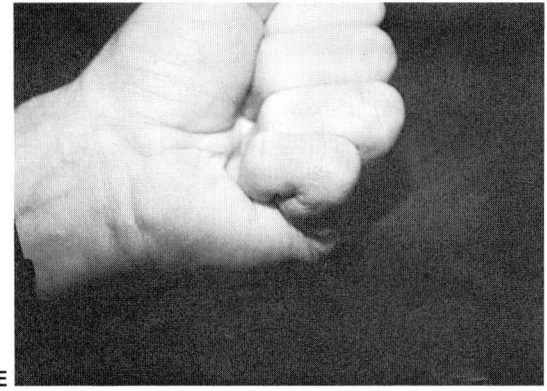

Fig. 32.11 A Cutaneous type; potential recurrence. **B** Dermofasciectomy. **C** Split thickness skin graft because of large defect. **D** and **E** At 2 years' follow up. No recurrence, no extension.

stiffness is more frequent after joint release attempts.

If the extension lag is acceptable, we do not attempt to release the joint. If it is unacceptable we release the joint but never to such an extent as to face a dorsal subluxation which may occur in spite of a flexed position, around 30° degrees.

Proximal interphalangeal joint contracture

Special attention should be paid to the release of interphalangeal joint contracture (Tonkin et al 1985). When the digital joint cannot be extended, after complete fasciectomy, a careful limited excision of the volar plate and of the volar collateral ligaments is sometimes recommended. In fact, it is always dangerous because postoperative joint

Distal interphalangeal joint extension

The attitude toward hyperextension of the distal interphalangeal joint is different. Excision of all the pathological tissue along the retinacular ligament should reduce the deformity. If not, tenotomy of the central slip of the extensor tendon over the distal interphalangeal joint is usually sufficient to achieve flexion. An incomplete result must be preferred to the risk of definite joint stiffness.

When the small finger is involved, amputation should be considered and discussed preoperatively with the patient as an acceptable substitute to a stiff finger.

RESULTS

In the preoperative consultation, we always warn patients that after the operation they will have to face 2–3 weeks of dressings followed by 2–3 weeks of active physical therapy and splinting and 6–8 weeks of reduced but persistent therapy and splinting. No evaluation of the result can be made before the third month, but some patients may achieve a good result in 4–6 weeks.

We categorize our results into three grades according to functional criteria and active range of motion:

1. *Good:* those who achieve at least 80% of normal movement and normal function with no pain.
2. *Bad:* those with 50% or less of normal movement with no function and a painful hand.
3. *Fair:* those with reduced movement and function but with no pain.

In a study of 254 fasciectomy operations between 1974 and 1980 (Iselin 1980) our overall results were as follows:

1. Good: 193 (76%).
2. Fair: 33 (13%).
3. Bad: 28 (11%).

Most unsatisfactory results were secondary to dystrophy.

In this same group we observed 26 recurrences (10%) after 3 years. We agree with Hueston that after 3 years, true recurrences are highly unlikely but extensions can occur much later. Tubiana (1986) has observed very late recurrences in about 30% of operated cases.

Recurrences usually occur in juvenile patients and in cutaneous types of the disease where our surgical choice is now dermofasciectomy. During the same study period (1974–1980) we operated on 62 recurrences by dermofasciectomy and only observed one new recurrence in a follow-up of 6–12 years (Iselin 1986).

MANAGEMENT OF THE FASCIA

FASCIOTOMY

PART 7
FASCIOTOMY
J. Colville

The typical patient developing DD who proved suitable for fasciotomy was a male of about 70 years who had a very slow progressive contraction of usually one finger of either or both hands, often present for between 5 and 10 years prior to presentation. Frequently this interfered with some recreational activity in his retirement, stimulating a request for treatment. Having been satisfied that in some instances fasciotomy alone can adequately treat DD, the following indications for fasciotomy were developed:

1. *Type of cord.* The superficial longitudinal fibres of the palmar fascia only are involved. This is determined from the superficial location of the cord which essentially must bow-string across the concavity of the palm and the base of the digit. It is the absence of deep connections such as oblique bands or septal involvement that allows bow-stringing.

    A further quality of the cord that is sought is its cord-like development. Ideally for a fasciotomy the Dupuytren's cord resembles a flexor tendon and retracts almost as easily as a tendon on division. A certain amount of flattening of the cord is however acceptable.
2. *The overlying skin.* In the normal hand there is a generous layer of specialized fat intervening between the skin and the next immediate structure, the superficial layer of the palmar fascia. Running through this fat, especially in the distal part of the palm, there is a pennate-type distribution of palmar fascial fibres from the main longitudinal

band to their insertions at intervals in the skin. On contraction these either approximate skin locally to the cord in the form of pits or if more generally dispersed, pull the cord out to a very close relationship to the overlying skin. Obviously since the object of fasciotomy is the distal retreat of the divided cord, it must be free from skin attachment to allow this.

Occasionally there is very little skin attachment to the well formed Dupuytren's cord but more frequently a moderate amount of skin attachment is observed. If the skin can be freed from the main Dupuytren's cord then this still allows a successful fasciotomy. Extensive skin involvement contraindicates fasciotomy and indeed quite often causes such a rigidity of the skin combined with the Dupuytren's complex that even if the superficial layer of the fascia only is involved the skin ridigity would prevent a successful outcome from cord division.

Occasionally we find that the skin of the palm has accumulated in corrugations and on release of the skin attachments to the Dupuytren's tissue, these corrugations of skin provide a useful reservoir of available skin for extension of the fingers.

All rules are made to be broken and in DD we accept that occasionally there are exceptions to the above requirements. This is mainly because of social or medical circumstances and particularly where the type of Dupuytren's disease comes close to qualifying for fasciotomy. Also, some elderly patients who were unwilling to come into hospital for a formal fasciectomy were agreeable to attend as outpatients for a relatively simple operation under local anaesthesia; on occasion this was agreed to on the definite understanding that the condition would probably recur over the next year or two. A similar prognosis was given to a few patients who were accepted for fasciotomy and who had other contraindications to general or even brachial anaesthesia. A few patients who had previous extensive surgery for carcinoma but who were sufficiently troubled by their hand contracture were also allowed fasciotomy for the temporary relief that this would provide. A very few elderly people (oldest 98 years) were treated by fasciotomy on the grounds that a modest improvement in hand function for a year or two was also worth the relatively small effort involved. All patients are warned that by its nature DD is a progressive condition and there is a distinct risk of recurrence.

PREPARATION OF THE FASCIOTOMY BLADE

A No. 11 Swann Morton blade is modified according to the design shown in Figure 32.12. The shank should be parallel and the cutting tip not more than 1 mm. This blade is mounted on a conventional handle and provides a rigid fasciotome which is easily orientated under the skin.

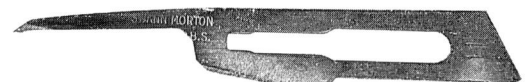

Fig. 32.12 No 11 Swann Morton blade modified for fasciotomy.

OPERATIVE TECHNIQUE

Fasciotomy is carried out as an outpatient procedure. A tourniquet was used initially but more recently has been discarded because the operation is relatively bloodless and furthermore is performed by touch rather than sight.

The surgeon is seated on the ulnar side of the hand. For anaesthesia, 2 ml of 2% plain Xylocaine is usually sufficient for local infiltration of a sufficient area of the palm to complete the operation; 1 ml is inserted 2 cm proximal to the distal palm crease around the cord and the remaining 1 ml between the distal palm crease and the base of the digit. Occasionally when a single simple cord extends through the proximal phalanx this was also divided by fasciotomy, in which case a further 1 ml is required for the proximal phalanx.

The finger is stretched and the mobility of the overlying skin assessed. Skin adherent to a cord proximal to the level of division does not restrict the distal retreat of the divided cord so there is no need to separate the skin proximal to the most proximal fasciotomy point. Distal to this point, however, the skin must allow free excursion of the divided cord. Therefore, before any part of the cord is touched the adhesions attaching the skin to the cord are divided. If the skin cannot be separated satisfactorily from the underlying cord then there is not much point in proceeding with the fasciotomy. The situation is not entirely lost, however, since freeing of the skin from the cord can still be done more distally, thus providing a situation where on fasciotomy more distally the divided cord is still permitted sufficient excursion to give a worthwhile improvement in extension. There is no point in doing the fasciotomy proximal to an area of skin still adherent to the cord.

The blade enters the palmar skin about 15 mm on the ulnar side of the cord and is advanced under the skin and swept through an arc represented by the length of blade insertion until the skin has been freed. Having visibly freed the skin from the longitudinally running cord at a proximal level, the same procedure is repeated more distally if necessary so that from the centre of the palm to the base of the digit the skin is freely mobile. The blade is then re-inserted into the proximal stab wound and turned vertically. With the relevant finger under tension, using the operator's other hand, the cord is gently scratched with the point of the blade. This is not a cutting procedure. The tense band can be scratched through until a gratifying snapping sensation is not only felt but also heard and the finger extends with continuing traction. This is repeated between the distal palm crease and the web crease level, obtaining further extension. At this level any corrugations of skin released by the preliminary separation of the skin and cord unfold. The limiting factor in fasciotomy at this stage is invariably skin tension and the additional skin provided by the unfolding of the corrugations helps considerably. Sometimes the skin may rupture where it has been adherent or in the distal palm crease fold where it is rather thin. On rupture a transverse separation of skin edges changes shape with further stretching to a longitudinally oriented narrow diamond-shaped defect that may be held in place by a suture if necessary. This very efficient means of transposing skin from a lateral to a longitudinal orientation has been referred to by the author as a 'diamond-plasty' and is particularly efficient in redistributing the skin to the advantage of the procedure.

Following the release of the contracture the hand is dressed conventionally and immobilized in a plaster of Paris gutter slab retaining as much extension improvement as possible. This is worn continuously for 1 week. The patient is next seen 1 week later when the dressings are removed and the wound is invariably dry and healed. A fresh lightly padded plaster of Paris slab is remade and applied snugly to the bare arm and forearm with the fingers in as much extension as possible. After a few minutes, when this has become sufficiently rigid, it is removed and carefully placed in a bag with one or two crepe bandages. The patient does not require further dressings and is given the new splint to take home carefully and instructed to bandage this to the hand and forearm each night before retiring. The patient is also instructed to report if either the plaster becomes damaged or if further extension is achieved, requiring a more closely fitting splint. One patient, a female with 120° contracture which had improved to a 45° contracture position, reported 3 weeks later with her finger almost completely extended.

Splintage is normally discarded after a period of 3 months. Invariably the patient can immediately start using the hand after the plaster has been removed at the first postoperative attendance.

In our series of 95 patients with 137 affected fingers (Colville 1983) plus quite a number following that publication, who have had fasciotomy performed, there has not been any instance of haematoma or infection nor has there been any evidence of permanent damage to digital nerves. Some patients mention tingling of the fingers for a number of weeks, presumably due to stretching of the nerves, but this invariably recovers.

In a few patients with a distal interphalangeal joint hyperextension defect associated with boutonniere deformity resulting from long-standing proximal interphalangeal joint flexion, it has proved useful to use the same fasciotome to divide the insertion of the distal joint extensor. This has the effect of allowing some distal joint flexion and also helps in recovery of active proximal interphalangeal joint extension by permitting the whole extensor apparatus to slip proximally. Hueston has suggested to me that the extensor tendon fasciotomy may be done obliquely, thus theoretically allowing a repair of the distal joint extensor in the lengthened position. This tenotomy is done under local anaesthesia and the patient is able actively to move the fingers at the time of operation and assist in guiding the operator as to the extent of extensor tendon division necessary to obtain the controlled 'mallet' effect.

RESULTS

In a prospective trial by the author of 137 fingers treated by fasciotomy with a minimum follow-up of 2 years, the average preoperative extension deficit was 102°. The immediate postoperative average deficit was 45°. At 3 months this had reduced to 31° by splintage. At 6 months there was some deterioration to a 50° extension deficit position. After 1 year this deficit had increased to 56° and after 3 years for 107 of those fingers the deficit had deteriorated to 75°.

The 20 best results had an average preoperative deficit of 104° with an immediate postoperative correction to 26° deficit. After 3 months this had reduced to 23° and this was maintained at 6 months. After 1 year the deficit was 30° and after 3 years it was 32°. In 9 of these cases there was less than 20° extension deficit after 3 years, and at least 2 of these had a 150° deficit preoperatively.

DISCUSSION

Obviously there is a type of DD that affects only the superficial layer of the palmar fascia and does so in a fashion that is not aggressive, that does not extend elsewhere and that once interrupted by fasciotomy does not seem to have any tendency to reform or reproduce the contracture. Unfortunately this applies only to a small percentage of those presenting with DD but it would seem to be worthwhile to identify such a patient and him or her by the more simple method of fasciotomy.

Astley Cooper (1822) referred to fasciotomy (see Chapter 1). Hawkins (1835) referred to a case of traumatic fasciotomy; rupture of the palm 'by a restive house'. in which he sewed a diagonal shaped palmar skin defect longitudinally. Fasciotomy has also been recommended by Adams (1878) and Macready (1890). Luck (1959) in an article on fasciotomy advocated removal of the nodule as well as division of the band as an essential part of the operation. Since the results of simple fasciotomy in well selected cases are good and since the essence or the treatment is its simplicity, it would be difficult to recommend Luck's added procedure which really converts this into a mini fasciectomy.

There are reservations about fasciotomy at the proximal phalangeal level (Tubiana & Thomine 1974). If the disease in the palm has been superficial and if this extends into the proximal phalanx as a superficial cord, and provided this is also bow-stringing from the proximal to the middle phalanx, this procedure is still safe at this level. The digital nerves are well posterior to the plane of the fasciotomy and if only the superficial band is involved there is no intertwining of the digital nerves around this.*

Bassot (1965) and later Hueston (1974) advocated enzymic fasciotomy but as far as I am aware this procedure has not gained popularity and is not really any more efficient in achieving a fasciotomy than the much more precise method of using a fasciotome for this purpose.

It is our opinion that in about 8% of patients a type of DD develops where the contracting cord is very similar to tendon. If this is found or if a similar situation can be created; if there is soft uninvolved fat available fo fill the gap between the distracted ends of the divided Dupuytren's cord and if these can be kept separate for a sufficient length of time there is a good prospect of a permanent and useful recovery of extension. In a disease as diverse in its manifestations as DD, there must be a number of different surgical approaches to the management of the condition and the author suggests that fasciotomy has a rightful

*Editor's note: This is not so. A pretendinous cord which is in continuity with a spiral cord can present as a single prominent cord passing from the palm into the finger. There will be contraction of both metacarpophalangeal and proximal interphalangeal joints and one or other neurovascular bundle will be displaced toward the midline.

but small place in the overall management of the condition.

PART 8
TWO-STAGE OPERATION
B. Nagay

INTRODUCTION

It is well accepted that one can expect about 80–85% excellent or good late results after operative treatment of DD. However, it seems reasonable to pay more attention to the 15–20% of patients with only satisfactory or sometimes even poor late results (Honner et al 1971; Rodrigo et al 1976; Nagay 1985).

In my practice I used to divide all patients with DD into four stages according to Iselin (Iselin 1972; Figs 32.13A–C, 32.14 A, B). However, the preoperative classification can not be limited to one of four stages. Occupation and associated conditions such as previous rheumatoid disease, chronic alcoholism, diabetes and epilepsy may also be of value in deciding on the type and extent of operative procedure.

SELECTION OF OPERATION

In the first stage of the disease operation is generally not advised. The main subjects for surgical treatment are in the second to fourth stages of the disease. The best indication for operation is the second stage of contracture (Hueston 1977) when the hand cannot be placed flat on the table (Fig. 32.13C). Equally good results may be obtained in the third stage, but in this and the fourth stage a slightly different surgical approach is proposed.

OPERATIVE TECHNIQUES — SKIN INCISIONS

The operative procedures for surgery of DD consist of two main types of intervention: closed or open fasciotomy and fasciectomy which may be regional (limited) or extensive (radical).

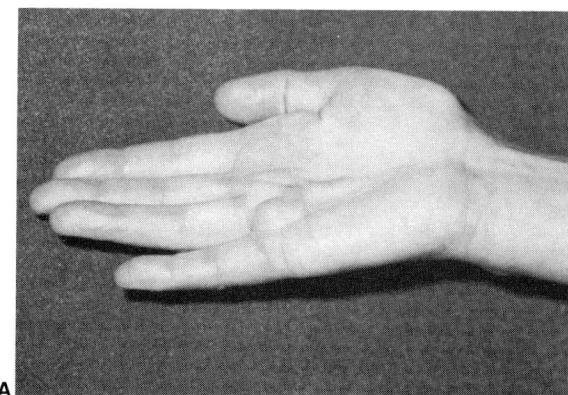
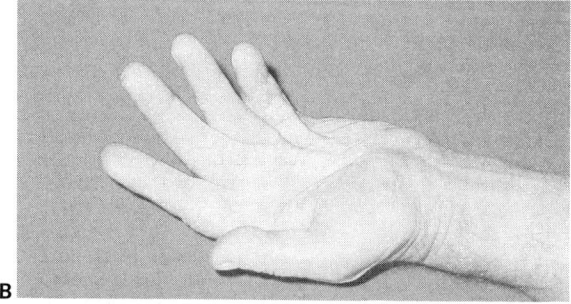
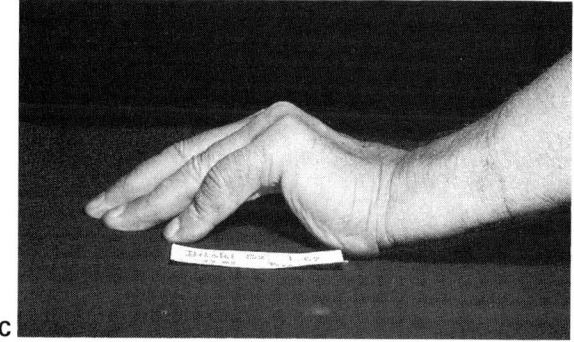

Fig. 32.13A–C The stages of DD.

Fasciotomy

For closed fasciotomy a small incision along the band in the palm is sufficient (Fig. 32.15, 32.16).

Open fasciotomy may be carried out by means of one or more transverse incisions within the palm and proximal part of the finger. The extension of the contracted finger enlarges the initial wounds which never need to be grafted. After fasciotomy,

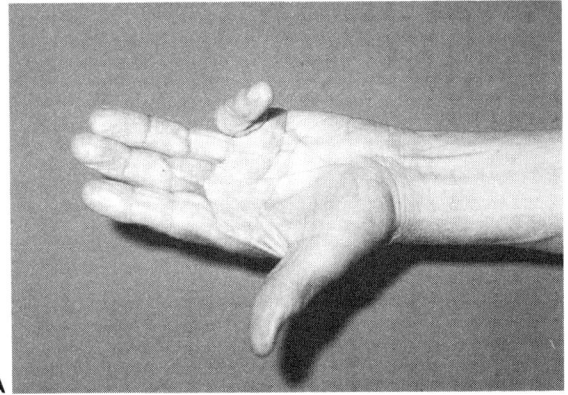
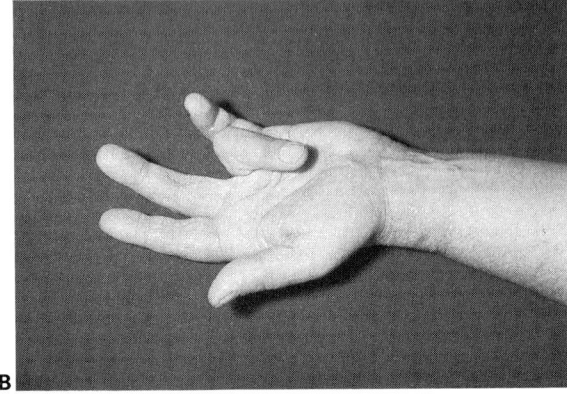

Fig. 32.14

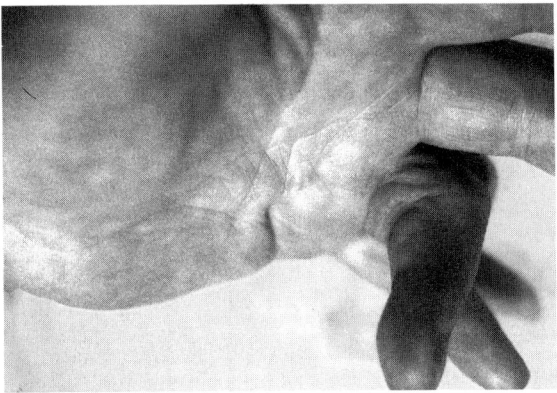

Figs 32.15, 32.16 Incisions for closed fasciotomy.

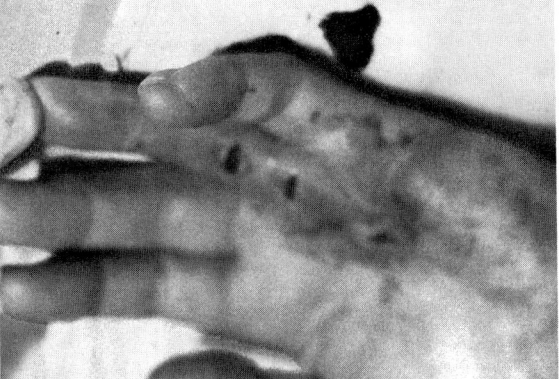

Fig. 32.16

the newly extended fingers must be splinted for at least 7 days; complete healing occurs within 12–20 days. Sometimes temporary Kirschnerpin arthrodesis may be advisable.

Fasciectomy

The extent of fasciectomy depends on the distribution of the contracted bands of palmar fascia. We confirm the opinion of Hueston (1961), Zachariae (1967), McFarlane (1983) and Buck-Gramcko (personal communication), that limited fasciectomy may give the same late results as an extensive one. Therefore we generally perform limited fasciectomy, however, in the area of operation, the excision of pathological tissues must be sufficiently radical i.e. including all transverse elements of palmar fascia and all — even small — digital bands. When the pathological changes extends to more than half of the palmar fascia, radical fasciectomy is advised.

On elevating skin flaps it is far better to leave some Dupuytren's tissue within the flaps rather than risk the worry of skin necrosis. For precise haemostasis after tourniquet release we exert gentle pressure on the operation area with wet, warm gauze pads, incorporating topical haemostatic agents such as adrenalin or thrombin.

When after excision of diseased fascia a large skin gap is created, a Wolfe graft may be inserted. We leave small gaps without any coverage and it is marvellous that excellent healing of these gaps occurs, similar to the open palm concept of McCash (1964).

The postoperative dressing holds the skin flaps against their bed for 4–7 days. In the first 3 days after operation we administer diuretics to diminish oedema of the operated hand together with elevation of the extremity. Thus we follow the method proposed by Reumert & Zachariae (1973).

RESULTS

In the last 25 years we have operated on a series of over 340 patients with all stages of DD. In analysing our treatment, excellent, good or fair results were achieved in nearly 90% of cases. However, further examinations done 1–15 years after operation revealed slightly poorer results. Complications may explain these findings.

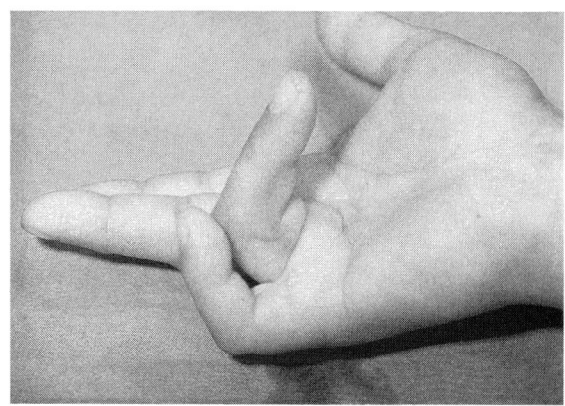

Fig. 32.17 Right hand: before fasciotomy.

Two-stage operation

Excluding such transient complications as haematoma, oedema and infection, there remains a group of patients with chronic dystrophic syndromes in the hand: pain, swelling, change of temperature, stiffness of joints and paraesthesiae. This syndrome, very similar to Sudeck's atrophy, may cause permanent disability.

Searching for a possible cause of the phenomenon described, we assume the possibility of existence in some individuals, especially in women, of a constitutional tendency to dystrophic reaction of the tissues following operative trauma. The presence of the above tendency cannot be predicted, but thick hands and extensive contractures in elderly patients may indicate this danger. Hence, since 1977 we have introduced a two-stage procedure in so-called 'bad cases' of DD (Nagay 1985).

In the first stage we usually perform open fasciotomy which rapidly eliminates finger contraction and constitutes a 'tissue test' before the next, more extensive operation.

In the second stage, if necessary, a fasciectomy is performed. This stage can be executed several months or years after primary intervention (Figs 32.17, 32.18).

Table 32.1 contains the results of such treatment of 60 patients and may support this proposed technique of treatment in selected cases.

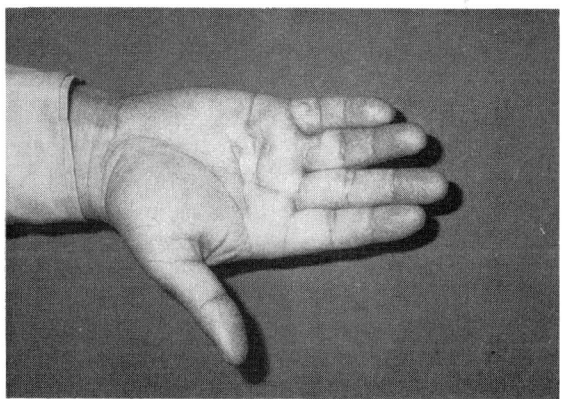

Fig. 32.18 Right hand: after fasciotomy and fasciectomy

Table 32.1 Two-stage operation for Dupuytren's disease in the years 1977–1985.

Stage of contracture (Iseline 1972)		Time between stages of intervention				Results
		6 months	6–12 months	1–3 years	Over 3 years	
Male (n=55)	III	2	8	8	3	Good
	IV	4	10	12	8	Fair
Female (n=5)	III	—	1	—	—	Good
	IV	2	2	—	—	Good
Total		60 cases with positive results				

340 DUPUYTREN'S DISEASE

LIMITED FASCIECTOMY

PART 9
VARIOUS TECHNIQUES
J. Varian

INTRODUCTION

Dupuytren's disease (DD) would be a simple condition to treat surgically were it not for a few problems, the solution of which makes it a challenge to the surgeon. The close anatomical association of the disease with nerves and with the skin of the hand predisposes to nerve injury and skin loss which are the main operative complications. The postoperative development of stiffness in the hand and recurrence of the disease following what initially would appear to be sucessful surgery is the main cause of unsatisfactory long-term results and a dissatisfied patient. The key to successful surgery for this condition is to avoid the development of these problems and to resolve them rapidly should any of them appear to be imminent.

OPERATIVE CONSIDERATIONS

Avoidance of skin loss

Once surgery has been decided upon and the decision made to proceed to a limited or extensive fasciectomy, rather than fasciotomy or local excision, one must consider which approach to make. If the disease is confined to the palm, it usually has a transverse distribution along the distal palmar crease and may cause contractures of the metacarpophalangeal joints of more than one finger. In these cases a transverse approach is recommended, making an incision along the distal palmar crease, being careful not to buttonhole the skin when raising the flaps, and leaving the wound open at the end of the operation. Where the disease has a longitudinal distribution down into one of the fingers most surgeons recommend a longitudinal approach. Where more than one finger is involved, only one finger incision is continued into the palm, and the palm can usually be cleared through that incision (Fig. 32.19).

Because a straight incision down the centre of the finger will lead to the development of a secondary scar contracture in all but the very old, the wound at the end of the operation must take the form of a zig-zag. The surgeon has two options — either to make a zig-zag incision at the outset, or convert the straight midline incision into a zig-zag with one or more Z-plasties. One should not be dogmatic about which of these techniques to use. The guiding factor must be the quality of circulation to the skin edges at the end of the operation so that secondary skin edge necrosis and delays in wound healing will be avoided. The thinnest subcutaneous tissue after fasciectomy is always found where the skin has been dissected off a nodule or off a superficial band.

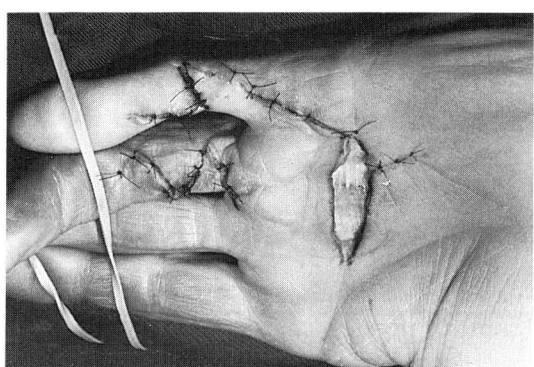

Fig. 32.19 Three principles shown in one case: **A** Zig-zag through the nodules in ring finger; only one finger incision carried into the palm. **B** Transverse incision in the palm left open.

Where the disease is early and active and nodules are prominent, the dissected skin will be thin and it is safer to make a zig-zag approach. The line of the incision should follow the nodules so that where possible the thinnest skin will be at the cut edge rather than in the base of the flap. It follows, therefore, that patterns of incision will vary according to the pattern of nodule formation. A regular even zig-zag up the finger is not necessary. This applies particularly to the palm where Z-plasty transposition is more difficult.

In contrast, where the disease manifests itself as a mature superficial longitudinal band, any zig-zag incision up that band will base each of the flaps on the thin skin over the band and prejudice the circulation in the flaps. It is better, therefore, in these cases to make a straight longitudinal incision up the band, which again leaves the thinnest skin at the skin edge, and to close with one or more Z-plasties in the finger (Fig. 32.20).

These two techniques may be combined so that frequently a straight longitudinal incision can be made in the finger and continued into the palm as a zig-zag, and closure will probably be with one Z-plasty in the proximal segment of the finger (Fig. 32.21). It is not necessary to make the Z-plasty so that it lies in the transverse crease in the finger. In fact the skin under the skin crease is often devoid of subcutaneous fat and has a poorer circulation than the skin between the creases. There is no reason why Z-plasties should not be made in the skin between the creases, and should be designed to use the best skin available.

Z-plasty is mandatory in cases where there is skin shortening. This can be measured by comparing the distance between the flexor creases of the affected finger with the distance between the same creases in the same finger of the other hand. The approach should always be such as to allow closure with a Z-plasty which will lengthen the skin. As a basic principle the skin incision should always be carried as far as the flexor crease beyond the last contracted joint. Multiple transverse incisions in the fingers are not recommended, as the operation involves considerable burrowing under the skin to remove the fascia. There is poor exposure causing a poor clearance of the disease and a high risk of nerve injury.

Avoidance of nerve injury

In primary fasciectomy there is really no excuse for damage to the digital nerves. In the management of recurrent disease the situation is often very much more difficult. In the primary case the nerve is never involved in the disease process. It may be moved out of its normal anatomical position by a contracting band. It may appear to penetrate a Dupuytren's nodule, but if the matter is investigated closely, it will be found that two cords have fused over the nerve and the nerve will be travelling in a tunnel underneath the nodule. Careful dissection should always allow the surgeon to preserve the nerves and this is particularly true if the dissection concentrates on the nerves rather than on the band.

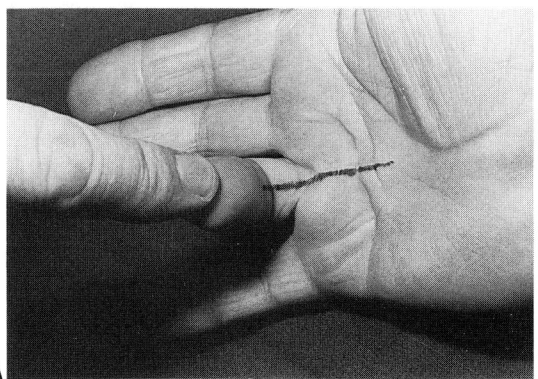
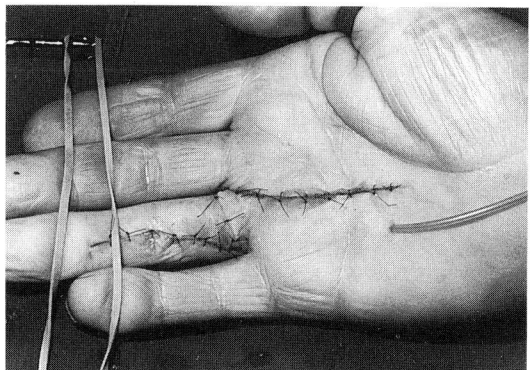

Fig 32.20A, B Superficial band and skin shortening requires Z-plasty.

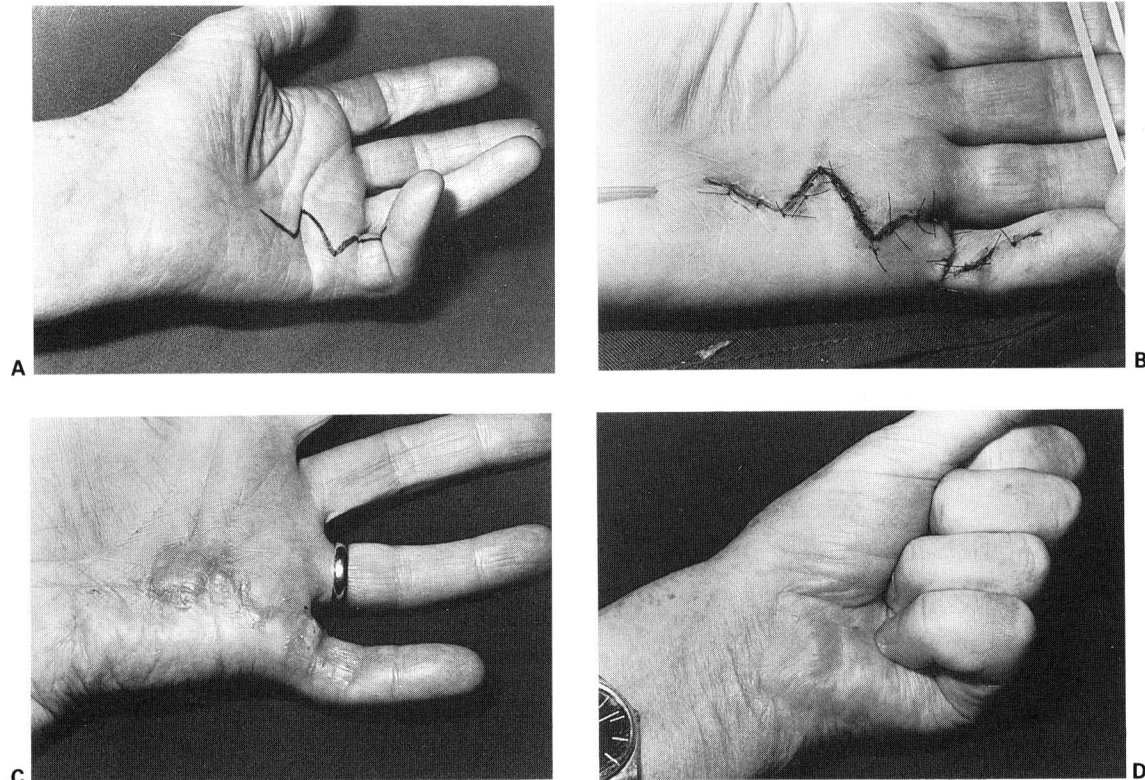

Fig. 32.21A–D Combination of Z-plasty in finger and zig-zag in the palm produces minimum problems and rapid return of good movement 4 weeks postoperatively.

Some points of anatomy are constant. The digital nerves in the palm remain under the transverse fibres of the palmar fascia. Therefore proximal to the distal palmar crease the band can be dissected with confidence, in the knowledge that the nerve does not wind around it. However just beyond the distal palmar crease, at the distal edge of the transverse fibres, the nerve can very sharply and suddenly appear to turn superficially over the top of the band and may be severed at this point by the unwary.

The relationship of the nerve to the band is then variable, depending on which band is prominent, at the palmar digital crease into the proximal segment of the finger. At this level it is the eccentric band that commonly has the nerve wound round it. Most bands causing contractures of the proximal interphalangeal joint have an attachment to the base of the middle phalanx beside the proximal edge of the A3 pulley. At this point, where the fascial band attaches to bone, the nerve is always superficial between the band and the skin. Frequently to get to that position it has passed under the band proximally. It is a common point of nerve damage. However note that at the terminal joint the same does not apply, and if there is a flexion contracture of that joint, the nerve lies deep to the band and the skin at the terminal skin crease.

Avoidance of injury to arteries

It is important not to forget the digital artery. This is particularly true when one is operating on recurrent disease as the other digital artery may have been damaged and diathermied or ligated at the previous operation. Usually, within the finger, the artery lies dorsal to the nerve. When the nerve sweeps over a band the artery always accompanies it, lying proximal to it.

Flexor sheath and joint release

The other tissues that require consideration at operation are the flexor tendon sheath and the interphalangeal joints. The sheath is not involved in the Dupuytren's process and should not be released in the primary fasciectomy. It may become involved in recurrent disease, particularly when part of the sheath has been excised during the initial operation. It is very important that the flexor sheath should be maintained intact if any consideration has been given to skin excision and grafting.

If the only remaining contracting tissue involves a joint, it will be in the proximal interphalangeal joint. The question is whether or not to release that joint. In the author's experience, if proximal interphalangeal joint release is carried out, one must be prepared for some loss of flexion.

Closure

Finally, the surgeon must consider the problem of haemostasis. Fasciectomy often involves one of the most widespread dissections of the flexor aspect of the hand. Meticulous haemostasis of all visible vessels during the period of dissection will considerably reduce the postoperative bleeding. If one is confident of this type of haemostasis and certain of circulation to the digit and skin flaps, then closure can be carried out prior to release of the tourniquet (*Editors' note*: see Chapter 31). However, one must always be aware that where there has been wide dissection in the palm, the cup of the palmar concavity can hold a considerable volume of haematoma. In these cases it is advisable either to leave the wound in the palm open or to put in a small drain. Where any skin grafting is being carried out it is mandatory to remove the tourniquet and secure haemostasis. The author prefers then to reinflate the tourniquet for the period of skin closure, and postoperative haematoma following this technique is very rare indeed.

In addition, it is important to remember that the concavity in the palm of the hand is triangular and the dressings should be cut into a triangle to fit that concavity when the hand is being dressed. Some form of splintage is essential for the immediate postoperative period and this is most readily achieved by a plaster volar slab (Varian 1975).

POSTOPERATIVE CONSIDERATIONS

Surgery for DD puts skin survival in doubt more than any other surgical procedure on the flexor aspect of the hand. It is advisable, therefore, always to redress the hand at 24 hours. Often at this time skin edge ischaemia can be noted and immediately relieved by removal of one or two appropriate sutures. It is important during the immediate postoperative period to note the amount of pain or discomfort of which the patient is complaining. A painful hand must be investigated and the surgeon must be satisfied that it is not a symptom of a tight bandage, ischaemia, haematoma, or infection, before administering large doses of strong analgesics. In contrast, absence of pain does not mean that a single Z-plasty flap may not be ischaemic.

Different surgeons will have their own routines with regard to postoperative mobilization but, by and large, all being well, it is better to commence mobilization early rather than late, this usually being on about the third postoperative day. Sutures are removed at 7–10 days and it is important to get the patient back to the clinic at about $2\frac{1}{2}$–3 weeks to pick off the scale and scab, which can, with dried out keratin, form an outer coat of sufficient strength to interfere with exercises and certainly make those exercises uncomfortable. If there is any evidence of incipient stiffness or undue complaints of pain without obvious cause, the physiotherapist and occupational therapist must be brought in to assist the patient early rather than late. The judicious use of serial splintage or lively splints can correct residual joint contracture, and should be instituted as soon as the skin has healed.

SPECIAL SITUATIONS

The 90/90/0 little finger contracture where the rest of the hand is good

Usually this can only be corrected to 0/90/0, which is more of a disability to the patient. The author's policy is to obtain permission to amputate if good correction proves impossible, and this is carried out through the metacarpal shaft. At amputation save the dorsal skin of the little finger and fold it as a flap into the palm.

Advancing contracture in the under 40-year-old

Always carry out dermofasciectomy.

The severely contracted hand which has already had several fasciectomies

Preoperatively, carefully examine for nerve damage and digital artery damage. Consider amputating the most contracted finger and using its dorsal skin to resurface the palm and/or open the palm transversely and insert a large full thickness skin graft.

The contracted terminal joint

Most commonly this is an extensor contracture due to involvement of Landsmeer's ligament in the contractile process, presenting like a boutonnière deformity. Consider the possibility of an extensor nodule of Dupuytren's disease (Hueston 1982).

Where there is a flexion contracture, the band is usually ulnar and superficial to the neurovascular bundle. There is sometimes a second band on the radial side which is not palpable until the ulnar band is removed. Ligament contracture in flexion (unlike the proximal interphalangeal joint) is not a problem.

PART 10
EVOLUTION OF A SURGICAL TECHNIQUE
L. Zachariae

In this chapter a description is given of how our present treatment of DD has evolved in the Department of Hand Surgery at Gentofte Hospital, Copenhagen.

PERSONAL EXPERIENCES

When I completed my surgical training in 1952 the only type of operation for DD was a radical fasciectomy, a rather heroic performance giving many postoperative sequelae. Therefore many hand surgeons felt that a less traumatic type of operation, the limited fasciectomy, should be the procedure of choice.

During the late 1950s and early 1960s two surgeons in our unit performed a more or less limited fasciectomy according to our different temperaments (Zachariae 1967, 1969). All operations were done through transverse incisions in the palm and longitudinal incisions on the sides of the fingers. In the extensive operation the entire palmar fascia was removed by careful dissection. Operation on the fingers was done only if they showed Dupuytren's changes, and the operation did not involve the first web space or the thumb. Limited fasciectomy involved removal of only that part of the fascia which showed fibrous thickening. Bands, if any, were divided and deep dissection was not performed.

From this material it was concluded that although the long-term results were very much alike after extensive and limited fasciectomy, the extensive fasciectomy was more difficult, complications more frequent and the postoperative course longer after this type of operation. The lack of subcutaneous tissue, which constituted the main cause of the poor result, was difficult to treat. Accordingly, limited fasciectomy was preferred. However there was a striking number of recurrences in the same area following limited fasciectomy.

The problem was therefore: how limited should a limited fasciectomy be? To solve this problem another follow-up study was performed some years later including 450 cases treated with limited fasciectomy.

The conclusion of these studies was that the operation for DD should be a limited fasciectomy, locally radical in order to avoid recurrence in the operated field, but at the same time so gentle as to avoid cicatricial contraction and postoperative fibrosis and dystrophy. In severe cases some form of plastic surgery on the skin, or perhaps a McCash (1964) procedure, was recommended.

PRESENT PROCEDURE

For many years there was no reason to change this technique. The results were good and the operations were performed by trained hand surgeons, but in 1969, when I became Chief of a new Department for Hand Surgery in Copenhagen, the situation changed. Some of the operations for DD had to be performed by surgeons in training. It has therefore been necessary to modify the treatment to fit these new circumstances.

Patients are admitted to hospital the day before operation so that their state of health can be evaluated. They are seen by the anaesthetist and the surgeon who is going to perform the operation. The most common patient is male, 50–70 years of age, with a localized cord in the palm extending to the ring or little finger or both, giving limitation of extension at the proximal interphalangeal or the metacarpophalangeal joint.

Most of the operations are performed under brachial or axillary block, only a few patients have general anaesthesia. The operations are performed in a bloodless field. The hand is simply elevated for 10 minutes before tourniquet pressure is ap-

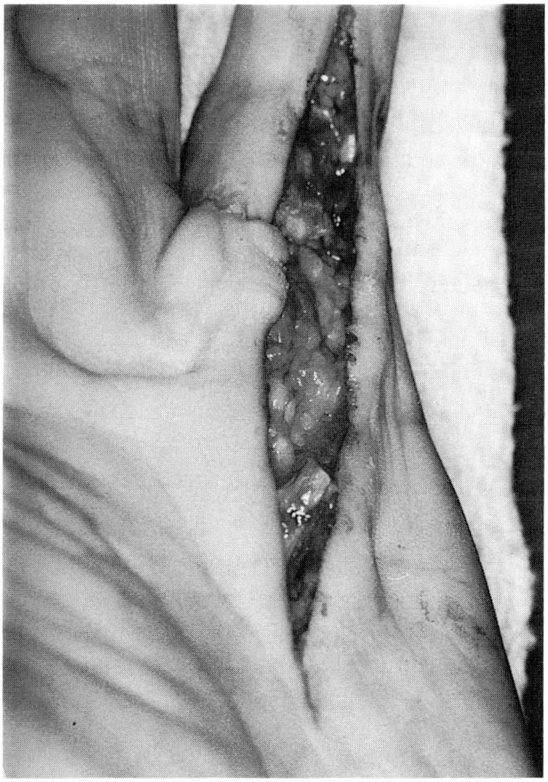

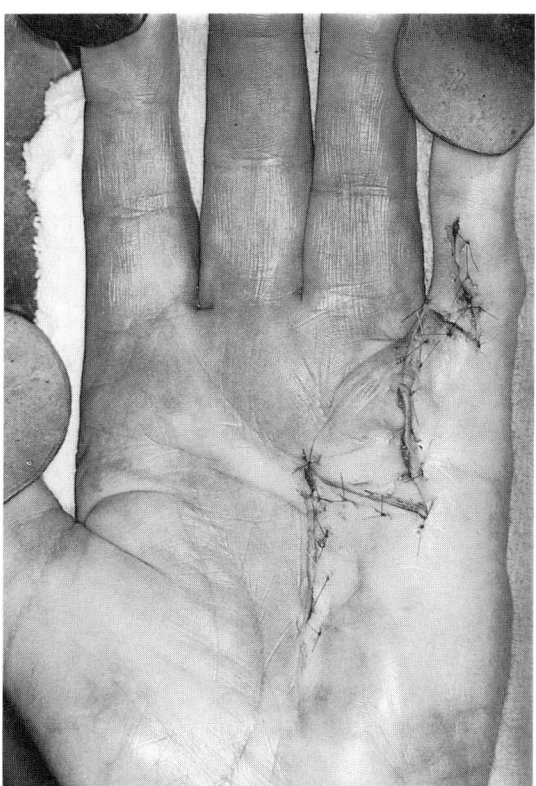

Fig. 32.22 Longitudinal incision along the cord.

Fig. 32.23 The sutured incision of Figure 32.22. Two Z-plasties have been made.

plied. No preliminary exsanguination of the hand is made, as blood remaining in the vessels aids their identification.

The skin incision is longitudinal following the cord from the proximal palm and extending beyond the distal crease of the involved finger. Before starting the operation two Z-plasties are planned, one in the palm and another in the finger (Figs 32.22 and 32.23). The angles are about 60° (Figs 32.24 and 32.25). This incision gives a good exposure and permits removal of the diseased fascia not only in the involved finger but also in the web spaces and the adjacent cords in the palm. It is easier to operate under the base of a triangular flap, as it is difficult to see under a concave incision.

The skin is dissected from the diseased fascia and the affected pretendinous cord is divided proximally in the palm and removed following the nerves and vessels during the dissection. The vertical septae are divided. At the level of the metacarpophalangeal joint the natatory ligaments are divided or partially excised. No special care is taken to avoid cutting the superficial transverse ligament of Skoog (1967). In the fingers the dissection is carried out following the neurovascular bundles, excising the fibrous tissue laterally as well as deep to them. The cord between the neurovascular bundles is removed. It often ends just distal to the proximal interphalangeal joint, where it is attached to the fibrous tendon sheath and must be cut free from this. It is important not to open the tendon sheath because bleeding alongside the tendons forms adhesions. There is always a plane of cleavage between the neurovascular bundles and the diseased fascia, even though it may be difficult to find around a severely contracted proximal interphalangeal joint.

Before skin closure, the tourniquet is removed and careful haemostasis is performed, all exposed

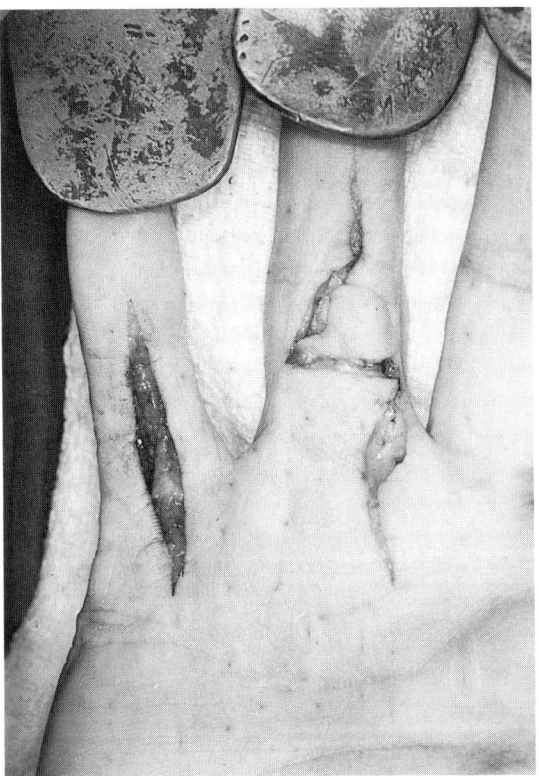

Fig. 32.24 Operation on two adjacent fingers. The primary longitudinal incision is made on the little finger and the Z-plasty on the ring finger.

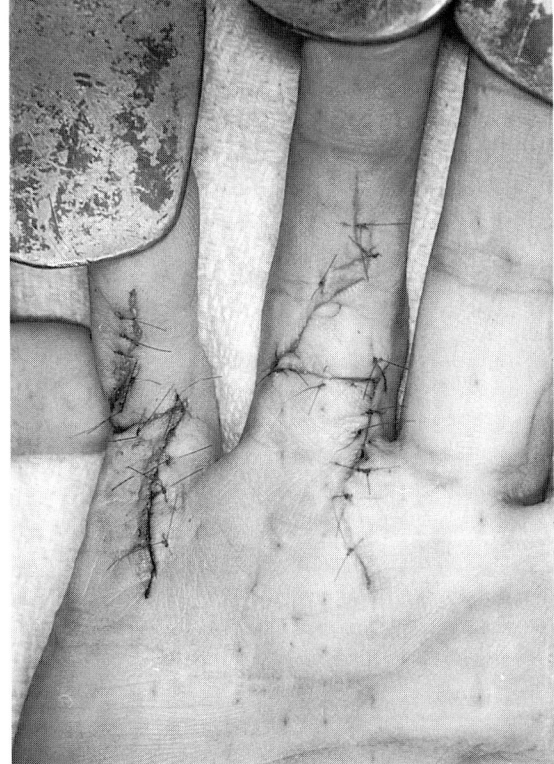

Fig. 32.25 Same hand as in Figure 32.24. The incisions are sutured.

small vessels having been ligated during the operation. The skin is then closed, transposing the Z-plasties. Skin closure is always obtained in this type of operation. If it is obvious before operation that there will be skin problems, we use the Mc-Cash (1964) open palm operation. A free skin graft is used in very few cases as it must be placed directly on the tendon sheaths or, even worse, on the tendon itself.

The skin is sutured with 5–0 monofilament, a compression gauze dressing is applied and a simple wooden splint placed on the palm and affected finger keeping it as extended as was obtained at operation.

The hand is elevated for 24 hours after the operation. The dressing is then changed to detect any haematoma. The splint is reapplied and the patient is allowed to go home and is informed to elevate the hand for the first 2 days and to move the shoulder, elbow and the free fingers. The splint and skin sutures are removed about 10 days after operation. The skin is usually healed by then but sometimes there are small defects that will heal in a few days. The patient is told how to move the hand and is seen at regular intervals until function is satisfactory. In uncomplicated cases physiotherapy is not necessary but regular visits are very important.

If there are difficulties in maintaining extension, a dynamic splint is used at night (Fig. 32.26). If the patient is unable to flex the fingers fully after 3–4 weeks, physiotherapy is instituted — earlier if there are signs of post-traumatic dystrophy.

Non-operative treatment of DD is very seldom used but if the only lesion is a local tender nodule in the palm possibly combined with a trigger finger, local injections of Lederspan may help for a time (Zachariae 1955).

SPECIAL CASES

Younger patients and active older patients may have a two-stage operation performed — the ulnar side of the palm and ring and little finger are operated upon first; some months later, when function of the hand is restored after the operation, the rest of the fibrosis is excised.

If it is obvious that skin covering cannot be

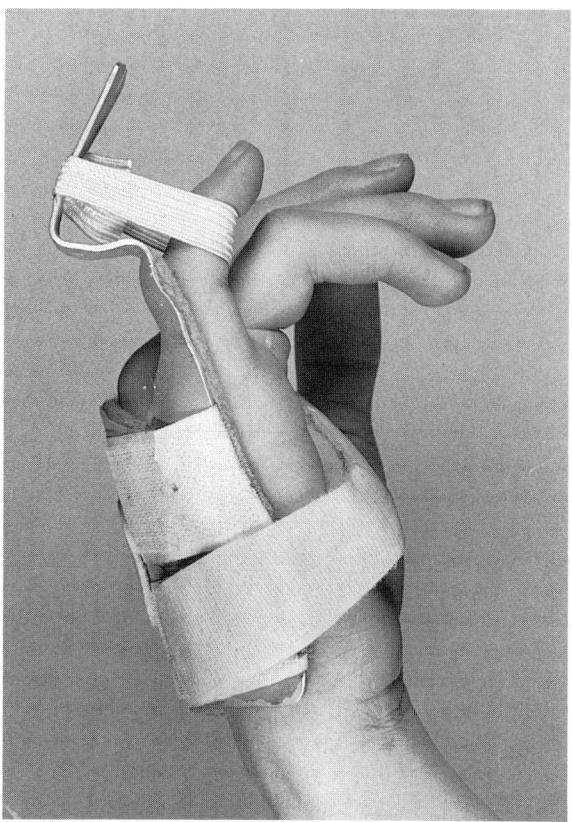

Fig. 32.26 Dynamic splint used in postoperative training.

achieved, the McCash (1964) open palm method is used with modifications (Jacobsen & Holst-Nielsen 1977).

Where extension in the proximal interphalangeal joint is not possible after the fibrosis is removed a partial excision of the fibrotic tendon sheath and sometimes a capsulotomy are indicated but these cases are often very difficult to rehabilitate postoperatively and some never regain full flexion capability. Amputation of a finger at the level of the proximal interphalangeal joint can be performed in selected cases.

Finally, a particular type of presentation will be mentioned: young patients with a very localized but often thick cord on the ulnar aspect of the fifth finger, sometimes only at the proximal interphalangeal joint but sometimes extending as far as the aponeurosis of abductor digiti V. In these cases a local fasciectomy is performed through a lateral incision as radically as possible. Recurrence in the operated field often occurs and the same operation may even have to be performed sometimes three or four times more. Some of these cases later develop widespread changes but in some of them no lesions are seen after local excision.

OUTPATIENT SURGERY

It has always been our practice to operate on patients with DD under cervical or axillary block or general anaesthesia. The patients have been in hospital for 24 hours after operation to have the hand elevated. During later years however, for economic reasons the waiting time for admittance to hospital has been 1 year or more which means that in many cases the lesion has deteriorated so that a more extensive operation than planned has been necessary. We have therefore tried to do some of the operations on an outpatient basis using intravenous regional anaesthesia.

The patients have been selected, the criterion being a fibrous cord in the palm extending to one finger giving a limitation of extension of less than 90° at the proximal interphalangeal joint. Furthermore the patients must be in good health. The results have been encouraging. In all cases the anaesthesia has been satisfactory and only 2 patients had discomfort from the cuff. There were no important postoperative complications, especially haematoma. We intend to continue this procedure with careful patient selection.

PART 11
COMMENTS ON TREATMENT
E. A. Rosenthal

PREOPERATIVE ASSESSMENT

Indications

Surgery is considered when DD impairs function or hand hygiene. Contractures are grouped into mild (<30°), moderate (30°–65°) and severe (>65°). Indications for surgery include: 30° contracture at the metacarpophalangeal or proximal interphalangeal joint; restricted thumb motion; thumb or finger web contracture, and intertrigo. DD without contracture and discomfort from nodules is not a surgical indication. Knuckle pads are sometimes tender but are not an indicator of progression or more aggressive DD (Mikkelsen 1977). Although connected to the extensor mechanism, they do not restrain finger flexion and may spontaneously regress following fasciectomy (Skoog 1963). I have not observed tethering of the extensor mechanism which required tendolysis (Addison 1984).

The surgical design

Skin quality, distribution of disease and severity of the contracture determine the surgical design. Two caveats deserve repeating: there is no such thing as a routine operation in treating DD (Tubiana 1974), and the experience of the operator influences the percentage of complications (Tubiana et al 1967).

Skin quality is the most important consideration in preoperative planning. Gelberman et al (1982) correlated skin grades with wound healing and flap necrosis. A modified classication has been a helpful guide during pre-operative planning.

Grade 1 — Mobile skin without dimples or blanching (Fig. 32.27A).
Grade 2 — Limited mobility; dimples; blanching with extension (Fig. 32.28A).
Grade 3 — Adherent skin; dimples; fissures; blanching at rest; tendon bowstringing (Fig. 32.28B).
Grade 4 — Intertrigo (Fig. 32.28C).

Separating disease from skin and shifting skin flaps is easier in grades 1 and 2; the prognosis for a Z-plasty or Y–V plasty is more favourable. Skin grafts in primary surgery for grades 1 or 2 are reserved for isolated moderate or severe contractures of the proximal interphalangeal joint and in the little finger with multiple digit disease, because of the less favourable outlook in this finger (Legge & McFarlane 1980).

Grade 3 adversely influences the prognosis for wound healing of local flaps. Transverse incisions are used in the ischaemic segments for primary

VARIOUS VIEWS AND TECHNIQUES 349

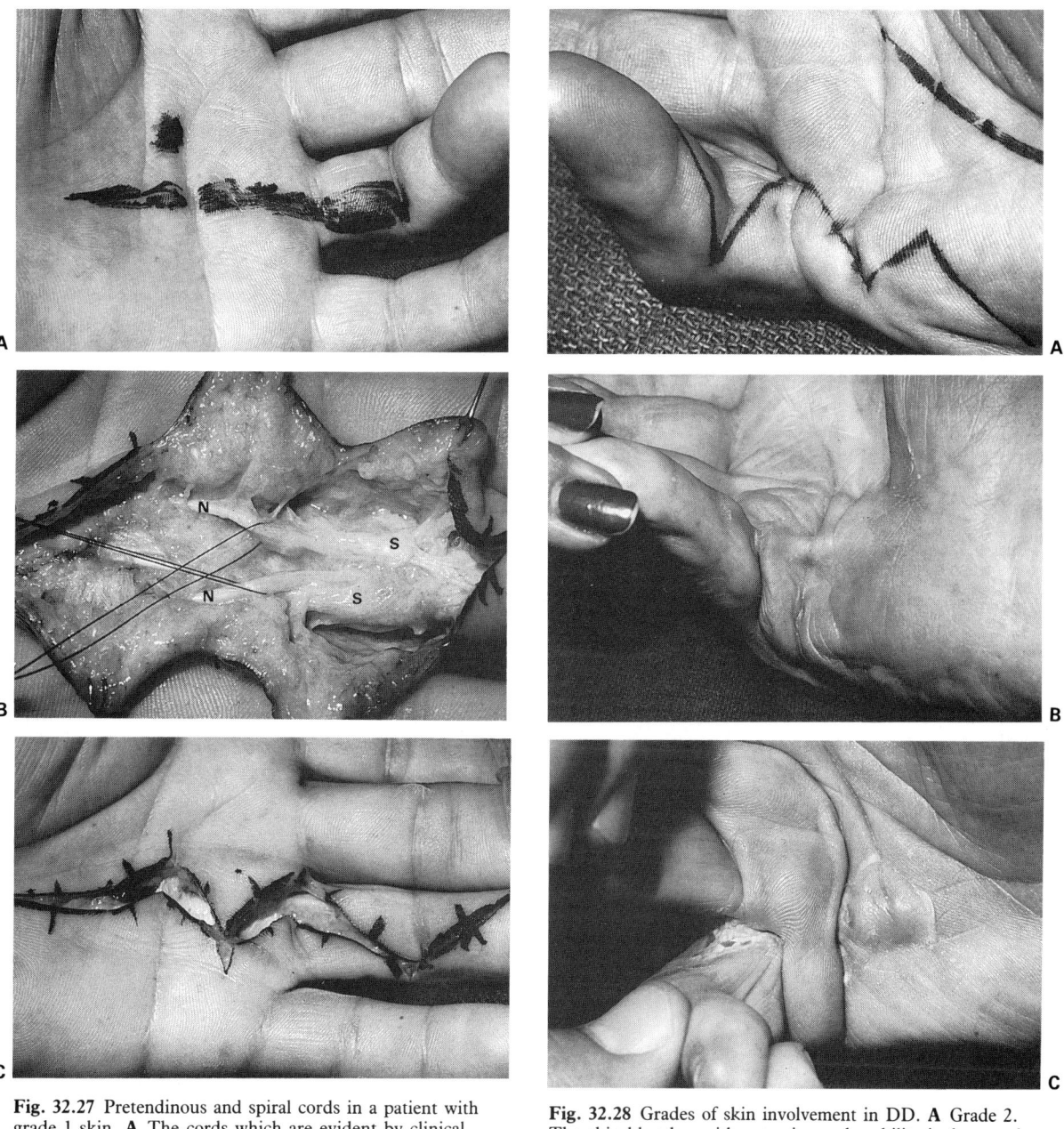

Fig. 32.27 Pretendinous and spiral cords in a patient with grade 1 skin. **A** The cords which are evident by clinical examination. **B** Both radial and ulnar digital neurovascular bundles — lifted by sutures — are displaced by the spiral cords. Displaced structures may not be apparent by clinical examination preoperatively. **C** Y–V plasty insertions begin proximally and progress distally. The length of the inset approximates one-third of each limb of the V. N = digital nerve; S = spiral cord.

Fig. 32.28 Grades of skin involvement in DD. **A** Grade 2. The skin blanches with extension and mobility is decreased; dimples are evident. Skin shifting with a Z and Y–V plasty has a favourable prognosis. **B** Grade 3. Skin is thin, adherent and may be blanched at rest. Skin shifting is more risky; a transverse open palm incision should be considered. **C** Grade 4. Intertrigo represents a contaminated wound environment. A limited open fasciotomy as the first stage of reconstruction is a cautious approach if skin hygiene cannot be improved due to contracture.

fasciectomy and recurrent disease; the open method is used in the palm and the digits are skin grafted. Severely involved palmar skin may be resected and replaced with a skin graft.

Full thickness skin grafts from the groin are favoured in primary surgery for isolated moderate or severe proximal interphalangeal joint contracture; primary surgery for advanced grade 3 palm or digit disease; the little finger in multiple digit disease, and for recurrent disease (Fig. 32.29).

Intertrigo (grade 4) should be cleared before surgery. Dacron batting between the contact surfaces and topical antifungal agents are helpful. A staged reconstruction with primary open fasciotomy is prudent when maceration and contaminated skin cannot be eradicated due to the deformity. An open fasciotomy is also a reasonable alternative in the poor-risk patient. Transverse incisions for both palm and digit are used in these circumstances.

Technical considerations

Fasciectomy through longitudinally oriented incisions is confined to the fascia which is contracted at the time of the operation. Preserving the integrity of fibres bordering excised fascia is important; severed fibres have been linked with recurring local contracture (Skoog 1967a). Displacement of digital neurovascular bundles by spiral cords cannot always be determined by palpation, but nevertheless must be anticipated (Fig. 32.27B). Variations in the configuration of digital disease and its intimacy with the neurovascular bundles necessitate direct access for precise excision (McFarlane 1974).

Fibre bundles which are adherent to skin may not be completely removed. Interposition of skin flaps or full thickness skin grafts which interrupt and re-orient both skin and residual fibre bundles is considered an important facet of surgical treatment.

Z-plasty

A linear palmar exposure is extended in the midline of the digit. The proximal palm Z-plasty is first designed and closed before designing the next more distal one. Flap shifting and skin closure are easier when the transverse limbs of Z-plasties are placed between flexion creases. Three are used for a single ray — two in the palm and one over the proximal phalanx. The length of the Z limbs in the digit should approximate the transverse diameter of the digit (Fig. 32.29).

Y–V plasty

The longitudinal zig-zag incision is centred over the pretendinous cord and midline of the finger; 90° apices are ideal. Reconstruction progresses from proximal to distal, one at a time. Flap advancements and change in digital position may

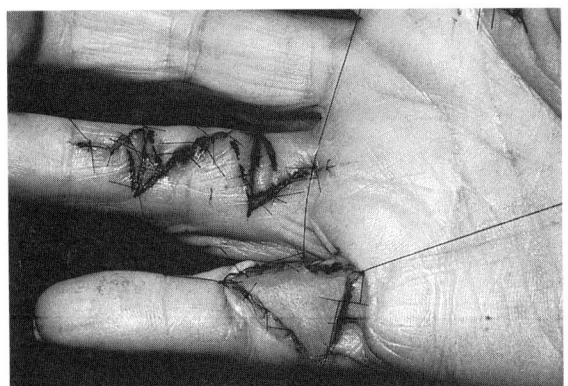
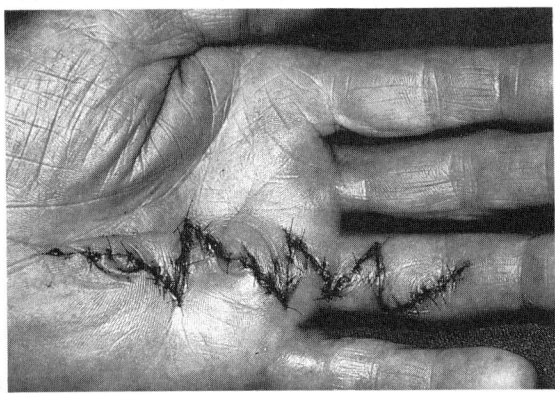

Fig. 32.29 Reconstructive methods for isolated proximal interphalangeal joint (PIPJ), single ray and multiple ray disease. **A** Isolated PIPJ contractures: Z-plasty is used when the skin is grade 1 or 2. Limbs of a Z-plasty approximate the transverse diameter of the digit. A full thickness skin graft is used for grade 3 skin and for PIPJ contracture of the little finger. **B** Single ray disease with metacarpophalangeal and PIPJ contractures: Z-plasties are designed between rather than on flexion creases; three are used when the disease extends to the middle phalanx.

shift skin margins unequally, which changes the site of the Y extension. The leg of the Y is ideally one-third the length of each of the equal sides of the V. Calculated lengthening is the square root of $2X/3$, where X is the length of each side of the V (Baker & Watson 1980). A Z-plasty may be inserted at the proximal or distal end of the reconstruction (Deming 1962; Watson et al 1975) but is usually not necessary (Fig. 32.27C).

SURGICAL TREATMENT

Metacarpophalangeal joint

Excision of the pretendinous cords with the vertical extensions proximal and distal to the superficial transverse palmar ligament permits extension of the metacarpophalangeal joint in most cases. The transverse fibres of the palmar aponeurosis are preserved. Prolonged, severe contracture of the metacarpophalangeal joint produces narrowing of the flexor fibro-osseous sheath and flexor tendons at the base of the proximal phalanx. The 'incarcerated' tendons resist proximal interphalangeal joint extension following fasciectomy (Littler 1977).

Proximal interphalangeal joint

The measure of success in correcting deformity of the proximal interphalangeal joint is the yardstick by which surgery for DD is judged. Some improvement is usually achieved; significant improvement poses a considerable challenge; full correction of severe ($>65°$) deformities is rare. Myostatic tightness resists extension. The intact extensor tendons can be attenuated over the dorsal condyles of the proximal phalanx by prolonged flexion of the proximal interphalangeal joint and may become functionally ineffective (Burkhalter & Carneiro 1979). The retrovascular cords adhere to the oblique retinacular ligaments, exaggerate proximal interphalangeal joint flexion and initiate distal interphalangeal joint extension (Tubiana & Thomine 1974). A classical boutonnière posture with proximal interphalangeal joint flexion and distal interphalangeal joint extension results when the stressed lateral bands dehisce dorsally and displace volarly.

Thorough excision of the restraining cords including their skin attachments is fundamental (Fig. 32.30). The flexor fibro-osseous sheath is not intentionally incised during primary fasciectomy. Surgical release of the volar plate or accessory collateral ligaments of the proximal interphalangeal joint, advocated for incomplete correction of the deformity after fasciectomy (Curtis 1974; Tubiana & Thomine 1974; King et al 1979; Schneider et al 1986), does not improve the functional result following a primary procedure if an adequate fasciectomy has been performed (Gosset 1974). The residual deformity following an adequate fasciectomy reflects alterations of the flexor and extensor tendons and joint capsule which are

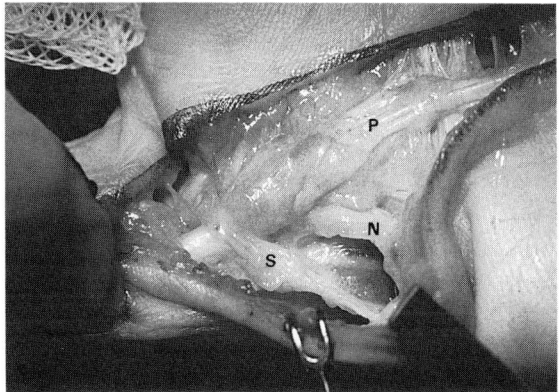

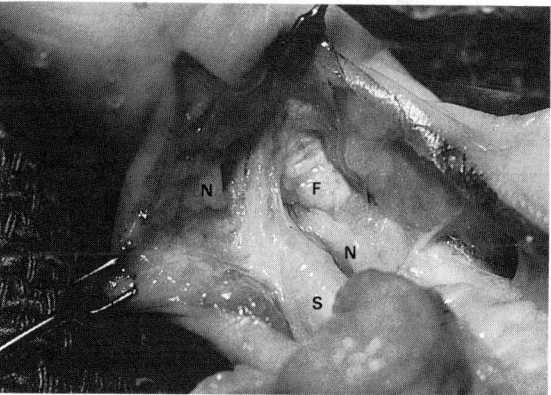

Fig. 32.30 Cords producing proximal interphalangeal joint contracture of little finger. **A** The ulnar digital nerve passes deep to the joined pretendinous and spiral cords. The spiral cord is continuous with the abductor digiti minimi. **B** The distal attachments of the spiral cord into the skin and flexor fibro-osseous sheath. F = flexor fibro-osseous sheath; N = ulnar digital nerve; P = pretendinous cord; S = spiral cord.

treated with judicious postoperative splinting. The proximal interphalangeal joint is not fixed with a Kirschner wire, but is immobilized in its resting corrected position with a bulky dressing of Dacron batting supported anteriorly with a plaster splint.

Incision of the flexor fibro-osseous sheath, volar plate release and resection of the accessory collateral ligaments may be required for secondary surgery following recurrent disease or an inadequate primary fasciectomy. The dorsal transposition flap (Harrison & Morris 1975) and cross-finger flap are alternative methods for surfacing finger defects with exposed flexor tendons. Cross-finger flaps are not recommended in younger patients with DD. A future fasciectomy in the donor digit might jeopardize the vascularity of a digit devoid of normal dorsal circulation (Hueston 1977).

The non-functional, fixed proximal interphalangeal joint flexion deformity with volar scarring which cannot reasonably be improved with further volar surgery is relieved by dorsal resection of the proximal interphalangeal joint with arthrodesis (Moberg 1973).

Amputation is offered for the rare digit which is ischaemic, insensate, painful or too severely deformed from previous surgery for anticipated improvement with another operation.

VARIATIONS

PART 12
SEGMENTAL APONEURECTOMY
J. P. Moermans

The almost proportionate relationship between the extent of the surgical procedure and the postoperative morbidity (Gonzalez 1985) and the high frequency of recurrences after all types of fasciectomies (Tubiana & Lecleroq 1985) made us look for a surgical treatment providing a simple postoperative course and longer relief of the contracture than usually achieved by simple subcutaneous fasciotomies.

In 1983 we began a prospective study of segmental aponeurectomy, a procedure we first heard about from Vilain (unpublished results) who uses a very similar technique. The basic postulate of this operation is that if we can create a permanent discontinuity in the retracted aponeurotic band without wide dissection of the fascia itself, then the retracted band whose tension has been eliminated will disappear or at least cease to act as a contracture. That possibility has been amply demonstrated for scar contractures and the idea extended to DD by McGregor (1985) among others. It is thus much more than a simple fasciotomy since we create a gap in the retracted aponeurosis.

SURGICAL TECHNIQUE

Anaesthesia and haemostasis

The operation is performed under pneumatic tourniquet and usually under regional intravenous anaesthesia.

Incisions

Small curved skin incisions about 1.5 cm long are staged along the retracted band in the palm and if necessary in the fingers, in such a way that if they were joined they would form a lazy S (Figs. 32.31A and 32.32A). They are preferably planned to allow the excision of the nodules since these seem to play the most significant role in the pathogenesis of the contracture (Hueston et al 1976; Badalamente et al 1983).

Dissection

The dissection between the skin and the underlying aponeurosis must be very carefully done close to the dermis to avoid any bridge of fascia. This also allows the re-expansion of the skin even if it is severely pitted. While an assistant pulls on the finger to keep the retracted tissue under tension, small pieces of fascia about 1 cm long are excised, beginning proximally without further skin undermining or wide fascia dissection. At the base of the first phalanx, this excision is usually difficult because of the neurovascular bundles. To diminish

VARIOUS VIEWS AND TECHNIQUES 353

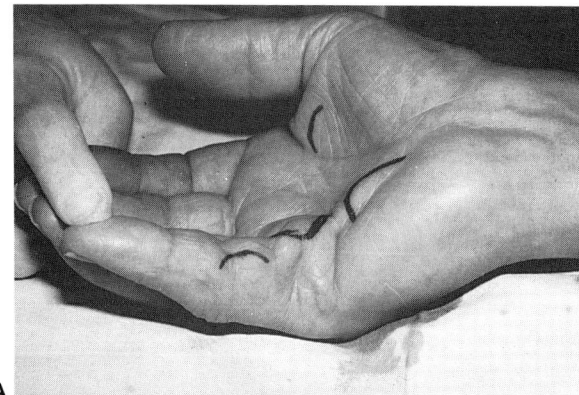

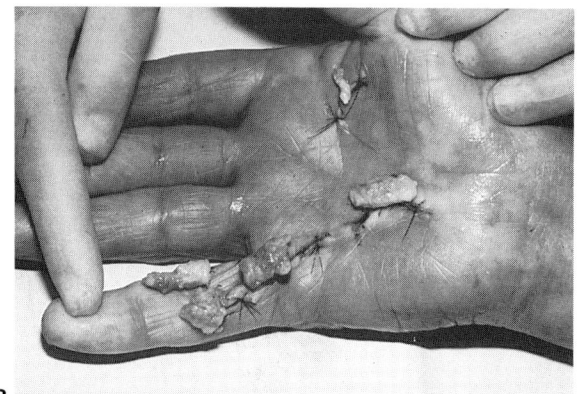

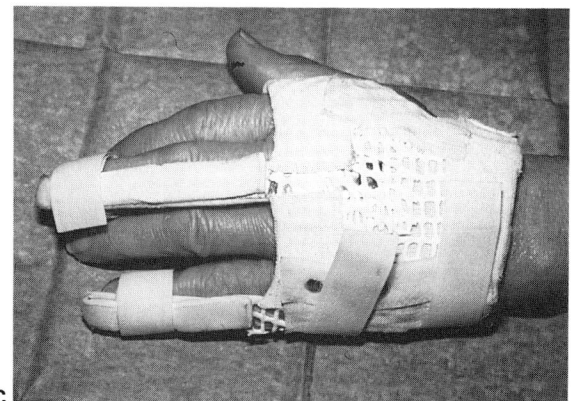

Fig. 32.31 A Staged curved skin incisions. **B** Segmental aponeurectomy. **C** Custom-made extension splint.

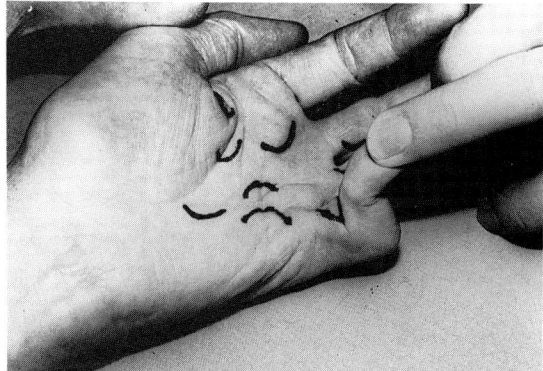

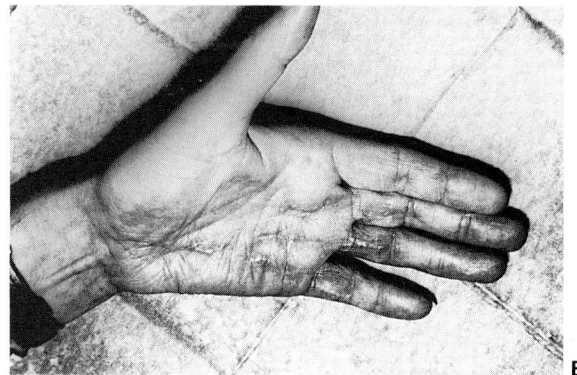

Fig. 32.32 A Staged curved skin incisions for DD affecting all rays. **B** Six weeks after the operation, the scars are still clearly visible but the patient has complete mobility.

the risks of damage of the digital nerves, it is always performed under maximum tension of the band, never using scissors but only a blade to wear away the tissue. At this point, complete extension of the fingers is usually achieved (Figs. 32.31B and 32.33A, B). In some cases a shortened volar joint capsule may restrict full extension at the proximal interphalangeal joint but this is best mobilized postoperatively and not by capsulotomy.

Skin closure

Since there is no wide dissection the skin can be sutured without drainage. Should a skin lengthening nevertheless be necessary it can be achieved by making a V–Y advancement using the pronounced curvature of the incision. A light pressure dressing is applied to the entire hand.

After-care

On the first postoperative day, active mobilization is started and a custom-made extension splint is applied. This should be worn continuously be-

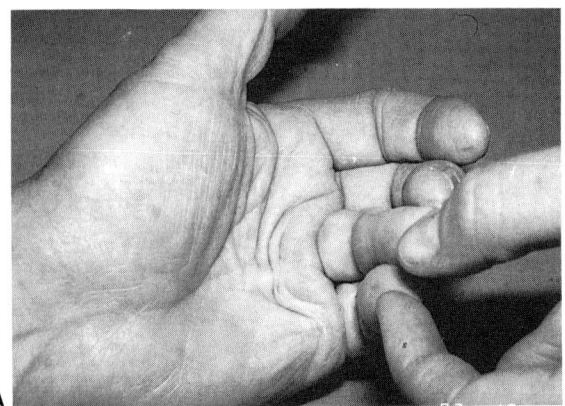

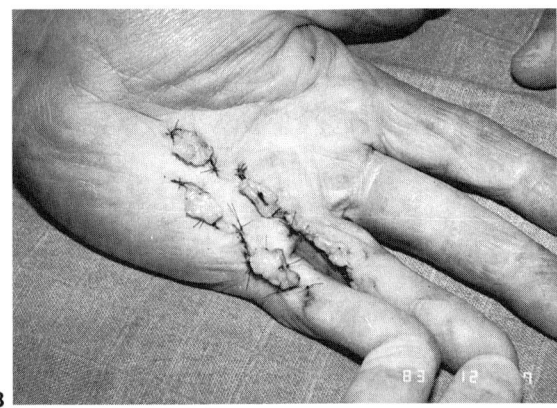

Fig. 32.33 A Contracture of rays 4 and 5 with obvious skin involvement. **B** After segmental aponeurectomy and V–Y advancement flap.

CLINICAL MATERIAL

We have studied our first 120 consecutive cases of DD treated by this method. Each hand was considered separately. There were 93 (77.5%) male and 27 (22.5%) female hands. Thirty-two of the 120 hands had previously been operated on the same or other rays. Of course during our study, more patients with a recurrence of the disease have been operated on but segmental aponeurectomy could not be used because of the abundance of scar tissue; dermofasciectomy with immediate skin grafting was performed instead.

To evaluate the results, pre- and postoperative mobility of the metacarpophalangeal and interphalangeal joints was measured. We also used the assessment formula proposed by Tubiana et al (1968) and the impairment of function assessment method of Swanson et al (1983), which we think is useful to show the functional impact of some possible complications like the postoperative loss of flexion.

PREOPERATIVE EVALUATION

The metacarpophalangeal joints ranged from 5 to 90°, while the proximal interphalangeal joints ranged from 5 to 110°. The average degree of contracture was 38.6° at the metacarpophalangeal level and 45° at the proximal interphalangeal level. Detailed data are given in Table 32.2.

Table 32.2 Pre- and postoperative contracture (in degrees)

Digit	Joint	n	Mean ±s.d. Preop	Mean ±s.d. Postop	Range Preop	Range Postop
I	MPJ	12	20.8 ± 12.6	1.8 ± 3.9	10–50	0–10
II	MPJ	6	17.5 ± 5.2	1.7 ± 4.1	10–25	0–10
	PIPJ	7	35.7 ± 10.2	13.6 ±14.4	25–55	0–30
III	MPJ	28	30.9 ± 16.3	0.7 ± 3.8	10–80	0–20
	PIPJ	17	30.0 ± 14.4	4.1 ± 9.4	5–50	0–30
IV	MPJ	72	38.8 ± 21.0	0.8 ± 3.9	10–90	0–25
	PIPJ	32	46.4 ± 28.1	13.8 ± 13.8	5–100	0–90
V	MPJ	54	48.5 ± 26.0	1.9 ± 6.6	5–90	0–35
	PIPJ	73	48.9 ± 25.6	17.5 ±22.4	10–110	0–90

MPJ = Metacarpophalangeal joint; PIPJ = proximal interphalangeal joint.

The average stage using Tubiana et al's (1968) formula was 3.6 (±2.5). The distribution is shown in Figure 32.34.

The average impairment of function was 7.6% (±6.5). The distribution is shown in Figure 32.35.

POSTOPERATIVE EVALUATION

All patients were regularly supervised until they had recovered complete range of motion or it was

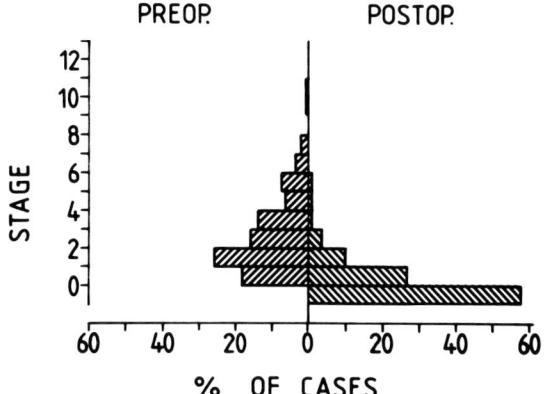

Fig. 32.34 Distribution of stages of contracture evaluated according to Tubiana et al (1968).

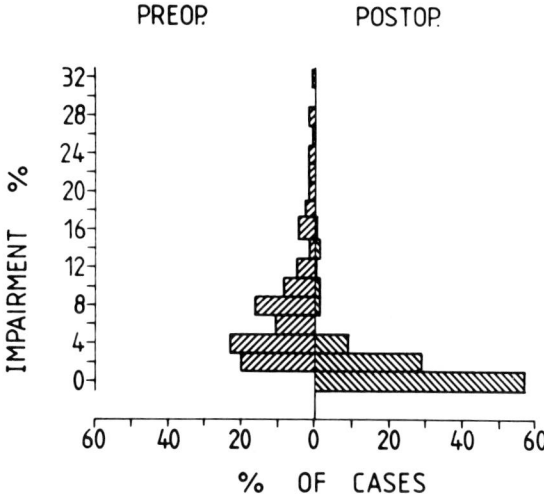

Fig. 32.35 Impairment of function.

felt that mobility would not improve any further. Most patients were under treatment for less than 6 weeks (range 2–30).

Complications

Haematomas

Three small haematomas developed without adverse consequences since they engendered neither infection nor skin necrosis.

Nerve lesions

Two collateral nerves were sectioned at the very beginning of our experience before we began using the safeguard described earlier. The lesions were identified during the operation and were immediately sutured.

Sympathetic dystrophy

Two patients developed a severe sympathetic dystrophy: they were treated for 30 weeks and were the only ones who lost some function.

Results

Detailed data shown in Tables 32.2 and 32.3 confirm the typical better prognosis of metacarpophalangeal contractures over proximal interphalangeal joint of the little finger. They compare favourably with those reported by McFarlane (1985).

Table 32.3 Improvement of contracture

Digit	Joint	n	Perfect	Improved	Same/worse
I	MPJ	12	75.0%	8.3%	16.7%
II	MPJ	6	83.3%	16.7%	
	PIPJ	7	42.9%	57.1%	
III	MPJ	28	96.4%	3.6%	
	PIPJ	17	82.4%	17.6%	
IV	MPJ	72	95.8%	4.2%	
	PIPJ	32	53.1%	46.9%	
V	MPJ	53	90.6%	9.4%	
	PIPJ	72	47.2%	51.4%	1.4%

MPJ = Metacarpophalangeal joint; PIPJ = proximal interphalangeal joint.

The average stage using Tubiana et al's (1968) formula was 0.7 (± 1.1). In 58% of cases a complete re-extension was obtained; 84% had a global extension deficit lower than 45° (stage 1) as shown in Figures 32.34 and 32.36.

The average impairment of function was 1.4% (± 2.9). In 92% of cases the impairment was less than 4%. The distribution is shown in Figures 32.35 and 32.37.

We calculated the percentage of improvement for the joint contractures, Tubiana et al's stage and the impairment of function (Fig. 32.36 and 32.37).

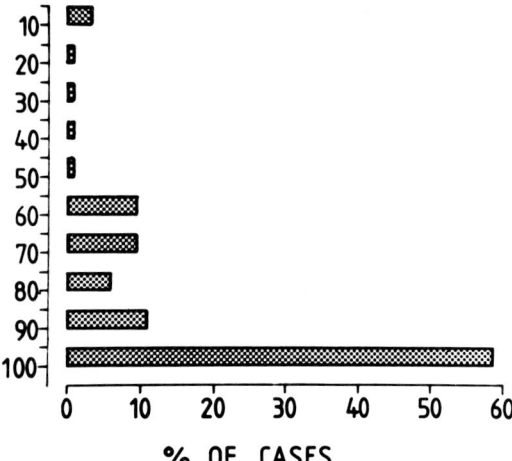

Fig. 32.36 Improvement in stages of contracture evaluated according to Tubiana et al (1968).

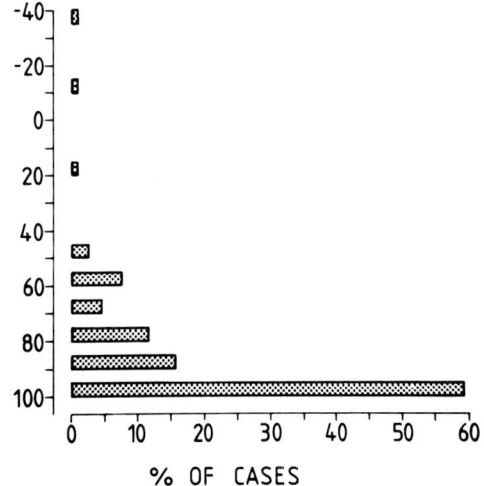

Fig. 32.37 Improvement in impairment of function.

This confirms the benefit of assessing the function since it is the only measure that reveals that the condition of 2 patients who developed a severe dystrophy was aggravated by the operation.

DISCUSSION

The results of surgery for DD have been assessed by a number of different methods and genuine comparison between procedures is extremely difficult. It is all the more so as many factors influence the results: the great variety in the severity of the disease, the operation performed, postoperative complications, especially haematoma, skin necrosis, sympathetic dystrophy, recurrence and extension of the disease. Trying to define the most appropriate procedure, some guidelines should be kept in mind:

1. The more aggressive the fasciectomy, the more numerous the complications, as Zachariae has already noted in 1967.
2. Fasciectomy in most patients is performed for the relief of finger flexion contracture, usually causing a low impairment of function. May operations carrying higher risks of complications and consequently of loss of function be proposed?
3. Although recurrences are frequent, DD is not cancer. Isn't a possibly higher number of recurrences acceptable if we bring down the postoperative complications?

Segmental aponeurectomy was studied as a possible way to achieve a complete correction of the contracture which cannot be obtained by simple fasciotomy, while trying to limit the postoperative discomfort and the sequelae of wide dissection. The early results we achieved in our first 120 cases are equal to or even better than those published for other techniques. Indeed, the overall complication rate was 5.8%, of which only 3.3% had long-term consequences compared with respectively 19% and 10% in the previously mentioned review of McFarlane (1985). In the same way, the overall improvement of contracture at the metacarpophalangeal level, as deduced from Table 32.3, was perfect in 93.7% of cases, improved in 6.3%, same or worse in 0%, compared with respectively 76.9, 18.3 and 4.8%. At the proximal interphalangeal level, our figures are 53.1, 46.1 and 0.8%, compared with 29.8, 51.7 and 18.5%.

These data enable us to have confidence in the technique. Nevertheless, it is only when the percentage of extensions and recurrences of disease are known that the real value of segmental aponeurectomy will be established.

PART 13
SKOOG'S SELECTIVE FASCIECTOMY
D. A. McGrouther

SKOOG'S TECHNIQUE

The operative approach which Skoog (1967) introduced is a limited and anatomically precise operation which he termed 'selective fasciectomy'. The essential details of this technique are, however, not always clearly appreciated. He made a plea in his writings that his method would not simply be remembered by a particular type of skin incision alone, but rather that the three essential principles of his approach were:

1. Preservation of the transverse fibres of the palmar aponeurosis intact to act as a safeguard in protecting the delicate anatomy of the deep palmar space during dissection. He first recognized in 1959 that the transverse fibres of the palmar aponeurosis (Chapter 12) were not involved in the disease although they were intimately attached to the contracture.
2. The neurovascular bundles were not isolated throughout their course, their exposure being mainly restricted to the bases of the digits. The delicate system of connective tissues was left as far as possible in place — this practice varies from that of Hueston (1963, 1982) who has advised progressive display of the neurovascular bundles throughout the dissection.
3. During the dissection the adjacent bordering longitudinal fibres should not be damaged as the healing process in severed longitudinal fibres may cause reappearance of the disease at that site.

To these may be added a fourth principle — minimizing lateral undermining and therefore the size of skin flaps by placing longitudinal incisions directly over the cords.

In performing Skoog's operation the starting point for the palmar incision is a transverse cut at the distal palmar crease. Separate longitudinal incisions are extended in each finger ray with Z-plasties in the digits to give wide exposure and skin lengthening. A proximal extension is made from the transverse palmar incision but offset from the distal cuts to give a discontinuity in the scar line.

The major benefit suggested by Skoog of the retention of the transverse fibres was the preservation of the underlying fibrous tunnel system for the tendons and neurovascular bundles. The retinacular function of these transverse fibres has been discussed (see Chapter 12). Healing time was said to be reduced and functional recovery quicker than after more radical operations. In addition the author considers that it is a worthwhile general principle to limit the extent of dissection (see below) to minimize the potential dead space and therefore the likelihood of haematoma and of recurrence. Should later intervention in the palm be necessary, the safe surgical landmark of the transverse fibres of the palmar aponeurosis can again be found and dissected free.

Skoog's advice of preserving the fat and areolar tissue around the neurovascular bundles as a discipline seems to minimize the disturbance to the anatomical and physiological mechanisms of the hand. The nerves are only uncovered at intervals, or more extensively if densely adherent in nodular areas. Dissection around the neurovascular bundles makes it likely that they will be intimately bound down in any recurrence.

Barclay (1972) used Skoog's operation and Borsetti & Nebiolo (1977) compared Skoog's operation with the more radical procedure of Mac-Indoe; they described a more rapid result with the former. The author's practice commenced by using Skoog's incision and preservation of the transverse fibres but without adequate information on Skoog's general philosophy. A conservative dissection approach was evolved independently and on referring to Skoog's writings, the author became aware that he had rediscovered the wheel, as it were — all the advice on conservative dissection was set out there. Since then the author has limited his surgical dissection further.

MINIMAL EXCISIONAL TECHNIQUE

The author's approach to the surgery of DD has

evolved over a period of years in response to experience, anatomical dissection, and the literature of surgery and pathogenesis. At the outset it is necessary for each patient to have a plan for the management of the skin, the fascia and the joints (Chapter 31). The author's current management of fascia is based on the following principles:

1. An anatomical approach.
2. Minimal dissection with minimal surgical trauma.
3. Fascial release by minimal excision.

The postoperative rehabilitation and splintage programme is viewed as being at least as important as the surgery.

Anatomical approach

The anatomy of the fascia is a precise and intimate three-dimensional network (Chapters 12 and 14) and a working knowledge of the principal features will be of great assistance to the surgeon, allowing a better understanding of the contracture pattern in each individual patient rather than treating each new hand as an amorphous block of Dupuytren's tissue from which nerves and arteries must be dissected. The ability to identify patterns of the disease should increase with experience.

In particular, the author has become aware of certain anatomical relationships which have been found to be useful during the operation. The most important of these is the one described by Skoog — in the mid-palm the neurovascular bundle will always lie deep to the transverse fibres of the palmar aponeurosis and these therefore act as a safe landmark. As these fibres extend as far distally as the distal palmar crease, it is possible to perform a very superficial dissection proximal to this skin crease without uncovering the neurovascular bundles.

A second safe surgical landmark is the system of natatory fibres as the nerve will always lie deep to these. This is not always of value however as these fibres can be involved in the contracture with resulting distortion and their recognition may therefore be difficult.

In the digit the transverse system of Grayson's ligaments are more difficult to define but lateral to the base of the middle phalanx they provide a system of anchorage for the neurovascular bundle.

The neurovascular bundle is therefore very likely to be held laterally in an undisplaced position at the base of the middle phalanx. This is to be considered as a useful guide in dissection rather than a *safe* rule and it is always necessary to identify the neurovascular bundle at this point.

An appreciation of the fascial anatomy on the radial side of the hand (Chapter 16) will also assist dissection in that area.

Minimal dissection

The distance to which different surgeons dissect proximally varies considerably, but it is now the writer's practice to dissect only as much as 1–1.5 cm proximal to the distal palmar crease. This proximal dissection is performed with a scalpel (number 15 blade) or a diamond knife. The transverse fibres can be identified by dissecting laterally from the Dupuytren's cord elevating the skin flap in a plane immediately next to the cord. The transverse fibres will be located in the spaces between the pretendinous longitudinal fibre bundles of adjacent rays. It is then easy to dissect beneath the cord with a scalpel in the plane between longitudinal and transverse fibres.

As one dissects distally from the distal free edge of the transverse fibres it is valuable to try to identify which anatomical fascial route the contracture is following (Chapter 14) to appreciate whether the cords may be superficial to or in the same plane as the nerves. It may be difficult to be certain at first and great care must be taken lest one should damage a nerve.

The author has tried to preserve the fat in the distal palm respecting Skoog's second principal. This can be achieved by following the fascia by gentle spreading (never cutting) alongside the cords with fine pointed tenotomy scissors. The fine rounded tips of this instrument are particularly designed for this type of dissection. This dissection will usually clarify whether the cords running distally are superficial or deep to the neurovascular bundle. It is only necessary to uncover the bundle at one, or perhaps two points within the web fat to identify the anatomy. The nerve may occasionally spiral around a cord in the web although the common site for this displacement is within the proximal segment of the digit. It has been the author's practice to follow the cords for a short distance and then to remove a short length of them extending from 1–1.5 cm proximal to the distal palmar crease and usually a similar distance distally. The cord should be fully dissected before it is divided as earlier release of tension makes dissection more difficult. In nodular areas it may be necessary to follow the bundle millimetre by millimetre. When the fascial cord is divided proximally and lifted off the transverse fibres the metacarpophalangeal joint will usually be completely released without further dissection. The resulting digital extension will allow a better view of the palmar surface of the digit facilitating further dissection. This is useful where there is a significant contracture of both metacarpophalangeal and proximal interphalangeal joints.

Hueston's technique of finding the fascial planes of the neurovascular bundles in the proximal palm and following the contracted cords through the hand has the advantage of progressively displaying the artery but the disadvantage that it requires a large dissection and produces an extensive longitudinal three-dimensional wound with a potential longitudinal dead space in which haematoma may collect.

Fascial release by minimal excision

The success of fasciotomy in some cases indicates that total longitudinal excision in a ray is not always necessary. Although the majority view would advise following a cord to its distal end, Skoog (1967) and Luck (1959) have compromised on this. If it is not necessary to excise all the involved fascia, the question may be asked whether it is necessary that the release of metacarpophalangeal and proximal interphalangeal joints should be in continuity.

The author has modified his philosophical approach to consider the primary objective of surgery to be the release of the joint contracture rather than total excision of the contracted fascia. The aim is to achieve a biomechanically stable internal wound, i.e. the separation of lengths of contracting fascia by fat, or skin grafts rather than by a contractile band of immature scar. The maintenance of the release is a 'tug-of-war' with the skin and internal wound healing processes, oedema, and complications such as reflex dystrophy on one side, and therapy, night splintage and the patient's own efforts on the other.

JOINTS

1. Metacarpophalangeal joint release is straightforward, being achieved by fascial release; the joint itself is uninvolved in the primary case.
2. Proximal interphalangeal joint release and the maintenance of its flexion and extension range is the true challenge of DD.

There are no absolute rules for the management of the contracted proximal interphalangeal joint. The central question is how much release has been achieved at operation by fascial dissection alone. With lesser degrees of persistent contracture after fasciectomy, perhaps up to 30°, it is best to accept the residual contracture and to try to maintain this range by postoperative splintage.

At the other end of the spectrum a severe proximal interphalangeal contracture is unlikely to respond to splintage and beyond a certain degree of flexion the mechanical advantage of the joint is poor. Moreover the patient may involuntarily tend to flex the digit out of the way. Arthrodesis is the author's preferred salvage procedure as it retains the digit and the width of the palm. Amputation at any level may serve to increase the patient's anxiety about the future should the next finger become involved in the disease process. The Dupuytren's patient seems to adapt readily to arthrodesis as he or she is used to stiff fingers.

It is in the intermediate range of residual proximal interphalangeal flexion contracture that the choice of treatment is most difficult (perhaps 30–70°). As the contracture increases in severity the tendency is to give splintage less consideration and move towards arthrodesis. The author has had disappointing results from soft tissue proximal interphalangeal joint release and has found the check-rein ligament to be a more amorphous structure than suggested by Watson et al (1979) or Bowers (1987). Nevertheless soft tissue release may be considered. It is the author's usual practice to warn the patient about the possibility of incomplete proximal interphalangeal joint release prior to operation and to obtain permission for arthrodesis if required.

In summary, a number of different treatment plans have been used for the management of flexion contracture in the digit:

1. *Skin good. Joint good.*
   a. A Z-plasty has been used for access, based on the proximal interphalangeal flexion crease (further distally than advised by MacIndoe) — the lateral limbs are elongated laterally at least as far as the mid lateral lines and the neurovascular bundles located and preserved laterally before the flaps are elevated. This technique avoids neurovascular bundle damage during flap elevation. The wide Z gives good exposure, allowing release of all the fascia. It is the author's practice to excise only 1 cm of each involved cord.
   b. Alternatively a transverse skin incision may be made avoiding damage to the neurovascular bundles, as described above. One centimetre of fascia is excised. Care must be taken to avoid opening the tendon sheath. The wound is left open (Beltran 1985) and early mobilization is commenced.
   c. The problem of opening the thin flexor tendon sheath at the proximal interphalangeal skin crease can be avoided by the technique of Gonzalez, dividing the skin transversely at the base of the finger rather than at the proximal interphalangeal joint level. The skin slides distally to a variable extent, partly or totally releasing the proximal interphalangeal joint.
   d. The author prefers to avoid longitudinal palmodigital dissection but occasionally this is necessary where there is difficulty identifying a neurovascular bundle at the proximal interphalangeal joint.
2. *Skin involved. Joint good.*
   A dermofasciectomy is indicated when the skin is significantly involved by disease or scarred by surgery.
3. *Joint stiff*
   Where release of skin and fascia does not enable full joint extension there are a number of approaches.
   a. Accept and splint.
   b. Proximal interphalangeal joint arthrodesis.
   c. Amputation only if specifically requested by the patient.

HAEMOSTASIS

Haemostasis is always performed with a bipolar coagulator. Wounds are closed as a general rule except where there is a minimal skin shortage or haemostasis is difficult.

POSTOPERATIVE CARE

A soft dressing is held loosely in the palm with an elasticated bandage and a plaster of Paris is applied to the palmar surface to support the wrist in the postoperative period (most operations are performed under supraclavicular block) and also to maintain corrected joints in an extended position (i.e. the palm and fingers are straight). The first dressing is removed at 3–5 days and mobilization is commenced. A thermoplastic night splint is made at this stage and worn initially day and night except during exercise periods. Daytime use is gradually reduced and the patient is reminded before, during and after surgery that he or she must wear a night splint all night, every night for 6 months and intermittently thereafter when the hand feels tight. All patients are seen by the therapist as a safety measure and those who are not progressing are selected for closer supervision and encouragement.

Surgeon, therapist and splint maker review the patients together and in the presence of other patients to encourage a competitive spirit to regain function and maintain correction.

PART 14
EXTENSIVE FASCIECTOMY
R. M. McFarlane

Although the technical details of operation in the palm are important in obtaining a good and long-lasting result, it is a fact that metacarpophalangeal joint contracture is easy to correct and recurrence and extension of disease in the palm do not often require further operation. In contrast, disease within the finger causes proximal interphalangeal joint contracture which is difficult to correct and sometimes is the site of recurrent contracture.

For these reasons I advocate an extensive operation in the finger, assuming that the patient is in good health and can enjoy the long-term benefits of operation.

THE INCISION

Even though most surgeons use some type of zig-zag incision, I prefer a midline longitudinal incision that begins in the mid-palm, but most importantly, extends to or just beyond the distal crease of the finger (Fig. 32.38). The disease that causes proximal interphalangeal joint contracture extends beyond this joint and therefore can only be exposed by an incision that extends well distal to the proximal interphalangeal joint. Furthermore, although uncommon, the disease may extend beyond the distal interphalangeal joint. Only by this distal exposure can the disease be seen and removed.

Initially I used a midline incision because it allowed me to turn skin flaps back to the mid lateral line on each side without disturbing the normal and pathological anatomy of the fascia. Having studied the fascia in this manner and described the diseased cords that contract the proximal interphalangeal joint, I continue to use this incision because the exposure provided is better than that obtained with a zig-zag incision.

The disadvantage of the zig-zag incision is that one cannot adequately remove diseased tissue near the base of a triangular flap without jeopardizing the blood supply to the flap. As a result the surgeon leaves the disease behind and recurrence is likely (Fig. 32.39).

The disadvantage of a midline incision is that it must be broken by Z-plasties in order to prevent postoperative scar contracture. If one is not confident in designing a Z-plasty then this incision should not be used. I do not design the Z-plasties at the beginning of the operation. It is much safer

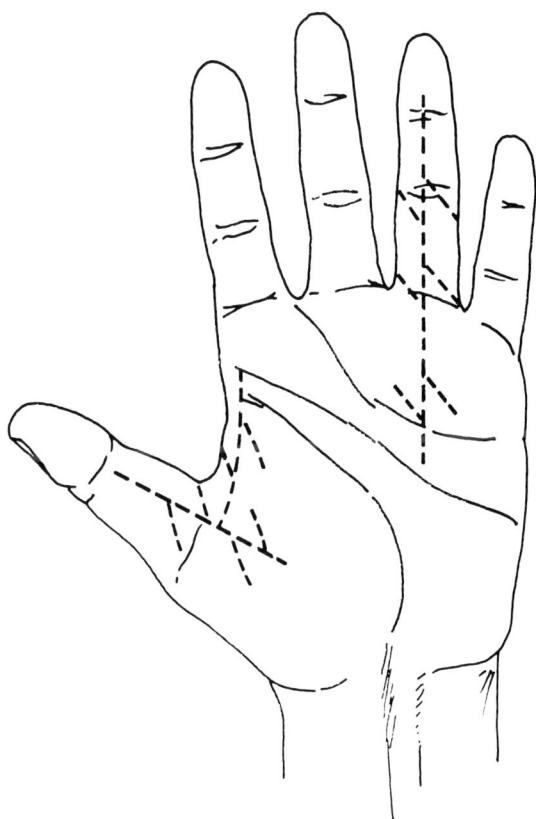

Fig. 32.38 Midline longitudinal incision to remove disease in the fourth ray. The incision extends just beyond the distal crease of the finger. The Z-plasties are designed after the fascia has been excised and are placed at or near the middle and proximal creases of the finger and the distal crease of the palm.

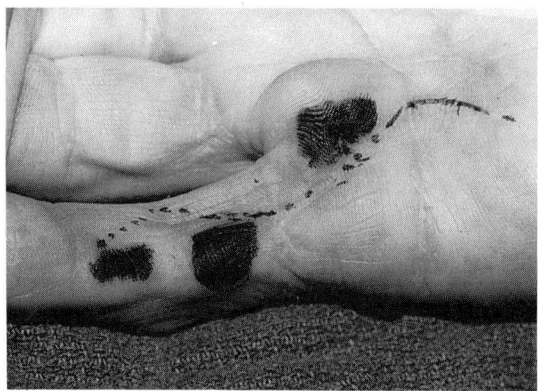

Fig. 32.39 This zig-zag incision did not permit removal of lateral cord tissue in the finger and as a result the patient developed recurrent contracture.

and more efficient to design them after the disease has been removed and the proximal interphalangeal joint is extended. Three Z-plasties are recommended (Fig. 32.38; see Fig. 32.42). One is placed near the distal crease of the palm, another near the proximal crease of the finger and a third near the middle finger crease. A Z-plasty is not required at the level of the distal interphalangeal joint because a midline scar across this joint does not contract. The Z-plasties can be moved a little proximal or distal in order to take advantage of well vascularized skin. The limbs of the Z-plasty need not extend to the mid lateral line. They are usually about 1.5 cm in length.

DISSECTION OF THE SKIN FLAPS

This is an important technical step in the operation. The skin should be dissected free of the underlying fascia. However one hopes to retain enough blood supply to the skin to assure its survival. To this end scalpel dissection and loupe magnification are essential to develop a plane of dissection just superficial to the diseased fascia. In the palm and distal finger a thick layer of superficial fascia can be left attached to the skin and thereby assure its vascularity. In the distal palm and the proximal segment of the finger the diseased fascia is intimately associated with the skin (Chapter 14). Nevertheless, with careful sharp dissection aided by magnification, a plane can be developed through which the skin can be separated from the diseased fascia. This skin will survive through its dermal circulation. The skin should be reflected to the mid lateral line on each side of the finger (Fig. 32.40).

EXPOSURE OF THE NEUROVASCULAR BUNDLES AND EXCISION OF THE FASCIA

Although it is interesting to dissect and follow the various cords that cause contracture of the proximal interphalangeal joint it is not necessary or advisable to do so. Rather the concept of performing a block dissection assures that all of the diseased and potentially diseased fascia will be removed. Carrying this analogy further, the first

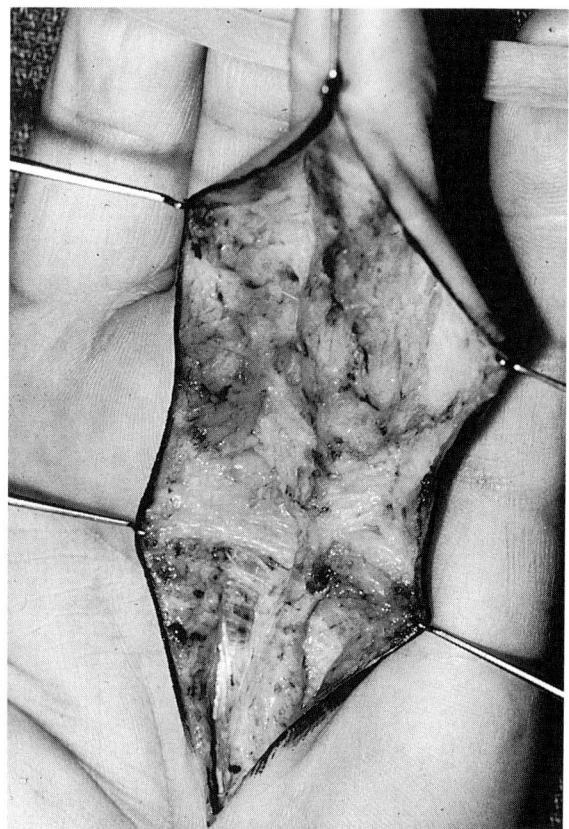

Fig. 32.40 Exposure of the fourth ray through a midline incision. The skin flaps are reflected to about the mid lateral line.

step in the excision is to expose both neurovascular bundles from the tip of the finger to the transverse fibres of the palmar aponeurosis in the mid-palm. The neurovascular bundle is found most readily near the distal crease of the finger so it is easiest to expose both bundles from distal to proximal. The artery is deep to the nerve and is best protected by keeping the nerve and artery within their fascial sheath rather then dissecting them separately. Unfortunately it is necessary to divide the palmar branches of both nerve and artery in this dissection but usually the dorsal branches can be spared.

A bipolar coagulator is used during the dissection and each small vessel is coagulated as it is encountered. With loupe magnification these vessels are seen easily. The branches of the digital artery should be coagulated about 3 mm from the artery so that the intima of the main vessel is not damaged. If haemostasis is attended to during the dissection there will be little or no bleeding when the tourniquet is released at the end of the operation.

Having exposed both neurovascular bundles they are not only free of danger of being cut but also any displacement of them has been overcome. It remains then to remove all of the fascia between the neurovascular bundles, as well as the fascia on either side and deep to the neurovascular bundles as a block dissection.

Beginning distally the fascia between the neurovascular bundles is very thin near the distal interphalangeal joint but will thicken and be adherent to the flexor tendon sheath and periosteum of the middle phalanx just distal to the proximal interphalangeal joint. It is usually possible to dissect this fascia off the tendon sheath but no harm is done by opening the sheath or removing a small amount with the fascia. The fascia is easily dissected off the tendon sheath over the proximal phalanx and into the palm.

Dissection of the diseased fascia lateral to the neurovascular bundle is more difficult because it is not only attached to the skin but passes deep to the neurovascular bundle. The bundle is best protected during this dissection by an assistant retracting it with a nerve hook. Again the dissection begins distally. As the web space is approached one should be sure that the natatory ligament is removed. Also the fascia may pass deeply to be in continuity with an interosseus tendon or attach to the side of the proximal phalanx near its base.

Finally one should examine the tissue deep to the neurovascular bundle to see if the retrovascular cord of Thomine is diseased. Almost always there is some thickened fascia near the proximal interphalangeal joint but occasionally this cord is very thickened and extends beyond the distal interphalangeal joint. The retrovascular cord is one cause of recurrent contracture at the proximal interphalangeal joint and should be removed even if it is not obviously diseased.

PROXIMAL INTERPHALANGEAL JOINT PROCEDURE

In patients with long-standing contracture at the proximal interphalangeal joint the joint will not fully extend even after an extensive fasciectomy. The surgeon has three choices:

1. Accept the residual contracture and hope that postoperative therapy and splinting will overcome it. Realistically one hopes that therapy and splinting will maintain the extension gained at operation rather than improve upon it.
2. Perform a soft tissue release. Occasionally a simple incision of the flexor tendon sheath over the proximal interphalangeal joint is all that is necessary to overcome residual contracture (Fig. 32.41). If this is not successful then excision of the attachment of the accessory collateral ligament to the volar plate, as advocated by Curtis (1954), or release of the palmar plate as suggested by Watson et al (1979) can be done. The release must be carried out bilaterally. I prefer the former procedure but whichever one is used it should not be extended beyond this simple release. Further soft tissue release in which the joint surfaces are exposed may overcome flexion contracture but carries the risk of loss of full flexion thereafter. I would not hold the PIPJ in extension with a K-wire.
3. If the residual flexion contracture is severe, that is, 60–90°, one must consider joint fusion, joint replacement, or amputation. I prefer joint replacement rather than fusion because the patient usually gains about 50° of movement within a range of 30–90° of flexion. I would only amputate the finger on the patient's insistence.

THE CLOSURE

The tourniquet should be released before closure to assure haemostasis but also to assess the viability of the skin flaps. Especially after dissection of recurrent disease one must assess the viability of the entire finger because one or other digital artery could have been damaged at the original operation. The Z-plasties are designed in areas of well vascularized skin (Fig. 32.42). If the triangular flap is of doubtful viability it can be managed as a full thickness skin graft and held in place with a bolus dressing.

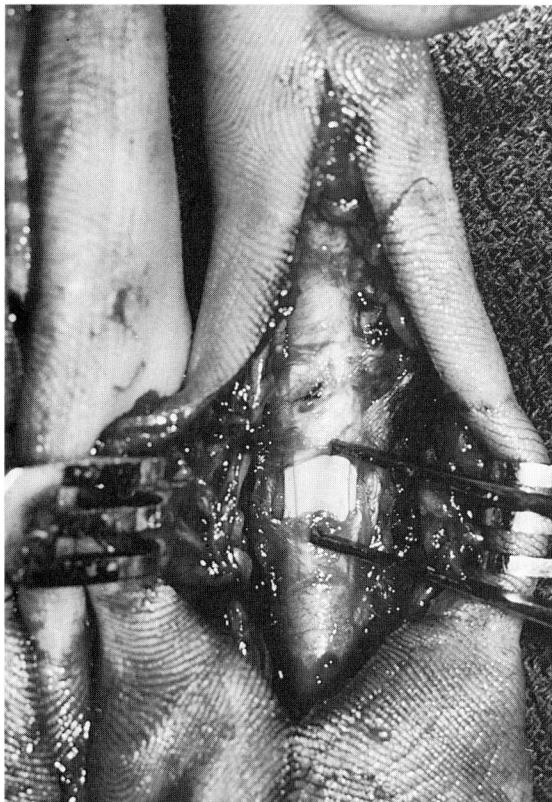

Fig. 32.41 Incision of the flexor tendon sheath as a first step in overcoming proximal interphalangeal joint contracture.

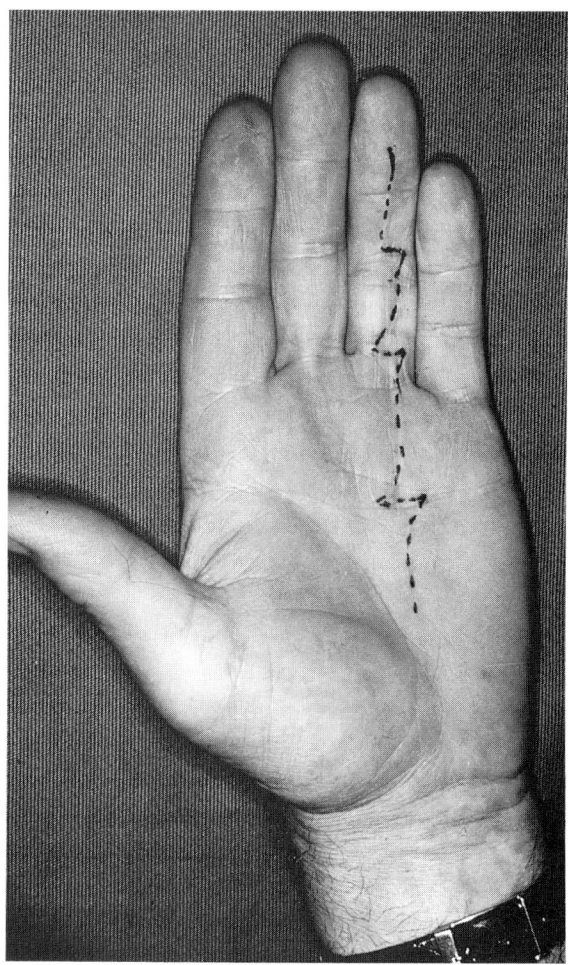

Fig. 32.42 The closure of the midline incision with three Z-plasties. The sides of the flaps are about 1.5 cm.

POSTOPERATIVE MANAGEMENT

The hand is immobilized in a bulky dressing and dorsal splint with the wrist in slight flexion to relax the palmar skin. The metacarpophalangeal joint is placed in about 30° flexion to facilitate proximal interphalangeal joint extension. The following day the dressing is removed and the therapist applies a thermoplastic splint with the wrist and hand in the same position. At the moment we are able to admit these patients to hospital the day before operation and they stay 1 or 2 days after operation. This is a luxury that may not last, but it permits observation of the patient and the hand for undue pain or swelling as well as adjustment of the splint and education of the patient in its use.

PART 15
DISTAL JOINT HYPEREXTENSION AND FLEXION
R. M. McFarlane

Distal joint contracture is not a typical feature of Dupuytren's disease (DD). Neither hyperextension nor flexion is rare but there is little direction in the literature about why they occur or how to treat them. Adams (1879) recognized both deformities, as shown in an illustration from his book (Fig. 32.43).

HYPEREXTENSION

This deformity never occurs without proximal interphalangeal joint flexion contracture but does occur in the absence of metacarpophalangeal joint contracture. It is usually a fixed deformity but occasionally it disappears as the patient flexes the finger. A fixed deformity is often corrected or at least improved if the proximal interphalangeal joint flexion contracture is corrected by fasciectomy. However the deformity may persist, regardless of a successful correction at the proximal interphalangeal joint.

Pathologically two types are seen. A rare type, described by Hueston (1985) and illustrated in Figure 32.44, has an unusually large plaque of Dupuytren's tissue over the middle phalanx. The size and location of the plaque prevent excursion of the extensor tendon and presumably Landsmeer's ligaments. It has only been seen in the little finger. Excision of the plaque should permit some distal interphalangeal joint flexion depending upon the duration of the deformity.

With the common type of hyperextension there is no dorsal disease but there is always severe proximal interphalangeal joint contracture (Fig. 32.45). This deformity is most common in the little finger, and is seen in the most severe form in this finger. It is not due to DD affecting dorsal structures. Rather it is due to volar disease

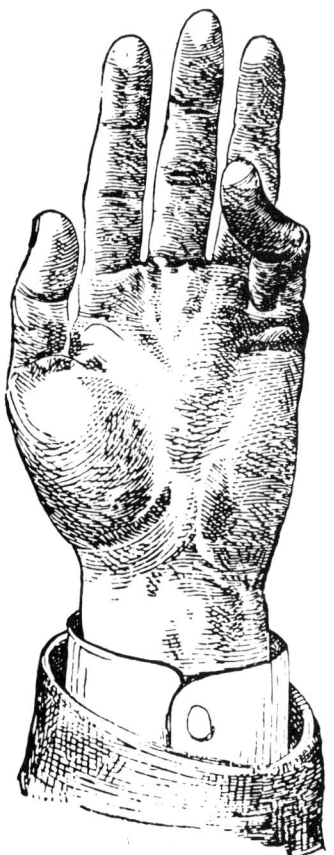
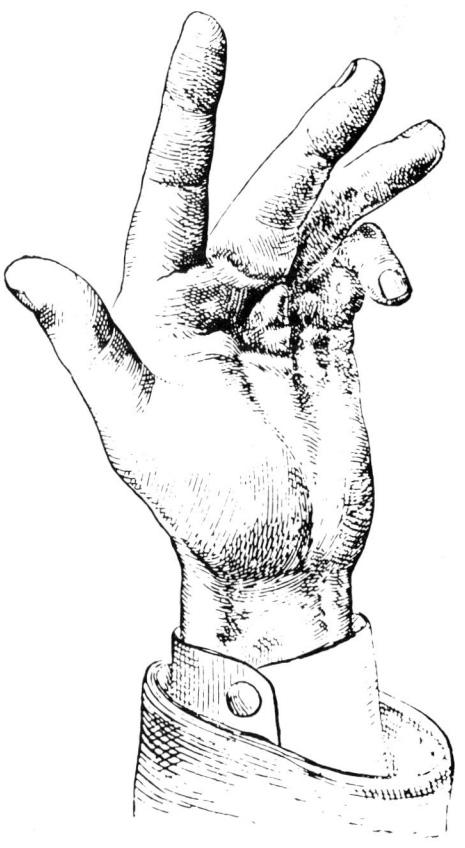

Fig. 32.43 From Adams (1879) showing two examples of severe disease in which the distal joint of the little finger is either flexed or hyperextended.

366 DUPUYTREN'S DISEASE

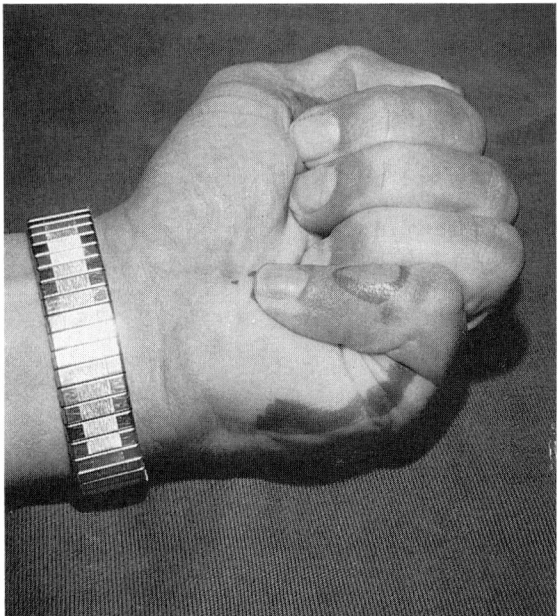

Fig. 32.44 An uncommon cause of distal interphalangeal joint hyperextension. This patient has severe bilateral disease with ectopic deposits of Dupuytren's tissue over the dorsum of the middle phalanx of both little fingers, which prevents distal interphalangeal joint flexion.

preventing normal excursion of the lateral bands and Landsmeer's ligaments in the region of the proximal interphalangeal joint. As described by Thomine (1972), the lateral and retrovascular cords are intimately associated with these structures at the proximal joint. With increasing flexion at the proximal interphalangeal joint these lateral structures become fixed (and the middle slip insertion attenuated) so that a boutonnière deformity develops. If the deformity persists after adequate fasciectomy it can be improved by tenotomy of the extensor tendon over the middle phalanx (Fig. 32.46).

FLEXION

Millesi (1967) reported distal interphalangeal joint flexion in 14 or 4.9% of his series of 287 patients. The little finger was most often involved and the contracture was usually accompanied by disease elsewhere in the same finger. Rarely the distal

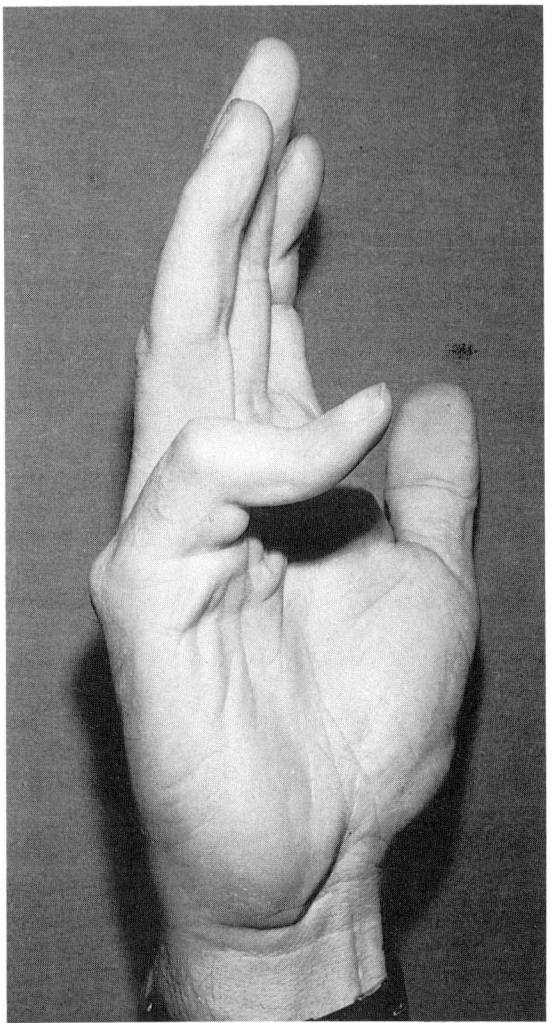

Fig. 32.45 The typical appearance of hyperextension at the distal interphalangeal joint. Both metacarpophalangeal and proximal interphalangeal joints are flexed. The patient has severe bilateral disease. The hyperextension deformity of this little finger was unchanged by extensive fasciectomy.

joint alone is involved, although it is not uncommon for the distal joint contracture to be the prominent feature. In Chapter 20 the data on distal interphalangeal joint contracture is shown in Profile A as well as other profiles. The success of correction of the distal joint contracture was between the good results at the metacarpophalangeal and less satisfactory results at the proximal interphalangeal joint.

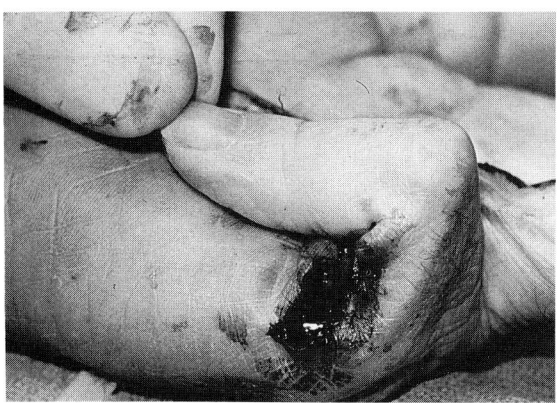 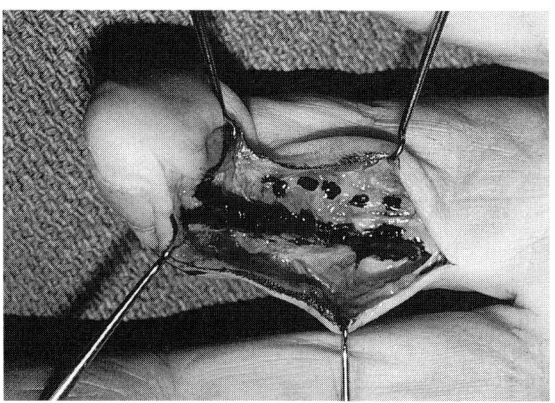

Fig. 32.46 The hyperextension at the distal joint was not corrected by extensive fasciectomy and correction of metacarpophalangeal and proximal interphalangeal joint flexion. An extensor tenotomy only temporarily corrected the hyperextension.

Fig. 32.47 This patient previously had an operation to correct metacarpophalangeal and proximal joint contractures of this left ring finger. He subsequently developed distal interphalangeal joint contracture which was mistakenly thought to be a mallet finger. The offending cord is shown lateral to the radial neurovascular bundle (dashed line). The cord was excised but the patient was left with 15° flexion contracture.

There is abundant normal fascia available to account for a diseased cord crossing the distal interphalangeal joint. The lateral digital sheet passes distally, lateral and volar to the neurovascular bundle to blend with the fascia of the distal pulp. Some fibres attach to the base of the distal phalanx and in so doing intermingle with the terminal branches of the artery and nerve. The retrovascular cord described by Thomine (1972) attaches to the base of the distal phalanx. The diseased cord is usually on one or other side of the finger and lateral to the neurovascular bundle, as shown in Figure 32.47. However it is in continuity with fascia that is deep to the neurovascular bundle. It is difficult to remove the diseased fascia distal to the distal interphalangeal joint where the fibres intermingle with the nerve and artery. For this reason it is difficult to obtain complete correction of the contracture, as attested by the results given in Chapter 31.

Injuries occur to patients with DD as well as others, so mallet finger and boutonnière deformity due to trauma can develop before or after the onset of their disease. Occasionally it is difficult to determine the cause of the deformity and thus plan the appropriate treatment.

… *E. J. Mackin and P. M. Byron*

Postoperative management

Despite good surgical treatment some patients recovering from surgery for Dupuytren's disease (DD) will develop complications unless a careful postoperative hand therapy programme is initiated. Some of these complications include persistent oedema, stiffness of the entire hand, haematoma and early recurrence of flexion contractures. The patient must understand that approximately one month of intensive postoperative therapy may be required if the good results attained at surgery are to be maintained and that night-time extension splinting may be necessary for 6 months or longer.

OPEN PALM TECHNIQUE

The open palm technique of McCash (1964) prevents haematoma and may contribute to the overall reduction of complications (Tubiana 1985). Therapy usually begins on the third to fifth postoperative day. Since the open palm technique allows free drainage of the wound, the whirlpool treatment assists in wound management. It is a good means of cleansing the wound and facilitates active motion.

A whirlpool bath or clear rinse procedure is used following the open palm technique. Betadine is added to the whirlpool. Niederhuber et al (1975) state: 'as an adjunctive modality in the treatment of many types of wounds, the therapeutic whirlpool provides the physiological benefits of heat to promote healing and the atraumatic removal of surface eschar and exudates where bacteria thrive'. They found that a combined treatment procedure of whirlpool agitation followed by a clean water rinse was more effective in removing bacteria than a procedure in which the part was not rinsed after removal from an agitated whirlpool bath. Bohannon (1982) produced further evidence of the value of rinsing contaminated ulcers, wounds or burns after removal from the whirlpool bath.

Whirlpool temperature is approximately 33–35°C. The patient's extremity is positioned with the elbow flexed so that the agitating water just covers the hand, thus avoiding the dependent position. Active flexion and extension exercises may be carried out in the bath. The risk of increasing oedema is decreased by having the patient remove the hand from the whirlpool and elevate it overhead where he or she performs active fist-making for 1 minute. This is repeated every 3–5 minutes (Byron and Muntzeri 1986).

The patient is asked to attend therapy twice a week for whirlpool, inspection of wounds and assessment of mobility. Between sessions with the therapist, the patient will carry out warm saline soaks at home, prepared with 1 tablespoon of table salt added to 2 litres of boiled water. This hypertonic solution is bactericidal. When the boiled water cools to a lukewarm temperature the patient may use it to soak the hand for 10–15 minutes. Home saline soaks may be repeated two to three times a day. Active motion of the hand is carried out during the soaks.

The patient is instructed in redressing the wound at home in the manner preferred by the surgeon. Generally dry sterile gauze dressings are used. They are changed after each whirlpool bath treatment or home saline soak. The crucial factor is to keep the granulating wound clean. A few patients may develop a superficial infection with an increase in the amount of daily exudate. This is treated with an antibiotic ointment which must be used sparingly in the very centre of the wound, since it might promote the formation of hypertrophic granulations. The ointment is applied after the saline soak or whirlpool bath. If granulations become exuberant, they respond to silver nitrate application (Fietti & Mackin 1984).

When resection into the digit is necessary, the dressing applied to the digit must not interfere with finger movement. Full active flexion/extension exercise must be possible within the confines of the dressing.

CLOSED PALM TECHNIQUE

As with the open palm technique, therapy usually begins on about the third postoperative day. The postoperative management for patients who have undergone the closed palm technique is essentially the same as for the open palm technique except that the whirlpool bath is not used as long as the sutures remain in the hand and digits. The wounds are kept dry. When the sutures have been removed — generally at 7–10 days — Betadine whirlpool baths may be initiated.

A postoperative complication of the closed palm technique is haematoma. Extensive operation in the palm followed by closure of the wound can result in the formation of a haematoma or blood clot, provoking inflammation and cellular response. If the edges of the wound become necrotic, infection is inevitable. The result is frequently swelling and stiffness of the hand.

Since immediate postoperative splinting is indicated to hold the patient's fingers in maximal extension during the period of wound healing, careful attention must be given to splint fabrication and the patient must have regular scheduled appointments. Should a haematoma begin to develop, causing additional swelling, the splint may no longer fit properly. If in addition the patient fails to attend therapy appointments, a constricting wrist strap can increase the oedema, resulting in more fibrosis, thicker scar and further problems.

SKIN GRAFTING

Skin grafts are closely monitored for vascularity during the early phase of healing. Generally, the volar plaster splint applied at surgery is removed and a lighter dressing is applied at the first postoperative visit. Care must be taken to apply the dressing so that it does not abrade or cause pressure to the graft during early mobilization. A palmar pan splint is fabricated to maintain extension (Fig. 33.1).

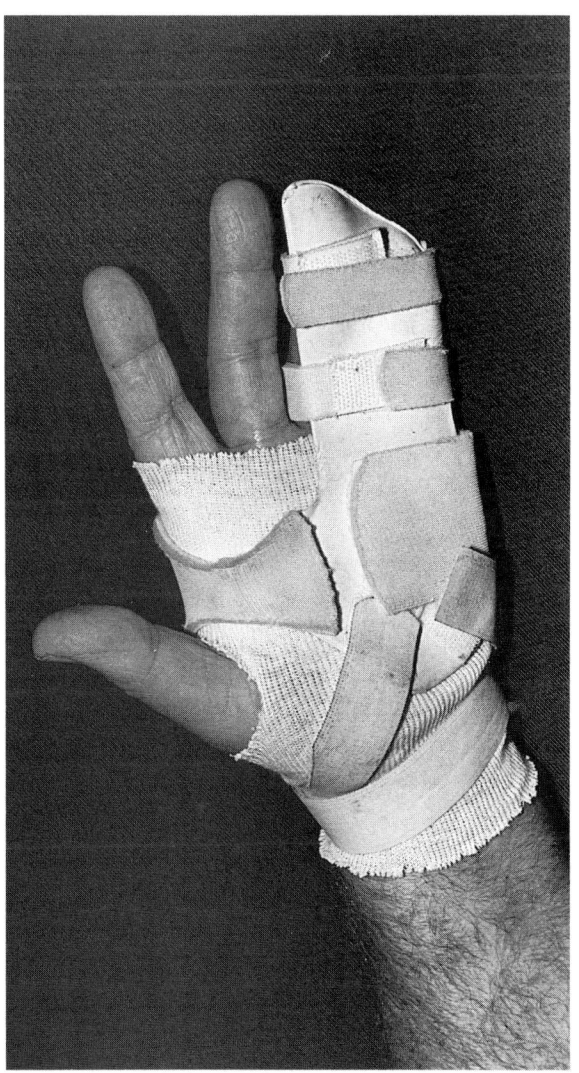

Fig. 33.1 The palmar pan splint is fabricated to provide pressure over the palmar incision and extension assist to involved digits. Uninvolved digits are free for active motion between exercise sessions.

EVALUATION

Since the postoperative Dupuytren's hand may change dramatically in as little as a few days due to the dynamics of the healing process, careful evaluation must be performed and documented from the first visit. The evaluation battery should include anterior and posterior range of movement, oedema and sensibility. Measurement of the fingernail to the distal palmar crease is taken, as this measurement relates to the function of grasp (Tonkin et al 1984). Measurement of the finger pulp to palm pulp in the hook position is also significant. Extension must also be closely monitored. Passive range of motion measures at each joint in both flexion and extension are taken.

Oedema is initially recorded using circumferential measurements taken with a tape measure. These measurements should be taken at specific landmarks to improve reproducibility. When the wounds are healed volumetric measurements replace circumferential measures. Volumetrics involve oedema measurement through water displacement. Oedema measures should be taken before and after treatment.

Sensibility may be affected as a result of DD surgery. The diminished sensation often recovers spontaneously but should be monitored as it may affect functional recovery.

CONTROL OF OEDEMA

Oedema is the first and most obvious reaction of the hand to injury after surgery. Most wounds have an excess of fluid content early in the healing process and this should not be a cause for alarm. It is the continuing oedema in the period 2 or 3 weeks postoperatively that presents itself as an ongoing complication and has long-term consequences. If oedema is allowed to persist in conjunction with immobilization, which is its advocate, gliding surfaces become adherent and the hand stiffens. Reflex sympathetic dystrophy is a severe complication of DD surgery and is to be suspected when oedema and stiffness are accompanied by pain.

Oedema is a common reaction in the hand disturbed by the complex surgical dissection required in many DD procedures. The importance of controlling oedema and thereby avoiding complications must be emphasized. Until good muscular activity is restored, we depend on gravity and external measures for the return of blood flow through the lymphatic and venous system. The patient's hand is maintained in a hand-over-heart position following surgery to minimize limb dependence and thus assist in oedema control. The elbow should not be acutely flexed as this will increase venous stasis. During sleep the hand should be elevated on pillows.

In cases of severe pitting oedema, intermittent compression with an intermittent compression unit is helpful in reducing swelling. The hand is placed in the sleeve with the fingers in extension. The extremity is elevated on a table or pillows to an angle of 30–45° to take advantage of the flow of gravity while the intermittent pressure is being applied. Use of external compression is not contraindicated in the presence of open wounds as long as sterile dressings are used. Felt pads can be positioned around pins to prevent pressure on them. The amount of pressure is adjusted to the condition. Initial treatment might be as low as 4 kPa for 30–60 minutes (to be effective unit pressure must exceed capillary pressure — 3.3 kPa — and be kept below the patient's diastolic pressure). After the mechanical massage by the intermittent compression unit, retrograde massage with lanolin may be applied by the therapist in a further attempt to push the extracellular fluid out of the hand. Care must be taken to avoid contaminating the wound area with lanolin. Coban wraps (Medical Product/3M, St Paul, MN) applied carefully to the digits and hand also assist in the reduction of oedema. Coban is applied distally to proximally and must be 'laid on'. Tightly applied Coban will interfere with the circulation of the fingers (Fig. 33.2). An Isotoner glove, which is an elasticized glove (Aris Isotener, New York, NY) may also be helpful in controlling oedema while allowing the patient to use the hand with minimal restriction. The tips of the glove may be cut off to allow sensory input.

We have found that an effective exercise that incorporates elevation and active motion is to have the patient elevate both arms over the head and make as firm a fist as possible 10 times each hour.

POSTOPERATIVE MANAGEMENT 371

in extension with the uninvolved hand, followed by proximal joint flexion with metacarpophalangeal joint extension.
3. Flexion of each finger to the thenar eminence.
4. Fist-making.
5. Finger abduction and adduction.
6. Finger extension.
7. Intrinsic extension.
8. Full wrist motion.

Ten repetitions of each exercise are carried out three to four times daily.

Severe proximal interphalangeal joint flexion contractures of the little finger frequently result in hyperextension of the distal joint, an attitude assumed by the digit to compensate for the proximal joint flexion (Gosset 1985). When these contractures are released at surgery, the surgeon's approach may be to hold the proximal interphalangeal joint in extension by K-wire fixation. Early active distal joint flexion must be emphasized to encourage tendon gliding and restore system alignment.

As motion improves, the exercise programme is modified, making the exercises more precise. Usually by the second postoperative week tendon gliding exercises can be initiated (Fig. 33.3). These exercises optimize flexor tendon motion and, as a result, joint motion (Wehbé & Hunter 1985). The flexor superficialis and profundus tendons glide over each other maximally when an attempt is made to form a hook. The wrist and metacarpophalangeal joints are held in extension and the interphalangeal joints are fully flexed. The flexor digitorum profundus attains its maximum excursion in respect to bone when an attempt is made to make a fist. The patient begins with the hook position, rolls the fingers in to make a full fist, returns to the hook position and then to full extension. The flexor digitorum superficialis attains its maximum excursion with respect to bone when the patient makes a straight fist. The wrist is in extension, the metacarpophalangeal and proximal interphalangeal joints are fully flexed and the distal joints are in extension. Each exercise must begin and end with the fingers and wrist in extension. Ten repetitions of each position are carried out three times a day.

The exercise programme can be modified by

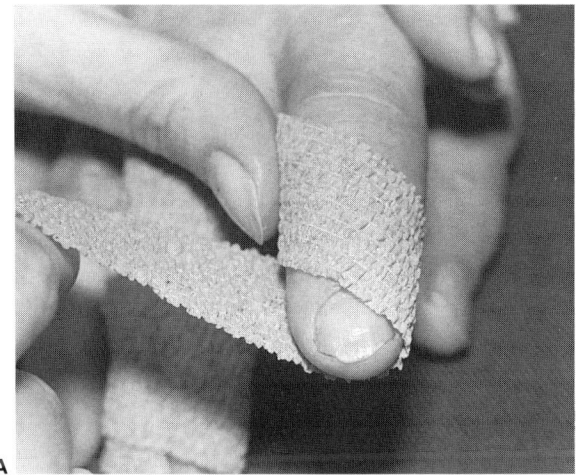

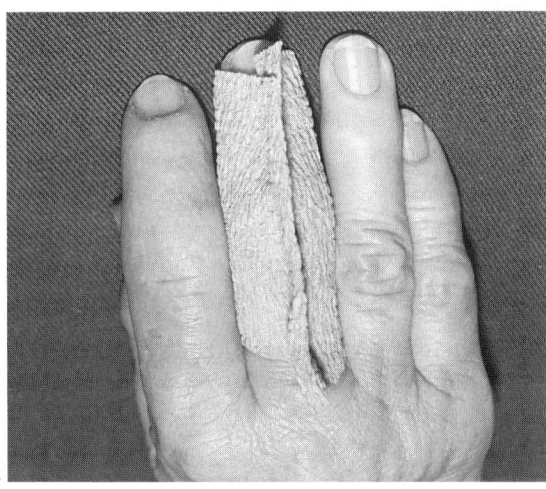

Fig. 33.2 Coban may be applied in figure-of eight fashion using, (**A**) 2.5 cm tape or (**B**) 7.5 cm tape pinched together to provide graded distal to proximal pressure.

This exercise can also be used to maintain good shoulder and elbow motion.

ACTIVE EXERCISES

Gentle basic active finger exercises are begun during the first postoperative visit. The active exercise programme includes:

1. Thumb opposition to each fingertip, abduction, and extension.
2. Finger blocking (distal joint flexion with the proximal and metacarpophalangeal joint held

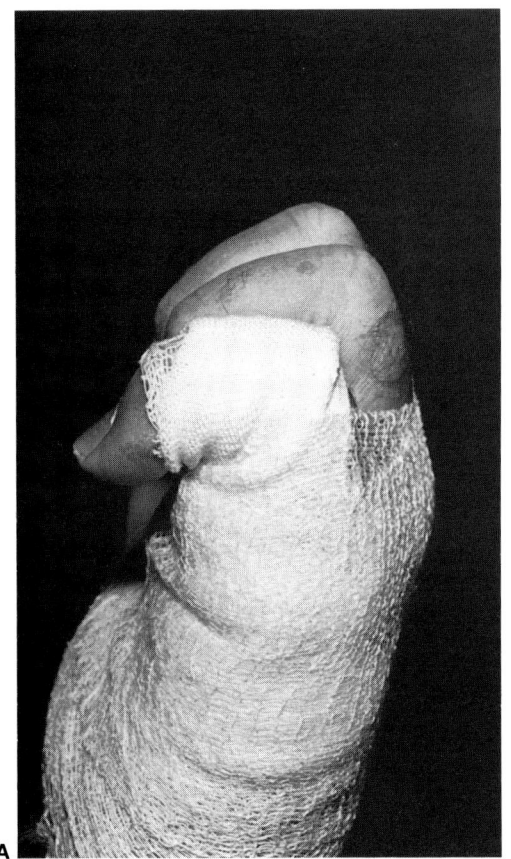 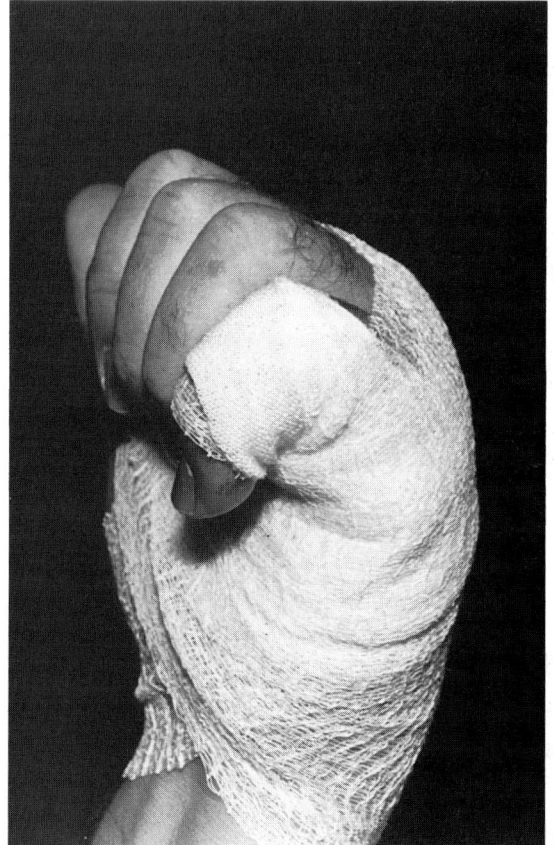

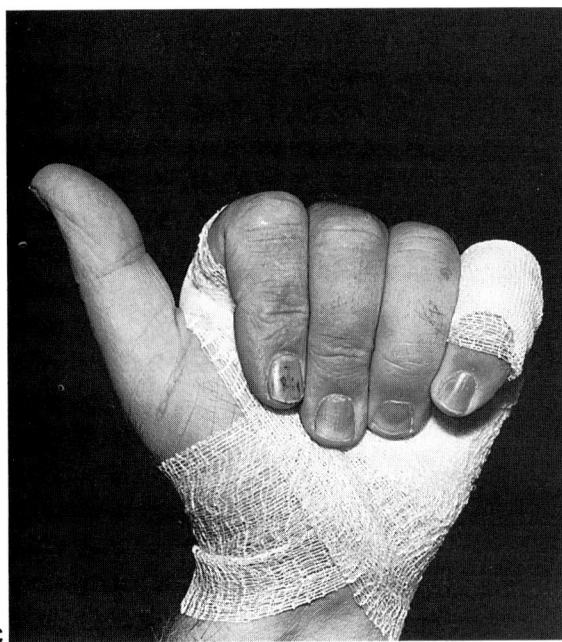

Fig. 33.3 The tendon gliding programme of (**A**) hook, (**B**) fist and (**C**) straight fist positions is used to optimize tendon excursion.

discontinuing 'easy' exercises and making others more difficult. For example, as finger extension progresses, the patient may be asked to cross the fingers, index over long, long over index, long over ring and so on. This exercise can be made even more difficult by asking the patient to pass a coin from finger to finger.

Putty squeezing may be instituted at 4–6 weeks post-operatively. Making a 'hot dog' from putty, i.e. repetitive squeezing of the putty (Fig. 33.4) using only the fingers, strengthens the grip and improves flexion. Exercises should never be overdone. Squeezing the putty 10 times intermittently during the day is a far better regime than doing it for 10 or 20 minutes continually, which might result in pain and oedema. Patients must be cau-

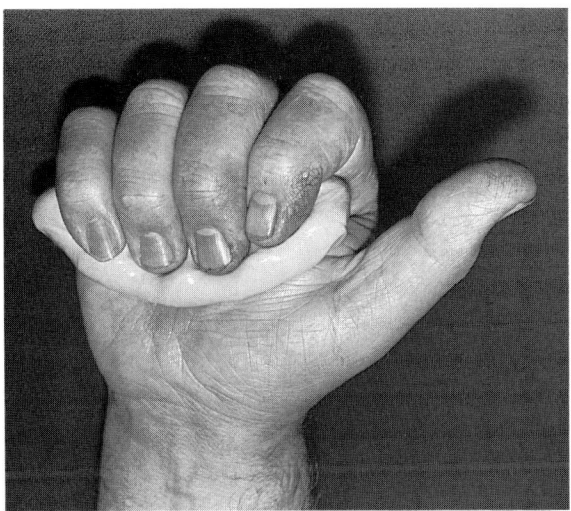

Fig. 33.4 The patient places the putty in the hand and squeezes it repetitively without reshaping it. This encourages a progressively tightened grip.

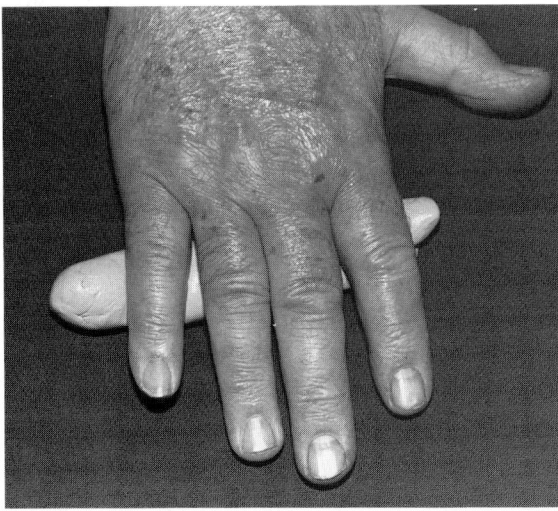

Fig. 33.5 Rolling the putty back and forth on a table encourages maximum finger extension. As the patient progresses a dowel may be used. This provides an even firmer stretch into extension.

tioned against this. Putty may also be used for extension exercises (Fig. 33.5).

Active hand use is encouraged in therapy via functional activities. While the palm is still open, light pick-ups and pinch activities may be initiated. When the wound closes, generally by 6–8 weeks, sustained grip activities, such as woodwork and leather-working help regain full function of the hand. Resistance is increased as tolerated.

SCAR MANAGEMENT

When the wound has healed, lanolin massage is helpful for softening of the scar and maintaining tissue mobility. The palm and digits should be massaged before each exercise session for approximately 10 minutes. A small, deep circular stroke is used for massage over the scar. After massage, excess lanolin should be removed to prevent skin maceration.

Silastic Elastomer (Dow, Midland, MI) is an effective adjunct in managing digital and palmar scars. Catalyst is added to the material and it is spread over the scar area (Fig. 33.6). Its advantage is its ability to conform to the entire scar area, thus producing a reusable mould with pressure over all areas of the scar. It can be applied before complete wound closure by placing a piece of non-adhering gauze over the wound and applying the Elastomer over it. Additional pressure is achieved with the palmar pan splint.

Occasionally, a patient may experience hypersensitivity over the healed area. This should be addressed through a programme of desensitization. Desensitization involves the stimulation of a hypersensitive area with textures that are normally not noxious. The stimulation is preferred for about 10 minutes each waking hour and proceeds

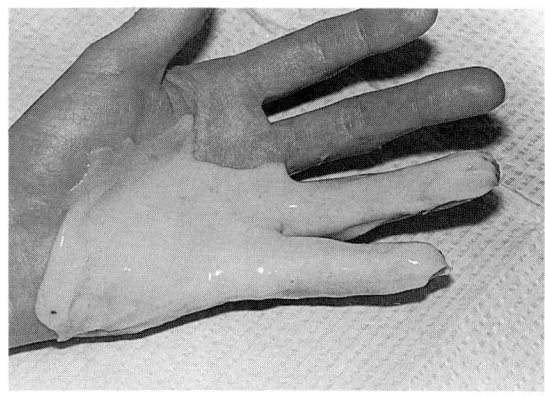

Fig. 33.6 Elastomer is worn at night under the palmar pan splint and may be secured with Coban if necessary.

through a predefined hierarchy, beginning with fur and progressing to vibration.

SPLINTING

Splinting is an important part of postoperative care. In a few patients with minimal disease and pliable skin and in whom good finger extension has been obtained, postoperative splinting may not be necessary; however, in all other patients a splint to maintain the extension of the digits gained in the operating room is fabricated at the initial therapy session. It is very important to know the intraoperative range of motion and the result the surgeon expects to obtain postoperatively. Neurovascular status is an important factor in splint application.

Splints must be carefully fitted and adjusted as necessary to hold the digits gently in extension during wound healing and not cause pain. A thermoplastic palmar pan splint (Fig. 33.1) holding the digits in extension is usually worn four times a day for 1 hour each time and all night. The surgeon and therapist may elect to change initial daytime splinting in specific cases. In severe cases where joint changes have already occurred, one finger, usually the little finger, will tend to flex again due to the fibrous retraction of the skin and proximal interphalangeal joint capsular and pericapsular structures.

In these cases, a splint designed specifically to address the proximal interphalangeal joint problem may be useful. To be effective, the static-

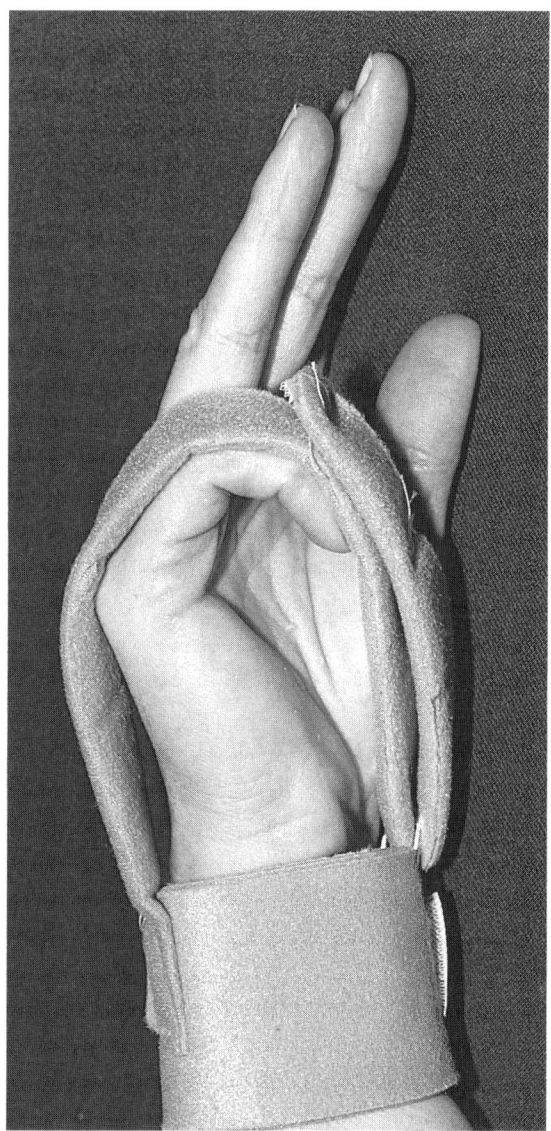

Fig. 33.8 The combination web strap is fabricated using Velcro. A long 2.5 cm wide strap is secured to a 5 cm wrist strap. A D-ring on the palmar side of the wrist strap stabilizes the finger strap as it is doubled back on itself.

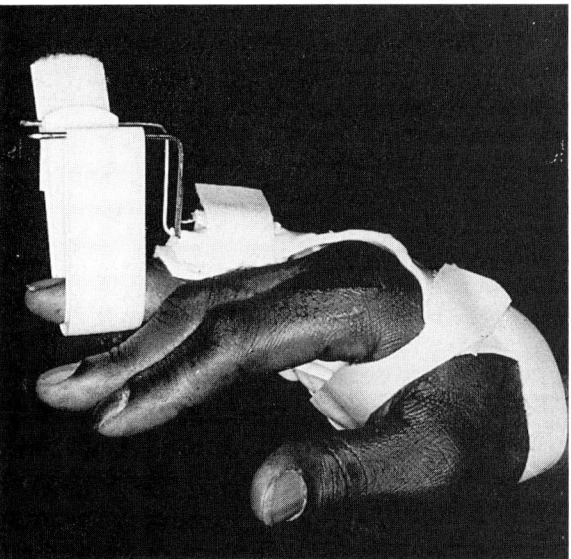

Fig. 33.7 If the proximal interphalangeal joint begins to develop a firmer end-feel the palmar pan splint may be replaced by a static adjustable proximal interphalangeal extension splint.

adjustable proximal interphalangeal extension splint (Fig. 33.7) requires good stabilization of the metacarpophalangeal joint. If this is not achieved, a pressure area will develop on the dorsal aspect of the proximal joint when extension force is applied. This splint is called static-adjustable because it employs a length of Velcro loop over the outrigger to provide the extension force. The Velcro provides a static pull. It may be adjusted to provide increased tension as tolerated by the patient between treatment sessions.

It is important to maintain flexion as well as extension. When flexion of the proximal interphalangeal joint is needed a web strap provides the necessary passive stretch (Fig. 33.8). The strap is worn over the proximal joint and behind the metacarpophalangeal joint. The strap is fabricated from a 2.5 cm wide webbing with a 2.5 cm wide buckle. The patient may begin wearing the strap for half an hour three times a day. The time the strap is worn may be increased gradually up to 2 hours three times a day.

When all the joints are stiff in extension a combination web strap or a flexion glove (Fig. 33.9) is indicated. Both are comfortable and easily adjusted. The combination web strap, however, is not effective in gaining the final degrees of proximal or distal interphalangeal joint motion. As flexion improves the combination web strap can be discarded and the web strap or distal joint elastic utilized. The length of time the combination web strap is worn is the same as for the web strap.

An elastic flexion strap is used to obtain distal joint flexion (Fig. 33.10). A piece of elastic with a

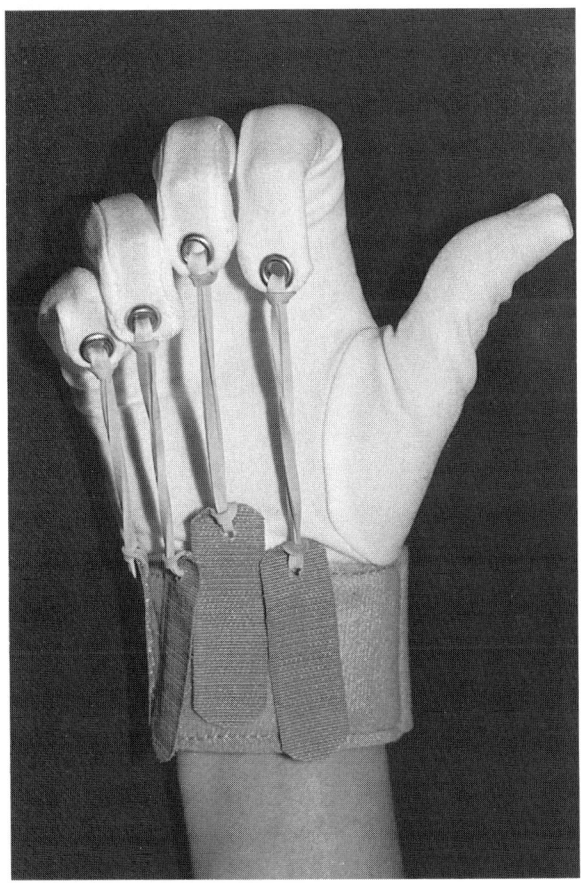

Fig. 33.9 The flexion glove is chosen when more than two digits require passive flexion and when all the joints of the involved digits are stiff.

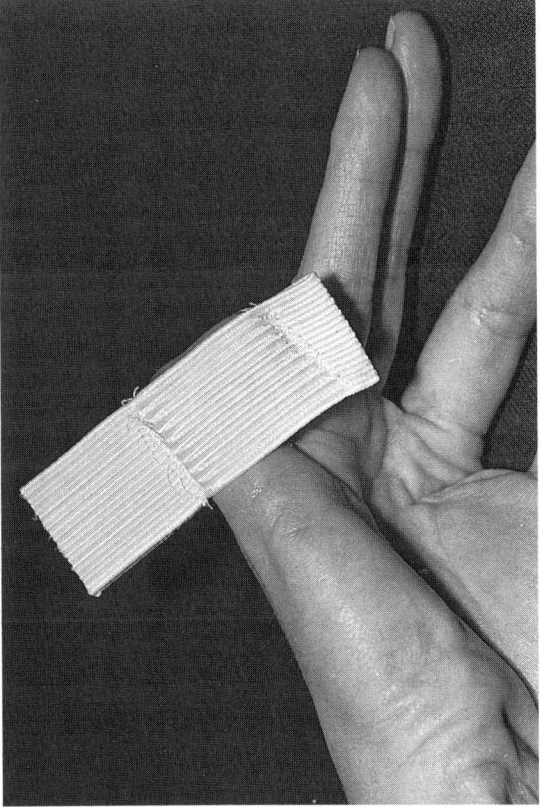

Fig. 33.10 When a distal interphalangeal joint elastic is used, care must be taken to not over-stretch the terminal extensor tendon, resulting in distal joint extension lag. These elastics are only used in the daytime splinting programme. Night splinting is always in extension.

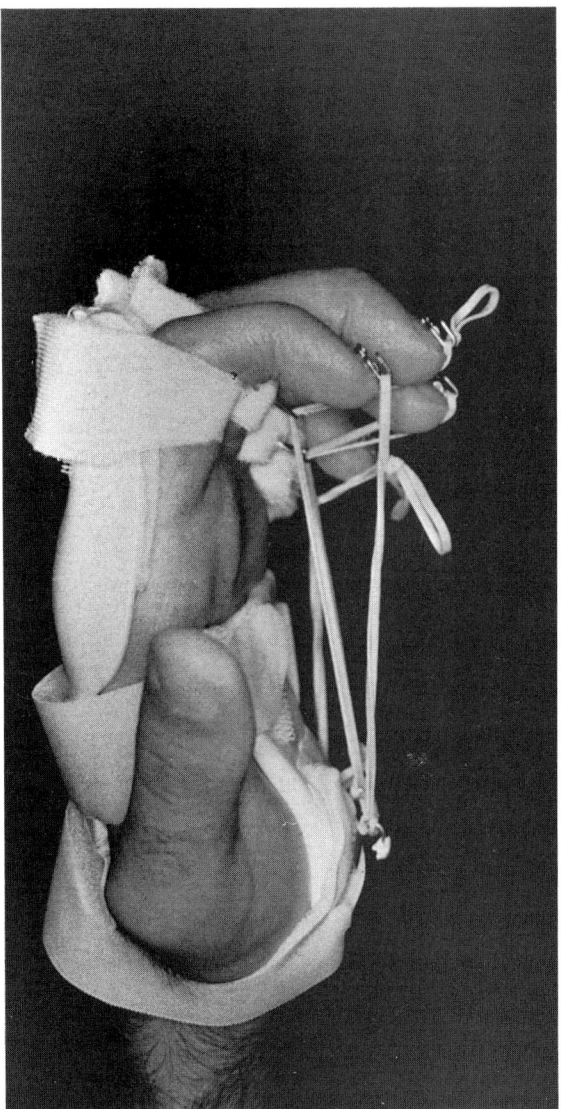

Fig. 33.11 The intrinsic stretcher splint has a dorsal thermoplastic base which maintains the metacarpophalangeal joint in extension. The interphalangeal joints may be brought into flexion using dress hooks and rubber band traction or elastic straps. The choice is determined by the degree of the contracture.

width of 2.5 cm and a length of approximately 10 cm is fitted around the patient's interphalangeal joints while they are held in maximum flexion. The elastic is marked where the two ends of elastic meet and the elastic is sewn together on that mark. The length of time it is worn is the same as described earlier for the web straps.

Because of prolonged positioning in metacarpophalangeal extension with interphalangeal joint and proximal interphalangeal joint flexion, intrinsic tightness may develop. The above splinting alternatives may not be specific enough to resolve this problem, as addressing it requires metacarpophalangeal extension with interphalangeal joint flexion. An intrinsic stretcher splint may be required in these cases (Fig. 33.11).

Specific instructions should be clearly written for the patient, describing the application of the splint and desired length of time each splint is to be worn. The patient must be instructed to look for changes in colour of the fingertips, increase in tingling, numbness, or swelling of the digit or hand as signs to decrease splint tension. Although passive flexion straps may be necessary to increase flexion, night splinting is always in extension.

CONCLUSIONS

The importance of a carefully supervised postoperative active motion exercise and splinting programme cannot be overemphasized. Gosset (1985) suggests that 50% of the result of the operation depends on active postoperative movement and that: 'without this, the best operation will be left with a functional deficit'.

R. M. McFarlane and D. A. McGrouther

34 Complications and their management

The results of treatment of Dupuytren's disease (DD) have improved greatly in recent years, primarily because of refinements in surgical technique. Nevertheless, there is still some reserve on the part of both physicians and patients to proceed to operation because of the possibility of postoperative problems. A long period of morbidity with pain, swelling and stiffness of the hand is of great concern to all parties. A certain morbidity is inevitable and will increase directly with the magnitude of the operation, as well as the work status of the individual. Fasciotomy, although not often performed during working age, would permit a sedentary worker to return to work immediately. Extensive fasciectomy could keep a manual worker off work for 3 months or more. Any deviation from a normal postoperative course will prolong the expected period of morbidity.

The complications arising from 1339 operations have been analysed statistically. The data are summarized in Tables 34.1 and 34.2 and reveal that even a selected group of experienced hand surgeons have postoperative problems (Tubiana et al 1967; Rank & Chang 1978). The demographic data in the profile fail to reveal differences such as age or sex that would identify a patient who might develop a complication. Also, the preoperative degrees of contracture at both metacarpophalangeal and proximal interphalangeal joints were no different. Further, the postoperative metacarpophalangeal joint angles were no different but the proximal interphalangeal joints angles, especially in the little finger, were much worse.

In Table 34.1 the features associated statistically with complications are listed and proved to be those of extensive disease and extensive operation.

Table 34.1 Factors associated with complications

Factor	p value
Bilateral disease	<0.005
Three or more rays involved	<0.005
Extensive fasciectomy in the finger	<0.01
Skin graft in palm or finger	<0.005
Proximal interphalangeal joint procedure	<0.005
General anaesthetic	<0.005

Table 34.2 Types of complications in 1339 operations

Complication	%
Infections	1.3%
Haematoma	2.2%
Skin loss	4.7%
Nerve injury	1.5%
Artery injury	0.8%
Gangrene of finger	0.1%
Loss of flexion	4.6%
Sympathetic dystrophy	4.2%
Other	2.7%
Overall	17%

Patients with three or more rays involved usually have an extensive fasciectomy which is probably performed under general anaesthesia and may be accompanied by a proximal joint procedure and/or skin grafting.

Thus, a complication not only causes a specific problem such as division of a digital nerve, but also prolongs morbidity and is associated with a less satisfactory result.

TYPES OF COMPLICATIONS

These are listed in Table 34.2. The overall rate was 17% which at first thought is high. However, one complication often leads to another so there are fewer patients involved than the complications listed.

Some of the complications of DD surgery arise from the operative intervention: division of nerve or artery, skin necrosis, haematoma or infection. They are hopefully avoidable in most instances by good judgement and careful technique, although occasionally even the most experienced and meticulous surgeon may have a problem, especially in the recurrent case where the anatomy may be more difficult to display. It seems wise, therefore, to provide the patient with some warning of potential hazards before proceeding.

Other complications are more related to disturbance of the physiology of the hand, such as oedema, reflex dystrophy and stiffness. There is great individual variation in these responses and the surgeon may only guess at their likelihood. It is difficult to predict before operation whether the hand or the patient will develop problems of this type. Where bilateral surgery has been performed, a disturbance of physiology may occur on only one side.

Varian (Chapter 32) has provided advice on operative treatment from the aspect of avoiding surgical complications and this places the correct emphasis on prevention rather than cure. Similarly, a careful postoperative review and rehabilitation programme may detect and control any early physiological changes.

Nerve and artery injury

The frequency of damage to the neurovascular bundles is probably greater than reported in Table 34.2. With the tourniquet inflated, it is difficult to see the digital artery. Damage to both structures is best avoided by dissecting with loupe magnification and keeping the nerve and artery together. The diseased fascia never passes between them.

Division or partial division of a nerve or vessel is less likely if the surgeon has a knowledge of neurovascular bundle displacement and the patterns of contracting cords (see Chapters 14 and 31). The operative field should be dry; almost all surgeons use an arm tourniquet, although a few rely on an elevated hand table alone. When a nerve or artery is divided it may be for one of the following reasons. The surgeon may be 'lost' — that is, unable to distinguish individual structures within a dense area of Dupuytren's tissue — where the anatomy is particularly difficult to display it is necessary to isolate the nerve and artery in a safe area proximally and distally and follow it through the involved area. When operating upon recurrent disease, the neurovascular bundle is adherent to scar tissue as well as Dupuytren's tissue. It is difficult, if not impossible, to dissect the nerve and artery cleanly and it may be prudent to leave a cuff of scar tissue around the bundle. However, at the first operation there is always a plane between the neurovascular bundle and the diseased fascia. This plane can always be developed by careful dissection.

Nerves may be accidentally divided quite simply by cutting down on to a cord without appreciating that a bundle may spiral across it; this is a particular risk in the proximal segment of the finger. The surgeon may mistake a well defined fascial cord for a nerve — an error possible even with loupe spectacles — then proceed with the dissection, protecting the 'false nerve' and excising all else, including the neurovascular bundle. A divided nerve is best repaired even in the elderly patient. Although sensation is unlikely to return, nerve suture may minimize trophic changes and cold intolerance. Nerve injury should be such a rare event that at the end of a long career in hand surgery, it should be possible to remember each case in startling detail!

When a digital artery has been divided, the integrity of the other artery should be checked by even more careful dissection, and the adequacy of perfusion assured on release of the tourniquet. If the finger remains white, an arterial repair or vein graft is required. The tourniquet should always be released before closure of the skin. Inadequate digital circulation is always apparent on release of the tourniquet and the surgeon should not be in the embarrassing position of discovering an ischaemic digit at the first dressing change.

Before operating upon a patient with recurrent disease, the status of the digital nerves and arteries should be determined. Loss of sensation on one or other side of a digit not only indicates division of a digital nerve but also the likely division of the digital artery. A digital Allen's test is difficult to perform in the scarred and contracted digit, but can give information on the status of the digital artery.

Infection, haematoma and skin loss

This triad followed 8% of operations. Infection alone is not a particular feature of DD but may occur following skin loss and is likely after haematoma. Haematoma is not uncommon in palmar wounds closed under tension. It cannot occur when the palm is left open and is unlikely to occur if a skin graft is applied.

Despite the most vigorous measures to stop bleeding some blood and fluid must inevitably collect in the dead space of operation — it is the amount of blood and its containment which are significant. Various measures have been used to limit the collection of blood. Elevation of the hand during operation, during the application of the dressing, and in the postoperative period, are widely used. The introduction of the bipolar coagulator to hand surgery has been one of the most significant advances in the technique of hand surgery. The widespread use of this instrument has led to much higher standards of wound haemostasis such that it is almost impossible to make treatment comparisons between the operations of today and 20 years ago.

Skin necrosis in DD has many contributory factors but one common cause — the inadequate design and elevation of skin flaps. Incisions should be made such that undermining is kept to a minimum and no flap should be designed such that a cord crosses its base. In the palm, the vessels that perforate the fascia to supply the skin can often be preserved. The thick palmar skin of Dupuytren's disease tolerates transposition poorly and even when designed by the most experienced plastic surgeon, Z-plasties are at some risk of tip necrosis. Closure under tension will impair the skin circulation further. Oedema and haematoma will aggravate this and these factors combine to predispose to infection. Small areas of skin loss should be allowed to heal by secondary intention while the hand is mobilized. Larger areas may require skin grafts or flaps.

Physiological disturbances

Operation upsets the physiological balance of the hand in a number of ways. There is always a degree of oedema, not only of the wound area, but of the entire hand. Delicate tissue handling, more limited operations and postoperative elevation help to control swelling. The best way to assure elevation of the hand is to admit the patient to hospital for at least 24 hours. Elevation of the hand and forearm above heart level on two pillows is satisfactory, although a commercially available foam rubber block is more efficient and is well accepted by patients (Fig. 34.1). Suspension by a bandage or roller towel is not recommended be-

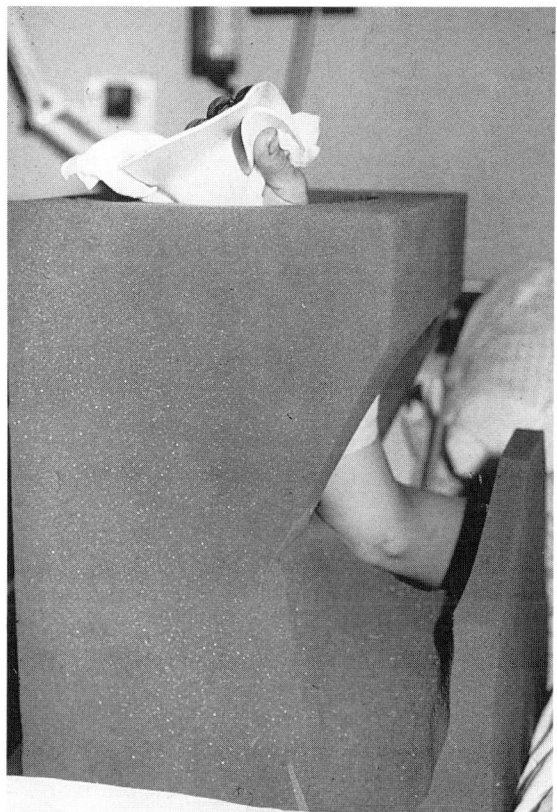

Fig. 34.1 A commercially available foam rubber block that accepts either right or left hand for elevation. Most patients find this position of the hand to be comfortable and some take the block home with them.

cause circumferential pressure at the wrist or elbow can occur. Today, many hand operations are performed on an outpatient basis, including those for DD. These patients should not be given a sling, but should be instructed to hold their hand high when walking and to elevate it on pillows when sitting or in bed for about 48 hours postoperatively.

Loss of flexion

One of the criteria of a good result is the return of finger flexion. It is prudent to record flexion preoperatively by measuring the distance of the fingertip to the distal crease of the palm because some patients are unable to flex the fingers fully before operation (see Chapter 20). Loss of flexion will accompany all other complications but occasionally it is seen in patients who otherwise have progressed well and in whom it is permanent and refractory to therapy.

Reflex sympathetic dystrophy

This complication was recorded in 4.2% of patients but, as shown in Table 34.3, the prevalence varied from 0.9% in the USA to 7.3% in Australia and even to 37% in France. Thus, the criteria for diagnosis must vary considerably. Zemel et al (1987) reported an incidence of 20% in females who were operated upon for DD: the incidence increased to 46% if the patient had an extensive fasciectomy, and to 58% if the patient had carpal tunnel syndrome. These authors prefer the term 'flare reaction', a term suggested by Howard (1959) to describe redness, oedema, pain and stiffness that appears 3–4 weeks postoperatively and often results in permanent stiffness of the fingers. This is indeed the picture of reflex sympathetic dystrophy. MacKinnon and Holder (1984) list their diagnostic criteria as follows: diffuse hand pain, diminished hand function, joint stiffness, and skin and soft tissue trophic changes. These authors recommend the use of three-phase radionuclide bone scanning to confirm the diagnosis and note that the diffuse increased tracer uptake in the delayed or third phase is diagnostic of reflex sympathetic dystrophy.

Diagnosis

There is a spectrum of severity of reflex sympathetic dystrophy. Lesser degrees are either transient or respond readily to treatment. If strict diagnostic criteria are used, especially a three-phase bone scan, the prevalence of this complication is probably about 4%. Reflex sympathetic dystrophy is the only complication that was more common in females. Following operation, it occurred in 7% of females and 3.5% of males ($p<0.025$). As shown in Table 34.4, it was more common following the treatment of extensive disease.

Table 34.3 Incidence of reflex sympathetic dystrophy by country

Country	n	%
USA	339	0.9%
Japan	128	1.6%
Canada	294	2.7%
Germany	108	4.6%
Australia	37	7.3%
France	147	37.0%

Table 34.4 Factors associated with reflex sympathetic dystrophy

Factor	p value
Female	0.02
Extensive disease	0.02
Extensive fasciectomy	0.02
Proximal interphalangeal joint procedure	0.02
General anaesthesia	0.02

Prevention

Although it may not be possible to prevent the onset of reflex sympathetic dystrophy, certain measures should be observed in all patients and certain patients should be watched closely. Elevation of the hand to prevent swelling and adequate analgesia to minimize anxiety and pain apply to all patients. Patients with extensive disease in whom an extensive operation is planned

Profile of complications: 198 patients with 221 hands and 294 complications

Family origin		Sex		Hand dominance		Hand involved		Occupation	
Northern European	87%	Male	83%	Right	97%	Right	15%	Manual	53%
Japanese	6%	Female	17%	Left	3%	Left	8%	Non-manual	47%
Southern European	3%					Both	77%		
Black American	1%	Other areas involved	29%			Associated diseases		Age at onset (years)	
Black African	1%	Family history	31%			Epilepsy	4%	Male	46.8 ± 15.0
American Indian	1%	Previous operation	24%			Diabetes	10%	Female	57.0 ± 15.5
						Alcoholism	13%	Age at operation (years)	
						Trauma	8%	Male	56.6 ± 11.3
								Female	61.6 ± 9.3

Hand profile				Operation profile					
					Palm	Fingers	Thumb	Anaesthesia	
Palm only	4%			Operation					
No palm	3%			Local	7%	9%	10%	Local	6%
One ray	27%			Regional	58%	42%	80%	Regional	37%
Two rays	29%			Extensive	35%	48%	10%	General	57%
Three or more rays	40%			Amputation		1%			
				Incision				Procedure at PIP joint	20%
Thumb and thumb web	31%			Longitudinal	72%	96%	76%		
Index finger	19%			Transverse	28%	4%	24%	Complications	100%
Middle finger	37%			Closure					
Ring finger	66%			Suture	63%	83%	85%	Therapy	83%
Little finger	78%			Open	14%	0%	0%	Splinting	55%
				Graft	23%	17%	15%		

Profile contd.

	Little finger			Ring finger			Middle finger			Index finger			Thumb		
	n	Pre	Post	n	Pre	Post	n	Pre	Post	n	Pre	Post	n	Pre	Post
MP joint	43	43.0 ± 26.2	5.8 ± 19.3	40	38.0 ± 20.2	4.0 ± 10.7	22	26.5 ± 15.9	3.6 ± 11.4	9	28.1 ± 19.6	6.7 ± 11.2	5	22.0 ± 7.5	12.0 ± 16.4
Outcome															
Perfect	81%	40.3 ± 25.7	0 ± 0	78%	35.7 ± 18.4	0 ± 0	87%	23.9 ± 13.1	0 ± 0	67%	19.7 ± 9.5	0 ± 0	60%	18.3 ± 2.9	0 ± 0
Improved	14%	54.2 ± 23.8	11.7 ± 4.1	20%	53.1 ± 19.8	18.9 ± 17.6	9%	45.0 ± 35.4	15.0 ± 7.1	33%	45.0 ± 26.0	20.0 ± 10.0	20%	35.0	30.0
Same/worse	5%	55.0 ± 49.5	90.0 ± 0	2%	5.0	10.0	4%	40.0	50.0				20%	20.0	30.0
PIP joint	54	56.5 ± 26.6	38.6 ± 26.6*	23	48.6 ± 28.9	23.4 ± 23.9	9	40.0 ± 24.5	28.3 ± 24.4						
Outcome															
Perfect	8%*	61.3 ± 22.5	0 ± 0	26%	31.7 ± 24.8	0 ± 0	22%	17.5 ± 10.6	0 ± 0						
Improved	48%	66.0 ± 21.4	29.2 ± 20.8	48%	68.6 ± 18.6	33.6 ± 21.7	45%	55.0 ± 20.8	30.0 ± 17.8						
Same/worse	44%	43.7 ± 27.3	55.3 ± 22.6	22%	21.6 ± 21.7	28.8 ± 26.4	33%	35.0 ± 26.5	45.0 ± 26.0						
DIP joint	11	29.2 ± 16.6	14.1 ± 15.5	4	36.3 ± 20.6	0 ± 0	2	35.0 ± 21.2	25.0 ± 35.4						
Outcome															
Perfect	36%	16.3 ± 13.1	0 ± 0	100%	36.3 ± 20.6	0 ± 0	50%	20.0	0 ± 0						
Improved	36%	40.0 ± 14.7	12.5 ± 6.5												
Same/worse	27%	28.3 ± 17.6	35.0 ± 8.7				50%	50.0	50.0						

Mean ± standard deviation.
Perfect = the flexion contracture was completely corrected; improved = the flexion contracture was less, but not completely corrected; same/worse = there was no correction or the flexion contracture was worse.
*The postoperative PIPJ V angle is greater and the outcome is worse ($p<0.001$) than in patients without complications. The same is true in the ring and middle fingers but there is not a significant difference.

should be admitted to hospital and kept there until the surgeon is satisfied that the postoperative course is uneventful. Nevertheless, it is surprisingly difficult to diagnose reflex sympathetic dystrophy early because it usually appears some 4–6 weeks after operation. In a personal series of 320 patients (RMM), 10 (3.2%) developed reflex sympathetic dystrophy. Four patients were diagnosed within 4 weeks of operation but 6 were diagnosed from 2 to 4 months after operation.

The surgeon should try to identify the patient who might develop reflex sympathetic dystrophy and take preventive measures. However, if one is to help patients with extensive disease, including females, an extensive operation is required. The incidence is only about 4% so it would seem reasonable to proceed with appropriate treatment in the assumption that this complication will not occur.

Treatment

The treatment of established reflex sympathetic dystrophy is difficult, prolonged and usually disappointing. Seven of 10 personal patients have permanent limitation of flexion and extension. The basis of our treatment is to admit the patient to hospital in order to receive intensive hand therapy. Adjunct measures (of unknown value in the individual patient) consist of stellate ganglion or guanethidine blocks, sedation, steroids and nifedipine, as recommended by Prough et al (1985). All of these measures are non-specific so treatment will remain empirical until the pathophysiology of reflex sympathetic dystrophy is understood.

CONCLUSIONS

To some extent, complications are predictable. They occur more often in patients with severe disease who require an extensive operation.

Complications compromise the result of treatment. Morbidity is prolonged, the correction of contracture at the proximal interphalangeal, but not the metacarpophalangeal joint, is less, and the patient often fails to recover full finger flexion.

D. A. McGrouther

35
Recurrence and extension

William Adams (1879) certainly appreciated that contracture might recur after operation and that the result of the operation depended not only on the surgical technique but also on the patient's rehabilitation effort. In the early 20th century the fashion was to express results as excellent (good), fair and poor. These were imprecise categories but at least this system indicated that surgical results form a spectrum with some patients achieving little or no benefit or even a deterioration in function following surgery. Many published results failed to separate palmar (metaphalangeal joint contracture) and digital disease (proximal interphalangeal joint contracture). This point was emphasized by Honner et al (1971) who recognized the different prognosis of the two joint contractures.

Longer-term results have usually been classified in terms of recurrence and extension of disease.

Gordon (1957) separated these processes by defining disease within the area operated upon as a recurrence: disease beyond the confines of the operative field was considered an extension.

The same conventions of definition were presented by Hueston (1963) and these have been generally accepted. It is necessary, however, to review these concepts.

RECURRENCE

Recurrence of flexion deformity may not necessarily indicate a process identical to the original contracture in DD.

Early deterioration in hand function, certainly within the first year after operation, and possibly during the second, may reflect a failure of recovery of range of joint motion with maturation of scar tissue on the palmer aspect in a shortened position rather than recurrence of the original disease process.

The aim of the primary operation is to release the joint contracture. Metacarpophalangeal joint release is generally successful; the joint is almost never involved and recurrent metacarpophalangeal joint contracture is therefore due either to contracture of skin, residual fascia or scar tissue, or to the resumption of a habitual flexed posture by the patient. This can be largely avoided by correct planning of incisions and adequate rehabilitation.

By contrast, recurrent proximal interphalangeal joint contracture is not unique to DD but is predisposed to by anatomical features of the joint and the digit. An entire text in this series has been devoted to its complexities (Bowers 1986). It is our lack of full understanding of the anatomy and mechanics of this joint which makes treatment difficult. Of the anatomical features, the region of the proximal edge of the volar plate has received much attention. To allow proximal interphalangeal joint flexion there is a complex folding of fascial structures in this area on joint flexion. Watson et al (1979) have described a check-rein ligament running from the lateral edge of the volar plate to the metacarpal neck; they divide this in order to overcome the joint contracture.

Restoration of normal anatomy and function in this area is difficult. Any dissection creates dead space which is likely to give rise to new scar tissue which in turn is likely to lead to progressive proximal interphalangeal stiffness in the weeks and months following surgery. If the biomechanical factors are analysed, there is a strong force flexing the proximal interphalangeal joint (flexor digitorum superficialis and flexor digitorum profundis) to its position of rest (mid flexed, more on the ulnar side of the hand). The extension force by contrast — the middle slip of the extensor apparatus — is weak, having a small moment of force about the joint's axis of rotation. In addition, following a prolonged period of flexion, the middle slip may be attenuated. Successful release of metacarpophalangeal flexion will weaken the middle slip action further since the extrinsic extensor acts more strongly with the metacarpophalangeal joint flexed.

The pattern of recurrent digital flexion is often quite different from that of the primary disease. In particular, both digital joints may be flexed, a pattern reminiscent of the 'intrinsic minus' digit. Landsmeer (1963) has shown how the digit requires a number of functional motors in order to balance its posture and allow motion of an intercalated chain of bones. Is there any evidence to suggest that an intrinsic minus mechanism may play a role in recurrent DD? Certainly the interossei and lumbricals have very small excursions (Woodburn and McGrouther 1988) and would be vulnerable to becoming adherent. Dissection deep in the palm or in the proximal segment of the digit might lead to fibrosis and tethering.

In the little finger the abductor band of DD is well recognized and may impair the intrinsic function. Certainly dissection in this area or division of the abductor tendon, although helping to relieve the initial contracture, may impair later intrinsic function with a progressive postoperative flexion deformity. Although this evidence is rather speculative, this mechanism does seem important in at least some Dupuytren's patients. The author has found at re-operation on such patients fibrosis and tethering of the intrinsic mechanism at various points. Swan neck deformity has been observed, apparently following mid palmer haematoma and a claw deformity is not unusual in the digits with associated fibrosis and tethering of the extensor apparatus in the proximal segment of the finger. It does seem therefore that a mechanism of intrinsic dysfunction may apply in some cases of recurrent Dupuytren's disease.

A progressive recurrence of contracture following DD surgery may therefore indicate a mechanical problem rather than necessarily a recurrence of DD. The patient's motivation combined with rehabilitation and splintage will have a strong influence on this sequence of events.

It is undeniable that many of these cases will have tight volar tissues but the resting length of the volar tissues may remodel to reflect a lack of active extension — both mechanisms probably develop together in the recurrent case.

EXTENSION

The concept of extension of disease is also imprecise. There may be difficulty in the individual case in deciding what is recurrence and what is extension. Is further disease in the same ray proximally or distally to be regarded as recurrence or extension? Also, the distinction between these processes may be difficult as operation on one digital ray may encroach on adjacent rays, precipitating the onset of the process there (Skoog 1967). Furthermore, the trauma of operation may accelerate the disease process elsewhere in the hand due to oedema, immobility and reflex sympathetic dystrophy.

Areas of the hand not operated upon may have much more pathological change than has been appreciated on external examination. This has been brought to the writer's attention by the recognition of knuckle changes (Chapter 15) and the opportunity to dissect a few hands with DD in the post-mortem room. The concept of the disease spreading, which is implied by the term 'extension', is not accurate. What actually happens is that 'disease' outside the operated area rises to clinical awareness so that its presence is obvious by external signs or by joint contracture.

Rather than an analysis of 'recurrence' or 'extension,' there seems a place for considering the number of hands which remain clear of signs of DD following a particular operative intervention. A comparison of this type has been made in published series in Table 35.1.

To judge the continuing progress of the disease in our own unit, two separate long-term reviews of samples of patients treated at Canniesburn

Table 35.1 Comparison of data regarding recurrence, extension and hands free of disease

Reference	No. of hands	Follow-up (years)	Type of operation	Recurrence	Extension	Hands clear of disease
Gordon (1957)	120	0–21	Limited	26%	9%	65%
Hueston (1961)	70	5–15	Limited	40%	40%	20%
Freehafer & Strong (1963)	51	1–7	Partial	2%	6%	
McFarlane & Jamieson (1966)	86	1	Limited	2%	1%	
Hakstian (1966)	73		McIndoe	34%	33%	49%
Dickie & Hughes (1967)	153	10	Radical	27%	37%	63%
Honner et al (1971)	138	1–9	Radical	41%	20%	
Rodrigo et al (1967)	65 (41)	2–6	Subtotal limited	63% (43%)	66%	
Rank & Chang (1978)	85	5–25	Limited	35%	45%	20%
Tonkin et al (1984)	154	1–7	Limited graft	54% 33%	28%	
Gonzalez (1985)	302	5	Graft	<10%		
Walton & McGrouther (1988)	200	1–19	all			0%

Table 35.2 Surgical experience in the treatment of DD at Canniesburn Hospital, Bearsden, Scotland, 1968–1987

	1978*	1987
Total patients	410	998
Total patients seen at follow-up	129	100
Total operations on patients followed up	261	272
Type of operation		
Open palm		27
Limited fasciectomy (with or without Z-plasty)	146	62
Total fasciectomy	6	
Amputation	18	
Free skin graft	15	
Fasciotomy and graft		25
Highly selective fasciectomy		72
Open fasciotomy		1
Proximal interphalangeal joint release		11
Miscellaneous		50
Number cured (no evidence of progression or recurrence)†		
2 years post-surgery	30	
5 years post-surgery	11(8.5%)	22%
5–10 years		10%
>10 years		0%

*From a study undertaken by Dr R. Gonzale
†In the uncured group, 185 joints lacked more than 30° of extension

Hospital have been undertaken (Gonzalez, personal communication; Walton & McGrouther, unpublished observations; Table 35.2).

Both studies indicated that many patients had had more than one operation on each hand. The types of operation which had been performed were changed, with a predominance of limited fasiectomy procedures performed before 1978 and more limited operation in the period 1978–1987. Few hands were soft and supple up to 5 years after operation and none were after 10 years.

The major conclusion of these studies was that surgery was *not curative* in DD in the west of Scotland. It is likely that the aim of our procedures must be redirected towards the release of contracture rather than an attempt at total excision of Dupuytren's tissue. Gonzalez has used the term 'control'. Careful study of the natural history of the disease suggests that it is progressive and ongoing in spite of our intervention — that our intervention merely delays the time course but does not arrest it. There was a high incidence of first, second, third and fourth recurrences. Many patients deteriorated after surgery but came to terms with recurrent flexion contracture and did not wish further treatment.

A further study has been undertaken to establish whether any of the operative approaches made a clear difference to the progression of DD.

A number of different operations had been performed, including limited fasciectomy, fasciotomy and skin grafting and the author's minimal excisional technique. The groups were composed by assessing the time to long-term review together with the time to further operations, if this had been required. In this series almost half of the hands treated by limited fasciectomy operations required a further operation after 2–7 (mean) years, whereas the minimal excision operations, with intensive therapy and prolonged splintage, had much fewer secondary procedures. Although the follow-up time of the latter was shorter, they seemed to have no poorer an outcome than the limited (more extensive) approach.

There was no evidence that a more radical operation within the range of procedures performed at Canniesburn Hospital would protect the patient from recurrence. It seems justifiable to perform the simplest possible operation to relieve the contracture and improve the function of the hand.

It is felt that the varying percentages of recurrence, extension and hands clear of disease simply reflect differences in the arbitrary criteria for definition of these terms.

36 The results of treatment

The severity and course of disease depend upon certain demographic factors, as discussed in Chapter 20. To some extent the type of operation is dictated by the severity of disease, but as shown in Chapter 32, most surgeons perform a certain type of operation by choice. The indications for the various surgical procedures are based upon personal concepts concerning the nature of the disease process and how it is best controlled. Hueston (1982) stated the reality of the situation: 'Fundamentally the patient produces the disease. The surgeon attempts to control it'.

METHODS OF EVALUATING RESULTS

In Chapter 20, the results of treatment were given according to various patient groups. In this chapter the results of treatment will be analysed according to the type of operation performed and, as before, early results will be evaluated according to the correction of contracture and late results according to the rate of recurrence and extension. Five factors have been evaluated:

1. Degree of correction of flexion contracture.
2. Outcome — *perfect* if full extension was obtained, *improved* if the flexion contracture was less and *worse* if the contracture was the same or greater.
3. Return of flexion after operation measured by the distance between the fingertip and the distal crease of the palm

   These three criteria were evaluated at 1 year after operation (±6 months) on the assumption that it could take this long to obtain a maximum result from operation. The worst results and the most difficult joint to correct was the proximal interphalangeal joint of the little finger. Often this joint alone was used to compare various aspects of treatment.

4. Recurrence — the appearance of disease within the area of operation.
5. Extension — the appearance of disease beyond the area of operation.

   These last two criteria were evaluated from 2 years (± 6 months) onward at yearly intervals. Adequate data were available for statistical analysis up to 5 years, but thereafter the numbers of patients were few.

RESULTS ACCORDING TO THE TYPE OF OPERATION

The type of operation performed in the palm and finger is often different; the type of incision and method of wound closure are not necessarily dictated by what is done to the diseased fascia. Therefore, this analysis considered these factors separately. Four types of operation were analysed:

1. A local operation which included subcutaneous and open fasciotomy whether closed by suture, skin graft or left open; also the Gonzalez operation.
2. A regional fasciectomy which removed the diseased fascia by a relatively localized excision.
3. An extensive fasciectomy in which the

surgeon attempted a more widespread removal of fascia, including fascia that appeared to be normal.
4. A dermofasciectomy which removed the overlying skin as well as the diseased fascia and where a full thickness skin graft was applied to the defect. This was usually an extensive operation, performed because of widespread disease. For many surgeons this is the treatment of choice for recurrent disease, but Hueston (Chapter 22) advocates this operation as a primary procedure when a strong diathesis is expressed by the patient.

Three types of wound closure were analysed:

1. By suture to obtain primary closure.
2. Left open after the method of McCash.
3. By skin graft, usually a full thickness skin graft.

The patient and operation profiles for the different types of operations and closures are provided in Profiles a–p at the end of the this chapter and are included for those surgeons who are interested in using these data to compare with their own series. The results are summarized in Tables 36.1–36.3.

In patients having a local operation, the preoperative contracture at the fifth metacarpophalangeal joint and the postoperative correction were greatest. Also, a perfect outcome at the fifth proximal interphalangeal joint was more frequent after a local operation both in the palm and in the finger. Regional fasciectomy was the most common procedure in the palm (to correct metacarpophalangeal joint contraction) whereas extensive fasciectomy was slightly more common in the finger (to correct proximal interphalangeal joint contracture). These figures suggest that factors other than preoperative angles dictated the type of operation performed and the most likely factor was the surgeon's preference.

In Table 36.2, a similar analysis considered the type of wound closure in the palm and in the finger. The statistically significant differences are of clinical value and application. At the metacarpophalangeal joint results were the same whether the wound was sutured, left open or skin-grafted. However, when the palm was left open, the proximal interphalangeal joint correction was much less and the outcome was less satisfactory than if the palmar wound was closed either by suture or skin graft. In the finger, the results were significantly better at the proximal interphalangeal joint when a skin graft was applied rather than the wound sutured. There were too few 'open fingers' for analysis.

In Table 36.3, the effect that the various operations and closures had on the ability of the patient to regain flexion to the distal crease of the palm is shown. These results should be considered with the data on the distal crease of the palm of Chapter 20 (p. 206). The distal crease of the palm is a good index of morbidity following an operation for DD. None of the results in Table 36.3 were significantly different from others, but there are trends that are of clinical value. One might expect a local operation to have little effect upon return of flexion and yet in the palm, the distal crease was similar to that following a regional fasciectomy although better than either extensive or dermofasciectomy. In the finger, a local operation was no better than a regional or extensive fascectomy and in the little finger, all three resulted in loss of flexion. Overall, the worst results were seen in the little finger.

In Tables 36.1 and 36.2, the rate of recurrence and extension is between 50 and 60% for all types of operation. This is further evidence that the biological activity rather than the type of operation dictates the ongoing process of the disease. The factors that exert a significant effect upon recurrence and extension are listed in Table 36.4. These are the diathesis factors of other areas involved, early onset of disease, extensive and radial side disease. The outcome of the operation had no bearing upon recurrence and extension.

Concerning outcome, Profiles q, r and s (see end of this chapter) were prepared to see if there were any features of the patients or their hands that would determine outcome. The significant features are listed in Table 36.5. The diathesis factors were not prominent, other than alcoholism and extensive disease. The type of operation did not affect the result but the type of closure had a significant effect. In the palm, the open palm procedure was more often associated with a worse result and a grafted palm with a perfect result. In the finger,

Table 36.1 A comparison of the results of treatment by type of operation

		Angles at MPJ V				Angles at PIPJ V			Perfect outcome (%)		Recurrence and extension (%)
	n	Pre	Post	Change	n	Pre	Post	Change	MPJ V	PIPJ V	
Palm operation											
Local	20	59.3±26.5[1]	9.3±18.9	50.0[4]	21	47.5±21.5	22.9±22.9	26.0	70	29[6]	50
Regional	146	43.9±25.3[2]	2.9±11.4	41.0	141	54.1±27.3	28.8±23.9	25.3	84	18	54
Extensive	19	48.3±20.8	1.8± 6.1	46.5	20	53.6±19.5	22.2±19.7	31.4	89	25	60
Dermofasciectomy	58	39.8±22.5[3]	2.4± 8.6	37.4[5]	49	50.2±24.0	24.5±19.4	25.7	89	16[7]	
Finger operation											
Local	18	48.2±36.4	4.7±14.4	43.5	28	50.0±22.1	23.2±22.7	26.9	83	28	61
Regional	90	47.6±25.0	3.2±13.8	44.4	94	54.8±28.3	25.0±25.7	29.8	84	23	59
Extensive	101	43.5±22.9	1.4± 4.5	42.1	134	51.6±23.1	30.1±20.6	28.5	89	13	54
Dermofasciectomy	1	50.0			2	50.0±28.3	35.0± 7.1	15.0			

Blanks indicate insufficient data (less than 10 observations).
Significant differences between groups: 1–2 $p<0.02$; 1–3 $p<0.005$; 4–5 $p<0.05$; 6–7 $p<0.05$.

Table 36.2 A comparison of the results of treatment by type of wound closure

		Angles at MPJ V				Angles at PIPJ V			Perfect outcome (%)		Recurrence and extension (%)
	n	Pre	Post	Change	n	Pre	Post	Change	MPJ V	PIPJ V	
Palm closure											
Suture	156	45.6±26.0	3.5±11.5	42.1	146	54.9±26.3	25.2±23.2[2]	29.7[2]	81	20[4]	56
Open	55	40.1±20.9	1.9± 6.5	38.2	49	46.5±25.9	34.8±20.5[1]	11.7[1]	91	8[3]	52
Graft	30	47.7±23.3	4.2±16.9	43.5	35	54.3±19.6	23.5±23.3[2]	30.8[2]	90	34[4]	47
Finger closure											
Suture	170	46.2±24.7	2.6±11.3	43.6	203	52.6±25.1	28.6±22.8	24.0[5]	86	17[7]	50
Open	6	49.5±31.2	2.5± 6.1	47.0	4	32.5±18.9	0.5± 1.0	32.0			
Graft	31	43.3±26.7	1.8± 5.4	41.5	47	56.2±23.3	23.8±24.5	32.4[6]	87	30[8]	

Blank spaces indicate insufficient data (less than 10 observations).
Significant differences between groups: 1–2 $p<0.01$; 3–4 $p<0.05$; 5–6 $p<0.05$; 7–8 $p<0.02$.

Table 36.3 A comparison of full flexion (at the distal crease of the palm) by type of operation and closure

	Full flexion preop (%)				Full flexion postop (%)			
	V	IV	III	II	V	IV	III	II
Palm operation								
Local	89	98	96	100	84	86	89	91
Regional	89	89	96	99	86	88	93	96
Extensive	96	97	98	98	79	90	90	91
Dermofasciectomy	97	98	98	99	80	89	90	93
Palm closure								
Suture	92	93	93	98	87	90	91	92
Open	95	92	95	94	78	87	89	91
Graft	92	94	95	95	81	83	89	91
Finger operation								
Local	91	96	100	—	72	80	80	—
Regional	91	88	91	79	79	85	91	79
Extensive	92	89	96	85	78	83	82	77
Dermofasciectomy	—	—	—	—	—	—	—	—
Fingerclosure								
Suture	87	79	87	72	77	76	85	60
Open	—	—	—	—	—	—	—	—
Graft	86	—	80	—	77	—	100	—

There are no significant differences.
Blank spaces indicate insufficient data (less then 10 observations).

Table 36.4 Variables contributing to recurrence and extension (R & E)

Variable	R & E	No R & E	p Value
Other areas involved	36%	21%	<0.001
Early onset of disease	40%	29%	<0.05
Three or more rays	33%	27%	<0.05
Index finger	14%	8%	<0.05
Middle finger	37%	28%	<0.05
Outcome			
Perfect	50%	50%	NS
Improved	44%	56%	NS
Worse	54%	46%	NS

NS = not significant.

Table 36.5 Variables contributing to a perfect or worse outcome at PIPJ V

Variable	Perfect	Worse	p Value
Alcoholism	8%	23%	<0.05
More than three rays	24%	42%	<0.05
Palm closure			
Open	9%	55%	<0.001
Graft	27%	9%	<0.05
Finger closure			
Primary	71%	87%	<0.05
Graft	29%	8%	<0.01
Complications	8%	36%	<0.01

skin grafts were more likely to provide a perfect result. Complications are bound to be associated with a worse result.

TIMING OF OPERATION

Metacarpophalangeal joint contracture can almost always be corrected, but because proximal joint contracture is so difficult to correct, it has been my view that the patient should be advised to have an operation as soon as the proximal joint begins to contract. The figures in Table 36.6 suggest that we should modify this view. When the preoperative joint angles are compared to the outcome of operation, the average degrees of preoperative flexion are less in those patients who had a worse outcome. Also, at the proximal interphalangeal joint of the little and ring fingers, the average preoperative joint angle associated with a perfect result was above 40°. Even at the metacarpophalangeal joint, lesser degrees of contracture are associated with a worse result.

The reasons for these figures are primarily surgical. With minimal joint contraction, the extent of disease is not obvious because cords are not well developed and it is easy to leave some of the disease behind. This is especially so at the proximal joint. Also, if an extensive fasciectomy is performed in the presence of minimal disease and slight contracture, the insult of the operation followed by scar contracture can combine to create a postoperative contracture greater than that which was present preoperatively.

On the basis of these results, one is cautioned

Table 36.6 The effect of preoperative joint angle on outcome

	Little finger	Ring finger	Middle finger	Index finger	Thumb
Metacarpophalangeal joint					
Perfect	43	34	28	21	22
Improved	55	53	31	45	35
Worse	31	22	25	17	10
Proximal interphalangeal joint					
Perfect	47	42	30		
Improved	63	64	50		
Worse	35	28	34		
Distal interphalangeal joint					
Perfect	21	30			
Improved	39	67			
Worse	23	10			

against operating upon early disease. It would seem best to wait until 30–40° of contracture is present either at the metacarpophalangeal or proximal interphalanged joint. For the same reasons, minimal disease elsewhere in a hand that requires an operation is best left alone. If, for instance, a little or ring finger is operated upon, minimal disease in the middle or index finger or thumb web should be left. The disease may not progress in those areas or, as shown in Table 36.6, the contracture can be made worse by removing it.

THE VALUE OF A PROXIMAL INTERPHALANGEAL JOINT PROCEDURE

In about 10% of operations, some type of procedure beyond excision of diseased fascia was performed at the proximal interphalangeal joint to overcome the flexion contacture. The patient, hand and operation profiles were analysed to determine what factors were associated with the surgeon's decision to perform this additional procedure. The significant factors are listed in Table 36.7. The only patient variable of significance was other areas involved. As one might expect, there was severe and aggressive disease in the hand. Complications were twice as frequent and these patients were more likely to have postoperative therapy and splinting.

Table 36.8 shows the results by correction of joint contracture and by outcome in joints with and without a proximal joint procedure. The former joints had a significantly greater preoperative flexion contracture whereas the postoperative contractures and the degrees of change were similar. The percentage of perfect, improved and

Table 36.7 Variables associated with a proximal interphalangeal joint procedure

Variable	P value
Other areas involved	<0.001
Three or more rays	<0.005
Radial side disease	<0.005
Previous operation	<0.001
Skin grafts	<0.005
Complications	<0.001
Therapy and splinting	<0.001

Table 36.8 The result at PIPJ V with and without a PIPJ procedure

Joint contracture	n	Preop	Postop	Change
PIPJ procedure	35	63.2±[1]25.1	32.4±26.9	30.8
No PIPJ procedure	126	49.5±[2]25.0	24.0±21.6	25.5

Significant difference 1–2: $p<0.003$.

Outcome	n	Perfect	n	Improved	n	Worse
PIPJ procedure	6	17%	23	66%	6	17%
No PIPJ procedure	24	19%	69	55%	33	26%

No significant differences.

worse outcomes were the same although the trend was for the proximal joint procedure to provide more improved and fewer worse outcomes.

The analysis suggests that a proximal interphalangeal joint procedure was only (and perhaps should only) be performed with severe disease and severe joint contracture. The procedure will not provide a better result but can gain a result that is similar to a less severe joint contracture treated without a proximal interphalangeal joint procedure.

POSTOPERATIVE THERAPY AND SPLINTING

The surgeons contributing to this study differed greatly in their use of both therapy and splinting but overall only 33% of patients received postoperative therapy and 42% were splinted. These are surprising figures in an era when hand therapy has emerged as an essential component of postoperative care. This study could not reveal the type of splint used (static or dynamic), the method (most of the time, at night only) or the duration of the splinting. The study did, however, distinguish between therapy provided by the surgeon, by a therapist and by a hand therapist and for this analysis, the results with no therapy were compared to those obtained when therapy was provided by a hand therapist.

Table 36.9 shows that splinting was used more often as the extent and severity of disease increased. When the disease was confined to the

Table 36.9 Postoperative splinting (Overall 42% were splinted)

Extent of disease		Severity of disease	
Palm only	12%	Previous operation	45%
One ray	41%	Complication	55%
Two rays	43%	Proximal interphalangeal joint procedure	59%
Three rays	47%	Sympathetic dystrophy	74%
Radial side	48%	None of above*	20%

*$p<0.001$.

palm, splinting was infrequent. Note, however, that when the operation attempted to correct a fifth proximal interphalangeal joint contracture (Tables 36.10 and 36.11), the majority of patients received therapy and were splinted.

Table 36.10 reveals that there was no difference in the pre- and postoperative angles in the splinted and not splinted groups, although there was a better change in angle in the latter group; 70% of the worse outcome group were splinted. Those results, coupled with those in Table 36.9, suggest that the most difficult cases to treat have biased the results against splinting. It would be incorrect to conclude that better results are obtained if splints are not used.

The analysis of postoperative therapy yielded similar results, as shown in Table 36.11. Although therapy and splinting fare poorly in the perfect and worse outcome groups, both modalities provided more improved results.

It appears from this analysis that most surgeons were selective in sending patients for splinting and therapy. Those patients had severe contractures and postoperative complications. If this course is followed, the results of splinting and therapy are bound to be unsatisfactory. I prefer to have all patients seen by a hand therapist. Most of these patients will be given a splint but how long the splint is worn during the day and night and the duration of splinting are different for every patient. I believe that therapy is more valuable then splinting. The quality of recovery is better when a skilled therapist is involved.

Table 36.10 The result at PIPJ V with and without splinting

Joint contracture	n	Preop	Postop	Change
Splinted	152	52.1±24.8	30.9±22.1	21.2[1]
Not splinted	117	55.4±26.1	22.3±23.1	33.1[2]

Significant difference 1–2: $p<0.001$.

Outcome	n	Perfect	n	Improved	n	Worse
Splinted	21	42%	83	57%	46	70%[1]
Not splinted	30	38%	63	43%	20	30%[2]

Significant difference 1–2: $p<0.025$.

Table 36.11 The result at PIPJ V with and without therapy

Joint contracture	n	Preop	Postop	Change
Hand therapy	84	46.2±25.1	32.1±24.0	14.1[1]
No hand therapy	51	52.2±20.7	22.7±18.5	29.5[2]

Significant difference 1–2: $p<0.003$.

Outcome	n	Perfect	n	Improved	n	Worse
Hand therapy		33%[1]		66%		74%[3]
No hand therapy		67%[2]		34%[2]		26%[4]

Significant difference 1–2: $p<0.005$; 3–4: $p<0.001$.

CONCLUSIONS

This statistical analysis has considered early results in terms of correction of joint contracture, outcome, and the return of finger flexion, and late results according to the prevalence of recurrence and extension of the disease. Early results were influenced by the severity of disease and the type of wound closure. Recurrence and extension were affected by diathesis factors, but not by the type of operation or the early result.

At the metacarpophalangeal joint, early and late results were uniformly good so this joint cannot be used to evaluate methods of treatment. In contrast, the results at the proximal interphalangeal joint varied with types of treatment.

There was no difference in the postoperative angles or outcome with the four types of operation, but there were significant differences with the types of wound closure. The open palm gave a less satisfactory result at the proximal joint than either suture or skin grafting, and skin grafting was better than suture in the finger. These results suggest that the palm should not be left open if a (severe) proximal interphalangeal joint contracture has been corrected and that skin grafts should be used often in the palm and fingers.

The overall results of treatment were good, but there is need for improvement at the proximal interphalangeal joint, especially of the little finger. These results were collected from the records of experienced surgeons and although not perfect, they can be considered to be the standard.

Profile a Palm operation: local fasciotomy/fasciectomy (93 patients and 109 hands)

Family origin		Sex		Hand dominance		Hand involved		Occupation	
Northern European	74%	Male	79%	Right	90%	Right	21%	Manual	69%
Japanese	22%	Female	21%	Left	10%	Left	13%	Non-manual	31%
Southern European	4%					Both	66%		
		Other areas involved	19%			Associated diseases		Age at onset (years)	
						Epilepsy	2%	Male	51.9±10.3
		Family history	28%			Diabetes	6%	Female	53.1±14.5
						Alcoholism	8%	Age at operation (years)	
		Previous operation	22%			Trauma	21%	Male	60.7±10.5
								Female	61.3±15.2

Operation profile

Hand profile				Palm	Little finger	Thumb	
Palm only	11%	*Operation*					
No palm	1%	Local	100%	76%	63%		
		Regional		15%	25%		
One ray	32%	Extensive		9%	12%		
Two rays	25%	Amputation					
Three or more rays	32%						
		Incision					
Thumb and thumb web	15%	Longitudinal	50%	62%	100%		
Index finger	15%	Transverse	50%	38%			
Middle finger	30%						
Ring finger	60%	*Closure*					
Little finger	66%	Suture	52%	66%	57%		
		Open	12%	8%	43%		
		Graft	36%	26%			

Anaesthesia

Local	24%
Regional	34%
General	42%
Procedure at PIP joint	5%
Complications	13%
Therapy	61%
Splinting	43%

Profile a contd.

	Little finger		Ring finger		Middle finger		Index finger		Thumb	
	n Pre Post		n Pre Post		n Pre Post		n Pre Post		Pre Post	
MP joint	20 59.3±26.5 9.3±18.9		22 33.2±19.4 3.9±12.0		16 29.1±21.1 5.9±13.1		2 12.5±10.6 10.0±14.1		5.0 5.0	
Outcome										
Perfect	70% 54.0±28.3 0± 0		82% 32.0±15.0 0± 0		81% 26.2±21.9 0± 0		50% 5.0 0± 0			
Improved	25% 74.0±19.2 25.0±21.2		14% 50.0±35.0 25.0±26.5		13% 42.5±17.7 27.5± 3.5					
Same	5% 60.0 60.0		4% 5.0 10.0		6% 40.0 40.0					
worse										
PIP joint	21 47.5±21.5 22.9±22.9		9 55.3±23.3 1.3± 4.0		2 35.0±21.2 5.0± 7.1		1 5.0 20.0			
Outcome										
Perfect	29% 61.3±22.8 0± 0		89% 54.7±24.8 0± 0		50% 50.0 0± 0		100% 5.0			
Improved	33% 52.9±19.1 29.3±27.3		11% 60.0 12.0		50% 20.0 10.0					
Same	38% 32.5±13.6 34.4±15.0									
worse										
DIP joint	6 31.5±23.2 6.7±12.1		1 65.0 0± 0		0					
Outcome										
Perfect	66% 36.0±28.5 0± 0		100% 65.0 0± 0							
Improved	17% 20.0 10.0									
Same	17% 25 30									
worse										

Profile b Palm operation: regional fasciectomy (650 patients and 729 hands)

Family origin		Sex		Hand dominance		Hand involved	
Northern European	88%	Male	85%	Right	95%	Right	19%
Japanese	9%	Female	15%	Left	51%	Left	11%
Southern European	3%					Both	70%
		Other areas involved	29%			Associated diseases	
		Family history	30%			Epilepsy	4%
		Previous operation	19%			Diabetes	8%
						Alcoholism	14%
						Trauma	14%

Occupation	
Manual	54%
Non-manual	46%
Age at onset (years)	
Male	48.3±12.7
Female	54.3±12.2
Age at operation (years)	
Male	57.6±10.9
Female	61.6±10.4

Operation profile

Hand profile			Palm	Little finger	Ring finger	Middle finger	Thumb
Palm only	6%	*Operation*					
No palm	2%	Local	100%	2%			3%
One ray	34%	Regional		61%			92%
Two rays	31%	Extensive		36%			5%
Three or more rays	29%	Amputation		1%			
		Incision					
Thumb and thumb web	24%	Longitudinal	77%	96%			100%
Index finger	11%	Transverse	23%	4%			
Middle finger	30%						
Ring finger	64%	*Closure*					
Little finger	67%	Suture	82%	93%			94%
		Open	14%	1%			
		Graft	4%	5%			6%

Anaesthesia	
Local	3%
Regional	45%
General	52%
Procedure at PIP joint	12%
Complications	16%
Therapy	74%
Splinting	40%

Profile b contd.

	Little finger			Ring finger			Middle finger			Index finger			Thumb		
	n	Pre	Post	n	Pre	Post	n	Pre	Post	n	Pre	Post	n	Pre	Post
MP joint	146	43.9±25.3	2.9±11.4	146	37.5±20.5	2.0± 6.6	59	27.8±15.2	2.3± 7.5	13	25.0±19.4	6.2±10.4	6	13.3± 6.1	7.5±12.5
Outcome															
Perfect	84%	41.7±23.9	0± 0	85%	35.2±19.4	0± 0	87%	27.0±13.7	0± 0	69%	20.0±13.7	0± 0	67%	13.8± 4.8	0± 0
Improved	13%	56.4±23.9	11.8± 7.1	14%	52.1±21.5	13.7±12.2	10%	35.8±25.2	12.2± 4.5	23%	45.0±26.0	20.0±10.0	33%	12.5±10.6	22.5±10.6
Same/worse	3%	31.3±39.7	48.7±47.1	1%	10.0	10.0	3%	25.0±21.2	30.0±28.3	8%	10.0	20.0			
PIP joint	141	54.1±27.3	28.8±23.9	74	45.9±27.1	14.6±17.1	21	35.1±18.6	16.3±17.4						
Outcome															
Perfect	18%	46.2±25.4	0± 0	43%	34.0±22.1	0± 0	43%	28.9±16.9	0± 0						
Improved	53%	66.7±21.5	30.4±18.0	45%	63.1±23.2	25.3±14.8	33%	44.3±16.4	22.9± 5.7						
Same/worse	29%	33.2±24.0	44.5±25.1	12%	22.8±17.7	26.9±17.5	24%	28.6±20.1	36.6±16.6						
DIP joint	18	26.2±18.7	11.2±12.9	8	22.5±28.7	7.3±15.9	1	10.0	0± 0						
Outcome															
Perfect	44%	13.8± 6.9	0± 0	76%	14.2± 9.7	0± 0	100%	10.0	0± 0						
Improved	39%	42.1±19.1	16.4± 6.9	12%	90.0	45.0									
Same/worse	17%	24.3±18.9	29.3±14.0	12%	15.0	15.0									

Profile c Palm operation: extensive fasciectomy (258 patients and 286 hands)

Family origin		Sex		Hand dominance		Hand involved		Occupation	
Northern European	87%	Male	89%	Right	98%	Right	15%	Manual	45%
Japanese	10%	Female	11%	Left	2%	Left	10%	Non-manual	55%
Southern European	3%					Both	75%		
		Other areas involved			33%	Associated diseases		Age at onset (years)	
						Epilepsy	2%	Male	45.9±12.5
		Family history			35%	Diabetes	7%	Female	56.6±10.0
						Alcoholism	8%	Age at operation (years)	
		Previous operation			20%	Trauma	9%	Male	56.1±10.6
								Female	63.6±8.9

Operation profile

Hand profile				Palm	Little finger	Thumb	Anaesthesia	
Palm only	3%				4%	5%	Local	3%
No palm	3%				46%	66%	Regional	70%
					50%	29%	General	27%
One ray	27%							
Two rays	34%						Procedure at PIP joint	8%
Three or more rays	36%			100%		100%		
		Incision					Complications	14%
Thumb and thumb web	24%	Longitudinal		82%	94%	88%		
Index finger	13%	Transverse		18%	6%	7%	Therapy	90%
Middle finger	38%	Closure				5%		
Ring finger	71%	Suture		81%	91%		Splinting	42%
Little finger	72%	Open		19%	3%			
		Graft			6%			

Profile c contd.

	Little finger				Ring finger				Middle finger				Thumb		Index finger			Thumb	
	n	Pre	Post	n	Pre	Post	n	Pre	Post	n	Pre	Post	n	Pre	Post	n	Pre	Post
MP joint	19	48.3±20.8	18.4± 6.1	15	40.9±20.6	2.3± 5.6	8	26.3±17.9	3.8± 8.8	0			4	30.0±14.1	0			
Outcome																		
Perfect	89%	48.6±19.3	0	80%	38.3±24.6	0	75%	28.3±19.7	0	0%			100%	30.0±14.1	0			
Improved	11%	45.0±42.4	17.5±10.6	20%	51.0±14.9	11.7± 7.2	25%	20.0±14.1	15.0±14.1	0%			0%					
Same/worse	0%			0%			0%			0%			0%					
PIP joint	20	53.6±19.5	22.2±19.7	10	53.2±23.8	25.3±26.3	1	40.0	0	1	45.0	15.0						
Outcome																		
Perfect	25%	36.0± 6.5	0	60%	47.5±17.5	0	0%			0%								
Improved	70%	59.4±19.7	27.4± 4	30%	76.3±17.0	20.0± 8.7	100%	40.0	0	100%	45.0	15.0						
Same/worse	5%	60.0	60.0	10%	18.0	20.0	0%			0%								
DIP joint	7	27.1±12.3	5.3± 9.3	3	38.0±40.1	6.7±11.5												
Outcome																		
Perfect	71%	22.4± 9.3	0	67%	15.0± 7.1	0												
Improved	29%	39.0±12.7	18.5± 4.9	33%	84.0	20.0												
Same/worse	0%			0%														

Profile d Palm operation: dermofasciectomy (73 patients and 74 hands)

Family origin		Sex		Hand dominance		Hand involved		Occupation	
Northern European	87%	Male	93%	Right	91%	Right	20%	Manual	37%
Japanese	10%	Female	7%	Left	9%	Left	7%	Non-manual	63%
Southern European	3%					Both	73%		
		Other areas involved	32%			Associated diseases		Age at onset (years)	
						Epilepsy	5%	Male	41.4±11.2
		Family history	17%			Diabetes	7%	Female	43.8± 3.0
						Alcoholism	11%	Age at operation (years)	
		Previous operation	34%			Trauma	7%	Male	52.5±10.4
								Female	57.2± 5.3

Operation profile

Hand profile				Palm	Little finger	Thumb		Anaesthesia	
Palm only	3%	Operation						Local	11%
No palm		Local			1%	18%		Regional	23%
		Regional			26%	27%		General	66%
One ray	27%	Extensive		100%	72%	55%			
Two rays	30%	Amputation			1%			Procedure at PIP joint	19%
Three or more rays	41%	Incision							
Thumb and thumb web	31%	Longitudinal			88%	100%		Complications	45%
Index finger	19%	Transverse			12%				
Middle finger	34%	Closure						Therapy	78%
Ring finger	62%	Suture			44%	55%			
Little finger	89%	Open			2%			Splinting	58%
		Graft		100%	54%	45%			

Profile d contd.

	Little finger			Ring finger			Middle finger			Little finger			Thumb	
	n	Pre	Post	n	Pre	Post	n	Pre	Post	n	Pre	Post	Pre	Post
MP joint	58	39.8±22.5	2.4± 8.6	59	35.5±18.1	2.3± 9.6	39	27.5±14.5	0.5± 2.3	11	23.5±10.6	0	20.5±10.2	22.5±28.7
Outcome														
Perfect	89%	40.5±22.8	0	92%	33.8±77.8	0	92%	28.3±14.4	0	100%	23.5±10.6	0	50% 17.5± 3.5	0
Improved	10%	37.5±22.0	15.3±11.1	7%	57.5± 9.6	19.5±17.8	3%	13.0	10.0	0%			25% 35.0	30.0
Same/worse	1%	20.0	50.0	1%	40.0	60.0	3%	10.0	10.0	0%			25% 12.0	60.0
PIP joint	49	50.2±24.0	24.5±19.4	30	48.9±25.9	14.6±17.1	8	44.6±30.8		3	25.0±17.3	15.0±15.0		
Outcome														
Perfect	16%	46.3±28.4	0	37%	39.1±20.3	0	16%	25.0± 0		33%	15.0	0		
Improved	65%	56.7±20.9	24.8±13.6	43%	66.3±21.8	38.8±22.3	68%	69.3±23.3	35.0±18.3	33%	45.0	30.0		
Same/worse	18%	30.6±21.1	45.6±21.2	20%	29.2±21.3	42.3±24.4	16%	15.0± 7.1	35.0±21.2	33%	15.0	15.0		
DIP joint	12	26.6±15.1	7.9±12.0	6	40.0±27.7	2.5± 6.1	1	20.0	0					
Outcome														
Perfect	58%	21.4±12.1	0	83%	45.0±27.8	0	100%	20.0	0					
Improved	25%	43.0±13.1	11.7± 7.6	0%			0%							
Same/worse	17%	20.0±14.1	30.0± 0	17%	15.0	15.0	0%							

Profile e Finger operation: local fasciotomy/fasciectomy (93 patients and 103 hands)

Family origin		Sex		Hand dominance		Hand involved		Occupation	
Northern European	87%	Male	78%	Right	94%	Right	27%	Manual	58%
Japanese	10%	Female	23%	Left	6%	Left	7%	Non-manual	42%
Southern European	3%					Both	66%		
		Other areas involved				Associated diseases		Age at onset (years)	
					28%	Epilepsy	2%	Male	48.9±12.0
		Family history			26%	Diabetes	4%	Female	52.7±12.6
						Alcoholism	14%	Age at operation (years)	
		Previous operation			23%	Trauma	14%	Male	57.8±11.8
								Female	62.0±13.0

Operation profile

Hand profile			Palm	Little finger	Thumb		Anaesthesia	
Palm only	3%	Operation					Local	26%
No palm	6%	Local	69%	93%	83%		Regional	36%
One ray	38%	Regional	20%	3%	17%		General	38%
Two rays	30%	Extensive	11%	3%				
Three or more rays	32%	Amputation		1%			Procedure at PIP joint	12%
		Incision						
Thumb and thumb web	19%	Longitudinal	60%	64%	100%		Complications	18%
Index finger	18%	Transverse	40%	36%				
Middle finger	40%	Closure					Therapy	65%
Ring finger	80%	Suture	58%	56%	50%			
Little finger	74%	Open	12%	7%	50%		Splinting	39%
		Graft	30%	37%				

Profile e contd.

	Little finger				Ring finger				Middle finger				Index finger				Thumb		
	n	Pre		Post	n	Pre		Post	n	Pre		Post	n	Pre		Post	n	Pre	Post
MP joint	18	48.2±36.4		4.7±14.4	16	32.3±15.1		0±0	6	37.7±25.7		0.8±2.0	1	20.0±0		0±0	2	15.5±14.8	2.5±3.5
Outcome																			
Perfect	83%	40.5±34.8		0±0	100%	32.3±15.1		0±0	83%	43.2±24.4		0±0	100%	20.0±0		0±0	50%	26.0	0±0
Improved	17%	86.7±10.4		28.3±27.5	0%				17%	10.0		5.0	0%				50%	5.0	5.0
Same/worse	0%				0%				0%										
PIP joint	28	50.0±22.1		23.2±22.7	15	62.8±24.7		7.7±18.3	3	36.7±15.3		10.0±10.0							
Outcome																			
Perfect	28%	55.1±23.3		0±0	73%	58.6±23.7		0±0	33%	50.0		0±0							
Improved	39%	58.2±21.5		27.7±21.4	27%	74.3±27.2		28.8±27.6	67%	30.0±14.1		15.0±7.1							
Same/worse	32%	35.6±15.7		38.3±18.4	0%				0%										
DIP joint	7	29.1±22.1		5.3±11.3	4	60.0±24.8		0±0	1	10.0±0		0±0							
Outcome																			
Perfect	72%	31.8±26.3		0±0	100%	60.0±24.8		0±0	100%	10.0		0±0							
Improved	14%	20.0±0		10.0±0															
Same/worse	14%	25.0±0		30±0															

Profile f Finger operation: regional fasciectomy (531 patients and 588 hands)

Family origin		Sex		Hand dominance		Hand involved	
Northern European	86%	Male	87%	Right	94%	Right	20%
Japanese	12%	Female	13%	Left	6%	Left	10%
Southern European	2%					Both	70%
		Other areas involved	27%			Associated diseases	
		Family history	27%			Epilepsy	4%
		Previous operation	22%			Diabetes	7%
						Alcoholism	9%
						Trauma	15%

Operation profile

Hand profile			Palm	Little finger	Thumb
Palm only	1%	Operation			
No palm	7%	Local	3%	1%	4%
		Regional	70%	95%	89%
One ray	34%	Extensive	27%	4%	7%
Two rays	36%	Amputation			
Three or more rays	29%	Incision			
Thumb and thumb web	21%	Longitudinal	79%	94%	100%
Index finger	13%	Transverse	21%	6%	
Middle finger	32%	Closure			
Ring finger	68%	Suture	81%	93%	89%
Little finger	72%	Open	11%	2%	
		Graft	8%	5%	11%

		Occupation	
		Manual	45%
		Non-manual	55%
		Age at onset (years)	
		Male	47.6±12.8
		Female	53.4±11.7
		Age at operation (years)	
		Male	57.1±11.0
		Female	60.9±9.6
		Anaesthesia	
		Local	3%
		Regional	55%
		General	42%
		Procedure at PIP joint	12%
		Complications	15%
		Therapy	85%
		Splinting	36%

Profile f contd.

	Little finger			Ring finger			Middle finger			Index finger			Thumb	
	n	Pre	Post	n	Pre	Post	n	Pre	Post	n	Pre	Post	n	Pre	Post
MP joint	90	47.6±25.0	3.2±13.8	80	43.7±22.3	4.2±10.6	24	32.1±18.9	2.6±5.6	1	60.0	20.0	3	13.3±2.9	0±0
Outcome															
Perfect	84%	46.4±23.5	0±0	74%	42.3±21.6	0±0	79%	30.0±16.9	0±0	100%	60.0	20.0	100%	13.3±2.9	0±0
Improved	12%	60.6±27.9	9.5±7.9	22%	52.8±22.2	14.0±13.2	21%	40.0±25.7	12.6±4.9						
Same/worse	3%	38.3±45.4	61.7±49.1	4%	18.3±18.9	26.7±28.9									
PIP joint	94	54.8±28.3	25.0±25.7	64	46.2±27.4	14.3±21.7	18	37.8±19.8	17.4±20.5						
Outcome															
Perfect	23%	43.6±25.9	0±0	50%	36.9±23.4	0±0	45%	30.0±14.6	0±0						
Improved	53%	66.5±23.4	28.2±20.7	34%	68.0±22.5	25.7±22.0	33%	52.5±16.7	29.2±16.9						
Same/worse	24%	33.2±19.2	47.4±19.8	16%	31.0±20.2	35.2±25.1	22%	25.8±21.2	34.5±20.9						
DIP joint	16	26.3±15.5	8.6±13.3	11	22.9±25.4	6.6±13.9	4	22.5±18.9	12.5±25.0						
Outcome															
Perfect	56%	19.1±11.8	0±0	73%	19.4±16.8	0±0	75%	13.3±5.8	0±0						
Improved	31%	39.0±11.4	15.0±19.4	9%	90.0	45.0									
Same/worse	13%	26.5±26.2	31.5±19.1	18%	10.0±7.1	14.0±1.4	25%								

Profile g Finger operation: extensive fasciotomy/fasciectomy (358 patients and 415 hands)

Family origin		Sex		Hand dominance		Hand involved		Occupation	
Northern European	92%	Male	86%	Right	97%	Right	11%	Manual	58%
Japanese	6%	Female	14%	Left	3%	Left	11%	Non-manual	42%
Southern European	2%					Both	78%		
		Other areas involved	35%			Associated diseases		Age at onset (years)	
						Epilepsy	3%	Male	47.5±13.1
		Family history	35%			Diabetes	8%	Female	57.4±11.1
		Previous operation	22%			Alcoholism	16%	Age at operation (years)	
						Trauma	8%	Male	57.9±11.9
								Female	63.3±10.1

Operation profile

Hand profile			Palm	Little finger	Thumb		Anaesthesia	
Palm only	1%	Operation					Local	2%
No palm	4%	Local	2%	2%	2%		Regional	49%
One ray	28%	Regional	60%	98%	71%		General	49%
Two rays	30%	Extensive	38%		27%			
Three or more rays	41%	Amputation					Procedure at PIP joint	14%
Thumb and thumb web	34%	Incision						
Index finger	13%	Longitudinal	73%	97%	100%		Complications	20%
Middle finger	36%	Transverse	27%	3%				
Ring finger	69%	Closure					Therapy	72%
Little finger	77%	Suture	69%	92%	92%		Splinting	59%
		Open	23%	2%	5%			
		Graft	8%	6%	3%			

Profile g contd.

		Little finger			Ring finger			Middle finger			Little finger			Thumb			Index finger	
	n	Pre	Post	n	Pre	Post	n	Pre	Post	n	Pre	Post	n	Pre	Post	n	Pre	Post
MP joint	100%	43.5±23.0	1.4± 4.5	64	40.2±18.7	1.8± 6.9	19	39.7±18.7	0				2	30.0±14.1	12.5±17.7			
Outcome																		
Perfect	89%	43.2±22.7	0	90%	39.1±18.4	0	100%	39.7±18.7	0				50%	40.0	0			
Improved	10%	48.8±26.2	12.2± 6.1	8%	57.6±12.6	17.6±15.9	0%						0%					
Same/worse	1%	5.0	20.0	2%	15.0	25.0	0%						50%	20.0	25.0			
PIP joint	134	51.4±23.2	30.0±20.8	58	49.6±25.4	22.4±19.9	17	40.1±24.1	22.1±19.3				6	39.2±15.6	13.3±11.7			
Outcome																		
Perfect	13%	43.1±19.5	0	31%	41.1±22.5	0	29%	28.0±15.2	0				34%	50.0	0			
Improved	60%	61.6±19.7	29.0±14.6	55%	60.5±22.4	31.2±14.0	48%	53.4±26.1	25.0±12.2				33%	47.5± 3.5	17.5±3.5			
Same/worse	27%	33.2±19.2	47.4±19.8	14%	24.7±19.9	37.4±21.0	23%	28.8±17.5	43.8±13.8				33%	20.0± 7.1	22.0±10.6			
DIP joint	25	27.9±16.8	9.1±10.7	7	34.1±26.7	2.9± 7.6	1	10.0	5.0				1	35.0	0			
Outcome																		
Perfect	52%	20.4±10.9	0	86%	25.8± 7.1	0							100%	35.0	0			
Improved	36%	41.3±18.2	15.8± 4.9	14%	84.0	20.0	100%	10.0	5.0									
Same/worse	12%	20.0±10.0	28.3± 2.9															

THE RESULTS OF TREATMENT

Profile h Finger operation: dermofasciectomy (77 patients and 81 hands)

Family origin		Sex		Hand dominance		Hand involved		Occupation	
Northern European	98%	Male	93%	Right	96%	Right	16%	Manual	42%
Southern European	2%	Female	7%	Left	4%	Left	6%	Non-manual	58%
						Both	78%		
		Other areas involved	33%			Associated diseases		Age at onset (years)	
						Epilepsy	4%	Male	41.7±9.9
		Family history	23%			Diabetes	6%	Female	44.0±6.3
						Alcoholism	10%	Age at operation (years)	
		Previous operation	41%			Trauma	11%	Male	53.6±8.9
								Female	55.0±5.1

Operation profile

Hand profile		Palm		Little finger		Thumb		Anaesthesia	
Palm only	9%	*Operation*						Local	15%
No palm		Local	1%		3%		40%	Regional	30%
One ray	43%	Regional	21%		13%		60%	General	56%
Two rays	26%	Extensive	78%		84%				
Three or more rays	31%	Amputation							
		Incision						Procedure at PIP joint	16%
Thumb and thumb web	27%	Longitudinal	53%		91%		100%		
Index finger	15%	Transverse	47%		9%			Complications	37%
Middle finger	23%	*Closure*							
Ring finger	47%	Suture	29%				60%	Therapy	83%
Little finger	91%	Open	5%				40%	Splinting	59%
		Graft	66%		100%				

Profile h contd.

	Little finger			Ring finger			Middle finger			Index finger			Thumb	
	n	Pre	Post	n	Pre	Post	n	Pre	Post	n	Pre	Post	Pre	Post
MP joint	1	50.0	0							11	23.5±10.6	0		
Outcome														
Perfect	100%	50.0±	0							100%	23.5±10.6	0		
Improved	0%									0%				
Same/worse	0%									0%				
PIP joint	2	55.0±28.3	35.0±7.1											
Outcome														
Perfect	0%													
Improved	100%	55.0±28.3	35.0±7.1											
Same/worse	0%													
DIP joint														
Outcome														
Perfect														
Improved														
Same/worse														

Profile i Palm closure: suture (794 patients and 896 hands)

Family origin		Sex		Hand dominance		Hand involved		Occupation	
Northern European	87%	Male	85%	Right	95%	Right	18%	Manual	51%
Japan	10%	Female	15%	Left	5%	Left	12%	Non-manual	49%
Southern European	3%					Both	70%		
								Age at onset (years)	
		Other areas involved	29%			Associated diseases		Male	47.5±12.7
						Epilepsy	3%	Female	55.2±11.4
		Family history	32%			Diabetes	7%		
						Alcoholism	10%	Age at operation (years)	
		Previous operation	20%			Trauma	14%	Male	55.2±11.4
								Female	62.3±10.6

Operation profile

Hand profile				Anaesthesia	
Palm only	6%	Palm		Local	5%
No palm	3%	*Operation*		Regional	54%
		Local	6%	General	41%
One ray	35%	Regional	68%		
Two rays	33%	Extensive	26%	Procedure at PIP joint	10%
Three or more rays	26%	Amputation			
		Incision		Complications	15%
Thumb and thumb web	21%	Longitudinal	89%		
Index finger	11%	Transverse	11%	Therapy	78%
Middle finger	31%	*Closure*			
Ring finger	63%	Suture	100%	Splinting	37%
Little finger	65%	Open			
		Graft			

Profile i contd.

	Little finger			Ring finger			Middle finger			Little finger			Thumb			Index finger			Thumb		
	n	Pre	Post	n	Pre	Post	n	Pre	Post	n	Pre	Post	n	Pre	Post	n	Pre	Post			
MP joint	156	45.6±26.0	3.5±11.5	157	34.8±19.3	2.1± 7.5	67	23.8±12.9	1.9± 5.9	14	14.3± 9.2	3.6±7.4	7	12.4±4.8	9.3±22.4						
Outcome																					
Perfect	81%	43.8±24.9	0± 0	86%	32.8±18.4	0± 0	87%	23.8±12.0	0± 0	79%	14.1±10.2	0±0	71%	14.0±4.2	0± 0						
Improved	16%	55.5±27.1	13.5±12.1	12%	51.3±19.9	13.3±11.5	10%	27.2±19.4	10.8± 2.0	7%	15.0	10.0									
Same/worse	3%	37.0±36.7	43.0±35.6	2%	18.3±18.9	26.7±28.9	4%	20.0±17.3	20.0±17.3	14%	15.0± 7.1	20.0±0	29%	8.5±4.9	32.5±38.9						
PIP joint	146	54.9±26.3	25.2±23.2	75	45.1±26.4	15.5±20.6	25	38.9±23.1	18.2±18.6												
Outcome																					
Perfect	20%	47.7±26.5	0± 0	45%	36.4±20.2	0± 0	40%	27.0±15.5	0± 0												
Improved	58%	63.2±22.4	27.3±18.0	39%	65.1±22.5	28.1±20.1	44%	54.7±20.6	30.0±12.4												
Same/worse	22%	35.6±24.1	43.1±26.3	16%	22.1±16.4	29.1±21.4	16%	20.0±17.8	31.3±20.2												
DIP joint	26	25.5±13.6	9.6±12.6	10	37.3±30.9	6.0±14.5	3	26.7±20.8	16.7±28.9												
Outcome																					
Perfect	50%	15.4± 7.5	0± 0	80%	36.9±28.0	0± 0	67%	15.0±7.1	0± 0												
Improved	38%	35.4±12.4	14.5± 7.2	10%	90.0	40.0															
Same/worse	12%	33.3±10.4	35.0±8.7	10%	15.0	15.0	33%	50.0	50.0												

THE RESULTS OF TREATMENT

Profile j Palm closure: open (128 patients and 174 hands)

Family origin		Sex		Hand dominance		Hand involved	
Northern European	90%	Male	90%	Right	95%	Right	16%
Japan	9%	Female	10%	Left	5%	Left	7%
Southern European	1%					Both	77%
		Other areas involved	35%			Associated disease	
		Family history	33%			Epilepsy	4%
		Previous operation	15%			Diabetes	10%
						Alcoholism	20%
						Trauma	12%
						Occupation	
						Manual	62%
						Non-manual	38%
						Age at onset (years)	
						Male	49.0±12.2
						Female	51.3±15.1
						Age at operation (years)	
						Male	57.6±10.5
						Female	62.0±10.2

Operation profile

Hand profile			Palm	Little finger	Thumb	Anaesthesia	
Palm only	2%	*Operation*				Local	2%
No palm	1%	Local	8%	8%	13%	Regional	47%
		Regional	60%	36%	65%	General	51%
One ray	18%	Extensive	32%	56%	23%		
Two rays	28%	Amputation				Procedure at PIP joint	11%
Three or more rays	52%	*Incision*					
Thumb and thumb web	34%	Longitudinal	24%	86%	100%	Complications	17%
Index finger	15%	Transverse	76%	14%			
Middle finger	43%	*Closure*				Therapy	77%
Ring finger	78%	Suture	100%	84%	81%	Splinting	62%
Little finger	88%	Open		11%	19%		
		Graft		5%			

Profile j contd.

	Little finger			Ring finger			Middle finger			Little finger			Thumb			Index finger		
	n	Pre	Post	n	Pre	Post	n	Pre	Post	n	Pre	Post	n	Pre	Post	n	Pre	Post
MP joint	55	40.1±20.9	1.9± 6.5	57	39.8±20.5	2.6±10.2	38	31.6±14.9	2.8± 8.7	12	34.0±14.8	4.2±10.0	2	13.3±6.1	20.0±17.3			
Outcome																		
Perfect	91%	38.5±21.0	0± 0	89%	38.1±19.8	0± 0	92%	30.7±13.7	0± 0	83%	28.8± 9.3	0± 0	50%	20.0	0± 0			
Improved	9%	56.0± 8.2	21.0± 8.2	11%	57.5±20.2	24.5±22.9	5%	42.5±38.9	14.0± 8.5	17%	60.0± 0.0	25.0± 7.1						
Same/worse	0%	0	0	0%			3%	40.0	50.0				50%	20.0	30.0			
PIP joint	49	46.5±25.9	34.8±20.5	29	48.0±26.6	17.9±18.9	6	26.3± 9.1	26.3±19.6									
Outcome																		
Perfect	8%	46.3±25.0	0± 0	41%	36.9±26.6	0± 0	17%	25.0	0± 0									
Improved	49%	62.2±21.7	32.9±16.2	48%	59.6±23.3	26.5±12.1	33%	25.0± 7.1	15.0± 7.1									
Same/worse	43%	28.6±18.4	43.7±19.3	10%	38.3±25.7	49.0±11.5	50%	27.7±13.3	42.7± 7.5									
DIP joint	9	24.8±23.6	10.3±12.7	3	13.3± 7.6	4.3± 7.5	0											
Outcome																		
Perfect	56%	21.0±14.3	0± 0	67%	17.0± 3.5	0± 0												
Improved	11%	80.0	20.0±	0%														
Same/worse	33%	12.7± 6.4	24.3± 6.0	33%	5.0	13.0												

Profile k Palm closure: graft (128 patients and 139 hands)

Family origin		Sex		Hand dominance		Hand involved		Occupation	
Northern European	84%	Male	86%	Right	93%	Right	24%	Manual	43%
Japan	12%	Female	14%	Left	7%	Left	6%	Non-manual	57%
Southern European	4%					Both	71%		
		Other areas involved	27%			Associated diseases		Age at onset (years)	
						Epilepsy	5%	Male	44.3±13.0
		Family history	17%			Diabetes	4%	Female	48.0±13.3
						Alcoholism	10%	Age at operation (years)	
		Previous operation	37%			Trauma	8%	Male	55.3±11.4
								Female	58.4±12.8

Operation profile

Hand profile				Palm	Thumb	Little finger	Thumb		
Palm only	8%			28%	17%			Anaesthesia	
No palm		Operation		19%	27%			Local	13%
One ray	29%	Local		53%	55%			Regional	22%
Two rays	24%	Regional			1%			General	64%
Three or more rays	39%	Extensive							
		Amputation						Procedure at PIP joint	19%
Thumb and thumb web	29%	Incision		40%	79%	10%			
Index finger	20%	Longitudinal		60%	21%	53%		Complications	34%
Middle finger	37%	Transverse				37%			
Ring finger	58%	Closure						Therapy	68%
Little finger	79%	Suture			49%	100%		Splinting	49%
		Open			1%				
		Graft		100%	50%	42%			

Profile k contd.

	Little finger			Ring finger			Middle finger			Index finger			Thumb		
	n	Pre	Post	n	Pre	Post	n	Pre	Post	n	Pre	Post	n	Pre	Post
MP joint	30	47.7±23.3	4.2±16.9	30	39.8±21.1	2.5± 5.8	18	34.8±22.0	4.7±10.2	0			5	25.5±12.5	3.0±6.7
Outcome															
Perfect	90%	47.3±21.4	0± 0	80%	37.8±19.7	0± 0	78%	35.8±23.4	0± 0				80%	30.0±14.1	0
Improved	7%	45.0±42.4	17.5±10.6	20%	51.3±25.2	12.5± 6.7	22%	31.3±18.4	21.3±11.1				20%	5.0	15.0
Same/worse	3%	20.0± 0	90.0												
PIP joint	35	54.3±19.6	23.5±23.3	20	58.3±24.3	12.3±18.6	6	55.0±16.7	27.5±36.6						
Outcome															
Perfect	34%	48.2±21.0	0± 0	60%	53.2±22.9	0± 0	50%	43.3± 5.8	0± 0						
Improved	52%	58.1±15.7	29.3±16.0	35%	72.7±18.5	32.1±17.9	16%	60.0	20.0						
Same/worse	14%	48.0±23.1	59.0±11.4	5%	18.0± 0	20.0	34%	70.0±21.2	72.5±17.7						
DIP joint	9	35.2±17.9	5.8± 8.9	6	35.7±31.9	3.3± 8.2	0								
Outcome															
Perfect	67%	34.0±21.8	0± 0	83%	26.0±23.8	0± 0									
Improved	33%	37.7± 9.3	17.3± 4.0	17%	84.0	20.0									
Same/worse															

THE RESULTS OF TREATMENT 405

Profile 1 Finger closure: suture (881 patients and 1017 hands)

Family origin		Sex		Hand dominance		Hand involved		Occupation	
Northern European	89%	Male	86%	Right	95%	Right	18%	Manual	50%
Japan	9%	Female	14%	Left	5%	Left	10%	Non-manual	50%
Southern European	2%					Both	72%		
		Other areas involved	32%			Associated diseases		Age at onset (years)	
						Epilepsy	4%	Male	47.3±12.9
		Family history	31%			Diabetes	7%	Female	54.9±11.4
						Alcoholism	12%	Age at operation (years)	
		Previous operation	23%			Trauma	12%	Male	57.1±11.1
								Female	62.8±9.7

Operation profile

Hand profile				Palm	Little finger	Thumb	Anaesthesia	
Palm only	2%	Operation					Local	4%
No palm	6%	Local	5%	6%	6%		Regional	53%
		Regional	65%	54%	80%		General	44%
One ray	32%	Extensive	30%	39%	14%			
Two rays	34%	Amputation		1%				
Three or more rays	32%						Procedure at	
		Incision					PIP joint	12%
Thumb and thumb web	26%	Longitudinal	78%	96%	100%			
Index finger	13%	Transverse	22%	4%			Complications	17%
Middle finger	34%							
Ring finger	67%	Closure					Therapy	79%
Little finger	73%	Suture	79%	96%	96%			
		Open	14%	3%	4%		Splinting	44%
		Graft	7%					

Profile 1 contd.

		Little finger		Ring finger			Middle finger			Thumb			Index finger			Thumb	
	n	Pre	Post	n	Pre	Post	n	Pre	Post	n	Pre	Post	n	Pre	Post	Pre	Post
MP joint	170	46.2±24.7	2.6±11.3	136	41.6±20.7	3.9± 9.4	42	36.5±18.4	1.5± 4.5	4	35.0±19.1	11.3±13.1	5	11 ±4.2	1.0±2.2		
Outcome																	
Perfect	86%	44.8±23.4	0± 0	81%	40.2±19.9	0± 0	80%	35.9±17.7	0± 0	50%	30.0±14.1	0± 0	80%	12.5±2.9	0±0		
Improved	12%	60.8±26.7	12.7±13.1	16%	55.5±19.4	15.4±13.6	12%	41.0±24.6	13.0± 4.5	25%	60.0	20.0	20%	5.0	5.0		
Same/worse	2%	32.5±38.9	51.3±45.2	3%	17.5±15.5	26.3±23.6	0%			25%	20.0	25.0					
PIP joint	203	52.6±25.1	28.6±22.8	115	47.1±26.6	16.9±20.1	34	37.7±19.0	20.0±20.0								
Outcome																	
Perfect	17%	46.9±25.3	0± 0	42%	37.5±20.9	0± 0	35%	29.6±13.4	0± 0								
Improved	55%	62.9±21.5	29.2±17.3	45%	64.2±23.0	28.6±18.2	44%	48.7±17.1	27.3±14.0								
Same/worse	28%	35.4±21.9	45.2±22.4	13%	22.2±15.5	30.6±20.3	21%	25.0±18.3	38.6±18.4								
DIP joint	39	26.4±16.4	10.2±12.8	15	34.9±30.3	5.3±12.6	6	18.3±16.0	9.2±20.1								
Outcome																	
Perfect	51%	16.6± 9.4	0± 0	81%	30.0±25.2	0± 0	66%	12.5± 5.0	0± 0								
Improved	36%	39.4±16.9	16.9± 8.5	13%	87.0± 4.2	32.5±17.7	17%	20.0	10.0								
Same/worse	13%	26.0±12.9	32.0± 7.6	6%	5.0	15.0	17%	40.0	45.0								

Profile m Finger closure: open (29 patients and 29 hands)

Family origin		Sex		Hand dominance		Hand involved		Occupation	
Northern European	79%	Male	90%	Right	88%	Right	24%	Manual	62%
Japan	21%	Female	10%	Left	12%	Left	14%	Non-manual	38%
						Both	62%		
		Other areas involved			28%	Associated diseases		Age at onset (years)	
		Family history			25%	Epilepsy	7%	Male	51.9±10.4
						Diabetes	10%	Female	59.0±12.7
		Previous operation			14%	Alcoholism	17%	Age at operation (years)	
						Trauma	21%	Male	58.2±2.5
								Female	70.0±6.9

Hand profile			Operation profile					Anaesthesia	
				Palm	Little finger	Thumb			
Palm only	34%		Operation					Local	10%
No palm	17%		Local	24%	33%	50%		Regional	72%
One ray	48%		Regional	36%	32%	50%		General	18%
Two rays			Extensive	40%	33%				
Three or more rays			Amputation		2%			Procedure at PIP joint	10%
Thumb and thumb web	24%		Incision						
Index finger	14%		Longitudinal	36%	49%	100%		Complications	0%
Middle finger	41%		Transverse	64%	51%				
Ring finger	66%		Closure					Therapy	72%
Little finger	86%		Suture	22%	18%				
			Open	70%	80%	86%		Splinting	52%
			Graft	8%	2%	14%			

Profile m contd.

	Little finger			Ring finger			Middle finger			Index finger			Thumb		
	n	Pre	Post	n	Pre	Post	n	Pre	Post	n	Pre	Post	n	Pre	Post
MP joint	6	49.5±31.2	2.5±6.1	4	32.5±18.9	0.5±1.0	4	21.3±11.1	2.0±4.0	0			0		
Outcome															
Perfect	83%	47.4±34.4	0±0	75%	36.7±20.8	0±0	75%	23.3±12.6	0±0						
Improved	17%	60.0±0.0	15.0	25%	20.0	2.0	25%	15.0	8.0						
Same/worse	0%			0%			0%								
PIP joint	7	49.6±35.8	25.3±16.9	4	60.5±35.9	15.5±31.0	2	31.5±16.3	26.5±23.3						
Outcome															
Perfect	0%			0%											
Improved	57%	71.8±29.8	23.8±9.5	75%	60.7±44.1	0±0	50%	20.0	10.0						
Same/worse	43%	20.0±15.0	27.3±26.8	25%	60.0	62.0	50%	43.0	43.0						
DIP joint	1	8.0	18.0	2	10.0±7.1	6.5±9.2	0								
Outcome															
Perfect	0%			50%	15.0	0±0									
Improved	0%			0%											
Same/worse	100%	8.0	18.0	50%	5.0	13.0									

Profile n Finger closure: graft (149 patients and 160 hands)

Family origin		Sex		Hand dominance		Hand involved		Occupation	
Northern European	91%	Male	90%	Right	97%	Right	19%	Manual	45%
Japan	5%	Female	10%	Left	3%	Left	5%	Non-manual	55%
Southern European	4%					Both	76%		
		Other areas involved			33%	Associated diseases		Age at onset (years)	
						Epilepsy	3%	Male	42.1±13.0
		Family history			26%	Diabetes	4%	Female	45.9±12.8
						Alcoholism	11%	Age at operation (years)	
		Previous operation			48%	Trauma	9%	Male	53.6±11.5
								Female	56.1±10.8

Operation profile

Hand profile			Palm	Little finger	Thumb	Anaesthesia	
Palm only	9%	Operation				Local	14%
No palm		Local	15%	20%	6%	Regional	35%
		Regional	31%	20%	53%	General	51%
One ray	39%	Extensive	54%	57%	41%		
Two rays	27%	Amputation		3%		Procedure at	
Three or more rays	34%					PIP joint	22%
		Incision					
Thumb and thumb web	27%	Longitudinal	56%	80%	100%	Complications	29%
Index finger	18%	Transverse	44%	20%			
Middle finger	32%					Therapy	76%
Ring finger	53%	Closure					
Little finger	84%	Suture	36%	18%	67%	Splinting	51%
		Open	7%				
		Graft	57%	82%	33%		

Profile n contd.

	Little finger			Ring finger			Middle finger			Index finger			Thumb		
	n	Pre	Post	n	Pre	Post	n	Pre	Post	n	Pre	Post	n	Pre	Post
MP joint	31	43.3±26.7	1.8±5.4	16	40.4±18.6	2.5±10.0	5	35.2±30.5	1.0±2.2	0			4	31.5±13.0	0±0
Outcome															
Perfect	87%	42.2±25.9	0±0	94%	40.5±19.2	0±0	80%	41.5±31.3	0±0				100%	31.5±13.0	0
Improved	13%	50.0±38.1	13.8±8.5	6%	20.0	2.0	20%	10.0	5.0						
Same/worse	0%			0%			0%								
PIP joint	47	56.2±23.3	23.8±24.5	18	60.4±22.5	17.9±25.6	6	57.0±31.4	23.3±33.1						
Outcome															
Perfect	30%	43.5±17.8	0±0	56%	58.3±25.7	0±0	50%	33.3±20.8	0±0						
Improved	60%	63.8±20.3	29.4±19.0	33%	65.0±22.2	32.2±20.2	33%	78.5±26.2	27.5±3.5						
Same/worse	20%	43.0±34.0	59.4±26.1	11%	57.5±3.5	65.0±14.1	17%	85.0	85.0						
DIP joint	10	36.9±14.8	4.5±7.2	5	35.0±24.7	0±0	0								
Outcome															
Perfect	70%	37.7±17.8	0±0	100%	35.0±24.7	0±0									
Improved	30%	35.0±5.0	15.0±0	0%											
Same/worse	0%														

Profile o No recurrence or extension (180 patients and 229 hands)

Family origin		Sex		Hand dominance		Hand involved		Occupation	
Northern European	82%	Male	88%	Right	95%	Right	23%	Manual	58%
Japan	17%	Female	12%	Left	5%	Left	12%	Non-manual	42%
Southern European	1%					Both	65%		
		Other areas involved	21%			Associated diseases		Age at onset (years)	
						Epilepsy	2%	Male	51.1±10.8
		Family history	27%			Diabetes	7%	Female	53.6±13.6
						Alcoholism	12%	Age at operation (years)	
		Previous operation	0%			Trauma	16%	Male	58.4±10.5
								Female	59.1±12.4

Operation profile

Hand profile			Palm	Little finger	Thumb	Anaesthesia	
Palm only	8%	*Operation*					
No palm	4%	Local	7%	5%		Local	6%
		Regional	68%	50%	84%	Regional	50%
One ray	34%	Extensive	25%	45%	16%	General	44%
Two rays	31%	Amputation					
Three or more rays	27%	*Incision*				Procedure at	
		Longitudinal	76%	93%	100%	PIP joint	7%
Thumb and thumb web	21%	Transverse	24%	7%			
Index finger	8%					Complications	19%
Middle finger	28%	*Closure*					
Ring finger	66%	Suture	80%	97%	95%	Therapy	79%
Little finger	67%	Open	15%	2%			
		Graft	5%	1%	5%	Splinting	41%

Profile p Recurrence or extension (158 patients and 219 hands)

Family origin		Sex		Hand dominance		Hand involved		Occupation	
Northern European	86%	Male	88%	Right	92%	Right	16%	Manual	48%
Japan	11%	Female	12%	Left	8%	Left	10%	Non-manual	52%
Southern European	3%					Both	74%		
		Other areas involved	36%			Associated diseases		Age at onset (years)	
						Epilepsy	3%	Male	47.2±12.3
		Family history	32%			Diabetes	9%	Female	56.7±10.4
						Alcoholism	12%	Age at operation (years)	
		Previous operation	0%			Trauma	15%	Male	55.6±10.9
								Female	61.1±10.3

Operation profile

Hand profile			Palm	Little finger	Thumb	Anaesthesia	
Palm only	5%	*Operation*					
No palm	4%	Local	4%	6%	15%	Local	3%
		Regional	65%	55%	85%	Regional	62%
One ray	31%	Extensive	31%	39%		General	35%
Two rays	32%	Amputation					
Three or more rays	33%						
		Incision				Procedure at	
Thumb and thumb web	21%	Longitudinal	78%	97%	100%	PIP joint	10%
Index finger	14%	Transverse	22%	3%			
Middle finger	37%					Complications	14%
Ring finger	63%	*Closure*					
Little finger	72%	Suture	83%	98%	100%	Therapy	73%
		Open	15%	1%			
		Graft	2%			Splinting	34%

THE RESULTS OF TREATMENT

Profile q Outcome at PIPJ V: perfect — 50 hands

Family origin		**Sex**		**Hand dominance**		**Hand involved**	
Northern European	85%	Male	88%	Right	94%	Right	32%
Japanese	11%	Female	12%	Left	6%	Left	6%
Southern European	4%					Both	62%
		Other areas involved	32%			**Associated diseases**	
						Epilepsy	2%
		Family history	36%			Diabetes	8%
						Alcoholism	8%
		Previous operation	20%			Trauma	18%

					Occupation	
					Manual	50%
					Non-manual	50%
					Age at onset (years)	
					Male	45.7±15.7
					Female	50.5±12.3
					Age at operation (years)	
					Male	56.2±11.9
					Female	61.2±13.0

Operation profile

Hand profile		Palm	Little finger	Thumb	Anaesthesia	
Palm only	4%				Local	4%
No palm	0%				Regional	51%
					General	36%
One ray	36%					
Two rays	36%					
Three or more rays	24%				**Procedure at PIP joint**	18%
Thumb and thumb web	28%	*Operation*				
Index finger	10%	Local	14%	16%		
Middle finger	20%	Regional	57%	46%	**Complications**	8%
Ring finger	42%	Extensive	29%	38%		
Little finger	96%	Amputation				
					Therapy	64%
		Incision				
		Longitudinal	100%	100%		
		Transverse				
					Splinting	40%
		Closure				
		Suture	64%	71%		
		Open	9%	0%		
		Graft	27%	29%		

Profile r Outcome at PIPJ V: improved — 145 hands

Family origin		Sex		Hand dominance		Hand involved		Occupation	
Northern European	88%	Male	78%	Right	97%	Right	17%	Manual	48%
Japanese	11%	Female	22%	Left	3%	Left	12%	Non-manual	52%
Southern European	1%					Both	71%		
		Other areas involved			31%			Age at onset (years)	
Associated diseases						Associated diseases		Male	49.0±13.4
		Male		Family history	27%	Epilepsy	5%	Female	51.4±12.7
						Diabetes	6%		
				Previous operation	26%	Diabetes	6%	Age at operation (years)	
						Alcoholism	16%	Male	58.2±10.4
						Trauma	12%	Female	61.1±11.1

Operation profile

Hand profile			Palm	Little finger	Thumb		Anaesthesia	
Palm only	1%	*Operation*					Local	5%
No palm	6%	Local	5%	8%			Regional	56%
One ray	40%	Regional	58%	35%			General	39%
Two rays	29%	Extensive	36%	57%				
Three or more rays	30%	Amputation					Procedure at PIP joint	21%
Thumb and thumb web	26%	*Incision*						
Index finger	10%	Longitudinal	100%	100%			Complications	18%
Middle finger	22%	Transverse						
Ring finger	47%	*Closure*					Therapy	85%
Little finger	99%	Suture	67%	78%				
		Open	19%	3%			Splinting	57%
		Graft	14%	19%				

Profile s Outcome at PIPJ V: same/worse — 66 hands

Family origin		Sex		Hand dominance		Hand involved		Occupation	
Northern European	89%	Male	77%	Right	95%	Right	15%	Manual	48%
Japanese	5%	Female	23%	Left	5%	Left	12%	Non-manual	52%
Southern European	2%					Both	70%		
Black American	6%								
		Other areas involved			29%	Associated diseases		Age at onset (years)	
						Epilepsy	3%	Male	47.9±13.6
		Family history			27%	Diabetes	12%	Female	49.7±16.1
						Alcoholism	23%	Age at operation (years)	
		Previous operation			30%	Trauma	12%	Male	57.0±12.7
								Female	61.7±13.2

Operation profile

Hand profile			Palm	Little finger	Thumb		Anaesthesia	
Palm only	2%	*Operation*					Local	9%
No palm	5%	Local	14%	14%			Regional	46%
		Regional	67%	32%			General	45%
One ray	32%	Extensive	18%	54%				
Two rays	24%	Amputation					Procedure at PIP joint	15%
Three or more rays	42%							
		Incision						
Thumb and thumb web	27%	Longitudinal	100%	100%			Complications	36%
Index finger	11%	Transverse						
Middle finger	38%							
Ring finger	36%	*Closure*					Therapy	82%
Little finger	98%	Suture	55%	87%				
		Open	36%	5%			Splinting	70%
		Graft	9%	8%				

D. Elliot

Bibliography of literature before 1900

Libraries

Each reference is indexed to the library or libraries in which it was found.
*1 Bibliothèque Interuniversitaire de Médecine,
    12 rue de l'Ecole de Médecine, 75006 Paris, France
*2 The Wills Library, Guy's Hospital Medical School,
    London Bridge, London SE1 9RT, UK
*3 John Rylands University Library of Manchester,
    University of Manchester, Oxford Road, Manchester M13 9PP, UK
*4 The Library of the Royal College of Physicians of Edinburgh,
    9 Queen Street, Edinburgh EH2 1JQ, UK
*5 The Library of the Royal College of Surgeons of England,
    35–43 Lincolns Inn Fields, London WC2A 3PN, UK
*6 The Library of the Royal Society of Medicine,
    1 Wimpole Street, London W1M 8AE, UK
*7 The Library, St Thomas's Hospital Medical School,
    St Thomas's Hospital, Lambeth Palace Road, London SE1 7EH, UK
*8 The Library of the Wellcome Institute for the History of Medicine,
    183 Euston Road, London NW1 2BP, UK
*9 Tyne and Wear Archives,
    Blandford House, Blandford Square, Newcastle upon Tyne NE1 4JA, UK
*10 National Library of Medicine,
    Bethesda, MD 20894, USA
*11 Science Library, University of Western Ontario,
    London, Ontario, Canada N6A 5B9
*12 Medical Library, McGill University,
    Montreal, Quebec, Canada H3G 1Y6
*13 William Boyd Library of the Academy of Medicine,
    288 Bloor West, Toronto, Ontario, Canada M5S 1V8
*14 University of Toronto Library,
    Toronto, Ontario, Canada M5S 1A5
*? These references have not been verified by the author.

Acknowledgements

I wish to thank the staff of the above libraries for their help in compiling this bibliography. In particular, I would like to acknowledge the considerable effort of Mme. Molitor (*1), Miss Cummings (*3), Miss Ferguson and Mr Milne (*4), Miss Griffiths and Mr Stewart (*6), and Miss Hibbott (*7) and thank them for their tolerance and good will. I would also like to thank Mrs Jeanette Botz, personal assistant to Dr R. M. McFarlane, for her help with the North American references.

Bibliography

Abbe R 1882 Dupuytren's contracture of the fingers. Illustrated Quarterly of Medicine and Surgery, New York 1: 41–42 *10
Abbe R 1886 On Dupuytren's finger-contraction — its nervous origin. Transactions of the New York Academy of Medicine 4: 239–259 *1, 3, 6, 11
reprinted in New York Medical Journal 1884 39: 436–440, 461–463 *6
abstracted in Medical Record, New York 1884 25: 470–472 *6
comments in discussion — Amidon, Gibney, Hamilton, Post, Ranney, Sayre and Weir
Abbe R 1888 Dupuytren's finger contraction. Further remarks on the theory of its nervous origin. Medical Record, New York 33: 236–239 *6
Adams W 1877 'Dupuytren's contraction' of the fingers. Medical Times and Gazette, London 1: 683 *3, 4
Adams W 1878 Contraction of the fingers (Dupuytren's contraction) and its successful treatment by subcutaneous divisions of the palmar fascia and immediate extension. British Medical Journal 1: 928–932
Adams W 1879 Observations on contraction of the fingers (Dupuytren's contraction). Churchill, London *4
Adams W 1881 Remarks on contraction of the fingers. Proceedings of the Medical Society of London 5: 132–133 *3, 4
comments in discussion — Fothergill, Gilbart-Smith, Owen and Watson
Adams W 1882 Dupuytren's contraction of the fingers in women. British Medical Journal 1: 84–85
Adams W 1885 On the treatment of Dupuytren's contraction of the fingers by subcutaneous division of the fascia and immediate extension. Congrès international périodique des sciences médicales, 1884, Copenhague. Compte-rendu des travaux de la section de chirurgie 2: 79–83 *?
Adams W 1890 Further observations on the treatment of Dupuytren's finger-contraction. Transactions of the Medical Society of London 13: 336–345 *3, 4

comments in discussion — Lockwood and Smith abstracted in British Medical Journal 1890 1: 722

Adams W 1891 On congenital contraction of the fingers and its association with 'hammer toe'; its pathology and treatment. Lancet ii: 165–168

Adams W 1892 On contractions of the fingers (Dupuytren's and congenital contractions) and hammer-toe. Churchill, London *4

Albinus B S 1734 Historia musculorum hominis. Haak & Mulhovium, Leiden, pp 472–475 *1

Alibert J L 1832 Monographie des dermatoses. Janet, Roux, Rignoux & Rey, Paris, pp 16–17 *1

Alibert J L 1833 Clinique de l'Hôpital St Louis, ou traité complet des malades de la peau. Cormon & Blanc, Paris, p 9 *4

Amat C 1886 Pathologie de la maladie de Dupuytren. Gazette Médicale de Paris 7s 3: 25–26, 39–40 *1, 4

Anderson W 1891 Lectures on contractions of the fingers and toes; their varieties, pathology and treatment. Lancet ii: 1–5, 57–59, 107–114, 161–163, 213–215, 279–282 translated in Wiener Medizinische Blätter 1891 14: 445–446, 462–464, 478–479 *4

Anderson W 1897 The deformities of the fingers and toes. Churchill, London, pp 4–43 *7

Annandale T 1865 The malformations, diseases and injuries of the fingers and toes. Edmonston & Douglas, Edinburgh, pp 234–244 *8

Avignon de Morlac J A 1832 Proposition du débridement de l'aponévrose-palmaire dans certains cas de rétraction permanente des doigts. Paris, thesis no. 1832/26 *1

Bähr F 1895 Kurze Bemerkung zu dem Artikel Bieganski's über die Dupuytrenische Contractur. Deutsche Medizinische Wochenschrift 21: 540 *1, 3, 6

Bailey S 1892 Dupuytren's finger contraction. American Practitioner and News, Louisville ns 14: 133–135 *1, 6, 12

Baillod J P 1877 Etude sur la rétraction de l'aponévrose palmaire. Paris, thesis no. 1877/138 *1

Bardeleben A 1872 Lehrbuch der Chirurgie und Operationslehre, vol 4. Reimer, Berlin, pp 722–728 *1

Bartholinus T 1668 Anatomy, vol 4, Chapter 9. Streater, London, p 166 *9

Baum 1878 Zur Lehre von Dupuytren's permanenter Fingercontractur. Centralblatt für Chirurgie 5: 129–134 *6

Bellamy E 1882 Note on the treatment of contracted fingers. Lancet ii: 439

Bérard A 1838 Main. In: Dictionnaire de médecine, vol 18. Béchet, Paris, pp 509–514 *1

Berger P 1892 Le traitement de la rétraction de l'aponévrose palmaire par une autoplastie (notice of a lecture only). Bulletin de l'Académie de Médecine 3s 27: 608 *1, 6

Bertrand C J H 1894 Contribution a l'étude de la rétraction de l'aponévrose palmaire (maladie de Dupuytren). Traitement par l'aponévrectomie. Nancy, thesis no. 1894/21 *1

Bieganski W 1895 Die spontane Contractur der Finger (Retractio aponeuroseos palmaris von Dupuytren) als ein trophischer Process centralen Ursprunges. Deutsche Medizinische Wochenschrift 21: 497–499 *6

Blum A 1882 Chirurgie de la main. Asselin, Paris, pp 126–133 *1

Bougery J M, Jacob N H 1839 Traité complet de l'anatomie de l'homme comprenant la médecine opératoire, vol 6. Delaunay, Paris, pp 134–135, plate 23 *6

Bouvier S H V 1836 Rétraction des doigts. Bulletin de l'Académie Royale de Médecine 1: 422–424 *1

Boyer A 1826 Traité des maladies chirurgicales, vol 11. Migneret, Paris, pp 55–56 *4

Brannis F 1846
see Tamplin 1846

Bryant T 1872 The practice of surgery. Churchill, London
1872 1st edi, pp 1015–1016 *5
1879 3rd edi, pp 323–324 *2

Buet 1832 Des diverses espèces de flexion permanente des doigts, et des moyens de les distinguer. Journal Complémentaire des Sciences Médicales 43: 172–177 *1, 3

Bulley F A 1864 Contraction of the fingers. The result of chronic rheumatic affection. Medical Times and Gazette, London 2: 218–219 *5

Bury J S 1882 Contraction of the palmar fascia. British Medical Journal 1: 189

Busch F 1882 Allgemeine Orthopädie, Gymnastik und Massage. In: v. Ziemssen H (ed.) Handbuch der allgemeinen Therapie, vol 5. Vogel, Leipzig, pp 91–96 *4
translated by Smith E N 1886
Busch: general orthopaedics, gymnastics and massage. In: von Ziemssen's handbook of general therapeutics, vol 5. Smith, Elder, London, pp 94–99 *4

Cardarelli A 1889 Sulla origine nevropatico del morbo del Dupuytren. Atti del Congresso della Associazione medica italiana, 1887, Pavia 2: 64–68 *?

Carter T A 1881 Dupuytren's contraction of the fingers. British Medical Journal 2: 1014

Caspari D 1896 Ueber den neuropathischen Ursprung der Aponeurositis palmaris. Archiv für Unfallheilkunde 1: 143–157 *1

Cayla A 1883 Diabète et rétraction de l'aponévrose palmaire. Gazette Hebdomadaire de Médecine et de Chirurgie 2s 20: 770 *1, 3, 6

Chassaignac E 1858 Rétraction de l'apnévrose palmaire traitée avec succès par l'excision. Bulletins de la Société de Chirurgie 8: 506 *1

Chassaignac E, Richelot G 1822
see Cooper 1822

Chevrot F 1882 Recherches sur la rétraction de l'aponévrose palmaire et son traitement chirurgical. Paris, thesis no. 1882/238 *1

Chomel A F 1813 Essai sur le rhumatisme. Paris, thesis no. 1813/63: 41 *1

Cline H Sr 1777 Notes on pathology and surgery. Manuscript 28, St Thomas's Hospital Medical School Library, London, p 185 *7

Cline H Sr 1787 Notes of Thomas Smart (student) from a lecture by Henry Cline Senior. Manuscript 29, St Thomas's Hospital Medical School Library, London *7

Cline H Jr 1808 Notes of John Windsor (student) from a lecture by Henry Cline Jr. Manuscript collection, John Rylands University Library of Manchester, Manchester, pp 486–489 *3

Cline H Jr 1834
see Windsor 1834

Cloquet J G 1842
see Denonvillier C P, Lacroix J B 1842

Cooper A P 1822 On dislocations of the fingers and toes — dislocation from contraction of the tendon. In: A treatise

on dislocations and fractures of the joints. Longman, London, pp 524–525   *5
translated by Chassaignac B, Richelot G 1837 Oeuvres chirurgicales complètes de Sir Astley Cooper. Béchet, Paris, pp 122–123   *1
Costilhes J 1885 De la rétraction de l'aponévrose palmaire (maladie de Dupuytren). Paris, thesis no. 1885/140   *1
Coulon M E 1896 Traitemente de la rétraction de l'aponévrose palmaire. La Presse Médicale, Paris 4: 306   *1
Cruvheilhier J 1849 Traité d'anatomie pathologique générale, vol 1. Baillière, Paris, pp 695–696   *1
D'Ambrosia A 1892 Retrazione dell'aponevrosi palmare, malattia di Dupuytren, contrattura di flessione delle dita della mano. La Riforma Medica, Napoli 3: 482–489   *1
Daniel J M 1891 Contractions of the palmar fascia. Maritime Medical News, Halifax 3: 48–51   *11
Deneffe V 1895 De la rétraction de l'aponévrose palmaire. Annales de la Société de Médicine de Gand 74: 175–179   *?
Denonvilliers C P, Lacroix J B 1842 Muséum d'Anatomie Pathologique de al Faculté de Medécine de Paris ou Musée Dupuytren, part 2, section II. Béchet & Labé, Paris, p 812   *1
Després 1880 Rétraction de l'aponévrose palmaire d'origine traumatique. Gazette Médicale de Paris 6s 2: 202–203   *1
Dieffenbach J F 1845 Die operative Chirurgie, vol 1. Brockhaus, Leipzig, pp 840–842   *1
Doane S see Dupuytren 1832a
Druitt R 1870 The surgeon's vade mecum. Renshaw & Churchill, London
1870 10th edi, pp 653–654   *2
1878 11th edi, pp 696–697   *6
Dupuytren G 1831 De la rétraction des doigts par suite d'une affection de l'aponévrose palmaire — description de la maladie — operation chirurgicale qui convient dans ce cas. Compte rendu de la clinique chirurgicale de l'Hôtel Dieu par MM les docteurs Alexandre Paillard et Marx. Journal Universel et Hebdomadaire de Médecine et de Chirurgie Pratiques et des Institutions Médicales 5: 349–365   *1, 3
reprinted 1939–1940 Medical Classics 4: 127–141   *6
translated (partially) by Koch S 1968 Plastic and Reconstructive Surgery 42: 262–265
Dupuytren G 1832a Leçons orales de clinique chirurgicale faites à l'Hôtel-Dieu de Paris par M. le Baron Dupuytren, chirurgien en chef, vol 1, 1st edn. Germer Baillière, Paris, pp 2–24, 517–530   *1, 8
Dumont, Bruxelles 1836 Brussels edn.   *6
reviewed by Forget M 1833 Transactions Médicales 11: 274–279   *1
translated by Doane A S 1833 Clinical lectures on surgery delivered at Hôtel-Dieu . . . Collins & Hannay, New York   *8
translated by Doane A S 1834 Lezioni verbali di clinica chirurgica . . . Paulo Lampato, Venice   *8
Dupuytren G 1832b Fascicule d'observations sur la rétraction des doigts. Clinique chirurgicale de l'Hôtel-Dieu de Paris (service de M. Dupuytren) par M. le docteur Alexandre Paillard. Journal Universel et Hebdomadaire de Médecine et de Chirurgie Pratiques et des Institutions Médicales 6: 67–76   *1

Dupuytren G 1832c–1834 Reports and further discussions/critiques of Dupuytren's work on retraction of the fingers.
Avignon de Morlac   Thesis 1832: see Avignon de Morlac   *1
Lemoine-Maujet   Thesis 1832: see Lemoine-Maujet   *1
Editorial   London Medical and Surgical Journal 1832 1: 266–268   *6
Vidal de Cassis   Gazette Médicale de Paris 1832 1s 3: 41   *1
Editorial   Gazette Médicale de Paris 1832 1s 3: 679–680   *1
Editorial   Gazette des Hôpitaux, Civils et Militaires 1833 7: 18–19   *1
Forget M   Transactions Médicales 1833 11: 77–79   *1
Guérin J   Gazette Médicales de Paris 1833 2s 1: 111–113   *1
Editorial   Lancet 1834 2: 222–225

Durel L 1888 Essai sur la maladie de Dupuytren (rétraction de l'aponévrose palmaire). Considerations nouvelles sur l'historique, l'étiologie et les procédés de traitement (procédé operatoire de M. Trélat). Paris, thesis no. 1888/227   *1, 4
Erichsen J E 1853 The science and art of surgery. Walton & Maberly, London, p 654   *2
Eulenburg A 1864 Einige Bemerkungen über die 'flectirten Finger-Contracturen'. Berliner Klinische Wochenschrift 1: 224–226, 234–237   *6
Eulenburg A 1870 Electrotherapeutische Mittheilungen. Berliner Klinische Wochenschrift 7: 196–198   *1
Eulenburg A 1883 Neuritis des N. ulnaris im Zusammenhange mit 'Strangcontracturen' der Finger. Neurologisches Centralblatt 2: 49–53   *1
Fasquelle A 1892 Contributions a l'étude du traitement chirurgical de la contracture de Dupuytren, dite rétraction de l'aponévrose palmaire. Lyon, thesis no. 1892/724   *1
Féré C 1897 Note sur la rétraction de l'aponévrose palmaire. Revue de Chirurgie 17: 797–804   *1, 3, 4, 6
Féré c 1899 Note sur la rétraction de l'aponévrose palmaire. Revue de Chirurgie 20: 272–277   *1, 3, 4, 6
Fergusson W 1842 A system of practical surgery. Churchill, London
1842 1st Edn, pp 202–204   *5
1870 5th Edn, pp 259–262   *6
Ferrari G 1883 Retrazione delle dita mignolo, anulare e pollice della mano sinistra; mignolo, anulare e medio della destra da contrattare del Dupuytren. Salute: Italia Medicina Genova 17: 1–3 (2s)   *?
Fisher F R 1885 The treatment of Dupuytren's contraction of the palmar fascia. British Medical Journal 1: 327
Fisher F R 1886 In Deformities of the Upper Limb. In: Ashhurst J (ed) The international encyclopaedia of surgery, vol 6. Macmillan, London, pp 1055–1059   *4
Forget M 1833 see Dupuytren 1833
Fort J A 1869 Des difformités congénitales et acquises des doigts. Paris, Concours pour l'Agrégation no. 1869/ -, pp 146–158   *1
Gangolphe M 1891 Traitement de la rétractopm de l'aponévrose palmaire par les sections multiples sous-cutanées. Mémoires et Comptes-Rendus de la Société des Sciences Médicales de Lyon 31 part 2: 214–217   *1

comments in discussions — Icard and Tripier reprinted in Lyon Médical 1891 68: 577–579 *1, 6

Gant F J 1878 The science and practice of surgery, vol 1, 2nd edn. Baillière, Tindall & Cox, London, pp 832–833 *6

Garrod A E 1893 On an unusual form of nodule upon the joints of the fingers. St Bartholomew's Hospital Report 29: 157–161 *6

Geck O 1889 Uber die Dupuytren'sche Fingercontractur. Bonn, thesis no. 1889/21 *1

Gemmel 1899 Drei Fälle doppelseitiger symmetrischer Contractur der Palmaraponeurose (Dupuytren) im Anschluss an Gicht. Deutsche Medizinische Wochenschrift 25: 286–287 *1, 3, 6

Gerdy P N 1852 Maladies générales et diathèses, vol 2. Victor Masson, Paris, pp 66–68 *1

Gersuny R 1884 Operation bei Kontraktur der Palmaraponeurose. Wiener Medizinische Wochenschrift 34: 969–971 *1, 3, 6

Gibney 1883 Adam's operation for Dupuytren's finger contraction. Medical Record, New York 23 and 24: 134 *1, 6
comment in discussion — Hunter

Gosselin 1877 Flexion incomplète et permanente de l'auriculaire due à l'existence d'une bride fibreuse. Gazette des Hôpitaux, Civils et Militaires 50: 649–650 *6

Goyrand G 1833 Nouvelles recherches sur la rétraction permanente des doigts. Mémoires de l'Académie Royale de Médecine 3: 489–496 *1, 3
critique by Sanson J, Breschet G 1833 Mémoires de l'Académie Royale de Médecine 3: 496–500 *1, 3
discussion following presentation of this critique reported in Gazette Médicale de Paris 1834 2s 2: 219 *1, 6
comments in discussion — Barthélemey, Cloquet, Dupuy, Lisfranc, Martin-Solon and Velpeau

Goyrand G 1835 De la rétraction permanente des doigts. Gazette Médicale de Paris 2s 3: 481–486 *1, 3, 6

Grapow M 1887 Die Anatomie und physiologische Bedeutung der Palmaraponeurose. Archiv für Anatomie und Physiologie, Leipzig Anatomische Abtheilung 2–3: 143–158 *1, 3, 6

Gray H 1890 Anatomy, 12th edn. Longmans, Green, London, p 439 *5

Guérin J 1833
see Dupuytren 1833

Guérin J 1842–1843 Discussion sur la ténotomie des fléchisseurs de la main. Bulletin de l'Académie Royale de Médicine 8: 129, 154, 230, 253, 341–349 (see p 357 Velpeau) *1, 6

Guinebault P 1897 Contribution á l'étude de la rétraction de l'aponévrose palmaire (maladie de Dupuytren). Paris, thesis no. 1897/117 *1

Hadlich
see Regis 1887

Hardie J 1884–1885 On the treatment of Dupuytren's contraction of the fingers. Medical Chronicle, Manchester 1: 9–16 *3, 4

Hardie J 1885 The treatment of Dupuytren's finger-contraction (letter). British Medical Journal 1: 681

Hawkins C 1835 Contraction of the fingers. London Medical Gazette 15: 814–815 *6

Hawkins C 1844 On contraction of the fingers of both hands. London Medical Gazette 34: 277–278 *6

Hedges C E 1896 The relation of gout and rheumatism to Dupuytren's contraction of the palmar fascia, with results of treatment by Adam's operation. St Bartholomew's Hospital Report 32: 119–144 *6

Helferich H 1880 Contractur der Fascia palmaris beider Hände. Aerztliches Intelligenz-Blatt 27: 161–162 *1

Helmuth W T 1887–1888 Contraction of the palmar fascia. Report of Helmuth House, New York 2: 47 *10

Heyfelder J 1845 Die Contractura digiti minimi manus sinist, aponeurotica. Das Chirurgische und Augenkranken-Clinicum der Universität Erlangen, pp 32–33 *4

Hoffa A 1989 Ein Beitrag zu den Erkrankungen der Plantarfascie. Centralblatt für Chirurgie 25: 166–167 *1

Holmes T
see Little 1862

Homans J 1887 A case of contracted fingers (Dupuytren's contraction) successfully operated upon after the method of Mr Adams (illustrated). Boston Medical and Surgical Journal 116: 177–179 *6

Howse H G 1892–1893 A case of Dupuytren's contraction affecting both hands. Clinical Journal, London 1: 307–308 *3, 6

Hutchinson J 1886 Simulation by muscular action of Dupuytren's contraction of the palmar fascia. British Medical Journal 1: 1097

Hutchinson J 1894–1897 Archives of Surgery
West, Newman, London
1894 5: 176, 333
1895 6: 180, 266
1896 7: 149, 285, 291, 335–343
1897 8: 170 *6

Jaerisch M 1898 Uber Dupuytren'sche Finkerkontrakturen. Halle a S., thesis no. 1898/- *1

Jeanpierre A 1882 Considerations sur la rétraction de l'aponévrose palmaire. Paris, thesis no. 1882/108 *1

Jobert de Lamballe A J 1849 Sur la flexion permanente des doigts. Gazette des Hôpitaux, Civils et Militaires 3s 1: 415–416 *1, 6

Keen W W 1881–1882 The etiology and pathology of Dupuytren's contraction of the fingers. Proceedings of the Philadelphia County Medical Society 4: 108–116 *10
reprinted in Philadelphia Medical Times 1882 12: 370–378 *6

Keen W W 1889 Dupuytren's finger contraction. Operation by removal of the contracting band by open wound. Immediate cure without reaction or pain. Proceedings of the Philadelphia County Medical Society 10: 258–261 *10

Keen W W 1890
see Gray 1890

Kingsbury G C 1891 Dupuytren's contraction of the palmar fascia treated by hypnotism. British Medical Journal 1: 62–63

Kirby J 1849 On an unusual affection of the penis. Dublin Medical Press 22: 209–210 *4, 6

Kisgen P 1889 Uber Dupuytren'sche Fingerkontrakturen. Wurzburg, thesis no. 1889/86 *1

Kocher T 1887 Behandlung der Retraktion der Palmaraponeurose. Centralblatt für Chirurgie 14: 481–487, 497 502 *3, 6
abstracted in Ricklin E 1887 Gazette Médicale de Paris 7s 4: 345–346 *1

Koenig F 1877 Lehrbuch der speciellen Chirurgie, vol 2. Hirschwald, Berlin, pp 703–706 *1

Lacroix C J 1868 Consedérations sur la flexion permanente des doigts et des moyens d'y remédier. Paris, thesis no. 1868/126 *1

Lane W A 1885–1886 Flexion of the fingers — Dupuytren's etc. and some senile changes in joints. Guy's Hospital Reports 43: 53–61 *6

Lancereaux E 1883 Traite de l'Herpétisme. Delahaye & Lacrosnier, Paris, pp 179–180 *1

Lange 1885 Zur Aetiologie der Dupuytren'schen Fingercontractur. Archiv für pathologische Anatomie und Physiologie und für klinische Medicin 102: 220 *1, 3, 6

Langhans 1887
 see Kocher 1887

Largilliére L S 1878 Essai de la rétraction de l'aponévrose palmaire. Paris, thesis no. 1878/247 *1

Le Bec 1887 Rétraction de l'aponévrose palmaire; dissection de la bride fibreuse. Gazette des Hôpitaux, Civils et Militaires 60: 488 *1, 3, 4, 6

Ledderhose G 1897 Zur Pathologie der Aponeurose des Fusses und der Hand. Archiv für klinische Chirurgie 55: 694–712 *1, 6

Le Dentu 1875 Main. In: Nouveau dictionnaire de médecine et de chirurgie pratique, vol 21 (LYC-MEC). Baillière, Paris, pp 358–361, plate III *1

Legueu F, Juvara E 1892 Des aponévroses de la paume de la main.
 Bulletins de la Société Anatomique de Paris 5s 6: 383–400 *1

Lemoine-Maudet J 1832 Dissertation sur la rétraction permanente des doigts, ayant pour cause la rétraction de l'aponévrose palmaire. Paris, thesis no. 1832/141 *1

Lepicard M 1889 Nerveux et arthritiques. Paris, thesis no. 1889/40, pp 64–66 *1

Little E M 1843–1844 Lectures on the deformities of the human frame, delivered at the Orthopaedic Institute, London during 1943 — lecture 11 (notice of lectures only). Lancet i: 852

Little E M 1862 Deformity from disease of the palmar fascia. In: Holmes T (ed) A system of surgery. Longman, Green, London
 1862 1st edn, vol 3, p 588
 1870 2nd edn, vol 3, pp 697–699 *6

Little E M 1880 Palmar hand and finger contraction. Abstract of the Transactions of the Hunterian Society, pp 29–36 *6
 comments in discussion — Adams, Baker, Bird, Davies-Colley, Lucas and MacKenzie

Lockwood C B 1886 Contractions of the digital and palmar fascia. Transactions of the Pathological Society, London 37: 556–559 *6

Macready J 1890 On the treatment of Dupuytren's contractions of the palmar fascia. British Medical Journal 1: 411–414

Madelung O W 1875 Die Aetiologie und die operative Behandlung der Dupuytren'schen Fingerverkrümmung. Berliner Klinische Wochenschrift 12: 191–193, 207–208 *6
 translated as first part of the causes and operative treatment of Dupuytren's contracture. (see Madelung 1876) abstracted in Dublin Journal of Medical Science 1876 62: 486–488 *6

Madelung O W 1876 The causes and operative treatment of Dupuytren's finger contraction. Trübner, London *5

Madelung O W 1877 Ueber die Operation der Dupuytren'schen Fingerverkrümmung. Report of Fünfter Congress, Berlin, 19–22 April 1876, Verhandlungen der Deutschen Gesellschaft für Chirurgie 5: 72–77 *1
 comments in discussion — Busch, König and Küster

Madelung O W 1886 Uber eine der Dupuytren'schen Palmarkontraktur entsprechende Erkrankung der Planta. Centralblatt für Chirurgie 13: 758 *3, 6

Maisonneuve 1840 Post-mortem report. Bulletins de la Société Anatomique de Paris 15: 77 *1

Malgaigne J F 1862 Leçons d'orthopédie. Delahaye, Paris, pp 7–13 *1

Mangiavillani G 1896 Sopra un caso di retrazione dell'aponevrose palmare. La Riforma Medica, Napoli 4: 254–259, 271–273, 284–287 *1

Maslieurat-Lagémard G E 1839 De l'anatomie descriptive et chirurgicale des aponévoroses et des membranes synoviales de la main, de leur application à la therapeutique et à la médecine opératoire. Gazette Médicale de Paris 7: 273–280 *1

Maslieurat-Lagémard G E 1840 Post-mortem report. Bulletins de la Société Anatomique de Paris 15: 106 *1

Mellet F L E 1835 De la flexion permanente des doigts. Manuel pratique d'orthopédie. Paris, De Just Rouvier et Lebouvier, pp 246–262

Menjaud A E 1861 De la rétraction spontanée et progressive des doigts dans ses rapports avec la goutte et le rhumatisme goutteux. Paris, thesis no. 1861/148 *1

Marker E 1897 Die Dupuytren'sche Fingerkontraktur. Berlin, thesis no. 1897/91 *1

Mills C K 1884–1885 A case of Dupuytren's contraction of the fingers.
 Proceedings of the Philadelphia County Medical Society 7: 14 *10
 reprinted in The Polyclinic (Philadelphia) 1884–1885 2: 36 *10
 reprinted in Maryland Medical Journal 1884–1885 2: 504–505 *13
 comments in discussion — Roberts and Angney reprinted in The Cincinnati Medical News 1884 8: 721–723 *10

Morel-Lavallée 1844 Thèse sur les rétractions accidentelles des membres. Paris Concours pour l'Agrégation no. 1844/t.2 no. 4 *1

Moser E 1894 Ueber Dupuytren'sche Fingercontracturen und deren Operationen. Berlin, thesis no. 1894/76 *1

Myrtle A S 1881 Dupuytren's contraction of the fingers. British Medical Journal 2: 894–895

Myrtle A S 1885 The treatment of Dupuytren's contraction of the palmar fascia. British Medical Journal 1: 378

Nélaton A 1859 Ele mens de pathologie chirurgicale. Germer Baillière, Paris
 1859 1st edn, vol 5, pp 937–940 *1
 1884 2nd edn, vol 6, p 1026 *4

Nicaise 1868 Flexion permanente des doigts; des causes anatomiques. Bulletins de la Société Anatomique de Paris 2s 13: 379–380, 428–429 *1, 6
 comments in discussion — Hénoque and Parmentier

Nichols J B 1899a A clinical study of Dupuytren's contraction of the palmar and digital fascia. American Journal of Medical Science, Philadelphia ns 117: 285–305 *1, 11

Nichols J B 1899b The histology of Dupuytren's contraction of the palmar fascia: report of microscopial examination in two additional cases. Medical News, New York 75: 491–493 *6

Paalzow 1899 Die Aponeurositis palmaris der Schuhmacher. Monatsschrift für Unfallheilkunde 6: 13–20 *1

Paget J 1875 On the minor signs of gout in the hands and feet. British Medical Journal 1: 665–666
Paillard A L M 1832
  see Dupuytren 1832
Paillard A L M, Marx M 1831
  see Dupuytren G 1831
Partridge 1854 Cast of the left hand of a middle-aged man and also a dissection of the same hand to show a contraction of the little finger. Transactions of the Pathological Society of London 5: 343 *5
Pavillon P
  see Velpeau 1841
Piechaud, Larauza 1894 Rétraction de l'aponévrose palmaire traitée et consedérablement ameliorée par l'application de boues thermales à Dax. Mémoires et Bulletins de la Société de Médicine et de Chirurgie de Bordeaux, pp 238–243 *1
Plater F 1614 Observationum in hominis affectibus, vol 3. König & Brandmyller, Basel, p 140 *8
Polaillon 1876 Main. In: Dictionnaire encyclopédique des sciences médicales 2s 4 (MAM-MAR) Asselin & Masson, Paris, pp 23–26, 104–110 *1
Polaillon 1886 Induration plastique du pénis — rétraction de l'aponévrose. L'Union Médicale de Paris 3s 42: 1–3 *1
Post A C 1876 On contraction of the palmar fascia and of the sheaths of the flexor tendons. Archives of Clinical Surgery 1: 43–56 *1, 14
  abstracted in Dublin Journal of Medical Science 1876 62: 486–488 *6
Reeves H A 1881 Remarks on the contraction of the palmar and planter fasciae. British Medical Journal 2: 1049
Reeves H A 1885a The rapid cure of Dupuytren's contraction by excision. British Medical Journal 1: 481
Reeves H A 1885b Bodily deformities and their treatment. A handbook of practical orthopaedics. H K Lewis, London, pp 353–372 *4
Régis E 1887 Un cas de maladie de Dupuytren dans la paralysie générale progressive. Association française pour l'Avancement des Sciences, Toulouse, part 2: 803–806 *1
  reprinted in Gazette Médicale de Paris 1887 7s 4: 582–583 *1
  abstracted in Hadlich 1887 Neurologisches Centralblatt 6: 558 *1, 3
Reid J 1836 Permanent flexion of the fingers from shortening and thickening of the palmar aponeurosis. Edinburgh Medical and Surgical Journal 46: 74–76 *5
Rémy C 1877 Endocardite végétante des valvules mitrale et tricuspide — rétraction de l'aponévrose palmaire par traumatisme. Bulletins de la Société Anatomique de Paris 4s 2: 275–277 *1
  reprinted in Le Progrès Médical 1877 5: 573–574 *1, 6
Richer P 1877 Rétraction de l'aponévrose palmaire. Bulletins de la Société Anatomique de Paris 4s 2: 124–129 *1
  reprinted in Le Progrès Médical 1877 5: 369–70 *1, 3, 6
  comments in discussion — Berger, Charcot, Després, Houel and Pozzi
Richet M A 1855 Traité pratique d'anatomie médico-chirurgicale. Chamerot, Paris, pp 852–854 *1
Riedinger J 1898 Bemerkungen zum Knochenbefund in der Plantarfascie. Centralblatt für Chirurgie 25: 693–696 *1, 3, 6
Rinne 1888 Ueber eine seltene Aetiologie der Dupuytren'schen Fingercontractur. Deutsche Medizinische Wochenschrift 14: 761–762 *6

abstracted in Verhandlungen der Medizinischen Vereine zu Greifwald (1888–89), Leipzig 1890, pp 42–44 *?
Rogues de Fursac A J B 1892 Traitement de la rétraction de l'aponévrose palmaire (maladie de Dupuytren) par l'autoplastic (méthode italienne modifiée). Paris, thesis no. 1892/368 *1
Roque P E 1872 De la rétraction de l'aponévrose palmaire. Paris, thesis no. 1872/414 *1
Rosch E 1891 Ueber die Dupuytren'sche Fingerkontraktur. Beiträge zur Caustik der Fingerkontraktur und ihrer Therapie. Strasburg, thesis no. 1891/- *4
Sabatier M L E 1849 Causes, diagnostic et traitement de la flexion permanente des doigts. Paris, thesis no. 1849/155 *1
Sanson L J, Breschet G 1833 *1, 3
  see Goyrand 1833
Sappey P C 1847 Manuel d'Anatomie Descriptive et de préparations anatomiques, vol 1. Germer Bailliére, Paris, pp 266–267 *1
Savory W 1894 A lecture on gout in some of its relations to surgery. Lancet i: 75–79
Schmidt A 1899 Ueber die Dupuytren'sche Palmarfasciencontractur. Wurzburg, thesis no. 1889/- *?
Schulz E 1879 Zur Aetiologie der Verkrümmung des vierten Fingers. Margurg, thesis no. 1879/- *?
Senator H 1898 Zwei Fälle von Tabes dorsalis — Tabesfuss und Tabes mit Dupuytren'scher Sehnencontractur. Berliner Klinische Wochenschrift 35: 633–636 *1, 3, 6
Sevestre A 1867 Note sur un cas de rétraction permanente des doigts.
Journal de l'Anatomie et de la Physiologie 4: 249–258, plates X and XI *1, 6
Smith E Noble 1882a The surgery of deformities. Smith, Elder, London, pp 91–94 *4
Smith E Noble 1882b
  see Busch 1882
Smith E Noble 1883 Some cases of lameness from abnormal conditions of the feet, chiefly from contractions of the muscles and fasciae. British Medical Journal 1: 1111–1112, 1168–1170
Smith E Noble 1885a Seventy cases of Dupuytren's contraction of the fingers. Proceedings of the Royal Medical and Chirurgical Society of London 1: 230–233 *6
  comments in discussion — Adams, Croft, Humphrey, Johnson and Walsham
  abstracted in British Medical Journal 1884 1: 603–604
  abstracted in Lancet 1884 1: 565
  reprinted in British Medical Journal 1885 1: 275–278
Smith E Noble 1885b The treatment of Dupuytren's contraction of the palmar fascia. British Medical Journal 1: 718
Souza-Leite 1886 Rétraction de l'aponévrose palmaire — de l'aponévrose plantaire. Rhumatisme articulaire aigu. Affection cardiaque. Le Progrès Médical 3: 816–818 *1, 3
Stephenson S H A 1885 Hereditary transmission of Dupuytren's contraction. British Medical Journal 1: 681
Stuparich 1898 Symmetrische Dupuytren'sche Contractur am kleinan Finger. Wiener Medizinische Presse 39: 57–58 *6
Tamplin R W 1846 Lectures on the nature and treatment of deformities. Longman, London, pp 256–267 *5
  translated in Brannis F 1846 Ueber Natur, Erkenntniss und Behandlung der Verkrümmungen. Förstner, Berlin *6
Tarnowski J 1887 Ueber die Retraktion der

Palmaraponeurose. Erlangen, thesis no. 1887/38 *1
Terrillon 1888 Rétraction de l'aponévrose palmaire des deux mains. Operation. Redressement des doigts. Bulletins et Mémoires de la Société de Chirurgie de Paris 14: 265–266 *1, 6
Testi A 1895 Contributo alla patogenesi della malattia di Dupuytren. Lavori dei Congressi di Medicina Interna, Milano 6: 234–241 *?
Topinard 1859–1863 Flexion permanente des doigts, spontanée et héréditaire (rétraction de l'aponévrose palmaire).
Recueil des Travaux de la Société Médicale d'Observation de Paris 2: 459–469 *6
Tranquilli E 1892 Due casi di retrazione dell'aponevrosi palmare (malattia di Dupuytren). Bulletino della Societa Lancisiana degli Ospedali di Roma 12: 162–173 *1
abstracted in Sperimentale Communicaz. e Riv. Firenze 1893 50: 100 *?
reprinted in Il Bolletino delle cliniche, Milano 1893 10: 294–300 *1
Trélat 1887 Rétraction de l'aponévrose palmaire (maladie de Dupuytren). Gazette des Hôpitaux Civils et Militaires 60: 27–28 *1, 3, 4
Trélat 1888
see Durel 1888
Velpeau A L M 1833 Traité complet d'anatomie chirurgicale. Méquignon-Marvis, Paris
1833 2nd edn, vol 2, pp 575–576 *1
1837 3rd edn, vol 2, pp 471–472, 486 = 487 *4
translated in Hancock H 1838 Velpeau's anatomy of the regions. Longman, London, pp 413, 420–421 *4
Velpeau A L M 1835 Sur la rétraction des doigts. Gazette Médicale de Paris 2s 3: 511 *1
Velpeau A L M 1841 Leçons orales de cliniques chirurgicales faites a l'Hôpital de la Charité. recueillies et publiées par M. le Docteur P. Pavillon, vol 3. Germer Baillière, Paris, pp 332–346 *1, 3, 4
Velpeau A L M 1842–1843
see Guérin 1842–1843
Verneuil 1857 Observations pour servir à l'histoire de la flexion permanente des doigts. Revue de Thérapeutique Médico-Chirurgicales, Paris 5: 225–230 *?
Vespa 1895–1896 Sulla mmalattia di Dupuytren. Bulletino della Societa Lancisiana degli Ospedali di Roma 16 fasc.1 *?
Vidal de Cassis 1832
see Dupuytren 1832c

Viger J 1883 De la rétraction de l'aponévrose palmaire chez les diabetiques. Paris, thesis no. 1883/57 *1
Vizioli R 1886 Casi di contrattura ereditaria ripetentesi in 3 generazioni. Giornale di Neuropatologia 4: 1 *?
abstracted in Sommer 1887 Neurologisches Centralblatt, Leipzig 6: 58 *1
Vogt P 1868 Verkrummung und Steifigkeit der Finger. In: v. Pitha, Billroth C A T (eds) Handbuch der allgemeine und speciellen Chirurgie, vol 4, part 2B, section 10. Enke, Stuttgart, pp 141–145 *1
Vogt P 1881 Die Chirurgischen Krankheiten der Oberen Extremitäten. Enke, Stuttgart, pp 88–101 *4
Warner E 1884 A case of Dupuytren's contraction. Boston Medical and Surgical Journal 111: 345–346 *6
Weinlechner 1879 Dupuytren'sche Fingercontractur an beiden Handen, vorwiegend linkerseits. Die von Prof. Busch empfohlene Trennung der Fascia palmaris nach Bildung eines dreieckigen Lappens hatte, weil an der Contractur die Sehnen selbst einen grossen Antheil nahmen, nur einen mässigen Erfolg. Bericht der K K Krankenalstalt Rudolph Stiflung in Wien in Jahr 1878, pp 458–459 *1, 6
Weinlechner 1880 Dupuytren'sche Verkrümmung des kleinen und Ringfingers. Operirt nach Busch, der Lappen gangranescirt und Patient vor Heilung der Wunde an Tuberculose gestorben. Bericht der K K Krankenalstalt Rudolph Stiflung in Wien in Jahr 1879, p 473 *1, 6
Weitbrecht J 1742 Ligamenta artuum superiorum sectio secundum in syndesmologia sive historia ligamentorum corporis humani. ex Typographia Acadamiae Scientarum, Petropolis, pp 43–44, 50 *1
Whelan B 1891 A case of Dupuytren's contraction. Transactions of the Michigan State Medical Society 15: 193–194 *11
Windsor J 1808
see Cline 1808
Windsor J 1834 Permanent contraction of the fingers. Lancet ii: 501–502 *1
Zahrtmann M K 1897 Om Patogenesen af Retractio palmaris (Dupuytren). Hospitalstidende, Kjøbenhaven 4R 5: 1037–1047 *1
Zimmermann 1898 Dupuytren'sche Contractur. Wiener Klinische Wochenschrift 11: 224 *1, 6
abstracted in Monatschrift für Unfallheilkunde 1898 5: 153 *1

References

Abbe R 1888 Dupuytren's finger contraction: further remarks on the theory of its nervous origin. Medical Record (New York) 33: 236–239

Abbott A C 1929 Dupuytren's contraction. A review of the literature and a report of a new technique in surgical treatment. Canadian Medical Association Journal 59: 250 cited by Skoog (1948)

Abercrombie M, Flint M H, James D W 1954 Collagen formation and wound contraction during repair of small excised wounds in the skin of rats. Journal of Embryology and Experimental Morphology 2: 264–274

Abercrombie M, Flint M H, James D W 1956 Wound contraction in relation to collagen formation in scorbutic guinea-pigs. Journal of Embryology and Experimental Morphology 4: 167–175

Abercrombie M, James D W, Newcombe J F 1960 Wound contraction in rabbit skin studied by splinting the wound margins. Journal of Anatomy (London) 94: 170

Adams W 1878 Contraction of the fingers (Dupuytren's contracture) and its successful treatment by subcutaneous divisions of the palmar fascia and immediate extension. British Medical Journal 1: 928

Adams W 1878 Contraction of the fingers (Dupuytren's contraction). Lancet 29: 928

Adams W 1879 Observations on contraction of the fingers. J & A Churchill, London

Addison A 1984 Knuckle pads causing extensor tendon tethering. Journal of Bone and Joint Surgery 66-B: 128

Akeson W H, Amiel D, LaViolette D 1967 The connective-tissue response to immobility: a study of the chondroitin-4 and 6-sulfate and dermatan sulfate changes in periarticular connective tissue of control and immobilized knees of dogs. Clinical Orthopaedics 51: 183–197

Albin R, Brickley D, Smith R, Glimcher M J 1975 Biochemical and structural studies of the palmar fascia in Dupuytren's Contracture. Journal of Bone Joint Surgery (America) 57: 585

Albinus B S 1734 Historia musculorum hominis. Leidae batavorum. Bibliotheque de Chirurgie, Paris

Ali I U, Mautner V, Lanza R, Hynes R O 1977 Restoration of normal morpohology, adhesion and cytoskeleton in transformed cells by addition of a transformation sensitive surface protein. Cell 11: 115

Allan P W 1977 The fibromatoses: a clinicopathologic classification based on 140 cases. American Journal of Pathology 1: 255

Anderson W 1897 The deformities of the fingers and toes. Churchill, London, pp 4–43

Annandale: 1865 The malformations, diseases and injuries of the fingers and toes. Edinburgh cited by Skoog (1948)

Anson B J, Ashley F L 1940 The mid palmar compartment, associated spaces and limiting layers. Anatomical Record 78: 389–407

Arafa M, Steingold R F, Noble J 1984 The incidence of Dupuytren's disease in patients with rheumatoid arthritis. The Journal of Hand Surgery 9B: 165–169

Arem J A, Madden J W 1976 Effects of stress on healing wounds; 1. Intermittent noncyclical tension. Journal of Surgical Research 20: 93–102

Arieff A J, Bell J 1956 Epilepsy and Dupuytren's contracture. Neurology 6: 115

Ariyan S, Krizek T J 1976 In defense of the open wound. Archives of Surgery 3: 293–296

Ariyan S, Enriquez R, Krizek T J 1978 Wound contraction and fibrocontractive disorders. Archives of Surgery 113: 1034–1046

Aron E 1977 Maladie de Dupuytren et alcoolisme chronique recherchéd'un lien pathogénique groupes HL-A. Semainedes Hopitauxde Paris 53: 139

Ashley F L 1953 A two-stage operation for Dupuytren's contracture. Plastic and Reconstructive Surgery 12: 79–85

Azzarone B, Failly-Crepin C, Daya-Grosjean L, Chaponnier C, Gabbiani G 1983 Abnormal behavior of cultured fibroblasts from nodule and nonaffected aponeurosis of Dupuytren's disease. Journal of Cellular Physiology 117: 353–361

Baarnhielm G 1905 Bidrag till den operative behandlingen afden Dupuytren'ska fingerkontrakturen. Hygiea 67: 719 cited by Skoog (1948)

Badalamente M, Stern L, Hurst L 1983 The pathogenesis of Dupuytren's contracture: contractile mechanisms of the myofibroblasts. Journal of Hand Surgery 8: 235

Bailey A J, Duance V C 1980 Editorial. Collagen in acquired connective tissue diseases: an active or passive role? European Journal of Clinical Investigation 10: 1–3

Bailey A J, Etherington D J 1980 Metabolism of collagen and elastin. In: Neuberger A (ed) Comprehensive biochemistry, vol 19B. Elsevier, Amsterdam, p 299

Bailey A J, Robins S P, Balian G 1974 Biological significance of the intermolecular crosslinks of collagen. Nature (London) 251: 105

Bailey A J, Bazin S, Sims T J, Le Lous M, Nicoletis C, Delaunay A 1975a Characterization of the collagen of

human hypertrophic and normal scars. Biochimica Biophysica Acta 405: 412
Bailey A J, Sims T J, Le Lous M, Bazin S 1975b Collagen polymorphism in experimental granulation tissue. Biochemica Biophysics Research Communications 66: 1160
Bailey A J, Sims T J, Gabbiani G, Bazin S, LeLous M 1977 Collagen of Dupuytren's disease. Clinical Science and Molecular Medicine 53: 499–502
Bailey A J, Light N D, Atkins E D T 1980 Chemical cross-linking restrictions on models for the molecular organization of the collagen fibre. Nature (London) 288: 408
Bailey A J, Sims T J, Light N D 1984 Crosslinking of type IV collagen. Biochemical Journal 218: 713
Baker G C, Watson H K 1980 Relieving the skin shortage in Dupuytren's disease by advancing a series of triangular flaps: how to design and use them. British Journal of Plastic Surgery 33: 1
Balletico M, Campailla E 1972 Studio elettroencefalografico della malattia di Dupuytren. Minerva Ortopedica 23: 57
Bandman E 1985 Myosin isoenzyme transitions in muscle development, maturation, and disease. International Review of Cytology 97: 97–131
Barclay T L 1972 Observations on Skoog's operation for Dupuytren's contracture. The Hand 4: 188–189
Barnard K, Gathercole L J, Bailey A J 1987a Basement membrane collagen — evidence for a novel molecular packing. FEBS Letters — in press
Barnard K, Light N D, Bailey A J 1987b Chemistry of the collagen cross-links. Biochemical Journal — in press
Barnes M J, Constable B J, Morton L F, Kodicek E 1971a Hydroxylysine in the N-terminal telopeptides of skin collagen from chick embryo and newborn rat. Biochemical Journal 125: 925
Barnes M J, Constable B J, Morton LF, Kodicek E 1971b Hydroxylysine in the N-terminal regions of the α_1 and α_2 chains of various collagens. Biochemical Journal 125: 433
Barnes M J, Constable B J, Morton L F, Royce P M 1974 Age-related variations in hydroxylation of lysine and proline in collagen. Biochemical Journal 139: 461
Bartal A H, Stahl S, Karev A, Lichtig C 1987 Dupuytren's contracture studied with monoclonal antibodies to connective tissue differentiation antibodies. Clinical and Experimental Immunology 68: 457
Bartholinus T 1668 Anatomy in four books and four manuals. Book 4, vol 90 Culpeper, London, p 166
Barton N J 1984 Dupuytren's disease arising from the abductor digiti minimi. Journal of Hand Surgery 9B: 265
Bassot J 1965 Traitement de la maladie de Dupuytren par exerèse pharmacodynamique isolée ou complétée par un temps plastique uniquement cutané. Lille Chirurgical 20: 38
Bauer M, Polaczek R, Hopfel-Kreiner I, Schlogel R 1985 Vascular and neuro-vascular changes and the aetiology of Dupuytren's disease. In: Hueston J T, Tubiana R (eds) Dupuytren's disease, 2nd edn. Churchill Livingstone, Edinburgh pp 106–113
Baur P S, Larson D L, Stacey T R 1975 The observation of myofibroblasts in hypertrophic scars. Surgery, Gynecology and Obstetrics 141: 22–26
Bazin S, Delaunay A, Nicoletis C, Delbet J P 1970 Biochimie des cicatrices humaines teneur en sialoglycoproteines et en mucopolysaccharides acides. Pathologie-Biologie (Paris) 18: 1071–1077

Bazin S, Le Lous M, Duance V C et al 1980 Biochemistry and histology of the connective tissue of Dupuytren's disease lesions. European Journal of Clinical Investigation 10: 9–16
Becchi G F, Olivieri M, Licitra G, Ghigliazza G B 1972 Valutazioni arteriografiche a pletismografiche nella malattia di Dupuytren. Rivista di Chirurgia della Mano 10: 232
Beckers-Bleukx G, Maréchal G 1985 Detection and distribution of myosin isozymes in vertebrate smooth muscle. European Journal of Biochemistry 152: 207–211
Bell E, Ivarsson B, Merrill C 1979 Production of a tissue-like structure by contraction of collagen lattices by human fibroblasts of different proliferative potential in vitro. Proceedings of the National Academy of Sciences USA 76: 1274–1278
Bellows C G, Melcher A H, Aubin J E 1981 Contraction and organisation of collagen gels by cells cultured from periodontal ligament, gingiva and bone suggest functional differences between cell types. Journal of Cell Science 50: 299–314
Bellows C G, Melcher A H, Bhargava U, Aubin J E 1982 Fibroblasts contracting three dimensional collagen gels exhibit ultrastructure consistent with either contraction or protein secretion. Journal of Ultrastructural Research 78: 178–192
Bellows C G, Melcher A H, Aubin J E 1982 Association between tension and orientation of periodontol ligament fibroblasts and exogenous collagen fibres in collagen gels in vitro. Journal of Cell Science 58: 125–138
Beltran J E 1985 Dupuytren's disease: the results of the open palm and digit technique. In: Hueston J T, Tubiana R (eds) Dupuytren's disease, 2nd edn. Churchill Livingstone, London, pp 142–148
Beltran J E, Jimeno-Urban F, Yunta A 1976 The open palm and digit technique in the treatment of Dupuytren's contracture. The Hand 8: 73–77
Benzonana G, Skalli O, Gabbiani G 1988 Correlation between the distribution of smooth muscle or non muscle myosins and α-smooth muscle actin in normal and pathological soft tissues. Cell Motility and the Cytoskeleton (in press)
Bereiter-Hahn J 1985 Architecture of tissue cells: the structural basis which determines shape and locomotion of cells. Acta Biotheoretica (Leiden) 34: 139–148
Berger P 1892 Traitement de la rétraction de l'aponévrose palmaire par une autoplastie. Bulletinde L'Académie de Médécine, Paris 56: 608 cited by Skoog (1948)
Berner P F, Frank E, Holtzer H, Somlyo A P 1981 The intermediate filament proteins of rabbit vascular smooth muscle: immunofluorescent studies of desmin and vimentin. Journal of Muscle Research and Cell Motility 2: 439–452
Bertrand J, Thomas J, Metman E H 1977 Maladie de Dupuytren et erythrose palmaire au cours des cirrhoses ethyliques. Semaine des Hôpitaux de Paris 53: 407
Bhatal P S 1972 Presence of modified fibroblasts in cirrhotic livers in man. Pathology 4: 139–144
Bhawan J, Bacchetta C, Joris U, Majno G 1979 A myofibroblastic tumor. Infantile digital fibroma (recurrent digital fibrous tumor of childhood). American Journal of Pathology 94: 19–29
Billig R, Baker R, Immergut M, Maxted W 1975 Peyronie's disease. Urology 6: 409–418

Birk D E, Trelstad R L 1985 Fibroblasts compartmentalize the extracellular space to regulate and facilitate collagen fibril, bundle and macro-aggregate formation. In: Reddi A H (ed) Extracellular matrix: structure and function. Alan R Liss, New York, pp 373–382

Bloom S, Cancilla P A 1969 Conformational changes in myocardial nuclei of rats. Circulation Research 24: 189–196

Bocanegra T S, King P, Vasey F B, Germain B F, Espinoza L R 1981 Dupuytren's contracture: a genetically predisposed disorder? Journal of Rheumatology 8: 1026–1027

Bocchi L, Orso C A, Lacovara V 1982 Rilievi sulla tecnica di Skoog nel trattamento della malattia di Dupuytren. Rivista di Chirurgia della Mano 19: 403

Bohannon R W 1982 Whirlpool versus whirlpool and rinse for removal of bacteria from a venous stasis ulcer. Physical Therapy, 62: 304–308

Bojsen-Moller F, Schmidt L 1974 The palmar aponeurosis and the central spaces of the hand. Journal of Anatomy 117: 55–68

Borden J 1974 The open finger treatment of Dupuytren's contracture. Orthopedia Review 3: 25

Borsetti G, Nebiolo R 1977 Surgical therapy of Dupuytren's disease: a comparison between two techniques (Italian). Rivista Italiana di Chirurgia Plastica 9: 71; Abstract Plastic and Reconstructive Surgery 61: 931

Bourgery J M 1834 Anatomie descriptive ou physiologique, vol 2. Paris, Libraire Anatomique, pp 127–128

Bowers W H 1986 The interphalangeal joints. Churchill Livingstone, Edinburgh, pp 2–13, 21–54

Bowser-Riley S, Bain A D, Noble J, Lamb D W 1975 Chromosome abnormalities in Dupuytren's disease. Lancet ii: 1282–1283

Boyes J H 1969 Dupuytren's contracture. The abductor minimi digiti band. In: Bürkle de la Camp H, Linder F, Trede M (eds) American College of Surgeons/Deutsche Gesellschaft für Chirurgie joint meeting Munich 1968. Springer Verlag, Berlin, p 349

Boyes J H (ed) 1971 Bunnell's Surgery of the Hand, 5th edn. p 231

Boyes J H, Jones F E 1968 Dupuytren's disease involving the volar aspect of the wrist. Plastic and Reconstructive Surgery 41: 205

Bradlow A, Mowat A G 1986 Dupuytren's contracture and alcohol. Annals of the Rheumatic Diseases 45: 304–307

Bray D, White J G 1988 Cortical flow in animal cells. Science 239: 883–888

Brett J G, Godman G C 1986 Cytoskeletal organisation affects cellular responses to cytochalasins: comparison of a normal line and its transformant. Tissue Cell 18: 175–199

Brickley-Parsons D, Eyre D R, Glimcher M J 1977 Direct evidence against natural reduction of aldehyde derived collagen crosslinks during maturation of collagen fibrils in vivo and in vitro. Transactions of the 23rd Annual Meeting of the Orthopaedic Research Society, 97

Brickley-Parsons D, Glimcher M J, Smith R J, Albin R, Adams J P 1981 Biochemical changes in the collagen of the palmar fascia in patients with Dupuytren's disease. Journal of Bone and Joint Surgery 63A: 787–797

Briedis J 1974 Dupuytren's contracture: lack of complications with the open palm technique. British Journal of Plastic Surgery 27: 218–219

Brouet J P 1986 Etude de 1000 dossiers de maladie de Dupuytren. In: Tubiana R, Hueston J T (eds) La maladie de Dupuytren, 3rd edn. Expansion Scientifique Francaise, Paris, pp 98–105

Brown J M, Flint M H 1982 Assessment of synthesis and degradation of glycosaminoglycan and plasminogen activator activity during tendon remodelling. Connective Tissue Research 9: 204

Brown J M, Flint M H 1983 Effects of removal of compressive forces on synthesis and degradation of GAG in fibrocatilagenous connective tissue. Connective Tissue Research 11: 241–242

Brunelli G 1982 Il morbo di Dupuytren. Trattamento chirurgico. Aponeurectomia sub-totale attrave: 50 incisione di Dieckmann Iselin. Rivista di Chirurgia della Mano 19: 297

Bruner J M 1949 The use of dorsal skin flap for the coverage of palmar defects after aponeurectomy for Dupuytren's contracture. Plastic and Reconstructive Surgery, 4: 599–565

Bruner J M 1951 Incisions for plastic and reconstructive (non-septic) surgery of the hand. British Journal of Plastic Surgery 4: 48

Bruner J M 1960 The selective treatment of Dupuytren's contracture with special reference to complications and indications for treatment. Transactions of the International Society of Plastic Surgeons 244–250

Bruner J M 1970 The dynamics of Dupuytren's disease. Hand 2: 172–177

Bruns R R, Press W, Engvall E, Timpl R, Gross J 1986 Type VI collagen in extracellular 100 nm periodic filaments and fibrils: identification by immunoelectron microscopy. Journal of Cellular Biology 103: 393

Buck R C 1953 Regeneration of tendon. Journal of Pathology and Bacteriology 66: 1–17

Buckingham B A, Uitto J, Sandborn C, Keens T, Kaufman F, Landin B 1981 Scleroderma-like syndrome in insulin-dependent diabetes: clinical and biochemical studies. Diabetes Care 2: 1027

Buckley I K, Porter K R 1967 Cytoplasmic fibrils in living cultured cells. A light and electron microscope study. Protoplasma 64: 349–380

Budtz-Olsen O E 1951 Clot retraction. Blackwell Scientific Publications, Oxford

Buell R, Wang N S, Seemayer T A, Ahmed M N 1976 Endobronchial plasma cell granuloma. A light and electron microscopic study. Human Pathology 7: 411–426

Bulfoni A 1980 Nevi vascolari, eritema palmare e contrattura di Dupuytren in corso di cirrhosi epatica alcoolica. Contributo clinostatistico. Archivo per le Scienze Mediche 137: 355

Bunnell S 1944 Surgery of the hand. JB Lippincott, Philadelphia

Burgess R C, Watson H K 1987 Stenosing tenosynovitis in Dupuytren's contracture. Journal of Hand Surgery 12A: 89

Burkhalter W E, Carneiro R S 1979 Correction of the attritional boutonnière deformity in high ulnar nerve paralysis. Journal of Bone and Joint Surgery 61A: 131

Burleigh M C 1977 Degradation of collagen by non-specific proteinases. In: Barrett A J (ed) Proteases in mammalian cells and tissues. North Holland Press, Amsterdam, p 285

Burridge K 1974 A comparison of fibroblast and smooth muscle myosins. FEBS Letters 45: 14

Burridge K 1981 Are stress fibers contractile? Nature 294: 691

Butler C, Madden J W, Davis W M, Peacock E E Jr 1977 Morphological aspects of experimental esophageal lye strictures: effect of steroid hormones, bougienage and induced lathyrism of acute lye burns. Surgery 81: 431–435

Butturini U 1950 Il trattamento della malattia di Dupuytren con l'acetato di alfatocoferolo. Minerva Medica 41: 1235

Byers H R, White G E, Fujiwara K 1984 Organization and function of stress fibers in cells in vitro and in situ: a review. In: Shay J W (ed) Cell and muscle motility. Plenum Press, New York, p 83

Byron P M, Muntzer E M 1986 Therapist's management of the mutilated hand. Hand clinics, hand rehabilitation. W B Saunders, Philadelphia, pp 69–79

Calatti A, Morelli E 1960 La nostra esperienza sul morbo di Dupuytren. Archivio di Ortopedia 73: 308

Callea F, Mebis J, Desmet V J 1982 Myofibroblasts in focal nodular hyperplasia of the liver. Virchows Archiv A (Pathology and Anatomy) 396: 155–166

Cammarn M R, Weckesser E C 1961 Dupuytren's contracture and diabetes. Proceedings of the 4th Congress de la Federation Internationale du Diabete 1: 445

Candiollo L 1956 Ricerche anatomiche sulla configurazione e sulla struttura dell'aponeurosi palmare superficiale nell'uomo. Zeitschrift für Anatomische Entwicklung der Gescn, 119: 500

Caplan A I, Fiszman M Y, Eppenberger H M 1983 Molecular and cell isoforms during development. Science 221: 921–927

Carlstedt C A 1987 Mechanical and chemical factors in tendon healing. Effects of indomethacin and surgery in the rabbit. Acta Orthopaedica Scandinavica 58 (suppl 224)

Caroli A, Vaccari A, Villani M, Botticelli A 1982 Le lesioni secondarie nel morbo di Dupuytren. Rivista di Chirurgia della Mano 19: 279

Carr T L 1970 A chemical–pathological study in Dupuytren's disease. The Hand 1: 50–55

Carr T 1974 Local radical fasciectomy for Dupuytren's contracture. The Hand 6: 40–49

Caster W C, Cabral A R 1985 Growth factors in human disease: the realities, pitfalls, and promise. Seminars in Arthritis and Rheumatism 15: 33

Castor C W, Ritchie J C, Williams C H et al. Composition and actions of a human platelet autocoid mediator. Arthritis and Rheumatism 22: 260–272

Caterson B, Lowther D A 1978 Changes in the metabolism of the proteoglycans from sheep articular cartilage in response to mechanical stress. Biochimica et Biophysica Acta 540: 412–422

Caughell K, McFarlane R, McGrouther D A, Martin A H 1987 Embryological development of the palmar aponeurosis and its relationship to the palmaris longus tendon (submitted for publication)

Caughell K A, McFarlane R M, McGrouther D A, Martin A H 1988 Developmental anatomy of the palmar aponeurium and its relationship to the palmans longus tendon. Journal of Hand Surgery 13A: 485–493

Cayla A 1883 Diabetes et rétraction de l'aponévrose palmaire. Iaz. Hebdanadaire de Médécine 20: 770

Ceruso et al 1987 Limited joint mobility: some observations about the possibility of surgical treatment. Journal of Hand Surgery

Chamley J H, Campbell G R, McConnell J D, Gröschel-Steward U 1977 Comparison of vascular smooth muscle cells from adult human, monkey and rabbit in primary culture and subculture. Cell and Tissue Research 177: 503–522

Chamley-Campbell J H, Campbell G R, Ross R 1979 The smooth muscle cell in culture. Physiological Reviews 59: 1–61

Chen W T, Hasagawa T, Hasegawa C, Weinstock C, Yamada K M 1985 Development of cell surface linkage complexes in cultured fibroblasts. Journal of Cell Biology 100: 1103

Chiandussi D, Mele R, Pittoni M, Polon A 1979 Aponeurectomia nel trattamento chirurgico del morbo di Dupuytren. La Chirurgia degli Organi di Movimento 65: 747

Chiu H F, McFarlane R M 1978 Pathogenesis of Dupuytren's contracture: a correlative clinical-pathological study. Journal of Hand Surgery 3: 1–10

Chow S P, Luk D K, Kung T M 1984 Dupuytren's contracture in Chinese. A report of three cases. Journal of the Royal College of Surgeons of Edinburgh 29: 49

Chung E B, Enzinger F M 1975 Proliferative fasciitis. Cancer 36: 1450–1458

Chung E B, Enzinger F M 1981 Infantile myofibromatosis. A review of 59 cases with localized and generalized involvement. Cancer 48: 1807–1818

Churg A M, Kahn L B 1977 Myofibroblasts and related cells in malignant fibrous and fibrohistiocytic tumors. Human Pathology 8: 205–218

Clarkson P 1961 The aetiology of Dupuytren's disease. Guy's Hospital Reports 110: 52

Clarkson P 1962 The radical fasciectomy operation for Dupuytren's contracture. A condemnation. Meeting of the Second Hand Club, Paris, May 23–26

Clarkson P 1966 Severe recurrent Dupuytren's contracture. British Society for Surgery of the Hand 370–371

Clarkson P, Pelly A 1962 The general and plastic surgery of the hand. Blackwell, Oxford, p 330

Cleland H, Morrison W A 1986 Dupuytren's disease in the thumb: two cases of a central cord. Journal of Hand Surgery 11B: 68

Cleland J 1878 On the cutaneous ligaments of the phalanges. Journal of Anatomy and Physiology 12: 526

Cline H 1777 Notes on pathology and surgery. Manuscript 28: 185, St Thomas's Hospital Library, London

Collinder B 1957 Survey of the Uralic languages. Almqvist & Wiksells, Uppsala

Colville J 1983 Dupuytren's contracture — the role of fasciotomy. The Hand 14: 162–166

Connolly W B 1974 Spontaneous healing and wound contraction of soft tissue wounds of the hand. The Hand 6: 26

Cooper A 1822 A treatise on dislocations and fractures of the joints, 1st edn. Longman, Hurst, Rees, Orme, Brown & Cox, London, pp 524–525

Cooper (ed) The craft of surgery. Little Brown, p 1302

Carrado E M, Messore L, Passaretti U, Lanza F, Napolitano F 1979 Malattia di Dupuytren. La Chirurgia degli Organi di Movimento 65: 741

Couch H 1938 Identical Dupuytren's contracture in identical twins. Canadian Medical Association Journal 39, 78: 225

Craik J E, McNeil I R R 1965 Histological studies on stressed skin. In: Kenedi R M (ed) Biomechanics and related bio-engineering topics. Pergamon Press, Oxford, pp 159–164

Craik J E, McNeil I R R 1966 Micro-architecture of skin and its behaviour under stress. Nature (London) 209: 931–932

Crisp A J, Heathcoate J G 1984 Connective tissue

abnormalities in diabetes mellitus. Journal of the Royal College of Physicians of London 18: 132

Critchley E M R, Vakil S D, Hayward H W, Owen V M H 1976 Dupuytren's disease in epilepsy: result of prolonged administration of anticonvulsants. Journal of Neurological Neurosurgery and Pyschiatry 39: 498

Crockett J E 1980 Adequate fasciectomy and the use of full-thickness skin gussets in the treatment of Dupuytren's contracture. Annals of the Royal College of Surgeons of England 62: 230–237

Crovella U 1982 Indagine statistica sulla malattia di Dupuytren in Piemonte. Rivista di Chirurgia della Mano 19: 261

Curtis R M 1954 Capsulectomy of the interphalangeal joints of the fingers. Journal of Bone and Joint Surgery 36A: 1219

Curtis R M 1970 Surgical restoration of motion in the stiff interphalangeal joints of the hand. Bulletin of the Hospital for Joint Disease 31: 1–6

Curtis R M 1974 Volar capsulectomy of the proximal interphalangeal joint in Dupuytren's contracture. In: Dupuytren's disease. Grune & Stratton, New York, p 135

Dahmen G 1968 Feingewebliche und submikroskopische Befunde beim Morbus Dupuytren. Zeitschrift für Orthopddische Chirurgie 104: 247

D'Andiran G, Gabbiani G 1980 A metastasizing sarcoma of the pleura composed of myofibroblasts. In: Fenoglio C M, Wolff M (eds) Progress in surgical pathology, vol II. Masson, New York, pp 31–40

Davis J S 1919 Plastic surgery, its principles and practice. London, p 673 cited by Skoog (1948)

David J E 1965 On surgery of Dupuytren's contracture. Plastic and Reconstructive Surgery 36: 277

Davis J S, Finesilver E M 1932 Dupuytren's contraction with a note on the incidence of the contraction in diabetes. Archives of Surgery 24: 933

de Campos Vidal 1972 Changes in the fibroblasts as revealed during fibrogenesis. Annales Histochimie (Paris) 17: 311–324

De la Caffinière J Y 1985 Travail manuel et maladie de Dupuytren. In:Tubiana R (ed) Maladie de Dupuytren. Expansion Scientifique Francais, Paris

Delbrück A, Schroder H 1983 Metabolism and proliferation of cultured fibroblasts from specimens of human palmar fascia and Dupuytren's contracture. The pathobiochemistry of connective tissue proliferation, II^2. Journal of Clinical Chemistry and Clinical Biochemistry 21: 11–17

Delbrück A, Zebe E, Bücher T 1959 Uber Verteilungsmuster von Enzymen des Energie-liefernden Stoffwechsels im Flugmuskel, Sprungmuskel und Fettkörper von Locusta migratoria und ihre cytologische Zuordnung. Biochemische Zeitschrift 331: 273–296

Delbrück A, Reimers E, Schönborn J 1981 A comparative study of the activity of lysosomal and main metabolic pathway enzymes in tissue biopsies and cultured fibroblasts from Dupuytren's disease and palmar fascia. Journal of Clinical Chemistry and Clinical Biochemistry 19: 931–941

Deming E G 1962 Y–V advancement pedicles in surgery for Dupuytren's contracture. Plastic and Reconstructive Surgery 29: 581

De Negri A 1972 La malattia di Dupuytren. Rivista di Chirurgia della Mano 10: 214

Desplas K, Meillere J 1932 Sur une technique operatoire concernant la maladie de Dupuytren. Bulletin et Mémoires de la Société Nationale de Chirurgie 58 :424 cited by Skoog (1948)

Dickie W R, Hughes N C 1967 Dupuytren's contracture: the value of hypotension in surgical correction. Plastic and Reconstructive Surgery 39: 600–602

Dickson W M 1928 Dupuytren's contracture after operation (discussion). Proceedings of the Royal Society of Medicine 21: 233

Dickie W R, Huges N C 1967 Dupuytren's contracture: the value of hypotension in surgical correction. Plastic and Reconstructive Surgery 39: 600–602

Diegelmann R F, Bryant C P, Cohen I K 1977 Tissue alpha-globulins in keloid formation. Plastic and Reconstruction Surgery 53: 418–423

Doillon C J, Hembry R M, Ehrlich H P, Burke J F 1987 Actin filaments in normal dermis during wound healing. American Journal of Pathology 126: 164–170

Donner L, de Lanerolle P, Costa J 1983 Immunoreactivity of paraffin-embedded normal tissues and mesenchymal tumors for smooth muscle myosin. American Journal of Clinical Pathology 80: 677–681

Donoff R B, Burke J F 1978 Abnormality of hypertrophic scar blood vessels. Journal of Surgical Research 25: 251–255

Donoff R B, Schweidt S 1982 The effect of skin grafting on the glycosidase activities and sulfated glycosaminoglycan content of healing wounds in rabbits. Journal of Surgery Research 33: 514–518

Drehmann 1913 Zur Operation der Dupuytren'schen Fingerkontraktur. Zentralblatt für Chirurgie 40: 19 cited by Skoog (1948)

Dresow B. Wiedenhöft G, Delbrück A 1986 The role of growth factor from human platelets in the pathogenesis of rheumatoid arthritis. In: Xth meeting of the Federation of European Connective Tissue Societies, Manchester 1986, Abstract 371

Dreyer C J 1961 Properties of stressed bone. Nature, (London) 189: 594–595

Duance V C, Restall D J, Beard H, Bourne F J, Bailey A J 1977 The location of three collagen types in skeletal muscle. FEBS Letters 79: 248

Duance V C, Shimokomaki M, Bailey A J 1982 Immunofluorescence localisation of type M collagen in articular cartilage. Bioscience Reports 2: 223

Dupuytren G 1831 De la rétraction des doigts par suite d'une affection de l'aponeurose palmaire. Journal Universel et Hebdomadaire de Médécine et de Chirurgie Practiques et des Institutions Médicales, Paris, 25: 349–365. Reprinted in Medical Classics 1939–1940 vol 4. Royal Society of Medicine, London, pp 127–141

Dupuytren G 1832 Lecons orales de clinique chirurgicale faites a L'Hôtel-Dieu. Balliere, Paris

Dupuytren G 1834 Permanent retraction of the fingers, produced by an affection of the palmar fascia. Lancet ii: 222–225

Durel L 1888 Essai sur la maladie de Dupuytren. Thèse, Paris cited by Skoog (1948)

Dvorak H F 1986 Tumors: wounds that do not heal. Similarities between tumor stroma generation and wound healing. New England Journal of Medicine 315: 1650–1659

Dylevsky I 1968 The origin and development of the palmar aponeurosis in human ontogeny. Sbornik Lekarsky 70: 353

Dylevsky I 1969 Critical comments on the so-called

developmental theory of Dupuytren's contracture. Sbornik Lekarsky 71: 289

Dylevsky I 1973 Phylogenetic development of the palmar aponeurosis. Folia Morphologica 21: 232

Early P F 1962 Population studies in Dupuytren's contracture. Journal of Bone and Joint Surgery 44B: 602–613

Eaton R G 1971 Joint injuries of the hand. Thomas, Illinois

Eckstein H 1922 Phalangenresektion zur Beseitigung von Fingerkontraktur. Zentralblatt für Chirurgie 49: 547

Eddy R J, Petro J A, Tomasek J J 1988 Evidence for the nonmuscle nature of the 'myofibroblast' of granulation tissue and hypertrophic scar. An immunofluorescence study. American Journal of Pathology 130: 252–260

Egawa T 1985 Dupuytren's contracture in Japan. Incidental study on outpatients in private practice of general orthopaedics. Journal of Japanese Society for Surgery of the Hand (in Japanese) 2: 536–539

Egawa T et al 1974 Dupuytren's contracture in Japan. Abstract of Japan US joint meeting of Hand Surgery, 94

Egawa T et al 1976 The incidence of Dupuytren's contracture in Japan: Survey in old people's homes. Central Japan Journal of Orthopaedic and Traumatic Surgery (in Japanese) 19: 984–986

Egawa T et al 1980 The incidence of Dupuytren's contracture in Japan: Survey in old people's homes. Seikeigeka (Orthopedic Surgery) (in Japanese) 31: 1699–1701

Egawai T, Horiki A and Senrui H 1985 Dupuytren's contracture in Japan. In: Hueston J T, Tubiana R (eds) Dupuytren's disease 2nd edn. Churchill Livingstone, Edinburgh p 100–103

Ehrlich H P, Brown H, White B S 1982 Evidence for type V and I trimer collagens in Dupuytren's contracture. Biochemical Medicine 28: 273

Einarsson F 1946 On the treatment of Dupuytren's contracture. Acta Chirurgica Scandinavica 93: 1–22

El-Labban N, Lee K W 1983 Myofibroblasts in central giant cell granuloma of the jaws: an ultrastructural study. Histopathology 7: 907–918

Engel J, Furthmayr H, Odermatt E et al 1985 Structure and macromolecular organization of type VI collagen. Annals of the New York Academy of Science 460: 25

Enzinger F M, Weiss S W 1983 Soft tissue tumors. C V Mosby, St Louis, pp 45–70

Enzinger F M, Lattes R, Torloni H 1970 Types histologiques des tumeurs des tissus mous. Classification histologique internationale des tumeurs no 3. World Health Organization Geneva, p 28

Etherington D J 1980 Proteinases in connective tissue breakdown. In: Evered D, Whelan J (eds) Protein degradation in health and disease. Ciba Foundation symposium 75. Excerpta Medica, Amsterdam, p 87

Eulenburg 1864 Einige Bemerkungenuber die flectirten Finger-contracturen. Berliner Klinische Wochenschrift 1: 224–226, 234–237

Eulenberg A 1883 Neuritis des Nervus ulnaris im Zusammenhange mit 'Strangcontracturen' der Finger. Neurologisches Centralblatt 3: 49

Evans R A 1986 The aetiology of Dupuytren's disease. British Journal of Hospital Medicine 36: 198–199

Evans J N, Kelley J, Low R B, Adler K B 1982 Increased contractility of isolated lung parenchyma in an animal model of pulmonary fibrosis induced by bleomycin. American Review of Respiratory Disease 125: 89–94

Evered D, Whelan J (eds) 1985 Fibrosis. Ciba Foundation symposium 114. Pitman, London

Eyre D R, Oguchi H 1980 The hydroxypyridinium crosslinks of skeletal collagens. Their measurement, properties and a proposed pathway of formation. Biochemical and Biophysical Research Communications 182: 403

Eyre D R, Paz M A, Gallop P M 1984 Crosslinks in collagen and elastin. Annual Review of Biochemistry 53: 717

Fahrer M 1980 The proximal end of the palmar aponeurosis. The Hand 12: 33

Fasquelle A 1892 Traitement chirurgical de la contracture de Dupuytren. Thèse Medicale, Lyon

Fere Ch, Francillon M 1902 Note sur la fréquence de la rétraction de l'aponévrose palmaire chez les aliènes. Revue de Médecine (Paris) 22: 539

Fergusson W 1846 A system of practical surgery. London, p 234

Ferrans V J, Roberts W C 1973 Structural features of cardiac myxomas. Histology, histochemistry and electron microscopy. Human Pathology 4: 111–146

Ferracint M 1941 La malattia di Dupuytren. Nistri-Lischi Editore, Pisa

Fietti V G, Mackin E J 1984 Open-palm technique in Dupuytren's disease. In: Hunter J M, Schneider L H, Mackin E J, Callahan A D (eds), Rehabilitation of the hand. C V Mosby Co, Springfield, pp 624–628

Fisher E R, Paulson J D, Gregorio R M 1978 The myofibroblastic nature of the uterine plexiform tumor. Archives of Pathology and Laboratory Medicine 102: 477–480

Fisher F R 1885 The treatment of Dupuytren's contraction of the palmar fascia. British Medical Journal 1: 327

Finlay J B, McFarlane R M 1981 A study of Dupuytren's tissue with the scanning electron miscroscope. Journal of Surgery 6: 482

Fisk G 1985 The relationship of manual labour and specific injury to Dupuytren's disease. In: Hueston J (ed) Dupuytren's disease, 2nd edn. Churchill Livingstone, Edinburgh

Fletcher C D M, Achu P, Van Noorden S, McKee P H 1987 Infantile myofibromatosis: a light miscroscopic, histochemical and immunohistochemical study suggesting true smooth muscle differentiation. Histopathology 11: 245–258

Fleischmajer R, Olsen B R, Kühn K 1985 Biology, chemistry and pathology of collagen. Annals of New York Academy of Science 460: 1

Flint M H 1971 The role of mucopolysaccharides in the healing and remodelling of split skin donor sites. Butterworths, Melbourne, pp 730–740

Flint M H 1972 The inter-relationships of mucopolysaccharides and collagen in connective tissue remodelling. Journal of Embryology and Experimental Morphology 27: 481–495

Flint M H 1981 Connective tissue organization. In: Tubiana R (ed) The hand, vol 1 Saunders, Philadelphia,

Flint M H 1983 The effect of physical forces on connective tissue. Connective Tissue Research 11: 338–339

Flint M H, Gillard G C 1980a Morphological changes following the release of pressure forces from the rabbit hind limb flexor digitorum profundus tendon. Connective Tissues Research 7: 200

Flint M H, Gillard G C 1980b The effect of wound

orientation on the healing of experimental rat wounds. Connective Tissue Research 7: 200

Flint M H, Lyons F 1975 The effect of heating and denaturation on the staining of collagen by the Masson trichrome procedure. Histochemical Journal 7: 547–555

Flint M H, Lyons F, Meaney M F, Williams D E 1975 The Masson staining of collagen — an explanation of an apparent paradox. Histochemical Journal 7: 529–546

Flint M H, Gillard G C, Merrilees M J 1980 The effects of local physical environmental factors on connective tissue organisation and glycosaminoglycan synthesis. In: Parry D A D, Creamer L K (eds) Fibrous proteins: scientific industrial and medical applications, vol 2. Academic Press, London, pp 107–119

Flint M H, Gillard G C, Reilly H C 1982 The glycosaminoglycans of Dupuytren's disease. Connective Tissue Research 9: 173–179

Flint M H, Craig A S, Reilly H C, Gillard G C, Parry D A D 1984 Collagen fibril diameters and glycosaminoglycan content of skin — indices of tissues maturity and function. Connective Tissue Research 13: 69–81

Foidart J M, Bere E W, Yaar M et al 1980 Distribution and immunoelectron microscopic localization of laminin, a noncollagenous basement membrane glycoprotein. Laboratory Investigation 42: 336

Fongo A 1982 Indicazioni e trattamento chirurgico del morbo di Dupuytren. Rivista di Chirurugia della Mano 19: 305

Fonzone Caccese L, Soldati O 1982 L'aponevrectosia selettiva secondo Skoog. Rivista di Chirurgia della Mano 19: 311

Fossati P, Delbart Ph, Derrien G 1975 La main diabétique. Lille Medical 20: 870

Frank E D, Warren L 1981 Aortic smooth muscle cells contain vimentin instead of desmin. Proceedings of the National Academy of Sciences USA 78: 3020-3024

Franke W W, Moll R 1987 Cytoskeletal components of lymphoid organs. I. Synthesis of cytokeratins 8 and 18 and desmin in subpopulations of extrafollicular reticulum cells of human lymph nodes, tonsils and spleen. Differentiation 36: 145-163

Franke W W, Schinko W 1969 Nuclear shape in muscle cells. Journal of Cell Biology 42: 326–331

Fraser R D B, MacRae T P, Miller A 1987 Molecular packing in type I collagen fibrils. Journal of Molecular Biology 193: 115

Fredet P 1932 A propos de la maladie de Dupuytren. Bulletin et Mémoires de la Société Nationale de Chirurgie 58: 440 cited by Skoog (1948)

Freehafer A A, Strong J M 1963 The treatment of Dupuytren's contracture by partial fasciectomy. Journal of Bone and Joints Surgery 45A: 1207–1216

Froscher W, Hoffman F 1983 Dupuytrensche Kontraktur and Phenobarbitaleir bei Epilepsies-patienten. Nervenarzt 54: 403

Froscher W, Hoffman F 1983 Dupuytren's contracture in patients with epilepsy: follow-up study. In: Oxley J, Janz D, Meinardi H (eds) Chronic toxicity of antiepileptic drugs. Raven Press, New York, p 147

Frost H M 1964 In: Lam C R (ed) The laws of bone structure. Charles C Thomas, Springfield

Frost H M 1988 Vital biomechanics. Proposed general concepts for skeletal adaptions to mechanical useage. Calcified Tissue International 42: 145–156

Fujimoto T, Singer S J 1986 Immunocytochemical studies of endothelial cells in vivo. I. The presence of desmin only, or of desmin plus vimentin, or vimentin only, in the endothelial cells of different capillaries of the adult chicken. Journal of Cell Biology 103: 2275–2786

Fujimoto T, Singer S J 1987 Immunocytochemical studies of desmin and vimentin in pericapillary cells of chicken. Journal of Histochemistry and Cytochemistry 35: 1105–1115

Fujimoto D, Akiba K, Nakamura N 1977 Isolation and characterisation of a fluorescent material in bovine Achilles tendon. Biochemical and Biophysical Research Communications 76: 1124

Furnas D W 1979 Dupuytren's contracture in a black patient in East Africa. Plastic and Reconstructive Surgery 64: 250–251

Gabbiani G, Majno G 1971 Presence of modified fibroblasts in granulation tissue and their possible role in wound contraction. Experientia 27: 549

Gabbiani G, Majno G 1972 Dupuytren's contracture: fibroblast contraction? An ultrastructural study. American Journal of Pathology 66: 131–138

Gabbiani G, Montandon D 1985 The myofibroblasts in Dupuytren's disease and other fibromatoses. In: Hueston J T, Tubiana R (eds) Dupuytren's disease, 2nd English edn. Churchill Livingstone, Edinburgh

Gabbiani G, Rungger-Brondle E 1981 The fibroblast. In: Glynn L E (ed) Handbook of inflammation, vol III: Tissue repair and regeneration. Elsevier, Amsterdam

Gabbiani G, Ryan G B, Majno G 1971 Presence of modified fibroblasts in granulation tissue and their possible role in wound contraction. Experimentia 27: 549–550

Gabbiani G, Hirschel B J, Ryan G B, Statkov P R, Majno G 1972 Granulation tissue as a contractile organ. A study of structure and function. Journal of Experimental Medicine 135: 719

Gabbiani G, Fu Y S, Kaye G I, Lattes R, Majno G 1972 Epithelioid sarcoma. A light and electron microscopic study suggesting a synovial origin. Cancer 30: 486–499

Gabbiani G, Majno G, Ryan G B 1973 The fibroblast as a contractile cell: the myofibroblast. In: Pikkarainen J, Kulonen K (eds) Biology of the fibroblast. Academic Press, New York, pp 139–154

Gabbiani G, Le Lous M, Bailey A J, Bazin S, Delauney A 1976 Collagen and myofibroblasts of granulation tissue. A chemical, ultrastructural and immunological study. Virchows Archiv B (Cell Pathology) 21: 133–145

Gabbiani G, Chaponnier C, Hüttner I 1978 Cytoplasmic filaments and gap junctions in epithelial cells and myofibroblasts during wound healing. Journal of Cell Biology 76: 561–568

Gabbiani G, Elemer G, Guelpa Ch, Vallotton M B, Badonnel M C, Hüttner I 1979 Morphologic and functional changes of the aortic intima during experimental hypertension. American Journal of Pathology 96: 399–422

Gabbiani G, Schmid E, Winter S et al 1981 Vascular smooth muscle cells differ from other smooth muscle cells: predominance of vimentin filaments and a specific α-type actin. Proceedings of the National Academy of Sciences USA 78: 298–302

Gabbiani G, Gabbiani F, Lombardi D, Schwatz S M 1983 Organization of actin cytoskeleton in normal and regenerating arterial endothelial cells. Proceedings of the National Academy of Sciences USA 80: 2361–2364

Gabbiani G, Kocher O, Bloom W S, Vandekerckhove J, Weber K 1984 Actin expression in smooth muscle cells of rat aortic intimal thickening, human atheromatous plaque, and cultured rat aortic media. Journal of Clinical Investigation 73: 148–152

Galambos J T, Hollingsworth M A, Falek A 1977 The rate of synthesis of glycosaminoglycans and collagen by fibroblasts cultured from adult liver biopsies. Journal of Clinical Investigation 60: 107–114

Gallagher J T, Gasiunas N, Schor S L 1980 Synthesis of glycosaminoglycans by human skin fibroblasts cultured on collagen gels. Biochemical Journal 190: 243–254

Garrod A E 1893 On an unusual form of nodule upon the joints of the fingers. St Bartholomew's Hospital Reports, 29: 157–161

Garrod A E 1904 Concerning pads upon the finger joints and their clinical relationships. British Medical Journal 2: 8

Gasperini E, Paparoni E 1969a Orientamenti sul trattamento della malattia di Dupuytren. La Clinica Ortopedica 21: 253

Gasperini E, Paparoni E 1969b Considerazioni sul trattamento chirurgico della mallatia di Dupuytren meniante aponeurectomia parziale e totale. La Clinica Ortopedica 21: 180

Gay S, Gay B 1972 1st der Dupuytren's kontraktur eine autoimmunerkrankung? Zentralblatt fur Chirurgie 97:728–733

Gelberman R H, Amiel D, Rudolph R M, Vance R M 1980 Dupuytren's contracture. Journal of Bone and Joint Surgery 62A: 425

Gelberman R H, Panagis J S, Hergenroeder P T, Zakaib GS 1982 Wound complications in the management of Dupuytren's contracture:a comparison of operative incisions. Hand 14: 248

Geldmacher J 1972 Die Eingriffe bei der Dupuytrenschen Kontraktur. Die Operationen an den Extremitaten. Springer Verlag, Berlin, pp 441–474

Gerritzen 1936 Operationserfolge der Dupuytren'schen Kontraktur unter Berucksichtigung der Unfall sweisen Entstehung. Zentralbla für Chirurgie 63: 161 cited by Skoog (1948)

Gersuny R 1884 Operation bei Kontraktur der Palmaraponevrose. Wiener Medizinische Wochenschrift 34: 969

Ghadially F N, Mehta P N 1971 Multifunctional mesenchymal cells resembling smooth muscle cells in ganglia of the wrist. Annals of the Rheumatic Diseases 30: 31–41

Ghadially F N, McNaughton J D, Lalonde J M A 1983 Myofibroblastoma: a tumor of myofibroblasts. Journal of Submicroscopic Cytology 15: 1055–1063

Gill A B 1919 Dupuytren's contracture, with a description of a method of operation. Annals of Surgery 70: 221

Gillard G C, Flint M H 1981 Collagen and proteoglycan organisation during post-natal development of tendons. Connective Tissue Research 8: 138

Gillard G C, Merrilees M J, Bell-Booth R G, Reilly H C, Flint M H 1977 The proteoglycan content and the axial periodicity of collagen in tendon. Biochemical Journal 163: 145–151

Gillard G C, Reilly H C, Bell-Booth P G, Flint M H 1977 A comparison of the glycosaminoglycans of weight-bearing and non-weight-bearing human dermis. Journal of Investigative Dermatology 69: 257–261

Gillard G C, Relly H C, Bell-Booth P G, Flint M H 1979 The influence of mechanical forces on the glycosaminoglycan content of the rabbit flexor digitorum profundus tendon. Connective Tissue Research 7: 37–46

Gillery P, Maquart F X, Borel J P 1986 Fibronectin dependence of the contraction of collagen lattices by human skin fibroblasts. Experimental Cell Research 167: 29–37

Gillies H 1945 Dupuytren's contraction. In: Turner G G (ed) Modern operative surgery, vol 2, 3rd edn. London, p 1655

Giocomelli F, Wiener J, Spiro D 1970 Cross-striated arrays of filaments in endothelium. Journal of Cell Biology 45: 188–192

Glasser S R, Julian J 1986 Intermediate filament protein as a marker of uterine stromal cell decidualization. Biology of Reproduction 35: 436–474

Glimcher M J, Shapiro F, Ellis R D, Eyre D R 1980 Changes in tissue morphology and collagen composition during repair of cortical bone in adult chicken. Journal of Bone and Joint Surgery 62A: 964

Gokel J M, Hübner G 1977 Intracellular 'fibrous long spacing' collagen in morbus Dupuytren's. Beiträge zur Pathologie 161: 176

Gold L I, Pearlstein E 1980 Fibronectin-collagen binding and requirement during cellular adhesion. Biochemical Journal 186: 551–559

Gonzalez R I 1969 Flexion deformities of the fingers. Current practice in Orthopaedic Surgery 4: 167–182

Gonzalez R I 1971 Dupuytren's contracture of the fingers. A simplified approach to the surgical treatment. California Medical West Journal of Medicine 115: 25

Gonzalez R 1971 Open fasciotomy and Wolfe grafts for Dupuytren's contracture. In: Hueston J T (ed) Transactions of the 5th international congress of plastic and reconstructive surgery. Butterworth, London, p 630

Gonzalez R I 1985 Open fasciotomy and full thickness skin graft in the correction of digital flexion deformity. In: Hueston J T, Tubiana R (eds) Dupuytren's disease, 2nd edn Churchill Livingstone. London

Gordon S D 1957 Dupuytren's contracture: recurrence and extension following surgical treatment. British Journal of Plastic Surgery 9: 286–288

Gordon S D 1964 Dupuytren's contracture; plantar involvement. British Journal of Plastic Surgery 17: 421–423

Gordon S, Anderson W 1961 Dupuytren's contracture following injury. British Journal of Plastic Surgery 14: 129

Gosset J 1966 Maladie de Dupuytren et anatomie des aponeuroses palmo-digitales. In: Maladie de Dupuytren (group d'etude de la main) l'Expansion Scientifique Francaise, Paris

Gosset J 1967 Maladie de Dupuytren et anatomie des aponevroses palmo-digitales. Annales de Chirurgie 21: 554

Gosset J 1972 Anatomie des aponeurosis palmodigitales. In: Tubiana R (ed) La maladie de Dupuytren, 2nd edn. Expansion Scientific Francais, Paris, p 11

Gosset J 1974 Dupuytren's disease and the anatomy of the palmodigital aponeuroses. In: Dupuytren's disease. Grune & Stratton, New York, p 11

Gosset J 1985 Dupuytren's disease and the anatomy of the palmodigital aponeuroses. In: Hueston J T, Tubiana R (eds) Dupuytren's disease, 2nd English edn. Churchill Livingstone, London, pp 13–26

Goyrand G 1833 Nouvelles recherches sur la rétraction permanente des doigts. Mémoires de l'Académie de Médécine 3: 489

Goyrand G 1834 Nouvelles recherches sur la rétraction

permanente des doigts. Memoires de l'Académie Royale de Médécine 3: 489–496
Grace D L, McGrouther D A Phillips H 1984 Traumatic correction of Dupuytren's contracture. Journal of Hand Surgery 9B: 59
Grapow M 1887 Die Anatomie and physiologische Bedeutung der Palmaraponeurose. Archiv für Anatomie and Physiologie 143: 2–3
Gray's Anatomy 1973 Warwick Rand Williams P (eds) 35th edn. Longman, Edinburgh
Grayson J 1940 The cutaneous ligaments of the digits. Journal of Anatomy 75: 164
Grenabo K J 1946 Nagra praktiskt viktiga detaljer vid behandlingen av Dupuytrens kontraktur. Nordisk Medicin 29: 96 cited by Skoog (1948)
Grillo H C 1963 Origin of fibroblasts in wound healing: an autoradiographic study of inhibition of cellular proliferation by local X-irradiation. Annals of Surgery 157: 453–467
Grimaud J A, Borojevic R 1977 Myofibroblasts in hepatic schistosomal fibrosis. Experientia 33: 890–892
Grinnell F, Lamke C R 1984 Reorganisation of hydrated collagen lattices by human skin fibroblasts. Journal of Cell Science 66: 51–63
Grinnell F, Billingham R E, Burgess L 1981 Distribution of fibronectin during wound healing in vivo. Journal of Investigative Dermatology 76: 181
Grodinsky M, Holyoke E A 1941 The fasciae and fascial spaces of the palm. Anatomical Record 79: 435
Guidry C, Grinnell F 1986 Contraction of hydrated collagen gels by fibroblasts: evidence for two mechanisms by which collagen fibrils are stabilised. Collagen and Related Research 6: 515–529
Guinebault P 1897 Contribution a l'étude de la rétraction de l'aponévrose palmaire. Thèse, Paris
Gunther O, Miosga R 1972 Dupuytrensche Kontractur als Diabetes–Spartkomplication. Zeitschrift fur Innere Medizin, 27: 77–82
Gurr E, Tizian C, Delbruck A, Berger A 1984 Glycosaminoglykone in der Dupuytren'schen kontraktur. Hand Chirurgie 16: 161–163
Gurr E, Mohr W, Pallasch G 1985a Proteoglycans from human articular cartilage: the effect of joint location on the structure. Journal of Clinical Chemistry and Clinical Biochemistry 23: 811–819
Gurr E, Pallasch G, Tunn S, Tamm C, Delbrück A 1985b High performance liquid chromatographic assay of disaccharides and oligosaccharides produced by the digestion of glycosaminoglycans with chondroitin sulphate lyases. Journal of Clinical Chemistry and Clinical Biochemistry 23: 77–87
Gurr E, Hafkemeyer P, Köller W, Delbrück A 1986 Glycosaminoglycans in human intervertebral disc. In: Xth meeting of the Federation of European Connective Tissue Societies, Manchester 1986, Abstract 297
Habuchi H, Kimata K, Suzuki S 1986 Changes in proteoglycan composition during development of rat skin. Journal of Biological Chemistry 261: 1031–1040
Haeseker B 1981 Dupuytren's disease and the sickle-cell trait in a female black patient. British Journal of Plastic Surgery 34: 438–440
Haimovici N 1978 Die Alloarthroplastik — Therapiealternative bei der arthrogenen Beugekontraktur der Finger bei Dupuytren'scher Krankheit. Handchirurgie 10: 135–148

Hakstian R W 1966 Long term results of extensive fasciectomy. British Journal of Plastic Surgery 140–149
Hall B J 1970 Cellular differentiation in skeletal tissue. Biological Reviews 45: 455–484
Hall A K, Behrman H R 1982 In: Lee J B (ed) Prostaglandins. New York, Elsevier Science, p 91
Hamamoto M, Ueba Y, Sudo Y, Sanada M, Yamamuro Y, Takeda T 1982 Dupuytrens contracture: morphological and biochemical changes in the palmar aponeurosis. The Hand 14: 237
Hamlin E 1952 Limited excision of Dupuytren's contracture. Annals of Surgery 135: 94
Hamlin E 1962 Limited excision of Dupuytren's contracture: a follow-up study. Annals of Surgery 155: 454–456
Handley C J, Lowther D A, McQuillan D J 1985 The structure and synthesis of proteoglycans of articular cartilage. Cell Biology International 9: 735–782
Hanya T, Tajima T, Takagi T et al 1984 Biochemical studies on the collagen of palmar aponeurosis affected with Dupuytren's disease. Tohoku Journal of Experimental Medicine 142: 437
Hardie J 1885 The treatment of Dupuytren's finger-contraction. British Medical Journal 1: 681
Harkness R D 1979 Mechanical properties of connective tissues in relation to function. In: Parry D A D, Creamer L K (eds) Fibrous proteins: scientific, industrial and medical aspects. Academic Press, New York
Harkness R D 1961 Biological functions of collagen. Biological Reviews of the Cambridge Philosophical Society 36: 399–464
Harris A K, Wild P, Stopak D 1980 Silicone rubber substrata: a new wrinkle in the study of cell locomotion. Science 208: 177
Harris A K, Stopak D, Wild P 1981 Fibroblast traction as a mechanism for collagen morphogenesis. Nature 290: 249
Harrison S H, Morris A 1975 Dupuytren's contracture: the dorsal transposition flap. The Hand 7: 145–149
Hawkins C 1835 Medical Gazette XV, 814
Hay D 1981 Cell biology of extracellular matrix. Plenum, New York
Heathcote J G, Cohen H, Noble J 1981 Dupuytren's disease and diabetes mellitus. Lancet i: 1420
Hedges C E 1896 The relation of gout and rheumatism to Dupuytren's contracture of palmar fascia. St Bartholomew's Hospital Report 32: 119
Hedman K, Johansson S, Vartio T, Kjellen L, Vaheri A, Hook M 1982 Structure of the pericellular matrix: association of heparan and chondroitin sulfates with fibronectin-procollagen fibers. Cell 28: 663–671
Hellgren L 1964 The prevalence of Dupuytren's contracture in Sweden. Paper read before the Scandinavian congress of rheumatologists in Lund, Sweden
Herman I M, D'Amore P A 1985 Microvascular pericytes contain muscle and nonmuscle actins. Journal of Cell Biology 101: 43–52
Herzog E G 1951 The aetiology of Dupuytren's contracture. Lancet i: 1305
Hessle H, Engvall E 1984 Type VI collagen — studies on its localization, structure and biosynthetic form with monoclonal antibodies. Journal of Biological Chemistry 259: 3955
Highton D I R, James D W 1964 The force of contraction of full-thickness wounds of rabbit skin. British Journal of Surgery 51: 462–466

Hill N A 1985 Current concepts review: Dupuytren's contracture. Journal of Bone and Joint Surgery 67-A: 1439–1443

Hoffmann-Berling H 1954 Adenosintriphosphat als Betriebsstoff von Zellbewegungen. Biochimica Biophysica Acta 14: 182–194

Hohmann G 1936 Zur orthopädischen Behandlung der Dupuytren'schen Fingerkontraktur. Munchen Medizinische Wochenschrift 83: 2088

Honda T, Matsunaga E, Katagiri K, Shinkai H 1986 The proteoglycans in hypertrophic scar. Journal of Dermatology 13: 326–333

Honner R, Lamb D W, James J I P 1971 Dupuytren's Contracture. Long term results after fasciectomy. Journal of Bone and Joint Surgery 53B: 240–246

Hoopes J E, Jabalex M E, Chi-Tsung S U, Wilgis S, Im M J C 1977 Enzymes of glucose metabolism in palmar fascia and Dupuytren's contracture. Journal of Hand Surgery 2: 62–65

Horrobin D F 1980 A biochemical basis for alcoholism and alcohol-induced damage including the fetal alcohol syndrome and cirrhosis: interference with essential fatty acid and prostaglandin metabolism. Medical Hypotheses 6: 929

Horwitz A, Duggan K, Buck C, Beckerle M C, Burridge K 1986 Interaction of plasma membrane fibronectin receptor with talin, a transmembrane linkage. Nature 320: 531

Horwitz T 1942 Dupuytren's contracture. Archives of Surgery, Chicago 44: 687

Houghton S, Holdstock G, Cockerell L, Wright R 1983 Dupuytren's contracture, chronic liver disease and IgA immune complexes. Liver 3: 220

Housley T, Tanzer M L, Henson E, Gallop P M 1975 Collagen crosslinking isolation of hydroxyaldol-histidine, a naturally occurring crosslink. Biochemical and Biophysical Research Communications 67: 824

Howard L D 1959 Dupuytren's contracture: a guide for management. Clinical Orthopaedics 15: 118

Hueston J T 1960 Baron Dupuytren. Medical Journal of Australia 1: 808

Hueston J T 1960 The incidence of Dupuytren's contracture. Medical Journal of Australia 2: 999–1002

Hueston J T 1961 Limited fasciectomy for Dupuytren's contracture. Plastic and Reconstructive Surgery 27: 569–585

Hueston J T 1962 Digital Wolfe grafts in recurrent Dupuytren's contracture. Plastic and Reconstructive Surgery 29: 342–344

Hueston J T 1962 Further studies on the incidence of Dupuytren's contracture. Medical Journal of Australia 1: 586

Hueston J T 1963 Dupuytren's contracture. E & S Livingstone, Edinburgh, pp 54–63

Hueston J T 1963 Recurrent Dupuytren's contracture. Plastic and Reconstructive Surgery 31: 66–69

Hueston J T 1964 Dupuytren's contracture: the trend to conservatism. Annals of the Royal College of Surgeons of England 134–151

Hueston J T 1968 Dupuytren's contracture and specific injury. Medical Journal of Australia 1: 1084

Hueston J T 1974 Enzymic fasciotomy and Aetiological questions in Dupuytren's contracture. In: J T Hueston, R. Tibiana (eds) Dupuytren's disease, 2nd edn. Churchill Livingstone, Edinburgh, pp 141–143

Hueston J T 1975 Dupuytren's contracture. In: Flynn T B (ed) Hand surgery, 2nd edn. Williams & Wilkins, Baltimore, pp 797–823

Hueston J T 1977 Dupuytren's contracture. In: Converse J M (ed) Reconstructive plastic surgery, 2nd edn. W B Saunders, Philadelphia, pp 3403–3427

Hueston J J 1982 Dorsal Dupuytren's disease. Journal of Hand Surgery 7: 384

Hueston J T 1982 Dupuytren's contracture. In: Flynn J E (ed) Hand surgery. Williams & Wilkins, Baltimore, pp 797–822

Hueston J T 1984 Current state of treatment of Dupuytren's disease. Annales de Chirurgie de la Main 3:812

Hueston J T 1984 Some observations on knuckle pads. The Hand 9B: 75–78

Hueston J T 1984 'Firebreak' grafts in Dupuytren's contracture. Australia and New Zealand Journal of Surgery 54: 277–281

Hueston J T 1985 The extensor apparatus in Dupuytren's disease. Annales de Chirurgie de la Main 4: 7

Hueston J T 1985 Dermofasciectomy: skin replacement in Dupuytren's disease. In: Hueston J T, Tubiana R (eds) Dupuytren's disease, 2nd edn. Churchill Livingstone, Edinburgh, pp 149–153

Hueston J T 1985 The management of ectopic lesions in Dupuytren's disease. In: Hueston J T, Tubiana R (eds) Dupuytren's disease. Churchill Livingstone, Edinburgh, pp 204–210

Hueston J T 1985a The role of the skin in Dupuytren's disease. Annals of the Royal College of Surgeons of England 167: 372–375

Hueston J T 1985b Overview of aetiology and pathology. In: Hueston J T, Tubiana R (eds) Dupuytren's disease, 2nd English edn. Churchill Livingstone, Edinburgh, pp 75–81

Hueston J T 1987 Dupuytren's contracture: medicolegal aspects. Medical Journal of Australia 147: 52

Hueston J T 1987a Editorial. Dupuytren's contracture and occupation. Journal of Hand Surgery (American) 12A: 657–658

Hueston J T 1987b Dupuytren's contracture: medicolegal aspects. Medical Journal of Australia 147: S2-11

Hueston J T, Hurley J V, Whittingham S 1976 The contracting fibroblast as a clue to Dupuytren's contracture. The Hand 8: 10

Hueston J T, Wilson W F 1973 Knuckle pads. Australian and New Zealand Journal of Surgery 42: 274–277

Hulmes D J S, Miller A, Parry D A D, Piez K A, Woodhead-Galloway J 1973 Analysis of the primary structure of collagen for the origins of molecular packing. Journal of Molecular Biology 79: 127

Hunter D, McLaughlin A I G, Perry K M A 1944 British Journal of Industrial Medicine 2: 10

Hunter J A, Ogdon C 1975 Dupuytren's contracture II: scanning electron microscopic observations. British Journal of Plastic Surgery 28: 19

Hunter J A, Ogdon C, Norris M G 1975 Dupuytren's contracture I — chemical pathology. British Journal of Plastic Surgery 28: 10–18

Hurst L C, Badalamente M A, Makowski J 1986 The pathobiology of Dupuytren's contracture: effects of prostaglandins on myofibroblasts. Journal of Hand Surgery (America) 11: 18–23

Hutchinson J 1917 Dupuytren's contraction of the palmar fascia. Lancet 95: 285

Hynes R O 1981 Fibronectin and its relation to cellular

structure and behaviour. In: Hay E D (ed) Cell biology of extracellular matrix. Plenum, New York

Hynes R O 1986 Fibronectins. Scientific American 5: 42

Hynes R O 1987 Integrins: a family of cell surface receptors. Cell 48: 549

Hunter T, Shanahan W R, Robertson G A, Stranc M F, Schroeder M L 1981 The distribution of histocompatibility antigens in patients with Dupuytren's contracture. Arthritis and Rheumatism 24: 1218–1219

Ipbuker A, Erkurt R 1965 Diabetes mellitus ve palmer fascia kontraktura (Dupuytren's contracture). Turk Tip Cemiyeti Mecmuasi 3L: 612

Iselin M 1954 Aspects chirurgicales de la maladie de Dupuytren. Revue de Rhumatisme 18: 316

Iselin M 1954b Maladie de Dupuytren. Concours Médicale 48: 4425

Iselin M 1955 Chirurgie de la main, vol 2. Livre de chirurgien. Masson, Paris

Iselin F 1972 Maladie de Dupuytren. Gazette Médicale de France 79: 6565–6572

Iselin F 1980 Traitement chirurgical de la maladie de Dupuytren. Entretiens de Bichat 1980 — Chirurgie. Expansion Scientifique Francaise, Paris pp 44–51

Iselin F 1983 Communication au 2ème Congrès International de Chirurgie de la Main Panel on Dupuytren's disease. Boston

Iselin M 1985 Dermofasciectomy for recurrent Dupuytren's disease. In: Hueston J T, Tubiana R (eds) Dupuytren's disease 2nd edn. Churchill Livingstone, London, pp 172–176

Iselin F 1986 Les dermofasciectomies pour les formes cutanées de la maladie de Dupuytren. In: La maladie de Dupuytren, Hueston J T, Tubiana R (eds) 3rd edn. Expansion Scientifique Francaise, Paris, pp 176–180

Irlé C, Kocher O, Gabbiani G 1980 Contractility of myofibroblasts during experimental liver cirrhosis. Journal of Submicroscopic Cytology 12: 209–217

Isenberg G, Rathke P C, Hülsmann N, Franke W W, Wohlfahrt-Bottermann K E 1976 Cytoplasmic actomyosin fibrils in tissue cultured cells. Direct proof of contractility by visualization of ATP-induced contraction in fibrils isolated by laser microbeam dissection. Cell and Tissue Research 166: 427–433

Iversen J 1909 Uber die traumatische Entstehung der Dupuytren'schen Kontraktur u. deren Lokalisation am Daumen. Inaugural Dissertation Kiel, cited by Skoog (1948)

Iwasaki H, Müller H, Stutte H J, Brennscheidt U 1984 Palmar fibromatosis (Dupuytren's contracture). Ultrastructural and enzyme histochemical study of 43 cases. Virchows Archiv A (Pathology and Anatomy) 405:41–53

Jacobsen K, Holst-Nielsen F 1977 A modified McCash operation for Dupuytren's contracture. Scandinavian Journal of Plastic and Reconstructive Surgery 11: 231–233

Jacubic J 1965 Early occurrence of Dupuytren's contracture. Acta Chirurgiae Ortopedicae et Traumatologiae Czechoslovaca 32: 527

Jahnke A 1960 Elektronenmikroskopische Untersuchungen uber die Dupuytrensche kontraktur. Zentralblatt fur Chirurgie 85: 2295

James J I P 1985 The genetic pattern of Dupuytren's disease and idiopathic epilepsy. In: Hueston J T, Tubiana R (eds) Dupuytren's disease. Churchill Livingstone, Edinburgh, p 94

James D W, Newcombe J F 1961 Granulation tissue resorption during free and limited contraction of skin wounds. Journal of Anatomy (London) 95: 247

James D W, Taylor J F 1969 The stress developed by sheets of chick fibroblasts in vitro. Experimental Cell Research 54: 107–110

Janssen P 1902 Zur Lehre von der Dupuytren'schen Fingerkontractur, mit besonderer Berücksichtigung der operativen Beseitigung und der patholgischen Anatomie des Leidens. Archiv für Klinische Chirurgie 67: 761–789

Jentsch F R 1937 Zur Erblichkeit der Dupuytrenschen Kontraktur. Der Erbarzt 4: 85

Jobert, Brandon 1846 Annales de thérapeutiques. Cited by Skoog (1984)

Joyce N C, DeCamilli P, Boyles J 1984 Pericytes, like vascular smooth muscle cells, are immunocytochemically positive for cyclic GMP-dependent protein kinase. Microvascular Research 28: 206–219

Joyce N C, Haire M F, Palade G E 1985a Contractile proteins in pericytes. I. Immunoperoxidase localization of tropomyosin. Journal of Cell Biology 100: 1379–1386

Joyce N C, Haire M F, Palade G E 1985b Contractile proteins in pericytes. II. Immunocytochemical evidence for the presence of two isomyosins in graded concentrations. Journal of Cell Biology 100: 1387–1395

Judd P A, Finnegan P, Curran R C 1975 Pulmonary sarcoidosis: a clinicopathological study. Journal of Pathology 115: 191–198

Juno T C, Hohmann J A, Gerneth A et al 1971 Diabetic hand syndrome. Metabolism 20: 1008

Kalberg W 1935 Zur Anatomie der Palmaraponeurose. 81: 149–159

Kanavel A B 1925 Infections of the hand. London, Baillière Tindall & Cox

Kanavel A B, Koch S L, Mason M L 1929 Dupuytren's contraction. Surgery, Gynecology and Obstetrics 48: 145–190

Kaplan E B 1938 The palmar fascia in connection with Dupuytren's contracture. Surgery 415–422

Kaplan E B 1965 Functional and surgical anatomy of the hand, 2nd edn. Lippincott, Philadelphia

Kaplan E B 1966 Functional surgical anatomy of the hand, 2nd edn. Lippincott, Philadelphia

Kawamoto S, Adelstein R S 1987 Characterization of myosin heavy chains in cultured aorta smooth muscle cells. A comparative study. Journal of Biological Chemistry 262: 7282–7288

Kay N R M, Slater D N 1981 Fibromatoses and diabetes mellitus. Lancet ii: 303

Keen W W 1906 A new method of operating on Dupuytren's contraction of the palmar fascia. American Journal of Medical Science 131: 23

Keen H, Ekde J M 1984 The geography of diabetes mellitus. British Medical Bulletin 40: 359

Kelly A P Jr, Clifford R H 1959 Subcutaneous fasciotomy in the treatment of Dupuytren's contracture. Plastic and Reconstructive Surgery 24: 505–509

Kempf I, Gonzalo-Vivar F 1962 Les formations fibroaponévrotiques de la region metacarpo-phalangiennes. Bulletin de l'Association des Anatomistes, Paris 18: 804

Kennedy L, Beacom R, Archer D B et al 1982 Limited joint mobility in type I diabetes mellitus. Postgraduate Medical Journal 58: 481

Ketchum L D 1971 Effects of triamcinolone on tendon

healing and function. A laboratory study. Plastic and Reconstructive Surgery 47: 471–482

Ketchum L D, Hixson P F 1987 Original communications. Dermofasciectomy and full-thickness grafts in the treatment of Dupuytren's contracture. Journal of Hand Surgery (American) 12A: 659–663

King E W, Exeter M H, Bass D M, Watson H K 1979 Treatment of Dupuytren's contracture by extensive fasciectomy through multiple Y-V plast incisions: short-term evaluation of 170 consecutive operations. Journal of Hand Surgery 4: 234

Kipikasa A 1968 Demographic study of the incidence of Dupuytren's contraction. Rozhledy v Chirurgii 47: 211

Kischer C W, Hendrix M J C 1983 Fibronectin (FN) in hypertrophic scars and keloids. Cell and Tissue Research 231: 29

Kischer C W, Shetlar M R 1974 Collagen and mucopolysaccharide in the hypertrophic scar. Connective Tissue Research 2: 205–213

Kischer C W, Speer D W 1984 Microvascular changes in Dupuytren's contracture. Journal of Hand Surgery 9A: 58

Kischer C W, Shetlar M R, Chvapil M 1982a Hypertrophic scars and keloids: a review and new concept concerning their origin. Scanning Electron Microscopy IV: 1699–1713

Kischer C W, Thies A C, Chvapil M 1982b Perivascular myofibroblasts and microvascular occlusion in hypertrophic scars and keloids. Human Pathology 13: 819–824

Kivirikko K 1970 Urinary excretion of hydroxyproline in health and disease. International Review of Connective Tissue Research 5: 93

Kivirikko K I, Myllylä 1984 Biosynthesis of collagen. In: Piez K A, Reddi A H (eds) Extracellular matrix biochemistry. Elsevier, New York, p 83

Kleinman H K, McGarvey M L, Hassell J R, Martin G R, Baron van Evercooren A, Dubois-Dalcq M 1984 The role of laminin in basement membranes and in the growth, adhesion, and differentiation of cells. In: Trelstad R L (ed) The role of extracellular matrix in development. Alan R Liss, New York, p 123

Knowles H B 1981 Joint contractures, waxy skin, and control of diabetes. New England Journal of Medicine 305: 217

Kocher T 1887 Behandlung der Retraktion der Palmaraponeurose. Centralblatt fur Chirurgie 14: 482–487, 497–502

Kocher O, Gabbiani G 1986 Cytoskeletal features of normal and atheromatous human arterial smooth muscle cells. Human Pathology 17: 875–880

Kocher O, Skalli O, Bloom W S, Gabbiani G 1984 Cytoskeleton of rat aortic smooth muscle cells. Normal conditions and experimental intimal thickening. Laboratory Investigation 50: 645–652

Kocher O, Skalli O, Cerutti D, Gabbiani F, Gabbiani G 1985 Cytoskeletal features of rat aortic cells during development. An electron microscopic, immunohistochemical, and biochemical study. Circulation Research 56: 829–838

Koenig F 1889 Lehrbuch der speciellen. Chirurgie, 5th edn. Berlin, p 178 cited by Skoog (1948)

Kosinski K 1940 Operativ-orthopädische Behandlung der Dupuytren'schen Kontraktur. Chirurgie Narzadow Ruchu 11: 283 abstracted in Zentralblatt für Chirurgie 67: 1939–1940

Krall L P, Zorilla E 1963 Disorders of the skin in diabetes. In: R S M Ling The genetic factor in Dupuytren's disease. The Journal of Bone and Joint Surgery 45B;709–718

Kreis T E, Birchmeier W 1980 Stress fiber sarcomeres of fibroblasts are contractile. Cell 22: 555–561

Krogius A 1920 Neue Gesichtspunkte zur Aetiologie der Dupuytrenschen Finger Kontraktur. Zentralblatt für Chirurgie 47: 914–918

Krogius A 1921 Studien und Betractungen uber die Pathogenese der Dupuytren'schen Fingerkontractur Acta Chirgica Scandinavica 54: 33

Krogius A 1922 Studien und Betractungen über die Pathogenese der Dupuytrenschen Fingerkontractur. Acta Chirurgica Scandinavica 54: 33

Kuczynski K 1972 Development of the hand and some anatomical anomalies. The Hand 4: 1

Lagacé R, Delage C, Boutet M 1975 Light and electron microscopic study of cellular proliferation in carcinoid heart disease. In: Roy P E, Rona G (eds) Recent advances in studies on cardiac structure and metabolism, vol 10. University Park Press, Baltimore, p 605

Lagacé R, Bouchard H L, Seemayer T A 1979 Desmoplastic fibroma of bone. An ultrastructural study. American Journal of Surgical Pathology 3: 422–430

Lagacé R, Schurch W, Seemayer T A 1980 Myofibroblasts in soft tissue sarcomas. Virchows Archives A, Pathology, Anatomy and Histology 389: 1–11

Lagacé R, Grimaud J A, Schürch W, Seemayer T A 1985 Myofibroblastic stromal reactions in carcinomas of the breast and variations of collageneous matrix and structural glycoproteins. Virchows Archiv A (Pathology and Anatomy) 408: 49–59

Laidlaw J P, Richens A 1982 Textbook of epilepsy, 2nd edn. Churchill Livingstone, Edinburgh, p 21

Lamb D W 1981 Dupuytren's disease. In: Lamb D W, Kuczynski K (ed) The practice of hand surgery. Blackwell, Oxford, p 476

Landsmeer J M F 1949 The anatomy of the dorsal aponeurosis of the human finger and its functional significance. Anatomical Record 104: 31–44

Landsmeer J M F 1963 The co-ordination of fingerjoint motions. Journal of Bone and Joint Surgery 45A: 1654–1622

Landsmeer J M F 1976 Atlas of anatomy of the hand. Churchill Livingstone, Edinburgh

Lane B P 1965 Alterations in the cytologic detail of intestinal smooth muscle in various stages of contraction. Journal of Cell Biology 27: 199–213

Lane L S 1981 The treatment of Dupuytren's contracture with flexor tendon sheath involvement — the sliding volar flap. Annals of Plastic Surgery 6: 20–23

Langanger G, Moermans M, Daneels J, Sobieszek A, DeBrabander M, DeMey J 1986 The molecular organization of myosin in stress fibers of cultured cells. Journal of Cell Biology 102: 200

Langvad-Nielsen A 1946 Dupuytren's kontraktur. Ogesk f Laeger 108: 530 (in Danish) cited by Skoog (1948)

Larkin J G, Frier B M 1986 Limited joint mobility and Dupuytren's contracture in diabetic, hypertensive, and normal populations. British Medical Journal 292: 1494

Larsen R D 1975 Dupuytren's contracture. In: Flynn (ed) Hand surgery, 2nd edn. Williams & Wilkins, Baltimore, p 571

Larsen R D, Posch J L 1958 Dupuytren's contracture with

special reference to pathology. Journal of Bone and Joint Surgery 40A: 773–792

Larsen R D, Takagishi N, Posch J L 1960 The pathogenesis of Dupuytren's contracture (experimental and further clinical observations). Journal of Bone and Joint Surgery 42A: 993–1007

Larson R D, Takagishi N, Posch J L 1960 The pathogenesis of Dupuytren's contracture. Journal of Bone and Joint Surgery 421: 993

Larson D L, Abston S, Willis B et al 1974 Contracture and scar formation in the burn patient. Clinics in Plastic Surgery 1: 653–666

Larson D M, Fujiwara K, Alexander R W, Gimbrone M A 1984 Heterogeneity of myosin antigenic expression in vascular smooth muscle in vivo. Laboratory Investigation 50: 401

Larson D M, Fujiwara K, Alexander R W, Gimbrone Jr M A 1984 Myosin in cultured vascular smooth muscle cells: immunofluorescence and immunochemical studies of alterations in antigenic expression. Journal of Cell Biology 99: 1582–1589

Lauro R, Verga G A 1970 Sulle recidive del morbo di Dupuytren. Rivista Italiana di Chirurgia Plastica 2: 239

Law P, McGrouther D A 1984 The dorsal wrinkle ligaments of the proximal interphalangeal joint. Journal of Hand Surgery 9B: 271–275

Lawson P M, Maneschi F, Kohner E M 1983 The relationship of hand abnormalities to diabetes and diabetic retinopathy. Diabetes Care 6: 140

Ledderhose G 1897 Zur Pathologie der Aponeurose des Fuses und der Hand. Archiv für klinische Chirurgie 55: 694

Legge J W H, McFarlane R M 1980 Prediction of results of treatment of Dupuytren's disease. Journal of Hand Surgery 5: 608

Legge J W, Finlay J B, McFarlane R M 1981 A study of Dupuytren's tissue with the scanning electron microscope. Journal of Hand Surgery 6: 482

Le Gros Clark W E 1958 The tissues of the body. Oxford University Press, Oxford

Legueu F, Juvara E 1892 Des aponeuroses de la paume de la main. Bulletins de la Société Anatomique de Paris 6: 383

Leung D Y M, Glagov S, Clark J M, Mathews M B 1975 Mechanical influences on the biosynthesis of extracellular macromolecules by aortic cells. In: Slavkin H C, Greulich R C (eds) Extracellular matrix influence on gene expression. Academic Press, New York, pp 633–645

Lewis W H 1901 The development of the arm in man. American Journal of Anatomy 1: 145

Lexer E 1931 Die gesamte Widereherstellungschirurgie, 2nd edn Leipzig, p 837

Light N D, Bailey A J 1980 The chemistry of collagen cross-links. Biochemical Journal 185: 373

Lilienfeld A M 1960 The distribution of diesase in the population. Journal of Chronic Diseases 11: 471

Ling R S M, 1963 The genetic factor in Dupuytren's idsease. Journal of Bone and Joint Surgery 45B: 709–718

Lipper S, Kahn L B, Reddick R L 1980 The Myofibroblast. Pathology Annual, Part 1: 409–441

Littler J W, 1974 Special points of technique in Dupuytren's contracture. In: Hueston J T, Tubiana R (eds) Dupuytren's Disease, 1st English edn. Churchill Livingsone, Edinburgh, p 97

Littler J W 1977 Stenosing digital tendovaginitis. In: Converse J M (ed) The hand and upper extremity; number 3 of reconstructive plastic surgery, 2nd Edn. Saunders, Philadelphia

Losapio P L, Setti E, Faldi F 1978 Morbo di Dupuytren: aponevrectonia selettiva, risultati a distanza. Rivist. Italiana di Chirugia Plastica 9: 397

Lotheissen G 1900 Zur operativen Behandlung der Dupuytren'schen Kontraktur. Zebtralblatt für Chirurgie 27: 761

Lubahn J O, Lister G G, Wolfe T 1984 Fasciectomy of Dupuytren's disease, comparison between the open-palm technique and wound closure. Journal of Hand Surgery 9a: 53

Luck J V 1959 Dupuytren's contracture — A new concept of the pathogenesis correlated with surgical management.

Lund M 1941 Dupuytren's contracture and epilepsy. Acta Psychiatrica et Neurologica Scandinavica 16: 465

Luppino T, Fiocchi R, Montorsi A 1974 Le vie di accesso nella malattia di Dupuytren: analisi critica dei moderni orientamenti ed ulteriori contributi. La Chururgia degli Organi di Novimento 63: 225

Lyons T J, Kennedy L 1985 Non-enzymatic glycosylation of skin collagen in patients with type I (insulin-dependent) diabetes mellitus and limited joint mobility. Diabetologia 28: 2

MacCallum P, Hueston J T 1962 The pathology of Dupuytren's contracture. Austrian & New Zealand Journal of Surgery 31: 241-253

Macready J 1890 On the treatment of Dupuytren's contraction of the palmar fascia. British Medical Journal 1: 411–414

MacDonald R A 1959 Origin of fibroblasts in experimental healing wounds: autoradiographic studies using tritiated thymidine. Surgery 46: 376–382

MacKinnon S E, Holder L E 1984 The use of three-phase radionuclide bone scanning in the diagnosis of reflex sympathetic dystrophy. Journal of Hand Surgery 9A: 556

Madden J W 1973 On 'the contractile fibroblast'. Plastic and Reconstructive Surgery 52: 291–292

Madden J W, Carlson E C, Hines J 1975 Presence of modified fibroblasts in ischemic contracture of the intrinsic musculature of the hand. Surgery, Gynecology and Obstetrics 140: 509–516

Madelung O W 1875 Die Aetologie und die operative Behandlung der Dupuytren'schen Finger ver Krummung. Berliner Klinische Wochenschrift 12: 191

Madelung O W 1876 The causes and operative treatment of Dupuytren's finger contraction. Trubner, London

Maeda K et al (1974) Treatment of Dupuytren's contracture and incidental difference between Caucasians and Japanese. Abstract of Japan US joint meeting of Hand Surgery. 95.

Maes J 1979 Dupuytren's contracture in an Oriental patient. Plastic and Reconstructive Surgery 64:251

Majno G, Shea S M, Leventhal M 1969 Endothelial contraction induced by histamine-like mediators. An electron microscopic study. Journal of Cell Biology 42: 647–672

Majno G, Gabbiani G, Hirschel B J, Ryan G B, Statkov P R 1971 Contraction of granulation tissues in vitro: similarity to smooth muscle. Science 173: 548–550

Manske P R, Lesker P A 1983 Palmar aponeurosis pulley. Journal of Hand Surgery 8: 259–263

Manson JS 1931 Heredity and Dupuytren's contracture. British Medical Journal 2: 11

Malins J M 1972 Diabetes in the population clinics. Endocrinology and Metabolism 1: 645

Mantero R, Ghigliazza G B, Bertolotti P, Roggero F 1966 La malattia di Dupuytren: il nostro orientamento terapeutico. Rivista di Chirurgia della Mano 4: 194

Marsano R 1965 Incisione cutanea spezzata nell'intervento di asportazione dell'aponeurosi palmare nella malattia di Dupuytren. Minerva Ortopedica 16: 302

Marsico B 1963 Sul trattamento Roentgen della malattia diDupuytren. Riforna Medica 77: 931

Maslieurat-Lagemard G-E 1839 De l'anatomie descriptive et chirurgicale des aponévroses et des membranes synoviales de la main, de leur application à la thérapeutique et à la medecine operatoire. Gazette Méicale de Paris 7: 273–280

Marin G R, Timpl R, Mühn K 1985 The genetically distinct collagens. Trends in Biochemistry 10: 285

May H 1948 Repair of cicatricial and Dupuytren's contractures of the hand. Plastic and Reconstructive Surgery: 439–450

McCash C R 1964 The open palm technique in Dupuytren's Contracture British Journal of Plastic Surgery 17: 271

McFarlane R M 1974 Pattern of the diseased fascia in the fingers in Dupuytren's contracture. Plastic and Reconstructive Surgery 54: 31

McFarlane R M 1982 In: Green D P, (ed) Operative hand surgery. Churchill Livingstone, New York, p 463

McFarlane R M 1983 The current status of Dupuytren's contracture. Journal of Hand Surgery 8/A: 703

McFarlane R M 1984 The anatomy of Dupuytren's disease. Bulletin of the Hospital for Joint Disease 44: 318

McFarlane R M 1985 Some observations on the epidemiology of Dupuytren's disease. In: Hueston J T, Tubiana R Livingstone, (eds) Dupuytren's disease, 2nd edn. Churchill London

McFarlane R M 1985 The anatomy of Dupuytren's disease. In: Hueston J T, Tubiana R (eds) Dupuytren's Disease, 2nd English edn. Churchill Livingstone, London, pp 55–72

McFarlane R M Jamieson W G 1966 Dupuytren's contracture. The management of 100 patients. Journal of Bone and Joint Surgery 48A: 1095–1105

McGregor I 1967 The z-plasty in hand surgery. Journal of Bone and Joint Surgery 49B: 448–457

McGregor I A, 1985 Pásciotomy and graft in the management of Dupuytren's contracture. In: Hueston J T, Tubiana R, (eds) Dupuytren's disease, 2nd edn. Churchill Livingstone, London.

McGrouther D A 1982 The microanatomy of Dupuytren's contracture. The Hand 13: 215–236

McIndoe A H, Beare R L B 1958 The surgical management of Dupuytren's contracture. American Journal of Surgery 95: 197

Meagher S W 1971 Wear and tear: a popular fallacy. Boston Bar Journal 15: 7

Meister P, Gokel J M, Remberger K 1979 Palmar fibromatosis — 'Dupuytren's contracture', a comparison of light electron, and immunofluorescence microscopic findings. Pathology and Research in Practice 164: 402

Mennen U 1983 Dupuytren's disease in Negros. Presented at Vail Symposium on Hand Surgery

Mennen U 1986 Dupuytren's contracture in the negro. Journal of Hand Surgery 110: 61–64

Mennen U, Grabe R P 1979 Dupuytren's contracture in a Negro: A case report. Journal & Hand Surgery 4: 451–453

Menzel EJ, Piza H, Zielinski C, Endler AT, Steffen C, Millesi H 1979 Collagen types and anti-collagen-antibodies in Dupuytren's disease. The Hand 2: 243–248

Merker E 1897 Die Dupuytren'sche Fingerkontraktur. Inaug Diss, Berlin, cited by Skoog (1948)

Merlo G, Ambroggio G P, Castagna B, Mosca A, Oberto E 1986 Fibrin/fibrinogen and fibrinolytic activity of the palmar fascia in Dupuytren's contracture. Journal of Hand Surgery (British) 11-B: 55–57

Merlo G, Ambroggio G P, Mosca A, Oberto E 1987 Possible role of palsminogen activator content of the palmar nodules in recurrrence of Dupuytren's contracture. Journal of Hand Surgery 12A: 1017–1019

Merrilees M J, Flint M H 1980 Ultrastructural study of tension and pressure zones in a rabbit flexor tendon. American Journal of Anatomy 157: 87–106

Merrilees M J, Gillard G C, Glint M H 1978 The tendon — a homeostatic unit tuned to mechanical forces. In: Sturges J M (ed) Ninth Internation Congress on Electron microscopy, Vol 2. Toronto, pp 658–659

Messina A 1982 La tecnica dell'aponevrectomia parziale o segmentaria. Rivista di Chirurgia della Mano 19: 317

Mey J, Grünwald J, Hauss WH 1980 Growth rate differences between arterial smooth muscle cells cultivated from rat impaired by short- or long-term hypertension respective. Artery 8: 348–354

Meyerding, H W, Black, J R, Broders A C 1936 The etiology and pathology of Dupuytren's contracture. Surgery, Gynecology and Obstetrics 582–590

Meyerding H W, Black J R, Broders A C 1941 The etiology and pathology of Dupuytren's contracture. Surgery, Gynecology & Obstetrics 72: 582–590

Michon J 1974 Operative difficulties and post operative complications in the surgery of Dupuytren's contracture. In: Hueston J T, Tubiana R (eds) Dupuytren's disease, 1st English edn. Churchill Livingstone, Edinburgh, p 101

Mikkelsen O A 1972 The prevalence of Dupuytren's disease in Norway. Acta Chirurgica Scandinavica 138: 695

Mikkelsen O A 1976 Dupuytren's disease — a study of the pattern of distribution and stage of contracture in the hand. The Hand 8: 265

Mikkelsen O A 1977 a Dupuytren's disease — initial symptoms, age of onset and spontaneous course. The Hand 9: 11

Mikkelsen O A 1977b Knuckle pads in Dupuytren's disease. The Hand 9: 301

Mikkelsen O A 1978 Dupuytren's disease — the influence of occupation and previous hand injuries. Hand 19: 1

Milford L 1968 Retaining ligaments of the digits of the hand. WB Saunders, W B and Company, Philadelphia

Miller E J 1976 Biochemical characteristics and biological significance of the genetically-distinct collagens. Molecular and Cellular Biochemistry 13: 165

Miller E J, Martin G R, Piez K A, Powers M J 1967 Characterization of chick bone collagen and compositional changes associated with maturation. Journal of Biological Chemistry 242: 5481

Millesi H 1959 Neue Gesichtspunkte in der Pathogenese der Dupuytrenschen Kontractur. Bruns' Beitrage zur klinischen Chirurgie 198: 1–25

Millesi H 1965 Zur Pathogenese und Therapie der Dupuytren'schen Kontraktur. Ergebnissc der Chirurgie und Orthopaedie 47: 51–101

Millesi H 1966 The clinical and morphological course of Dupuytren's disease. In: Maladie de dupuytren. Expansion Scientifique, Paris, p 47

Millesi H 1967 Uber die Beugekontraktur des distalen Interphalangealgelenkes im Rahmen einer Dupuytrenschen Erkrankung. Bruns' Beitrage zur Klinischen Chirurgie 214: 400

Millesi H 1974 The Clinical and morphological course of Dupuytren's disease. In: Hueston J T, Tubiana R (eds) Dupuytren's disease. Churchill Livingstone, London, p 49

Millesi H 1981 Dupuytren's contracture. In: Handchirurgie, vol 1. Georg Thieme Verlag, Stuttgart, pp 15.1–15.57

Millesi H 1985 The clinical and morphological course of Dupuytren's disease. In: Hueston J T, Tubiana R (eds) Dupuytren's disease, 2nd English edn. Churchill Livingstone, Edinburgh, pp 114–121

Mitchell J, Woodcock-Mitchell J, Reynolds S, er al 1989 Alpha smooth muscle actin in parenchymal cells of bleomycin injured rat lung. (in press)

Moberg E 1973 Three useful ways to avoid amputation in Dupuytren's contracture. Orthopedic Clinics of North America 4: 1001

Moermans J P, Duchateau J 1984 La maladie de Dupuytren: résultats d'une technique simplifiee. Revue Médicale de Bruxelles 5: 467–471

Mohr W, Vosbeck G 1985 Untersuchungen zur Proliferation und [^{3}H]-Prolin-Inkorporation von Zellen der Palmarfibromatose (Morbus Dupuytren) Zeitschrift für Rheumatologie 44: 226–230

Mollica Q, Restuccia G, Gensini A 1980 La malattia di Dupuytren: orientamenti clinici e terapeutici. Giornae Italiano di Ortopedia e Traumatologia 6: 213

Mollica Q, Restuccia G, Branciforti B 1982 Il trattamento della malattia di Dupuytren secondo la tecnica di Tubiana: valuatione dei primi 50 casi operati. Rivista di Chirurgia della Mano 19: 413

Montenero P, Colletti A, Fabbri G 1965 Maladie de Dupuytren et diabète. Journées Annuelles di Diabétologie de l'Hôtel-Dieu 6:/75

Morelli E 1982 Trattamento delle recidive e delle complicanze tardive nel morbo di Dupuytren. Rivista di Chirurgia della Mano 19: 349

Morinaga H, Katsuna T, Mizuoka J, Takara K, Oniki Y, Morimoto K 1979 Present state of Dupuytren's contracture in Japan. Journal of the Japanese Orthopaedic Society 3: 1747

Moschella F, Soma P F, D'Arrigo M 1982 Utilita della termografia nella malattia di Dupuytren in fase iniziale. Rivista di Chirurgia della Mano 19: 399

Moser E 1894 Ueber Dupuytren'sche Fingercontracturen und deren Operationen. Inaug Diss, Berlin cited by Skoog 1948

Moss N S, Benditt E P 1970 Spontaneous and experimentally induced arterial lesions. I. An ultrastructural survey of the normal chicken aorta. Laboratory Investivation 22: 166–183

Mosse P R L, Campbell G R, Wang Z L, Campbell J H 1985 Smooth muscle phenotypic expression in human carotid arteries. I. Comparison of cells from diffuse initimal thickenings adjacent to atheromatous plaques with those of the media. Laboratory Investigation 53: 556–562

Mourao P A S, Machado-Santelli G M 1978 Sulphated glycosaminoglycans of cells grown in culture: dermatan sulphate disappearance in successive fibroblast subcultures. Cell Differentiation 7: 367–374

Mumenthaler M 1961 Die Ulnarisparesen (Quoted in Viljanto J, Seppala PO, Lehonen A 1971, Annals of Rheumatic Diseases 30: 423)

Murphy G, Reynolds J J 1985 Current views of collagen degradation. Bioessays 2: 55

Murrell G A, Francis M J, Bromley L 1987a Free radicals and Dupuytren's contracture. British Medical Journal 295: 1373–1375

Murrell G A C, Pilowsky E, Murrell T G C 1987b A hypothesis on the resolution of Dupuytren's contracture with allopurinol. Speculations in Science and Technology 10: 107–112

Nagay B 1985 Die zweizeitige operative Behandlung der Dupuytrenschen Kontraktur. Handchirurgie-Mikrochirurgie-Plastische Chirurgie 17: 143–144

Nagay B 1985 Dupuytren's contracture — contemporary views on the etiopathogenesis and clinic of the disease. Materia Medica Polona 17: 251–256

Nagle R B, Kneiser M R, Bulger R E, Benditt E P 1973 Induction of smooth muscle characteristics in renal interstitial fibroblasts during obstructive nephropathy. Laboratory Investigation 29: 422–427

Napier J R 1965 Functional aspects of the anatomy of the hand. In: Pulvertaft R G (ed) The hand. Butterworth, London

Nardoni A, Baldissera A, Iacono M, Copetti R, Cella R 1981 Malattia di Dupuytren prospettive etiopatogenetiche attuali. Minerva Medica 72: 859

Navas-Palacios J J 1983 The fibromatoses. An ultrastructural study of 31 cases. Pathology Research and Practice 176: 158–175

Nazari B 1966 Dupuytren's contracture associated with liver disease. Journal of Mount Sinai Hospital of New York 33: 69

Nelaton 1908 Société de Chirurgie, séance du 24 juin. Bulletin et Mémoires de la Société des Chirurgiens de Paris 34: 803

Nezelof C 1985 Histological aspects of Dupuytren's disease. In: Hueston J T, Tubiana R (eds) Dupuytren's disease, 2nd English edn. Churchill Livingsone, Edinburgh, pp 82–85

Niederhuber S S, Stribley R F, Koepke G H 1975 Reduction of skin bacterial load with use of therapeutic whirlpool. Physical Therapy 55: 482

Nieminens M 1986 Resection of the palmaris longus tendon in surgery for Dupuytren's contracture. Annales Chirurgeicae er Gynecologyical 75: 164

Nissenbaum M, Kleinert H E 1980 Treatment considerations in carpal tunnel syndrome with coexistent Dupuytren's disease. Journal of Hand Surgery 5: 544

Noble J, Harrison D H 1976 Open palm technique for Dupuytren's contracture. The Hand 8: 272–278

Noble J, Heathcote J G, Cohen H 1984 Diabetes mellitus in the aetiology of Dupuytren's disease. Journal of Bone and Joint Surgery 66B: 322–325

Novotny G E K, Pau H 1984 Myofibroblast-like cells in human anterior capsular cataract. Virchows Archiv A (Pathology and Anatomy) 404: 393–401

Nyberg L M, Bias W B, Hochberg M C, Walsh P C 1982 Identification of an inherited form of Peyronie's disease with autosomal dominant inheritance and association with Dupuytren's contracture and histocompatibility B7 cross-reacting antigens. Journal of Urology 128: 48–51

Oehlecker F 1930a Uber Dupuytren'sche Fingerkontraktur. Zentralblatt für Chirurgie 57: 1102

Oehlecker F 1930b Uber Dupuytren'sche Fingerkontraktur. Beitrage zur Klinlsane Chirurgie 149: 333

Ohtani H, Sasano N 1980 Myofibroblasts and myoepithelial cells in human breast carcinoma. An ultrastructural study. Virchows Archiv A (Pathology and Anatomy) 385: 247–261

Olivetti G, Anversa P, Melissari M, Loud A V 1980 Morphometric study of early postnatal development of the thoracic aorta in the rat. Circulation Research 47: 417–424

Operti F 1979 La malattia di Dupuytren. Ortopedia e Traumatologia dell'Apparato Motore 24: 15

Orbach E 1934 Die funktionelle Behandlung des Dupuytren'schen Fingerkontraktur. Archiv für Orthopaedische und Unfall Chirurgie 34: 572

Orlando J C, Smith J W, Goulian D 1974 Dupuytren's contracture: a review of 100 patients. British Journal of Plastic Surgery 27: 211–217

Osborn M, Weber K 1983 Tumor diagnosis by intermediate filament typing: a noval tool for surgical pathology. Laboratory Investigation 48: 372–394

Outhwaite J M, Merry P, Allen R E, Blake D R 1988 Free radicals and Dupuytren's contracture. British Medical Journal 296:

Owens G K, Loeb A, Gordon D, Thompson M M 1986 Expression of smooth muscle-specific α-isoactin in cultured vascular smooth muscle cells: relationship between growth and cytodifferentiation. Journal of Cell Biology 102: 343–352

Paeslack V V 1962 Dupuytrensche Kontractur und Diabetes mellitus. Schweizerische Medizinische Wochenschrift 92: 349

Paget J 1875 Abstract of clinical lectures delivered at St Bartholomew's Hospital. II On the minor signs of gout in the hands and feet. British Medical Journal 1: 665–6

Pal B, Griffiths I D 1987 Association of limited joint mobility with Dupuytren's contracture in diabetes mellitus. Journal of Rheumatology 14: 582–585

Palmar L A, Southworth J L 1945 Bridge operation for Dupuytren's contracture. American Journal of Surgery 68: 351

Palmen A J 1932 Die Sageplastik, eine unter anderen fur Dupuytren'sche Fingerkontraktur und Syndactylie geeignete Schnittfuhrung. Zentralblatt für Chirurgie 59: 1377

Palmer G 1933 Maladie de Dupuytren. Rétraction de l'aponévrose palmaire. Gazette del'Hôpital 106: 1369

Panciera C, D'Antonio G F, Tamaro C 1980 La aponevrectomia selettiva secondo Skoog nella cura della malattia di Dupuytren. Rivista di Chirurgia della Mano 17: 207

Parker H G 1979 Dupuytren's contracture as a cause of stenosing tenosynovitis. Journal of the Main Medical Association 70: 147

Parrini L, Brunelli G 1959 Considerazoini sulla terapia chirurgica della malattia di Dupuytren. Archivio di Ortopedia 72: 1089

Parry A D 1988 The molecular and fibrillar stucture of collagen and its relationship to the mechanical properties of connective tissue. Biophysical Chemistry 29: 195–209

Parry D A, Flint M H, Gillard G C, Craig A S 1982 A role for glycosaminoglycans in the development of collagen fibrils. Federation of European Biochemical Societies Letters 149: 1–7

Parsons D, Adams S, Smith R, Glimcher M J 1985 Collagen polymorphism in Dupuytren's disease. Transactions of the 31st Annual Meeting of the Orthopaedic Research Society, 116

Pastremoli A 1968 Sul trattamento della malattia di Dupuytren mediante roentgenterapia superficiale con tubo a finestra di Berillio. Bollettino delle Scienze Mediche 140: 142

Patel J-C 1961 Constatations du microscope electronique dans la maladie de Dupuytren. Presse Medicale 69: 793

Peiser 1917 Freie Fettransplantation bei der Behandlung der Dupuytren'schen Fingerkontraktur. Zentralblatt für Chirurgie 44: 6

Pennington S N, Smith C P, Strider J B 1979 Alterations in prostaglandin catabolism in rats chronically dosed with ethanol. Biochemical Medicine 21: 246

Pereira R S, Black C B, Turner S M, Spencer J D 1986 Antibodies to collagen types I-VI in Dupuytren's contracture. The Journal of Hand Surgery 11: 58-60

Pietrogrande V, Malotti A 1955 Considerazioni sulla retrazione dell'aponeurosi palmare. Ortopedia e Traumatologia dell'Apparato Motore 23: 321

Piez K A, Reddi A H 1984 Extracellular matrix biochemistry. Elsevier, New York

Piulachs P, Mir Y Mir 1952 Considerations sobre la enfermedad de Dupuytren. Folia Clinica Internacional II: 415–416

Plasse JS 1979 Dupuytren's contractures in a black patient. Plastic and Reconstructive Surgery 64: 250

Plewes L 1956 Sudek's atrophy of the hand. Journal of Bone and Joint Surgery 38B: 195

Pojer J, Radivojevic M, Williams F 1972 Dupuytren's disease its association with abnormal liver function in alcoholism and epilepsy. Archives of internal Medicine 129: 561

Pool J C F, Cromwell S B, Benditt E P 1971 Behavior of smooth muscle cells and formation of extracellular structures in the reaction of arterial wall to injury. American Journal of Pathology 62: 391–414

Postacchini F, Natali P G, Accinni L, Ippolito E, De Martino C 1977 Contractile filaments in cells of regenerating tendon. Experientia 33: 957–959

Povysil C, Matejovsky Z 1979 Ultrastructural evidence of Myofibroblasts in pseudomalignant myositis ossificans. Virchows Archiv A (Pathology and Anatomy) 381: 189–203

Powell B W E M, McLean N R, Jeffs J V 1986 The incidence of palmaris longus tendon in patients with Dupuytren's disease. Journal of Hand Surgery 11B: 382

Prough D S, McLeskey C H, Poehling G G et al 1985 Efficacy of oral nifedipine in the treatment of reflex sympathetic Dystrophy. Anaesthesiology 62: 796

Rabinowitz J L, Ostermann L J R, Bora F W, Staeffen J 1983 Lipid composition and de novo lipid biosynthesis of human palmar fat in Dupuytren's disease. Lipids 18: 371–374

Rafter D, Kenny R, Gilmore M, Walsh C H 1980 Dupuytren's contracture — a survey of a hospital population. Journal of the Irish Medical Association 73: 227

Ramos C V, Gillepsie W, Narconis R J 1978 Elastofibroma. A pseudotumor of myofibroblasts. Archives of Pathology and laboratory Medicine 102: 538-540

Ramstedt 1933 Zur Operation der Dupuytren'schen Fingerkontraktur. Zentralblatt für Chirurgie 60: 2214

Rank B K, Chang L 1978 Dupuytren's contracture — late results. Australian and New Zealand Journal of Surgery 53B: 240

Ravid M, Dinai Y, Sohar E 1977 Dupuytren's disease in diabetes mellitus. Acta Diabetologica Latina 14: 170–174

Reeves H A 1885 The rapid cure of Dupuytren's contraction by excision. British Medical Journal 1: 481

Reichel 1937 Dupuytren'sche Fingerkontraktur als Folge von Verletzung des Nervus ulnaris. Deutsche Zeitschrift für Chirurgie 138: 466

Reid T, Flint M H 1974 Changes in glycosaminoglycan content of healing rabbit tendon. Journal of Embryology and Experimental Morphology 31: 489–495

Reumert T, Zachariae L 1973 Continued investigation into the effect of diuretics upon oedema of the hand following operation for Dupuytren's contracture: bumetanide leo. Acta Orthopedica Scandinavica 44: 410–416

Rhomberg H P 1967 Dupuytrensche Kontraktur und interne Erkrankamgen. Wiener Klinische Wochenschrift 79: 792

Riches D W H 1988 The multiple roles of macrophages in wound healing. In: Clark R A F_b, Henson P M (eds) The molecular and cellular biology of wound repair. Plenum, New York, pp 213–239

Richer P 1877 Rétracim de l'aponévrose plamain. Progrés médicale 5: 369

Richet A 1873 Traité pratique di'anatomie medico-chirurgicale, 4th edn. Paris, p 725

Rigby B J 1977 Thermal transitions in the collagenous tissues of poikilothermic animals. Journal of Thermal Biology 2: 89–93

Rinaldi E, Orso C A 1974 Difficolta chirurgiche nei reinterventi per malattia di Dupuytren. Rivista di Chirurgia della Mano 11: 176

Ritter C 1930 Zur operativen Behandlung der Dupuytren'schen Fingercontractur. Deutsche Zeitschrift für Chirurgie 227: 554

Robbins T H 1981 Dupuytren's contracture: the deferred z-plasty. Annals of the Royal College of Surgeons of England 63: 357–358

Roberts F P 1981 Dupuytren's contracture: a vibration injury. Journal of the Society of Occupational Medicine 31: 148

Robins S P, Bailey A J 1972 Age-related changes in collagen: the identification of reducible lysine-carbohydrate condensation products. Biochemical and Biophysical Research Communications 46: 76

Rodrigo J J, Niebauer J J, Brown R L, Doyle J R 1971 Treatment of Dupuytren's contracture. Long-term results after fasciotomy and fascial excision. Journal of Bone and Joint Surgery 58A: 380–387

Rodrigo J J, Niebauer J J, Brown R L, Doyle J R 1976 Treatment of Dupuytren's contracture. Long-term results after fasciotomy and fascial excision 58-A: 380–387

Rosenberg L, Buckwalter J A 1986 Articular cartilage biochemistry. In: Kuettner K E, Schleyerbach R, Hoscoll V C (eds) Workshop conference Hoechst-Werk Albert. Raven Press, New York, pp 39–57

Rosenbloom A L, Frias J L 1974 Diabetes mellitus, short stature and joint stiffness. A new syndrome. Clinical Research 22: 92A

Rosenbloom A L, Silverstein J H, Lezotte D C, Richardson K, McCallum M 1981 Limited joint mobility in childhood diabetes mellitus indicates increased risk for minor microvascular disease. New England Journal of Medicine 305: 191

Ross R, Everett N B, Tyler R 1970 Wound healing and collagen formation. VI. The origin of the wound fibroblast studied in parabiosis. Journal of Cell Biology 44: 645–654

Roth P B 1920 Dupuytren's contraction in a man aged 31. Annals of Surgery 134: 186

Routier 1908 Rétraction de l'aponévrose palmaire. Opération sans suture sans autoplastie. Bulletin et Mémoires de la Société des Chirurgiens de Paris 34: 860

Rovner A S, Thompson M M, Murphy R A 1986a Two different heavy chains are found in smooth muscle myosin. American Journal of Physiology 250: C861–C870

Rovner A S, Murphy R A, Owens G K 1986b Expression of smooth muscle and nonmuscle myosin heavy chains in cultured vascular smooth muscle cells. Journal of Biological Chemistry 261: 14740–14745

Rowe D W, Starman B J, Fujimoto W Y, Williams R H 1977 Abnormalities in proliferation and progein synthesis in fibroblast cultures from patients with diabetes mellitus. Diabetes 26: 284

Rowley D I, Couch M, Chesney R B, Norries S H 1984 Assessment of percutaneous fasciotomy in the management of Dupuytren's contracture. Journal of Hand Surgery 9B: 163–164

Royce P M, Barnes M J 1977 Comparative studies on collagen glycosylation in chick skin and bone. Biochimica Biophysica Acta 498: 132

Rudnick P A, Anderson P S 1962 Diabetes mellitus in Hiroshima, Japan. Diabetes 11: 533

Rudolph R, Guber S, Suzuki M, Woodward M 1977 The life cycle of the myofibroblast. Surgery, Gynecology and Obstetrics 145: 389–394

Rudolph R, Abraham J, Vecchione T, Guber S, Woodward M 1978 Myofibroblasts and free silicon around breast implants. Plastic and Reconstructive Surgery 62: 185–186

Rudolph R, McLure W J, Woodward M 1979 Contractile fibroblasts in chronic alcoholic cirrhosis. Gastroenterology 76: 704–709

Rungger-Brändle E, Gabbiani G 1983 The role of cytoskeletal and cytocontractile elements in pathologic processes. American Journal of Pathology 110: 361–392

Russ R 1908 The surgical aspects of Dupuytren's contraction. American Journal of Medical Science 135: 856

Rüssel J D, Witt W S 1976 Cell size and growth characteristics of cultured fibroblasts isolated from normal and keloid tissue. Plastic and Reconstruction Surgery 57: 202–212

Ryan G B, Cliff W J, Gabbiani G et al 1974 Myofibroblasts in human granulation tissue. Human Pathology 5: 55–67

Sadun R, Ronconi P 1982 Aspetti strutturali ed ultrastrutturali della malattia di Dupuytren. Rivista di Chirurgia della Mano 19: 269

Sakamoto M, Sakamoto S, Brickley-Parsons D, Glimcher M J 1979 Collagen synthesis and degradation in embryonic chick bone explants. Journal of Bone and Joint Surgery 61: 1042

Sakkas L, Demaine A G, Welsh K I, Panayi G S 1987 Immunoglobulin gene polymorphisms are associated with the susceptibility to rheumatoid arthritis. Tissue Antigens (in Press)

Salaghi M 1902 Della contrattura di Dupuytren o retrazione dell'aponeurosi palmare. Archivio di Ortopedia 19: 32

Salvi V 1973 Personal experience with McCash's 'open palm' technique for Dupuytren's contracture. The Hand 5: 161

Salvi V, Porrino F 1982 La tecnica 'a palmo aperto' secondo McCash nel trattamento della malattia di Dupuytren. Rivista di Chirurgia della Mano 19: 323

Sanmartino A 1957 Lîneamenti di patologia della malattia di Dupuytren. Rilievi istologici, oscillografici, fotopletismografici. La Chirurgia degli Organi di Movimento 45: 59

Sanson L-J 1834 Rapport sur le mémoire du docteur G. Goyrand a l'Académie: 'Nouvelles recherches sur la rétraction permanente des doigts'. Mémoires de l'Académie Royale de Médécine 3: 496–500

Santoni Rugiu P 1969 Le fibre trasversali dell'aponeurosi palmare e la loro importanza nel trattamento chirurgico della contrattura di Dupuytren. Rivista Italiana di Chirurgia Plastica 1: 83

Santoni-Rugiu P 1982 Il trattamento chirurgico della contrattura di Dupuytren. Rivista di Chirurgia della Mano 19: 331

Sappino A P, Skalli O, Jackson B, Schürch W, Gabbiani G 1988 Smooth-muscle differentiation in stromal cells of malignant and non-malignant breast tissues. International Journal of Cancer 41: 707–712

Schmid E, Osborn M, Rungger-Brändle E, Gabbiani G, Weber K, Franke W W 1982 Distribution of vimentin and desmin filaments in smooth muscle tissue of mammalian and avian aorta. Experimental Cell Research 137: 329–340

Schmidt A 1889 Ueber die Dupuytren'sche Palmarfasciencontracture. Inauq diss, Wurzburg

Schmidt D 1983 Connective tissue disorders induced by antileptic drugs. In: Oxley J, Janz D, Meinardi H (eds) Chronic toxicity of antiepileptic drugs. Raven Press, New York, p 115

Schneider B 1970 Mathematische Grundlagen der medizinischen Diagnostik. In: Ehlers C Th, Holberg N, Proppe A (eds) Werkzeug der Medizin. Springer Verlag, Berlin, pp 160–182

Schneider T 1964 Dupuytren's contracture in diabetes mellitus, abstracted. Excerpta Medical International Congress Series 74: 75

Schneider T 1971 Diabetic neuropathy. Hand lesions. In: E R Pfeiffer (ed) Handbook of Diabetes mellitus. JF Lehman Verlag, Munich pp. 614–616

Schneider L H, Hankin F M, Eisenberg T 1986 Surgery of Dupuytren's disease: a review of the open palm method. Journal of Hand Surgery 11A: 23

Schroder C H 1934 Die Vererbung der Dupuytren'schen Fingerkontraktur. Archiv für Rassen-und Gesellschafts-Biologie 28: 353

Schürch W, Seemayer T A, Lagacé R 1981 Stromal myofibroblasts in primary invasive and metastatic carcinomas. A combined immunological, light and electron microscopy study. Virchows Archiv A (Pathology and Anatomy) 391: 125–139

Schürch W, Lagacé R, Seemayer T A 1982 Myofibroblastic stromal reaction in retracted scirrhous carcinomas of the breast. Surgery, Gynecology and Obstetrics 154: 351–358

Schürch W, Seemayer T A, Lagacé R, Gabbiani G 1984 The intermediate filament cytoskeleton of myofibroblasts: an immunofluorescence and ultrastructural study. Virchows Archiv A: Pathology Anatomy 403: 323–336

Schürch W, Skalli O, Seemayer T A, Gabbiani G 1987 Intermediate filament proteins and actin isoforms as markers for soft tissue tumor differentiation and origin. I.Smooth muscle tumors. American Journal of Pathology 128: 91–103

Scolz O 1953 Zur Entstehung der Dupuytrenschen Kontraktur. Zentralblatt für Chirurgie 61: 104

Scott J E 1984 The periphery of the developing collagen fibril. Biochemical Journal 218: 229–233

Scott J E, Hughes E W 1986 Proteoglycan-collagen relationships in developing chick and bovine tendons. Influence of the physiological environment. Connective Tissue Research 14: 267–278

Scott J E, Orford C R, Hughes E W 1981 Proteoglycan-collagen arrangements in developing rat tail tendon. Biochemical Journal 195: 573–581

Seemayer T A, Lagace R, Schurch W, Thelmo W L 1980 The myofibroblast: biologic, pathologic and theoretical considerations. Pathology Annual 15: 443

Seemayer T A, Lagacé R, Schürch W 1979a On the pathogenesis of sclerosis and nodularity in nodular sclerosing Hodgkin's disease. Virchows Archiv A (Pathology and Anatomy) 385: 283–291

Seemayer T A, Lagacé R, Schürch W, Tremblay G 1979b Myofibroblasts in the stroma of invasive and metastatic carcinoma. A possible host response to neoplasia. American Journal of Surgical Pathology 3: 525–533

Seemayer T A, Lagacé R, Schürch W, Thelmo W L 1980 The myofibroblast: biologic, pathologic, and theoretical considerations. Pathology Annual 12: 491–492

Seemayer T A, Schürch W, Lagacé R 1981 Myofibroblasts in human pathology. Human Pathology 12: 491–492

Seemayer T A, Schürch, Lagacé R 1982 The myofibroblast and defence against neoplasia: a hypothesis. Survey of Immunologic Research 1: 268–273

Serafini-Fracassini A, Smith J W 1974 Glycosaminoglycans and proteaglycans. In: (eds) The structure and biochemistry of cartilage. Churchill Livingstone, Edinburgh, pp 64–112

Sergovich F R, Botz J S, McFarlane R M 1983 Nonrandom cytogenetic abnormalities in Dupuytren's disease. New England Journal of Medicine 308: 162–163

Sharpe D N, Scott P J, Flint M H, Donald J 1980 Arterial connective tissue changes and distribution of ^{125}I-labelled low density lipoprotein in hypertensive pigs. Atherosclerosis 35: 393–411

Shaw M H 1951 The treatment of Dupuytren's contracture. British Journal of Plastic Surgery 4: 218–233

Shaw M H, Eastwood D S 1965 Dupuytren's contracture: a selective approach to treatment. British Journal of Surgery 18: 164–170

Shetlar M R, Shetlar C L 1977 The hypertrophic scar: location of glycosaminoglycans within scars. Burns 4: 14–19

Shum D T, McFarlane R M 1988 Histogenesis of Dupuytren's disease; an immunohistochemical study of 30 cases. Journal of Hand Surgery 13A: 61–66

Singer I I 1979 The fibronexus: a transmembrane association of fibronectin-containing fibers and 5 nm microfilaments in hamster and human fibroblasts. Cell 16: 675

Singer I I, Kawka D W, Kazazis D M, Clark R A F 1984 In vivo co-distribution of fibronectin and actin fibers in granulation tissue: immunofluorescence and electron microscope studies of the fibronexus at the myofibroblast surface. Journal of Cell Biology 98: 2091–2106

Singer I I, Kazazis D M, Kawka D W 1985 Localization of the fibronexus at the surface of granulation tissue myofibroblasts using double-label immunogold electron microscopy on ultrathin frozen sections. European Journal of Cell Biology 38: 94–101

Singer I I, Scott S, Kawka D W, Hassell J R 1987 Extracellular matrix fibers containing fibronectin and basement membrane heparan sulphate proteoglycan coalign with focal contacts and microfilament bundles in stationary fibroblasts. Experimental Cell Research 173: 558–571

Skalli O, Gabbiani G 1988 The biology of the myofibroblast relationship to wound contraction and fibrocontractive disease. In: Clark R A F, Henson P M (eds) The molecular and cellular biology of wound repair. Plenum, New York, pp 373–402

Skalli O, Ropraz P, Trzeciak A, Benzonana G, Gillessen D, Gabbiani G 1986a A monoclonal antibody against α-smooth muscle actin: a new probe for smooth muscle differentiation. Journal of Cell Biology 103: 2787–2796

Skalli O, Bloom W S, Ropraz P, Azzarone B, Gabbiani G 1986b Cytoskeletal remodeling of rat aortic smooth muscle cells in vitro: relationships to culture conditions and analogies to in vivo situations. Journal of Submicroscopic Cytology 18: 481–493

Skalli O, Vandekerckhove J, Gabbiani G 1987 Actin isoform pattern as a marker of normal or pathological smooth-muscle and fibroblastic tissues. Differentiation 33: 232–238

Skalli O, Schürch W, Seemayer T et al 1989a Myofibroblasts from diverse pathological settings are heterogeneous in their content of actin isoforms and intermediate filament proteins. Laboratory Investigation (in press)

Skalli O, Pelte M F, Peclet M C et al 1989b α-smooth muscle actin, a differentiation marker of smooth muscle cells, is present in microfilamentous bundles of pericytes. Journal of Histochemistry and Cytochemistry (in press)

Skinner H L 1941 Dupuytren's contraction. Operative correction by use of tunnel skin graft. Surgery 10: 313

Skoog T 1948 Dupuytren's contraction with special reference to aetiology and improved surgical treatment, its occurrence in epileptics. Note on knuckle pads. Acta Chirurgica Scandinavica 96 (suppl 139)

Skoog T 1957 Dupuytren's contracture. Post Graduate Medicine 21: 91

Skoog T 1963 The pathogenesis and etiology of Dupuytren's contacture. Plastic and Reconstructive Surgery 31: 258–267

Skoog T 1967 The superficial transverse fibres of the palmar aponeuroses and their significance in Dupuytren's contracture. Surgical Clinics of North America 47: 443

Skoog T 1967 Dupuytren's contracture: pathogenesis and surgical treatment. Surgical Clinicals of North America 47: 433–444

Skoog T 1967b The transverse elements of the palmar aponeurosis in Dupuytren's contracture. Scandinavian Journal of Plastic and Reconstructive Surgery 1: 51

Skoog T 1985 Dupuytren's contracture: pathogenesis and surgical treatment. In: Hueston J, Tubiana R (eds) Dupuytren's disease, 2nd edn. Churchill Livingstone, London, pp 184–192

Slack C, Flint M H, Thompson B M 1982 Glycosaminoglycan synthesis by Dupuytren's cells in culture. Connective Tissue Research 9: 263–269

Slack C, Thomson B M, Flint M H 1983 Embryonic tendons in organ culture — an in vitro system for the study of effects of mechanical forces on connective tissue metabolism. Connective Tissues Research 11: 349–350

Slack C, Bradley G, Beaumont B, Poole A, Flint M 1986 Changes in the morphology and synthetic activity of cultured rat tail tendon. Cell Tissue Research 245: 359–368

Small J V, Sabieszek A 1980 The contractile apparatus of smooth muscle. International Review of Cytology 64: 241–306

Smith N 1884 Seventy cases of Dupuytren's contraction of the fingers. British Medical Journal 1: 602–604

Smith N 1885 Seventy cases of Dupuytren's contraction of the fingers. Proceedings of the Royal Medical Chirurgical Society of London 1: 230

Snedecor G W, Cochran W G 1967 Statistical methods 6th edn. Iowa State University Press, Ames

Sodek J 1976 A new approach to assessing collagen turnover by using a micro-assay. Biochemical Journal 160: 243

Spencer J D, Welsh K I 1984 Histocompatibility antigen patterns in Dupuytren's contracture. The Journal of Hand Surgery 9B: 276–278

Spina G M, Tessari L 1960 Alcuni rilievi istochimici to tema di malattia di Dupuytren. Archivio di Ortopedia 73: 882

Spitzy H 1916 Behandlung von Hand und Fingerkontrakturen mit kunstlicher Fettumscheidung. Zeitschrift für Orthopaedische Chirurgie 35: 550

Spring M, Fleek H, Cohen B D 1970 Dupuytren's contracture: warning of diabetes. New York State Journal of Medicine 70: 1037–1041

Stack H G 1971 The palmar fascia and the development of deformities and displacements in Dupuytren's contracture. Annals of the Royal College of Surgeons of England 48: 230

Stack H G 1973 The palmar fascia. Churchill Livingstone, Edinburgh

Stackebrandt H 1932 Die Hereditat bei der Dupuytrenschen Kontraktur, darge an 5 Stammbaumen. Inaug.-Diss., Munster

Stamenkovic I, Skalli O, Gabbiani G 1986 Distribution of intermediate filament proteins in normal and diseased human glomeruli. American Journal of Pathology 125: 465–475

Stanisavljevic S, Pool R 1962 The paratendinous apparatus of the digits. Journal of Bone and Joint Surgery 44B: 910

Stein A, Wang M K H, Macomber B W, Rajpal R, Heffernan A 1960 Dupuytren's contracture a morphologic evaluation of the pathogenesis. Annals of Surgery 151: 577–580

Stern B D, Mechanic G L, Glimcher M J, Goldhaber P 1963 The resorption of bone collagen in tissue cultures. Biochemica Biophysica Research Communication 13: 137

Stewart H D, Innes A R, Burke F D 1985 The hand complications of Colles' fracture. Journal of Hand Surgery 10B: 103

Stiller D, Katenkamp D 1975 Cellular features in desmoid fibromatosis and well-differentiated fibrosarcomas. An electron microscopic study. Virchows Archiv A (Pathology and Anatomy) 369: 155–164

Stopak D, Harris A K 1982 Connective tissue morphogenesis by fibroblast traction. 1. Tissue culture observations. Developmental Biology 90: 383–398

Strawich E, Glimcher M J 1983 Differences in the extent and heterogeneity of lysyl hydroxylation in embryonic chick cranial and long bone collagens. Journal of Biological Chemistry 258: 555

Strickland J W, Bassett R L 1985 The isolated digital cord in Dupuytren's contracture: anatomy and clinical significance. Journal of Hand Surgery 10: 118–24

Sthuler T, Stankovic P 1977 Epilepsie und Dupuytren'sche Kontraktur — Syntropie zweier Krankheiten. Hand Chirurgie 9: 219

Su C 1970 Dupuytren's contracture. Its association with alcoholism and cirrhosis. Archives of Internal Medicine 126: 278–281

Su C K, Patek A J 1970 Dupuytren's contracture: its association with alcoholism and cirrhosis. Archives of Internal Medicine 126: 278

Summerskill W H J, Davidson C S, Dible J H et al 1960 Cirrhosis of the liver a study of alcoholic and nonalcoholic patients in Boston and London. New England Journal of Medicine

Swanson A B, Hagert C G, Swanson G 1983 Evaluation of impairment of hand function. Journal of Hand Surgery 8: 709

Tait B D, MacKay I R 1982 HLA phenotypes in Dupuytren's contracture. Tissue Antigens 19: 240–241

Tajana G, Montagnani S, Marotta M et al 1982 Caratterizzazione strutturale di miofibroblasti isolati de pazienti affetti da contrattura di Dupuytren. Rivista di Chirurgia della Mano 19: 373

Tamkun J W, DeSimone D W, Fonda D et al 1986 Structure of integrin, a glycoprotein involved in the transmembrane linkage between fibronectin and actin. Cell 46: 271

Tasca G, Franzi P G, Salvatore P 1969 Aponeurectomia selettiva per morbo di Dupuytren. Ospeduli d'Italia Chirurgia 20: 293

Taxy J B 1977 Juvenile nasopharyngeal angiofibroma. An ultrastructural study. Cancer 39: 1044–1054

Telhag H, Lindberg L 1972 A method of inducing osteoarthritic changes in rabbits' knee. Clinical Orthopaedics 86: 214–223

Tessari L, Parrini L 1959 Osservazioni biochimiche sul morbo di Dupuytren. Archivio di Ortopedia 72: 435

Thaxter T H, Mann R A, Anderson C E 1965 Degeneration of immobilized knee joints in rats; histological and autoradiographic study. Journal of Bone and Joint Surgery 47-A: 567–585

Then Bergh H 1939 Konkordantes Vorkommen von Dupuytren'scher Fingerkontraktur bei 3 Zwillingpaaren. Allgemeine Ztschrift für Psychiatrie und ihre Grenzgebnis 112: 327

Thieme 1989 Journal of Hand Surgery (in press).

Thomine J M 1965 Conjonctif d'enveloppe des doigts et squelette fibreux des commissures interdigitales. Annales de Chirurgie Plastique 10: 194

Thomine J M 1972 Le fascia digital. In: Tubiana R (ed) La maladie de Dupuytren, 2nd edn. Expansion Scientific Francais, Paris, p 1

Thurston A J 1987 Conservative surgery for Dupuytren's contracture. Journal of Hand Surgery 12-B: 329–334

Timpl R, Wiedermann H, van Delden V, Furthmayr H, Kühn K 1981 A network model for the organization of type IV collagen in basement membrane. European Journal of Biochemistry 120: 203

Tipton C M, Shild R J, Flatt A E 1967 Measurement of ligamentous strength in rat knees. Journal of Bone and Joint Surgery 49-A: 63–72

Tipton C M, James S L, Merger W, Tcheng T-K 1970 Influence of exercise on strength of medial collateral knee ligaments of dogs. American Journal of Physiology 218: 894–901

Tipton C M, Matthes R D, Maynard J A, Carey R A 1975 The influence of physical activity on ligaments and tendons. Medicine and Science in Sports 7: 165–175

Toccanier-Pelte M F, Skalli O, Kapanci Y, Gabbiani G 1987 Characterization of stromal cells with myoid features in lymph nodes and spleen in normal and pathologic conditions. American Journal of Pathology 129: 109–118

Tomasek J J, Schultz R J, Episalla C W, Newman S A 1986 The cytoskeleton and extracellular matrix of Dupuytren's disease 'myofibroblast': an immunofluorescence study of a nonmuscle cell type. Journal of Hand Surgery 11a: 365

Tomasek J J, Schultz R J, Haaksma C J 1987 Extracellular matrix cytoskeletal connections at the surface of the specialized contractile fibroblast (myofibroblast) in Dupuytren's disease. Journal of Bone and Joint Surgery: in press

Tonkin M A, Burke F D, Vavian J P W 1984 Dupuytren's contracture: a comparative study of fasciectomy and dermofasciectomy in 100 patients. Journal of Hand Surgery 9-B: 156–162

Tonkin M A, Burke F D, Varian J P W 1985 The proximal interphalangeal joint in Dupuytren's disease. Journal of Hand Surgery 10B: 358–364

Toole B P, Lowther D A 1968 Dermatan sulphate-protein: isolation and interaction with collagen. Archives of Biochemistry and Biophysics 128: 567–578

Trelat M 1888 Essai sur la maladie de Dupuytren cited by Skoog (1948)

Tremblay G 1979 Stromal aspects of breast carcinoma. Experimental and Molecular Pathology 31: 248–260

Tricomi E 1907 Su tre asportazioni totali di ambedue le aponeurosi palmari per malattia del Dupuytren. Archivio di Ortopedia 24: 1

Tsukuda T, McNutt M A, Ross R, Gown A M 1987 HHF35, a muscle actin-specific monoclonal antibody. II. Reactivity in normal, reactive, and neoplastic human tissues. American Journal of Pathology 127: 389–402

Tubiana R 1963 Les temps cutanées dans le traitement chirurgical de la maladie de Dupuytren. Annales de Chirurgie Plastique 8: 157–168

Tubiana R 1964 Le traitement sélectif de la maladie de Dupuytren. Revue de Chirurgie Orthopaédique 50: 311–333

Tubiana R 1967 Les conceptions actuelles du traitement chirurgical de la maladie de Dupuytren. In: Orthopédie et traumatologie, Conférences d'enseignement. Expansion Scientifique, Paris, p 7

Tubiana R 1974 The principles of surgical treatment of Dupuytren's contracture: In: Dupuytren's disease. Grune & Stratton, New York, p 71

Tubiana R 1985 Overview on surgical treatment of Dupuytren's disease. In: Hueston J T, Tubiana R (eds) Dupuytren's disease, 2nd edn. Churchill-Livingstone, Edinburgh, pp 129–130

Tubiana R 1986 Traitment des récidives. In: Tubiana R, Hueston J T (eds). La maladie de Dupuytren, 3rd edn. Expansion Scientifique Francaise, pp Paris, 149–153

Tubiana R, De Frenne H 1976 Localisation de la maladie de Dupuytren à la partie radiale de la main. Chirurgie 102: 989–993

Tubiana R, Leclerco C 1985 Recurrent Dupuytren's disease. In: Hueston J T, Tubiana R (eds) Dupuytren's disease, 2nd edn. Churchill Livingstone, London

Tubiana R, Thomine J M 1974 Surgical treatment of Dupuytren's contracture: technique of fasciotomy and fasciectomy. In: Dupuytren's disease. Churchill-Livingstone, Edinburgh, pp 85–92

Tubiana R, Thomine J M, Brown S 1967 Complications of surgery in Dupuytren's contracture. Plastic and Reconstructive Surgery 39: 603

Tubiana R, Michon J, Thomine J M 1968 Scheme for the assessment of deformities in Dupuytren's disease. Surgical Clinics of North America 48: 979

Tubiana R, Simmons B P, De Frenne H A R 1982 Location of Dupuytren's disease on the radial aspect of the hand. Clinical Orthopaedics and Related Research 168: 222–229

Tubiana R, Simmons B P, De Frenne H A 1985 Dupuytren's disease on the radial side of the hand. In Hueston J T, Tubiana R (eds) Dupuytren's disease, 2nd edn. Churchill Livingstone, London, pp 131–133

Tunn S 1985 Doctoral thesis. Hannover, FRG

Tunn S, Gurr E, Delbrück A, Buhr T, Flory J 1988 The distribution of unsulphated glycosaminoglycans in palmar fascia from patients with Dupuytren's disease and healthy subjects. Journal of Clinical Chemistry and Clinical Biochemistry 26:7–14

Tyler J A 1985 Chondrocyte-mediated depletion of articular cartilage proteoglycans in vitro. Biochemical Journal 225: 493–507

Urushizaki Y, Seifter S 1985 Phosphorylation of hydroxylysine residues in collagen synthesized by cultured aortic smooth muscle cells. Proceedings of the National Academy of Science USA 82: 3091

Ushijima M, Tsuneyoshi M, Enjoji M 1984 Dupuytren type fibromatoses. A clinicopathologic study of 62 cases. Acta Pathologica Japonica 34: 991–1001

van Bockxmeer F M, Martin C E, Constable I J 1985 Models for assessing scar tissue inhibitors. Retina 5: 239–252

VandeBerg J S, Gelberman R H, Rudolph R, Johnson D, Sicurello P 1984 Dupuytren's disease: comparative growth dynamics and morphology between cultured myofibroblasts (nodule) and fibroblasts (cord). Journal of Orthopaedic Research 2: 247

Vandekerkchove J, Weber K 1978a At least six different actins are expressed in a higher mammal: an analysis based on the amino acid sequence of the amino-terminal tryptic peptide. Journal of Molecular Biology 126: 783–802

Vandekerckhove J, Weber K 1978b Mammalian cytoplasmic actins are the products of at least two genes and differ in primary structure in at least 25 identified positions from skeletal muscle actins. Proceedings of the National Academy of Sciences 75: 1106–1110

Vandekerckhove J, Weber K 1981 Actin typing on total cellular extracts. A highly sensitive protein-chemical procedure able to distinguish different actins. European Journal of Biochemistry 113: 595–603

Varian J P W 1975 The ridged plaster volar slab. The Hand 7: 78

Varian J P W 1985 Full thickness skin grafting in the management of recurrent Dupuytren's disease. In: Hueston J T, Tubiana R (ed) Dupuytren's disease, 2nd edn. Churchill Livingstone, Edinburgh, pp 154–157

Verga G A, Galassi G P, Ferrari M 1972 Aspetti angiologici della malattia di Dupuytren. Rivista Italiana di Chirurgia Plastica 3: 299

Viale G, Doglioni C, Iuzzolino P et al 1988 Infantile digital fibromatosis-like tumour (inclusion body fibromatosis) of adulthood: report of two cases with ultrastructural and immunocytochemical findings. Histopathology 12: 415–424

Viger J 1883 De la rétraction de l'aponévrose palmaire chez les diabétiques. Thèse, Paris

Vigliani F, Rodighiero G C 1964 La validità dell'aponeurectomia subtotale nella cura del morbo di Dupuytren. Rivista di Chirurgia della Mano 2: 67

Viglian F, Rodighiero G C 1965 La malattia di Dupuytren. Cappelli Editore, Bologna

Viidik A 1967 The effect of training on the tensile strength of isolated rabbit tendons. Scandinavian Journal of Plastic and Reconstructive Surgery 1: 141–147

Viidik A 1968 Elasticity and tensile strength of the anterior cruciate ligament in rabbits as influenced by training. Acta Physiologica Scandinavica 74: 372–380

Viidik A 1979 Biomechanical behaviour of soft connective tissues. In: Akkas N (ed) Progress in biomechanics. Sijthoff & Nordhoff, Alpen Aan den Rijn, pp 75–113

Viidik A, Danielsen C C, Oxlund H 1982 On fundamental and phenomenological models, structure and mechanical properties of collagen, elastin and glycosaminoglycan complexes. Biorheology 19: 437–451

Vogel K, Heinegard D 1985 Characterisation of proteoglycans from adult bovine tendon. Journal of Biological Chemistry 260: 9298–9306

Vogel K G, Paulsson M, Heinegard D 1984 Specific inhibition of type I and type II collagen fibrillogenesis by the small proteoglycan of tendon. Biochemical Journal 223: 587–597

Vogel K, Keller E, Lenhoff R, Campbell K, Koob T 1986 Proteoglycan synthesis by fibroblast cultures initiated from regions of adult bovine tendon subjected to different mechanical forces. European Journal of Cell Biology 41: 102–112

Vogt P 1881 Die chirurgischen Erkrankungen der oberen Extremitat. Deutsche Chirurgie Lieferung 64: 88

Volpato B, Setti E, Leidi P 1982 La nostra esperienza in merito a novanta casi di malattia di Dupuytren operiti con la technica a palmo aperto. Rivista di Chirurgia della Mano 19: 419

von der Mark K 1982 Localisation of collagen types in tissue. International Review of Connective Tissue Research 9: 265

Von Siemen H 1936 Zur operation der Palmarkontraktur (Dupuytrensche Fingerkontraktur). Deutsche Zeitschrift für Chirurgie 246: 693

Von Stapelmohr S 1947 Om 14 ars Dupuytren - operatimer a Norrkopings lasarett. Svenska lak Tidning 44: 81 (in Swedish) cited by Skoog (1948)

Wada S, Toda S, Omori Y, Yamakido M, Blackard W G 1964 The clinical features of diabetes mellitus in Japan as observed in a hospital outpatient clinic. Diabetes 13: 485

Wagner S 1932 Ergebnisse der operativen Behandlung bei Dupuytrunscher Kontraktur. Beitraege Zur Klinische Chirurgie 155: 271

Watson H K, Gonzales F 1988 Simultaneous carpal tunnel and Dupuytren's surgery. To be published

Watson H K, Bass D, Deming E G 1975 Current management of Dupuytren's contracture utilizing the Deming Y-V-Z advancement incision. Journal of Bone and Joint Surgery 57A: 726

Watson H K, Light T R, Johnson T R 1979 Checkrein resection for flexion contracture of the middle joint. Journal of Hand Surgery 4: 67–71

Watson J D 1984 Fasciotomy and z-plasty in the management of Dupuytren's contracture. British Journal of Plastic Surgery 37: 27–30

Weathers D R, Campbell W G 1974 Ultrastructure of the giant-cell fibroma of the oral mucosa. Oral Surgery 38: 550–561

Webb-Jones A 1965 Dupuytren's contracture: the results of radical fasciectomy. British Journal of Plastic Surgery 18: 377–384

Weber R 1967 Biochemical and cellular aspects of tissue involution in development. Experimental Biology and Medicine 1: 63–76

Weckesser E C 1964 Results of wide excision of the palmar fascia for Dupuytren's contracture. Annals of Surgery 160: 1007–1013

Weeds A 1982 Actin-binding proteins — regulators of cell architecture and motility. Nature 296: 811–816

Wegmann T, Geiser W 1964 Die dupuytrensche Kontraktur der Hand as internistisches Problem: Untersuchungen zur Aetiologie. Helvetica Medical Acta 1: 6

Wehbé M, Hunter J M 1985 Tendon gliding. Orthopaedic Review 14: 416–418

Weiss C, Smith R, Glimcher M, Trahan C, Altmann K 1976 Morphological studies in Dupuytren's contracture. Transactions of the Orthopaedic Research Society 1: 220

Weitbrecht I 1742 Syndesmologia sive historia ligamentorum. Corporaris humani petropoli. Faculté de Mé decine, Paris

White S 1984 Anatomy of the palmar fascia on the ulnar border of the hand. Journal of Hand Surgery 9B: 51

White G E, Gimbrone M A, Fujiwara K 1983 Factors influencing the expression of stress fibers in vascular endothelial cells in situ. Journal of Cell Biology 97: 416–424

Willingham M L, Yamada K M, Yamada S S, Pouyssegur J, Pastan I 1977 Microfilament bundles and cell shape are related to adhesiveness to substratum and are dissociable from growth control in cultured fibroblasts. Cell 10: 375

Wilson W F 1972 Shearer's knuckles. Australian and New Zealand. Journal of Surgery 42: 192–193

Wirman J A 1976 Nodular fasciitis, a lesion of myofibroblasts. An ultrastructural study. Cancer 38: 2378–2389

Woessner J F Jr 1968 Biological mechanisms of collagen resorption. In: Gould S (ed) Treatise on collagen, vol 2. Biology of collagen. Academic Press, London

Wolfe S J, Summerskill W J M, Davidson C S 1956 Thickening and contraction of the palmar fascia (Dupuytren's contracture) associated with alcoholism and hepatic cirrhosis. New England Journal of Medicine 235: 559–563

Wollf J L 1892 Das Gesertz der Transformation der Knochen, A. Hirschwald, Berlin

Wong A, Pollard T D, Herman I M 1983 Actin filament stress fibers in vascular endothelial cells in vivo. Science 219: 867–869

Woo SL-Y, Ritler M A, Amiel D et al 1980 The biomechanical and biochemical properties of swine tendons. Long-term effects of exercise on the digital extension. Connective Tissue Research 7: 177–183

Woo SL-Y, Gomez M A, Woo Y-K, Akeson W H 1982 Mechanical properties of tendons and ligaments. Biorheology 19: 397–408

Woodburn K, McGrouther D A 1988 Tendon excursions of the interossei and superficial hypothenar muscles: an anatomical study. Journal of Hand Surgery 13B; 415–420

Woodcock-Mitchell J, Adler K B, Low R B 1984 Immunohistochemical identification of cell types in normal and in bleomycin-induced fibrotic rat lung: cellular origins of interstitial cells. American Review of Respiratory Disease 130: 910–916

Wood Jones F 1941 The principles of anatomy as seen in the hand, 2nd edn. Baillière, Tindall & Cox, London

Woolf M 1920 In a discussion on Dupuytren's Contracture. Proceedings of the Royal Society of Medicine 13: 114

Woolley D E, Evanson J M (eds) 1980 Collagenase in normal and pathological connective tissue. John Wiley, Chichester

Woyke S, Domagala W, Olszewski W, Korabiec M 1974 Pseudosarcoma on the skin. An electromicroscopic study and comparison with fine structure of the spindle-cell variant of squamous cell carcinoma. Cancer 33: 970–980

Wurster-Hill D H, Brown F, Park J P, Gibson S H 1988 Cytogenic studies in Dupuytren's contracture. American Journal of Human Genetics 43: 285

Yamada K M 1983 Cell surface interactions with extracellular materials. Annual Review of Biochemistry 52: 761

Urushizaki Y, Seifter S 1985 Phosphorylation of hydroxylysine residues in collagen synthesized by cultured aortic smooth muscle cells. Proceedings of the National Academy of Science USA 82: 3091

Ushijima M, Tsuneyoshi M, Enjoji M 1984 Dupuytren type fibromatoses. A clinicopathologic study of 62 cases. Acta Pathologica Japonica 34: 991–1001

van Bockxmeer F M, Martin C E, Constable I J 1985 Models for assessing scar tissue inhibitors. Retina 5: 239–252

VandeBerg J S, Gelberman R H, Rudolph R, Johnson D, Sicurello P 1984 Dupuytren's disease: comparative growth dynamics and morphology between cultured myofibroblasts (nodule) and fibroblasts (cord). Journal of Orthopaedic Research 2: 247

Vandekerkchove J, Weber K 1978a At least six different actins are expressed in a higher mammal: an analysis based on the amino acid sequence of the amino-terminal tryptic peptide. Journal of Molecular Biology 126: 783–802

Vandekerckhove J, Weber K 1978b Mammalian cytoplasmic actins are the products of at least two genes and differ in primary structure in at least 25 identified positions from skeletal muscle actins. Proceedings of the National Academy of Sciences 75: 1106–1110

Vandekerckhove J, Weber K 1981 Actin typing on total cellular extracts. A highly sensitive protein-chemical procedure able to distinguish different actins. European Journal of Biochemistry 113: 595–603

Varian J P W 1975 The ridged plaster volar slab. The Hand 7: 78

Varian J P W 1985 Full thickness skin grafting in the management of recurrent Dupuytren's disease. In: Hueston J T, Tubiana R (ed) Dupuytren's disease, 2nd edn. Churchill Livingstone, Edinburgh, pp 154–157

Verga G A, Galassi G P, Ferrari M 1972 Aspetti angiologici della malattia di Dupuytren. Rivista Italiana di Chirurgia Plastica 3: 299

Viale G, Doglioni C, Iuzzolino P et al 1988 Infantile digital fibromatosis-like tumour (inclusion body fibromatosis) of adulthood: report of two cases with ultrastructural and immunocytochemical findings. Histopathology 12: 415–424

Viger J 1883 De la rétraction de l'aponévrose palmaire chez les diabétiques. Thèse, Paris

Vigliani F, Rodighiero G C 1964 La validità

dell'aponeurectomia subtotale nella cura del morbo di Dupuytren. Rivista di Chirurgia della Mano 2: 67

Viglian F, Rodighiero G C 1965 La malattia di Dupuytren. Cappelli Editore, Bologna

Viidik A 1967 The effect of training on the tensile strength of isolated rabbit tendons. Scandinavian Journal of Plastic and Reconstructive Surgery 1: 141–147

Viidik A 1968 Elasticity and tensile strength of the anterior cruciate ligament in rabbits as influenced by training. Acta Physiologica Scandinavica 74: 372–380

Viidik A 1979 Biomechanical behaviour of soft connective tissues. In: Akkas N (ed) Progress in biomechanics. Sijthoff & Nordhoff, Alpen Aan den Rijn, pp 75–113

Viidik A, Danielsen C C, Oxlund H 1982 On fundamental and phenomenological models, structure and mechanical properties of collagen, elastin and glycosaminoglycan complexes. Biorheology 19: 437–451

Yamauchi M, London R E, Guenat C, Hashimoto F, Mechanic G L 1987 Structure and formation of a stable histidine-based trifunctional cross-link in skin collagen. Journal of Biological Chemistry 262: 11428

Yodaiken R E 1979 The basal lamina (basement membrane) of diabetic capillaries. Advances in Microcirculation 8: 37

Yost J 1955 Dupuytren's contracture. A statistical study. American Journal of Surgery 90: 568

Zachariae L 1955 Hydrocortisone acetate in the treatment of Dupuytren's contraction and allied conditions. Acta Chirurgica Scandinavica 109: 421

Zachariae L 1967 Extensive versus limited fasciectomy for Dupuytren's contracture — how limited should a limited fasciectomy be? Scandinavian Journal of Plastic and Reconstructive Surgery 1: 150

Zachariae L 1969 Dupuytren's contracture. How limited should a limited fasciectomy be? Scandinavian Journal of Plastic and Reconstructive Surgery 3: 145

Zachariae L, Vilh J, Olesen E 1970 The electroencephalogram in patients with Dupuytren's contracture. Scandinavian Journal of Plastic and Reconstructive Surgery 4: 35

Zancolli E A 1979 Structural and dynamic bases of hand surgery. J B Lippincott, Philadelphia, pp 3–36

Zancolli E A, Zancolli E R 1984 Congenital ulnar drift and camptodactyly produced by malformation of the retaining ligaments of the skin. Bulletin of the Hospital for Joint Disease Orthopaedic Institute 2: 558

Zaworski R E, Mann R J 1979 Dupuytren's contracture in a black patient. Plastic and Reconstractive Surgery 63: 122–124

Zemel N P, Balcomb T V, Stark H H et a l 1987 Dupuytren's disease in women: evolution of long-term results after operation. Journal of Hand Surgery 12A: 1012

Zimman O A, Robles J M, Lee J C 1978 The fibrous capsule around mammary implants: an investigation. Aesthetic and Plastic Surgery 2: 217–234

Zimmerman 1898 Wissenschaftl Verein der k and k. Militerazte der Garrison Wien. Demonstration. Wiener Klinische Wochenschrift 11: 224

Zimmet P 1983 The global epidemiology of diabetes mellitus. Tohoku Journal of Experimental Medicine 141: 41

Index

A₁ pulley of flexor tendon sheath in DD, 294
Abductor digiti minimi, tendon of, 177, 178, 273, 384
Actin
　fascia shortening involving, 83
　in myofibroblasts/tractofibroblasts, 87, 93–4, 94–7, 97, 98, 107, 108
　as a marker of origin, 41–2, 43
Adhesion plaques, 107, 108
Aetiology of Dupuytren's disease, 84–5, 99–103, 275–89
Age
　at operation, in surgical patients, 222–38, 381, 394–412
　of DD occurrence, 99–100, 269
　　Japanese population study, 240, 242, 244
　　Norwegian population study, 191–2, 198, 199
　of DD onset, 269
　　assessment for surgery regarding, 293
　　Norwegian population study, 192, 199
　　in surgical patients, 209, 212–13, 222–38, 293, 381, 394–412
Aged, residential institutions for the, in Japanese epidemiological study, 240–1
Aggravating factors, 247–9, 261–2
Aging, vascular related phenomenon of, 257
Alcoholism, DD associated with, 204–5, 220, 253–5
　assessment for surgery regarding, 293–4
Aldimine cross links in collagen, 63, 64, 75
Alibert, J. L. (Baron), 4
American surgical patients, data on, 222–3
Amputation
　with distal interphalangeal joint hyperextension, 333
　with proximal interphalangeal joint contractures and deformities, 310, 352

Anaesthesia, 352
　surgical data regarding, 222–38, 381, 394–412
Anatomy, normal and pathological, 117–83
Ankyrin, 107
Anoxia, tissue, 147, 286–7
Antibiotic ointments, 369
Aponeurectomy, segmental, 307, 352–6
Aponeurosis, palmar, 119, 121–2, 123–5
　anatomy and development, 119, 121–2, 123–5, 139
　collagen in
　　in DD, 15, 67, 69
　　in normal conditions, 15, 66–7, 67, 69
　function, 119
　load bearing in relation to, 139
　longitudinal fibres of, 131
　　damage during dissection, 357
　　rupture, 248
　proximal tension upon, DD related to, 119
　repair of trauma, DD related to, 46
　transverse fibres of, 128, 130, 174
　　surgical approaches to preserving, 357
Aponeurotic type of Dupuytren's disease, 328
Arteries, surgical problems regarding, 180, 378–9
Arthritis, rheumatoid see Rheumatoid arthritis
Arthroplasty, Swanston's replacement, 310
Asian patients, epidemiological studies of, 210, 226, 239–45
Assessment/evaluation of patient, 249, 293–4 see also Examination
　clinical, 249
　postoperative, 354–6, 370
　preoperative, 293–4, 348–51, 354
Atrophy, Sudek's, 248
Australian surgical patients, data on, 230

Bands
　clinical diagnosis, 189
　pretendinous see Pretendinous fibres/fascial bands
Barbiturate medication, DD associated with, 203
Bartholinus, T., 127
Baths, whirlpool, 368–9, 369
Bilateral disease, 233, 270
　prevalence, 209
　surgical data, 233
Biology of Dupuytren's disease, 11–116
Black (Negro) persons, DD occurrence in, 247, 281
Blanching sign, 188–9
Blood vessels, myofibroblasts originating from, 43–4
Boutonnière deformity with distal interphalangeal joint hyperextension, 335–6, 366
Boyer, A., 4, 7
British surgical patients, data on, 229

Callus formation, internal, 23–4
Canada
　occurrence of DD in, 224, 247
　surgical patient data from, 224–5
　West German surgical patient data and, comparisons, 211
Capsulectomy with proximal interphalangeal joint contractures, 310
Carcinomas
　myofibroblasts in, 33
　stroma of, wound healing related to, 45
Care, postoperative see Postoperative care
Carpal tunnel release, 294
Carpal tunnel syndrome, 294
Cartilage, joint, glycosaminoglycans in, 49
Cause (aetiology) of Dupuytren's disease, 84–5, 99–103, 275–89

443

Cell(s), 31–47
  biology, 31–47
  contraction and, 107–9
  growth kinetics in DD, 52
Celts, DD occurrence in, 247
Central cord, 162
  in thumb, 161, 175
Central core fibres,
    division/tearing/rupture/dehiscence,
    22, 23, 284–5
Chest, flaps from, 304
Chomel, A. F., 4
Chondroitin sulphate
  in DD, distribution/levels, 17, 18,
    19, 52, 53, 54, 151–2
  in normal connective tissue, 16, 49,
    50
Chromosome abnormalities in DD
    tissue, 289
Cirrhosis, alcoholic, DD and, 254
Claw deformity, DD and, distinction,
    190
Cleft-like spaces, diagnostic
    significance, 266
Cleland's ligament, development and
    anatomy, 122–3, 157–8, 178
Cline, Henry (Jr), 3
Cline, Henry (Sr), 1–3, 3
Closed palm technique, postoperative
    management, 369
Coagulator used in haemostasis, 362–3
Collagen, 15, 58–85
  antibodies to, in DD, 102–3
  biological and clinical implications
    of changes in biochemical
    characteristics of, 79–85
  cross-linking, 61–4
    in DD, 68–9, 75–7
  deposition and localization in DD,
    58, 69–71
  fibrous, 59–60
  fibrous long-spacing, 66
  filamentous, 60–1
  general properties and
    characteristics, 15
  glycosylation, 66, 286
  metabolism, 58–64, 286
    anabolic (synthetic), 61–4, 111–12
    catabolic (degradative), 64,
      111–12
  in cultures fibroblasts from
    diabetics, 257–8
  non-fibrous, 60
  organization in DD, 72–85
  polymorphism, 77–8
  remodelling, in DD, 109, 111–12
  structure, 59–64
    changes in DD, 64–6, 72–4
  type I
    in DD, 78
    in normal tissue, 15, 59, 66, 77
  type II, in normal tissue, 59
  type III
    in DD, 19, 67, 69, 71, 73–4

  in normal tissue, 15, 59–60, 66,
    77
  type IV, in normal tissue, 60
  type V
    in DD, 57, 69, 71, 78
    in normal tissue, 60
  type VI
    in DD, 68, 71
    in normal tissue, 60–1
  type IX in normal tissue, 60
  in wound healing, 44
Collagen fibres
  characteristics/distribution, 14, 16,
    25
  in connective tissue remodelling
    studies, 112
  in DD
    in involutional stage disease, 36
    shortening, 73, 74
    fat pad loss affecting, 148–9
    forces on, 150, 152–3, 284
    interconnecting bonds between
      Dupuytren's
      nodules/tractofibroblasts and,
      93, 97
    tearing/shredding/severing, 150–1,
      153
Collagen fibrils in DD, shortening,
    73, 74
Collagenases, 64
Collagenous tissue in DD, 66–71
  biochemical changes, 66–71
  structural changes, 64–6
Colles' fracture, 272
Compensation for Dupuytren's
    disease, 261–4
Complications (postoperative), 355,
    377–86
  factors associated with, 377
  with open palm technique, 301–2,
    311, 368
  surgical data regarding, 222–38,
    394–412
  treatment, 382
Compression of postoperative
    swellings, 370
Compressive forces, fibrotic tissue and
    the effects of, 148
Connective tissue (palmar), 13–24
  composition, 15
  continuum, 14, 138
    loss of biomechanical properties,
      24
  glycosaminoglycans and
    proteoglycans in see
    Glycosaminoglycans;
    Proteoglycans
  microvascularity, increased, 146–7
  remodelling/responsiveness, 14–15,
    110–16, 282–9
  shortening mechanisms, 72–4, 80–4,
    104–5
Contractile forces, intracellular,
    requirements for generation of,
    86

Contraction, 104–7
  cellular basis of, 107–9
  contracture and, distinction, 72,
    104–5
  muscle/muscle cell, 72, 104
  wound see Wound-healing
Contracture(s) see also specific types
    and Contractures; Fascia
  causes, 189–90
  contraction and, distinction, 72,
    104–5
  development, 109–16
  diabetic hand with, 256
  differentiation of various, 3, 7
  management, 115–16, 296, 304–10
    see also Treatment; Surgery
  signs preceding, 187
  as surgical indicators, 294
Cooper, Astley, 2, 3, 3–4, 7, 9
Cords (contracting), 156, 157–8,
    159–65, 174–5
  central see Central cord
  clinical diagnosis, 189
  combinations of, 165
  dissection/excision, 351, 358–9
  interphalangeal joint-associated see
    Interphalangeal joint
  lateral, 156, 162
  pretendinous, 174–5
  retrovascular, 157–8, 164–5, 351, 367
  spiral, 156, 162–4, 165
  surgical indications related to type
    of, 333
  ulnar side, 179–81
Counselling on outcome of treatment,
    246
Country
  of origin of surgical patients, 202
  surgical data relating to, 208–11,
    222–30
Course/outcome of DD
  counselling on, 246
  postoperative, 205–8 see also Surgery
    data regarding, 388–90, 410–12
  spontaneous, Norwegian population
    study, 193–6, 200
Cross-finger flaps, 304, 326, 352
Crush injury, DD related to, 269,
    271, 272
Cutaneous type of Dupuytren's
    disease, 328
Cytogenetics of DD tissue, 289
Cytoskeleton of myofibroblast, 36–45,
    87–90

Dehiscence, central/intrafascial, 22–3,
    140, 284–5
Dehydro-dihydroxylysinonorleucine
    crosslinks, 68
Dehydro-hydroxylysinonorleucine
    crosslinks, 68
Dermal fibres see Fibres
Dermal pits/dimples, 136, 137, 188–9

Dermal ridges, 137
Dermatan sulphate
  in DD, 17, 18, 19, 52, 53, 54
  in normal connective tissue, 16, 49, 50
Dermofasciectomy, 205, 211, 324–8, 331
  finger, 401
  indications, 331
  rationale, 328
  results, 388, 389, 397, 401
Desensitization of hypersensitive postoperative areas, 373–4
Desmin, as a marker of myofibroblast origin, 41, 43, 87
Desmin-positive cells, 30, 43
Development of palmar fascia, 119–26
Diabetes mellitus, DD associated with, 100, 187, 204, 219, 255–8, 270
  assessment for surgery in, 294
Diagnosis
  of Dupuytren's disease
    clinical, 187–90
    differential, 190, 268–73
    histological, 266–8
    in Japanese epidemiological study, 240
    in Norwegian epidemiological study, 191
  scar tissue, 266–73
Diamond-plasty, 335
Diathesis, Dupuytren, 246–52, 269–70
  strength/degree of
  numerical grading of, 249, 250–2
  treatment determined by, 249, 326–7
Digit(s) *see also* Finger; Thumb
  dermofasciectomy, 401
  fascia, 155–6
  fasciectomy, 309, 398–401
  open methods in, 301, 314–20
  palm and, junction of the, anatomy, 156
  skin flaps for, 302–4
  surgical results recorded by, 222–38, 381, 394–407
Digital artery, surgical problems regarding, 180, 378–9
Digital nerve, surgical problems regarding, 179–80, 378–9
Digital sheet, lateral, 156
Dimples (or pits), dermal/skin, 136, 137, 188–9
Diseases, DD-associated, 101, 202–5, 253–60
  assessment for surgery regarding, 293–4
  surgical data recording, 222–38, 381, 394–412
Dissection, in segmental aponeurectomy, 352–3
Disuse as an aggravating factor, 247
DNA metabolism, fascia tissue, 51–2

Dupuytren, G., 3, 4–9, 127
Dystrophy, sympathetic, postoperative, 355, 380

Elastic fibres, 26
Elastomer, silastic, 373
Elderly people's homes visited in Japanese epidemiological study, 240–1
Electroencephalogram in DD patients, 259, 277
Embryological development of palmar fascia, 120–3
Enzyme activities
  collagen degrading, 64
  collagen synthesizing, 61
  in DD tissue, 55–6
Enzymic fasciotomy, 336
Epidemiology of Dupuytren's disease, 99–101, 185–273
Epilepsy, DD associated with, 203, 219, 258–9, 270
Ethnicity *see* Race
Evaluation *see* Assessment
Examination, clinical, 249 *see also* Assessment
Excision of fascia *see* Fascia
Exercises, postoperative, 322, 323, 370–1, 371–3
Extension (position of), full, in open palm and digit technique, 320
  see also Hyperextension
Extension (=spread) and extent of DD, 384–6
  diathesis related to, 250, 384
  in surgical patients, 205
  treatment results assessing, 384–6, 388, 390, 408–9
  long-term, 207
Extension splint, 374, 375
Extensor mechanism/apparatus, 168–71, 310
Extent of disease *see* Extension
Extracellular material (at surfaces of Dupuytren's tractofibroblast), filamentous, 92–7
  location, 93–7
  structure, 93
Extracellular matrix (palmar fascia)
  in DD, 91–2
    at different stages, 33–6
    metabolism, 54–6
    normal metabolism, 50
Eye colour, DD occurrence related to, 247

Family history of Dupuytren's disease, 101–2
  diathesis assessment relating to, 249
  in a Norwegian population, 199
  surgical data recording, 222–38, 381, 394–412

in surgical patients, 201–2, 293
Family origin *see* Race
Fascia
  clinical signs of Dupuytren's disease, 189
  continuous, theory of, 123
  contracted *see* Fascia, contracted
  excision, 357–9, 362–3
    minimal, 357–9
  finger (anatomy), 125, 155–67
    diseased, 158–67
    surgery regarding, 358
  layers, 123
  management, 296, 304–9, 311, 333–67
  palmar *see* Fascia, palmar
  thumb, 172
  web space, 172, 173
Fascia, contracted
  management, 296, 304–9
  skin grafts to separate, 302
Fascia, palmar, 48–57, 119–26
  collagen in *see* Collagen
  in DD, 51–7, 74–8, 80–1, 135, 277
    shortening mechanisms, 72–4, 80–4, 104–5
  development and anatomy, 119–26, 135
  extracellular matrix *see* Extracellular matrix
  function, 137
  glycosaminoglycans and proteoglycans in, 48–57
  history of contractures in, 1–9
  terminology, 120
  tissue culture, 79
Fascia cells, metabolism *see* Metabolism
Fascial bundles *see also* Fibre bundles
  longitudinal/superficial longitudinal, 139–40
  connective tissue remodelling in, 112–13
  thickening, 21, 22, 149, 151
  wound-healing studies relating to, 22
Fasciectomy, 306–9, 321–4, 329–31, 338–9, 357–65
  DD and other complications after, 248, 294
  dermo- *see* Dermofasciectomy
  digital, 309, 398–401
  extensive, 360–5
    results, 387–8, 389, 396, 400
  in Italy, 278, 279
  limited/partial/regional/local, 205, 306–7, 321–4, 327, 338
    results, 387, 389, 394, 395, 398, 399
  variants, 307
  open, 339
  selective, 357
  total/radical/extensive, 205, 278, 307–9, 327

disadvantages and criticisms, 308–9
in two-stage operations, 338–9, 339–40
Fasciotomy, 304–6, 329, 333–7, 394, 395
closed, 304–6, 337
enzymic, 336
extensive, results, 400
finger, 398
history, 1, 3, 7, 304–6
local, results, 394, 398
open, 305, 337–8
subcutaneous, 306
technique, 334–6
Fasciotomy blade, 334
Fat
palmar
in alcoholics, 254
surgery preserving, 358
subcutaneous, operations on, 304
Fat pads, 138, 139–40, 140–50 passim
viscoelastic properties of, 286
Feet, soles of the, examination, 249
Females, DD occurring in, 99–100, 202, 210–11, 232 see also Sex
Japanese population study, 240, 242, 244
Norwegian population study, 191–2, 197, 198, 199
surgical data, 202, 211–12, 231
Fetal development of palmar fascia, 120–3
Fibre(s)
central core, division/tearing/dehiscence/rupture, 22, 23, 284–5
collagen see Collagen fibres
dermal, 136
types, 25–6
elastic, 26
fibrofatty loculi in relation to, 143–54
interfascial, rupture, 284
intrafascial, rupture, 283, 284
longitudinal, 131–4
damage during dissection, 357
of the palmar aponeurosis see Aponeurosis
perforating, 133–4
pretendinous see Pretendinous fibres
reticulum, 25
stress, 88, 90–1
surgical techniques regarding, 350
transverse, of the palmar aponeurosis see Aponeurosis
vertical, 135
Fibre bundles, 65–6 see also Fascial bundles
anatomy and development, 140
in central rupture/dehiscence, 22–3, 140
connective tissue remodelling in, 111–12, 113–14

shortening, 74
surgical techniques regarding, 350
thickening, 149, 151
Fibroblast(s)
contractile and non-contractile, differences between, 108
cultured, 83–4
of diabetics, 257–8
in fibrosarcoma and in DD, comparisons, 288
stress fibres of, 90
in wound contraction model studies, 31–2, 83–4
immature, 33
mature, 36
myo- see Myofibroblasts
myofibroblasts originating from, 42, 43, 44, 86–7
proliferation, 267–8, 286
in scar tissue, as opposed to DD, 267–8
traction by, 107
tracto- see Tractofibroblast
Fibroblastic tumour, non-metastasizing, 288
Fibrocytes, 36
Fibrofatty subcutaneous/subdermal tissue or loculi, 138, 139–40, 140–54
fascial fibres in relation to, 143–54
Fibromatosis
DD as a, 288
myofibroblasts in, 32–3
Fibronectin, surface/extracellular, 91, 91–2, 92, 93, 95–7
fascia shortening involving, 83
Fibronexus, 32, 97
Fibrosarcoma and DD, cultured fibroblasts from, comparisons, 288
Fibrosis in DD
development, 71, 105
of fat pads, 145–6, 146–7, 148–9
consequences, 148–9
regression, possible approaches resulting in, 71
Fifth (little) finger
disease affecting, 179, 181
postoperative results with, 222–38, 381, 390, 391, 394–407, 410–12
metacarpal fracture, 272–3
Finger(s) see also Digits
fascia see Fascia
fifth/little see Fifth finger
index, disease affecting, postoperative results with, 222–38, 381, 394–407
joints see Joints
locked trigger see Trigger finger
mallet (deformity), DD and, differentiation, 363
middle, disease affecting, postoperative results with,

222–38, 381, 394–407
most frequently affected, Norwegian population study of, 193, 194, 195, 200
normal and pathological anatomy, 155–71
results of surgery on, 398–401, 406–7
ring, disease affecting, postoperative results with, 222–38, 304–407, 381
Fingertip, distal crease of palm to, postoperative distance from, 206
Fire-break skin grafts, 116, 327
Flaps, skin, 238–50, 302–4, 362
Flexion
interphalangeal joint see Interphalangeal joint
loss, postoperative, 380
prolonged, posture of, causes, 189–90
recurrent, pattern of, 384
regained
in open palm and digit technique, 320
surgical results related to, 388, 390
Flexion contractures, 273
correction, 209, 352, 367
differential diagnosis, 7
Japanese epidemiological study of, 245
Flexion deformity, fixed proximal interphalangeal joint, 352
Flexion glove, 375
Flexion strap, 375–6
Flexor carpi ulnaris tendon, disease over distal end of, 182
Flexor tendon sheath, adherence to A_2 pulley of, in DD, 294
Fodrin, 107
Foot, sole of the, examination, 249
Forceful use of tool handles, DD related to use of, 261–2
Fracture, DD related to, 269, 271, 272–3
French surgical patients, data on, 227
Full thickness skin grafts, 285, 326, 327
in dermofasciectomy, 326, 327, 328

Gender see Sex
Genetic/inheritable factors in Dupuytren's disease, 101–2, 103, 280–1 see also Cytogenetics
with epilepsy, 259
mode of transmission of, 280–1
Norwegian population study of, 199
in surgical patients, 201–2
Germany, radical fasciectomy in, 309
Glucose tolerance test in DD patients, 257

Glyceraldehyde-phosphate dehydrogenase activity in DD tissue, 54–5
Glycoproteins, extracellular matrix, 91
Glycosaminoglycans (mucopolysaccharides), 15–19, 49–57
  in DD, 17–19, 51–7, 151–2
  metabolic changes, 111
  in normal connective tissue, 15–17, 48–51
Glycosylation, collagen, in DD, 66, 286
Gosset, spiral band of, 133, 156 *see also* Spiral cords
Goyrand, G., 9, 127–8
Grafts (skin), 116, 302, 321–33
  DD recurrence with, 328
  fire-break, 116, 327
  full thickness *see* Full thickness skin grafts
  indications, 302, 348
  postoperative management, 369
  in preventing DD recurrence, 285
  surgical data related to, 404, 406
Granulation tissue
  fibronectin role in, 92
  histopathology, 29–30
  myofibroblasts in, 45
Grayson's ligament
  in contractures, 162
  development and anatomy, 122–3, 157, 178
  surgery regarding, 358
Growth factors, 289
Guérin, J., 8

Haematomas, postoperative, 355, 369, 379
Haemostasis with various operations, 352, 360, 362–3
Hand *see also* parts of hand
  development, 120–3
  dominant (handedness)
    disease related to, 196–8, 200
    surgical data recording, 222–38, 381, 394–412
  previous injury, DD occurrence related to, 198, 200, 205, 248, 261, 265–73, 277
  radial side of, anatomy, 172–5
    pathological, 174–5
  ulnar side of, anatomy, 176–83
    pathological, 179–83, 273
Health status in assessment for surgery, 294
Heparan sulphate, in normal connective tissue, 48, 49
Heredity in Dupuytren's disease *see* Genetic factors
Hexosyhydroxylysine levels in palmar fascia in DD, 76
Hexosylysine/hexosyl-lysine levels in collagen in DD, 68
  in palmar fascia in DD, 76
Histochemical studies in DD, 277
Histocompatibility antigens, DD in relation to, 101, 102
Histopathology
  in Dupuytren's disease, 25–30, 266–8
    collagenous tissue, 64–5
  of nodule development, 149–54
  of scar tissue, 266
History
  of Dupuytren's disease and its treatment, 1–9, 277, 295–6, 304–6
  family *see* Family history
  of palm anatomy, 127–8, 140–3
  of skin incision procedures, 295–6, 297–300
HLA locus products, DD in relation to, 101, 102
Honeycomb technique, 296, 311–14
  advantages, 313–14
Hunter, John, 1
Hunter, William, 127
Hyaluronic acid/hyaluronates
  collagen fibres and the effects of decreases in, 148–9
  in DD, distribution/levels, 17, 18, 19, 52–3
  in normal connective tissue, 15, 49
Hydroxyaldohistidine cross links in collagen, 61, 63, 64
Hydroxylysine (in fascia/collagenous tissue)
  in DD, 75, 76, 78–9
    glycosylated, 66, 75
  in normal tissue, 75, 76, 78
    glycosylated, 75, 76
Hydroxylysinohydroxynorleucine crosslinks, 75, 76, 77, 79
Hydroxylysinonorleucine crosslinks, 75, 77
Hydroxymerodemosine crosslinks, 77
3-Hydroxy-pyridinoline crosslinks in collagen, 61
Hyperextension, distal interphalangeal joint
  boutonnière deformity with, 335–6, 366
  surgery for, 332–3, 335–6, 365–6
Hyperextension injury, 273
Hypersensitive postoperative areas, desensitization of, 373–4
Hypertrophic scarring
  collagen in, 19, 69
  fibronectin role in, 92
  nodules and, similarities between, 149–50
Hypothenar fat pads, 141

Incisions (operative), 295–302, 311–21
  in fasciectomy, 330, 361–2
  longitudinal, 296–301
  in segmental aponeurectomy, 352
  transverse, 301–2, 312, 316
  in two-stage surgery, 337–9
Infections
  DD and, distinction, 190
  postoperative, 379
Inheritable factors in Dupuytren's disease *see* Genetic factors
Injury/trauma
  to hand, 265–73
    DD distinguished from, 190
    previous/single, DD occurrence related to, 198, 200, 205, 248, 261, 265–73, 277
    repetitive, 262–3
    work-related, 261–3
  myofibroblast responses to, 32
  to palmar aponeurosis, Dupuytren's disease related to repair of, 46
Integrin, 97
Interconnecting bonds between contractile cells, 92–7
Intermediate filament proteins, as markers of myofibroblast origin, 41
Interphalangeal joint
  contractures *see* Interphalangeal joint contractures
  cords *see* Interphalangeal joint cords
  fifth proximal, outcome (with surgery) of disease affecting, 390, 391, 411, 412
  flexion, 367
    distal, 367
    fixed proximal, 352
    (hyper)extension, distal *see* Hyperextension
  procedures, proximal, value, 391
  release, proximal, 359
  splints, 374, 375, 375–6
Interphalangeal joint contractures, distal, 162, 165, 181
  surgery, 363
    results, 206, 207, 222–38, 381, 394–407
    timing, 390
Interphalangeal joint contractures, proximal, 162, 164, 164–5, 167, 181, 309–10, 332, 366
  in limited fasciectomy with skin grafts, problems relating to, 323
  surgery, 165, 206, 207, 309–10, 323, 351–2, 359, 363–4, 366, 383
    indications, 332
    results with, 206, 207, 222–38, 381, 383, 394–407
    timing, 390, 391
Interphalangeal joint cords
  distal, prognosis with, 180–1
  proximal
    prognosis with, 181
    surgery, 351

Intertrigo, 350
Involutional stage in DD, 27–8
  cellular and extracellular composition, 36
Iselin and Dieckmann's technique, 278
Italy, aetiology and treatment in, 277–9

Japan, epidemiological studies in, 239–45
  of surgical patients, 210, 226
Joint(s), finger *see also* specific joints
  in diabetic hands, 257–8
  mobility, limited, 257–8
    DD and, distinction, 190
  release, 359–60
  surgical results recorded by, 222–38, 381, 394–407
  swelling over, 169 *see also* Knuckle
Joint cartilage, glycosaminoglycans in, 49

Keratan sulphate, in normal connective tissue, 49
Knuckle, changes in, 168–71
Knuckle pads, 168, 169, 170, 270
  diabetic hand with, 256
  examination for, 249
  Norwegian population study of, 198–9, 200
  in surgical patients, 202, 251, 252
  as a surgical indicator, 348

Laceration, DD related to, 269, 271, 272
Lacroix, C. J., 6–7, 7
Laminin, extracellular matrix, 91, 92
Landsmeer's ligaments, 156, 160
Lanolin massage of wounds, 373
Lateral cords, 156, 162
Lateral digital sheet, 156
Lesion, palmar, genesis, 136–54
Ligaments
  anatomy, 122–3, 128–30, 156
  Cleland's, 122–3, 157–8, 178
  development, 122–3
  Grayson's *see* Grayson's ligament
  Landsmeer's, 156, 160
  natatory (Schwimmband; superficial transverse palmar), 122–3, 128–30, 174, 178, 358
  surgery regarding, 358
  transverse metacarpal, 128, 130
Limb, upper, development, 120–1
Limited joint mobility, DD and *see* Joint
Load bearing, 138–9, 284
Locked trigger finger *see* Trigger finger
Longitudinal structures in the hand, 131–4
Lysine, hydroxylation *see* Hydroxylysine

Lysosomal enzyme activities in DD tissue, 55–6

McCash techniques, 301, 320 *see also* Open palm technique
Madelung, O. W., 140–1, 141
Males, DD occurring in, 99–100, 201–11, 202, 231 *see also* Sex
  Japanese population study, 240, 242, 244
  Norwegian population study, 191–2, 197, 199
  surgical data, 202, 211–12, 231
Mallet finger deformity, DD and, differentiation, 363
Manual work, DD and, 197, 244, 248–9, 261–4
Marx, M., 5, 5–6
Maslieurat-Lagemard, G. E., 134–5, 140
Massage of wounds with lanolin, 373
Masson staining (of collagen fibres)
  green, 153
  red, 152, 153
Meissner's corpuscles, 25
Men *see* Males
Meniscus, glycosaminoglycans in, 49
Mercedessternformige incision, 309
Mesenchymal origin, DD as a benign tumour of, 46, 286
Metabolism
  collagen *see* Collagen
  fascia cells
    in DD, 55–7
    normal, 50–1
Metacarpal, fifth, fracture, 272–3
Metacarpal ligament, transverse, 128, 130
Metacarpophalangeal fat pads, 141
Metacarpophalangeal joint
  amputation at level of, 310
  surgery for deformities affecting, 351, 359, 383, 384
    results, 206, 207, 222–38, 381, 383, 384, 394–407
    timing, 390, 391
Microangiopathy, diabetic, DD combined with, 257
Microfilaments, actin, in myofibroblast/tractofibroblast cytoskeleton, 87, 93–4, 94–7, 97, 98, 107, 108
Microtendon, 140
Mobility
  joint *see* Joint
  palmar structures relating to, 138–9
Mucopolysaccharides *see* Glycosaminoglycans
Myofibroblasts, 29–30, 31–47, 72, 80 *see also* Tractofibroblast
  contractile properties, 105–7
  cytoskeleton of, 36–45, 87–90

  definition/ultrastructure/role in wound contraction, 31–2
  derivation/origin, 36–45, 86–90
  fascia shortening process involving, 82–4
  as a misleading term (in DD), 87, 92, 97, 106–7
  in pathological conditions, 32–3
  prostaglandins and, 254–5
  stress fibres in, 90
Myosin
  fascia shortening involving, 83
  in myofibroblast, 88–90
    as markers of origin, 41–2, 86, 88–90
  in stress fibres of cultured fibroblasts, 90

Natatory ligament, development and anatomy, 122–3, 128–30, 174, 178, 358
Natural history (spontaneous course) of DD, Norwegian population study, 193–6, 200
Negro (black) persons, DD occurrence in, 247
Neoplasia, stromal response to, myofibroblasts in, 33 *see also* Quasineoplastic proliferative conditions
Neoplasms *see* Tumours
Nephropathy, diabetic, DD related to, 101
Nerve(s), surgery and surgery-related problems regarding, 179–80, 355, 358, 378–9
Nerve end organs in palmar skin, 25
Neuropathy, diabetic, DD associated with, 257
Neurovascular bundles, surgery regarding, 357, 358, 359, 362–3
Nodules/nodular tissue
  Dupuytren's, 136, 149–54, 270, 273
    at proximal crease of thumb, 174
    cellular and extracellular composition, 33–6
    collagen/collagenous tissue in, 19
    definition, 136
    diabetic hand with, 256
    diagnosis, 187, 188, 266
    in different disease stages, 33–6
    formation/development, 22–4, 149–54, 283
    glycosaminoglycans/proteoglycans in, 19, 53
    interconnecting bonds between collagen fibres/tractofibroblasts and, 93
    myofibroblasts in, 46–7
  non-Dupuytren's, 273
Norway, epidemiological studies, 191–200

Occupation *see* Work
Oedema, postoperative, control, 370
Old people's homes visited in Japanese epidemiological study, 240–1
Oncogenes, 289
Onset of DD, age of *see* Age
Open digit/finger techniques, 301, 314–20
Open palm and digit technique, 314–20
Open palm technique, 278, 279, 301, 320–1
  disadvantages/complications, 301–2, 311
Open wound release, 304
Operative techniques *see* Surgery
Oriental patients, epidemiological studies of, 210, 226, 239–45
Outcome *see* Course
Outpatients
  Japanese study of DD incidence in, 241–2
  surgery, 348
Oxo-imine cross links in collagen, 61, 64

Pads
  fat, 138, 139–40, 140–50 *passim*
  knuckle *see* Knuckle pads
Paillard, A. L .M., 5, 5–6
Palm
  anatomy, 127–35, 137–8, 156
  closed (technique), postoperative management, 369
  digits and, junction of the, 156
  distal, longitudinal fibres of, 131–4
  open (technique) *see* Open palm technique
  proximal, longitudinal fibres of, 131
  results of surgery on, 394–7, 402–4
  skin flaps for, 302
Palmar, definition of the term, 127
Palmar crease, distal, 138
  fingertip to, postoperative distance, 206
Palmar fascia *see* Fascia
Palmar lesion, genesis, 136–54
Palmar pan splint, 369, 374
Palmaris longus muscle, function and anatomy, 119, 125, 126
Palmaris longus tendon
  absence, 122
  development and anatomy, 119, 122
  presence, 122
Paralysis, interosseous, 190
Pathogenesis of Dupuytren's disease, 21–4, 45–6, 136–54, 275–89
Pathological change, tissue threshold of resistance to, 263
Pathology
  anatomical, 119–83

  in Italy, 277, 278
  histo- *see* Histopathology
Patients, 'good' and 'bad', 328–9
Perforating fibres, 133–4
Perivascular fibroblastic activation, 147
Peyronie's disease, 281
Phenobarbitone-treated patients, DD in, 259
Physiological disturbances, postoperative, 379–80
Pits, dermal/skin, 136, 137, 188–9
Plasminogen activator degradative cascade, 110
Plater, Felix, 1
Population studies in Norway, 191–200
Postoperative assessment of patient, 354–6, 370
Postoperative care/management, 331, 360, 368–76, 391–2
  in dermofasciectomy, 331
  in fasciectomy, 331, 360, 364–5
    with skin grafts, 322–3
  in segmental aponeurectomy, 353–4
  value/results of, 391–2
Pounding with the hand, DD associated with, 262
Preoperative assessment of patient, 249, 293–4, 348–51, 354
Pretendinous cords, disease of, 174–5
Pretendinous fibres/fascial bands, 140, 173–4
  longitudinal, 131, 139, 284
  superficial, 131–3, 284
    fat pad loss affecting, 148–9
Prevalence of DD in Norwegian population study, 191–2, 199
Procollagen synthesis, 61
Prognosis of DD on ulnar side of hand, 182
Progression of disease *see also* Stage
  in Japanese old people's home subjects, 240, 242
  postoperative, 208
Proliferative stage in DD, 27, 33–6
  cellular and extracellular composition, 33–6
Prostaglandins, myofibroblasts and, 254–5
Proteins, myofibroblast cytoskeletal, 41–4
Proteoglycans, 15–19, 49–57
  in DD, 17–19, 51–7
  in normal connective tissue, 15–17, 49–57
Provoking (aggravating) factors, 247–9, 261–2
Putty squeezing exercises, 372
Pyridinoline levels in collagen in DD, 69, 77

Quasineoplastic proliferative conditions, myofibroblasts in, 32–3

  wound-healing and tumour stroma generation in relation to, 45–6

Race (and family origin), DD
  occurrence related to, 100, 201–2, 239, 246–7, 269–70
  surgical data recording, 222–38, 381, 394–412
Radial side of hand *see* Hand
Rat tail tendon fibre bundles, connective tissue remodelling studies employing, 111–12
Rays, number involved
  epidemiological study of, 212, 235, 236
  surgical data relating to, 235, 236
  surgical incisions relating to, 300
Recurrence of DD, 248, 249, 323–4, 325–6, 333, 383–4, 385
  avoiding/preventing, 248
  dermofasciectomy in, 325–6, 328
  full thickness skin grafts in, 285, 326
  diathesis related to, 250
  with fasciotomy, 306
  in Italy, 278
  in limited fasciectomy with skin grafts, 323–4
  treatment of, 323–4
  treatment results assessing, 385, 388, 390, 408–9
  long-term, 207
Reflex sympathetic dystrophy, postoperative, 380
Reid, J., 6
Repair (biological process of) *see also* Wound-healing
  aberrant, 23–4
  myofibroblasts in, 32
  to torn/shredded collagen fibres, 151
  of trauma to palmar aponeurosis, Dupuytren's disease related to, 46
Repetitive trauma, 262–3
Residual stage in DD, 28
  cellular and extracellular composition, 36
Reticulin staining in DD *passim*, 64–5
Reticulum fibres, 25
Retrovascular cord (of Thomine), 157–8, 164–5, 351, 367
Rheumatoid arthritis
  assessment for surgery regarding, 293–4
  DD occurrence related to, 101, 102–3
Rupture, fibre, 285–6
  central core, 22, 23, 283, 284–5
  interfascial, 284
  intrafascial, 283, 284
  longitudinal, of palmar aponeurosis, 248

Sarcomas, myofibroblasts in, 33 *see also* Fibrosarcoma
Scar tissue
  histopathology, 266
  hypertrophic *see* Hypertrophic scarring
  postoperative, management, 373–4
Schwimmband (natatory ligament), development and anatomy, 122–3, 128–30, 174, 178, 358
Scleroderma, DD and, distinction, 190
Septa
  fibrous, 143, 144
  oblique, 143, 144
  vertical, 122, 143, 144
Sesamoids, cartilaginous, 16
Severity of disease in surgical patients, 212
Sex (gender) *see also* Females; Males
  assessment for surgery regarding, 293
  DD occurrence related to, 99–100, 202, 211–12
    Japanese population study, 240, 242, 244
    Norwegian population study, 191–2, 199
    surgical data recording, 222–38, 381, 394–412
Signs, clinical, of Dupuytren's disease, 187–90 *see also* Symptoms
Silastic Elastomer, 373
Skin
  in assessment for surgery, 294
  biopsy, in limited joint mobility, 257–8
  clinical signs of Dupuytren's disease affecting, 188–9, 249
  closure *see* Wound
  deficiencies, skin grafts to heal, 302
  excision, elective, 302
  flaps, 302–4, 348–50, 362
  gaps, in two-stage operations, management, 339
  glycosaminoglycans in, 49
  grafts *see* Grafts
  knuckle, wrinkled, 168–9
  loss/necrosis, postoperative, 379
  palmar
    histopathology, 26–30
    normal, 25–6
  pits/dimples, 136, 137, 188–9
  surgical indications related to nature of overlying, 333–4, 348
  surgical management, 295–304, 311–33
Skoog's technique (selective fasciectomy), 279, 307, 357–60
Smooth muscle antigens, 30
Smooth muscle cells
  cells akin to, 29, 30
  myofibroblasts originating from, 43, 44, 86–7

Soles of the feet, examination, 249
Spectrin, fibroblast, 107
Spiral band of Gosset, 133, 156
Spiral cords, 156, 162–4, 165
Splinting, 374–6, 391–2
  in closed palm technique, 369
  in fasciotomy, 335
  in limited fasciectomy with skin grafts, 323
  in open palm and digit technique, 320
  surgical data regarding, 222–38, 381, 394–412
  value/results of, 391–2
Squeezing exercises, 372
Stages of Dupuytren's disease (different/various), 27–8, 33–6 *see also* Extent; Progression; Severity
  cellular and extracellular composition in, 33–6
  Norwegian population study of, 193–6, 197
  occupation related to, 197
  selection of operation related to, 337
Stenographic pad, holding a, DD associated with, 262
Stress fibres, 88, 90–1
Stretcher splints, intrinsic, 376
Stretching, forcible, of shortened tissues, 114
Stroma, tumour
  myofibroblasts in, 33
  wound healing and quasineoplastic proliferative conditions in relation to generation of, 45–6
Subcutaneum (palmar)
  histopathology, 26–30
  normal, 25–6
Sudek's atrophy, 248
Sulphate group-carrying glycosaminoglycans/proteoglycans, 16
Surgery, 291–412 *see also* Treatment
  assessment of patient for, 249, 293–4, 348–51, 354
  complications *see* Complications
  history, 3, 4, 7, 8–9, 278
  indications, 331–3, 336, 348
  in Italy, 278, 278–9
  nerves and arteries considered in, 179–80, 355, 378–9
  Norwegian population study of need for, 198, 200
  outpatient, 348
  overview, 295–310
  previous, patients undergoing, 213, 222–38, 238, 381, 394, 407
  procedures/techniques, 311–67
    frequency of, 210
    new, 278
    two-stage, 337–40
    types of, 205, 387–8
  recurrence following *see* Recurrence

  results, 205–7, 223, 225–8, 333, 336, 339–40, 355–6, 381, 387–412
    grading, 333
    methods of evaluating, 387
    timing, 295, 390–1
  in ulnar border disease, prognosis, 182
Surgical patients, epidemiology of, 201–38
Sutures, surgical data related to, 402, 405
Swann-Morton blade no. 11 modified for fasciotomy, 334
Swanston's replacement arthroplasty, 310
Swellings
  over finger joints, 169
  postoperative, compression of, 370
Sympathetic dystrophy, postoperative, 355, 380
Symptoms, Norwegian population study of initial, 192 *see also* Signs

Talin, 107
Tendinous sheath, palmar, 130
Tendon *see also* Microtendon
  of abductor digiti minimi, 177, 178, 273, 384
  of flexor carpi ulnaris, disease over distal end of, 182
  glycosaminoglycans in, 49
  rat tail, fibre bundles of, connective tissue remodelling studies employing, 111–12
  wound-healing studies with division of, 22
Tenosynovitis, DD and, distinction, 190
Tension, proximal, upon palmar aponeurosis, DD related to, 119
Tethering
  diabetic hand with, 256
  of knuckle skin wrinkles, 169
Thenar fat pads, 141
Thomine, retrovascular cord of, 157–8, 164–5, 351, 367
Thumb
  central cord in, 161, 175
  fascia, 172
  postoperative results with disease affecting, 222–38, 381, 394–407
Tissues
  anoxia, 147, 286–7
  threshold of resistance to pathological change, 263
Tolbutamide test in DD patients, 257
Tools, DD related to use of, 261–3
Traction, 105–7
Tractofibroblast (Dupuytren's), 87, 92, 107
  filamentous extracellular material *see*

Extracellular material interconnecting bonds between collagen fibres/Dupuytren's nodules and, 93, 97
Transmembrane linkages, 97
Transverse structures in the hand, 128, 129
Trauma *see* Injury/trauma
Treatment (of DD), 291–412
 finger fascia anatomy in the, 155
 history, 3, 4, 7, 8–9, 278
 in Italy, 278, 278–9
 new techniques, 278
 operative *see* Surgery
 of postoperative complications, 382
 results, 205–7, 223, 225–8, 333, 336, 339–40, 355–6, 381, 387–412
Trigger finger (locked), 294
 DD and, distinction, 190
Tubiana's technique, 278
Tumours/neoplasms
 benign, DD as a, 46, 286, 288–9
 myofibroblasts in, 32–3
 stroma *see* Stroma
Twin studies of Dupuytren's disease, 102, 280
Types of Dupuytren's disease, 211–13, 328

Ulnar digital artery, surgery regarding, 180
Ulnar digital nerve, surgery regarding, 179–80
Ulnar side of hand *see* Hand
United States, surgical patients in, data on, 222–3

Vascular alterations in palm of DD patients, 277, 278
Vascular disease, diabetic, DD combined with, 257
Vascular origin of myofibroblasts, 43–4
Vascularity of fibrofatty compartments, increased, 146–8
Vater-Pacinian corpuscles, 25
Vertebral disc, glycosaminoglycans in, 49
Vertical fibres, 135
Vidal de Casis, 7–8
Viking disease, DD as a, 247
Vimentin, as a marker of myofibroblast origin, 41, 43, 87
Vinculin, 107
Vitamin E levels in DD, 277
Volar flap, sliding, 304
Volkmann's ischaemic contracture, DD and, differentiation, 3

Web space
 contracted, 175
 fascia, 172, 173
Web strap, 374, 375
West German surgical patients, data on, 228
 Canadian data and, comparisons, 211
Whirlpool baths, 368–9, 369
Women *see* Females
Work (occupation)
 assessment for surgery regarding, 293
 disease related to hours outside, 285
 disease related to, 196–8, 244, 248–9, 261–4

Japanese population study of, 244
Norwegian population study of, 196–8
total stage of, 197
surgical data recording, 222–38, 381, 394–412
Wound
 closure/care/management, 205, 331
 in fasciectomy, 322, 330, 331, 364
 in open palm and digit technique, 320
 in open palm technique, 320–1
 in segmental aponeurectomy, 353
 surgical results related to, 388, 389, 390, 402–7
 complications, incision-related, 301–2
Wound-healing/contraction, 105–6, 151 *see also* Repair
 myofibroblasts in, 31–2, 32, 45, 105–6
 tendon division in studies of, 22
 tumour stroma generation and quasineoplastic proliferative conditions in relation to, 45–6
Wrinkle skin on knuckles, 168–9

Y-to-V advancement/plasty, 296, 350–1

Z-plasty, 250, 296, 300, 319, 360
 in fasciectomy, 330, 361–2
 fasciotomy and, 306
Zig-zag incisions, 296, 312–13
 disadvantages, 296–300
 in fasciectomy, 330, 361